The Central Nervous System

The Central Nervous System

FIFTH EDITION

Per Brodal, MD, PhD

Intitute of Basic Medical Sciences

University of Oslo

Oslo, Norway

UNIVERSITY OF NOTTINGHAM
JAMES CAMERON-GIFFORD LIBRARY

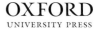

OXFORD
UNIVERSITY PRESS

OXFORD
UNIVERSITY PRESS

Oxford University Press is a department of the University of Oxford. It furthers
the University's objective of excellence in research, scholarship, and education
by publishing worldwide.Oxford is a registered trade mark of Oxford University
Press in the UK and certain other countries.

Published in the United States of America by Oxford University Press
198 Madison Avenue, New York, NY 10016, United States of America.

First Edition published in 1992
Second Edition published in 1998
Third Edition published in 2004
Fourth Edition published in 2010

100782+09X

Library of Congress Cataloging-in-Publication Data
Brodal, Per, author.
The central nervous system / by Per Brodal. — 5th edition.
p. ; cm.
Includes bibliographical references and index.
ISBN 978–0–19–022895–8 (alk. paper)
I. Title.
[DNLM: 1. Central Nervous System—physiology. WL 300]
QP370
612.8′2—dc23
2015031169

9 8 7 6 5 4 3 2 1
Printed by CTPS, China

Contents

Introduction

A BIRD'S EYE VIEW OF THE NERVOUS SYSTEM

What are the main tasks of the nervous system? This question is not easily answered—our brains are necessary for most of what we associate with being a human. At a superior level, we need the brain to create our reality: it makes it possible for us to select, sort, and interpret the overwhelming amount of information we receive from our bodies and the environment. The brain furthermore enables our control of behavior in accordance with our interpretations of reality. This control concerns behavior in a wide sense: one aspect is control and maintenance of the body and its inner milieu; another is our interaction with our surroundings and other human beings through actions and speech. A third aspect is our inner, subjective, mental reality that others can only partially know. In early childhood, plastic changes of brain circuits form the basis of our ability to create order and predictability, without which we would be unable to relate successfully to our environment and ourselves.

The essential building block of the nervous system is the **neuron** (nerve cell), specialized for rapid conveyance of signals over long distances and in a very precise manner. Together, billions of neurons in the brain form complicated and highly organized networks for **communication** and **information processing**.

The nervous system receives a wealth of information from an individual's surroundings and body. From all this information, it extracts the essentials, stores what may be needed later, and emits a command to muscles or glands if an answer is appropriate. Sometimes the answer comes within milliseconds, as a **reflex** or automatic response. At other times it may take considerably longer, requiring cooperation among many parts of the brain and involving **conscious processes**. In any case, the main task of the nervous system is to ensure that the organism adapts optimally to the environment.

The nervous system is equipped with sense organs, **receptors** that react to various forms of sensory information or stimuli. Regardless of the mode of stimulation (the form of energy), the receptors "translate" the energy of the stimulus to the language spoken by the nervous system, that is, **nerve impulses**. These are tiny electric discharges rapidly conducted along the nerve processes. In this way signals are conveyed from the receptors to the regions of the nervous system where information processing takes place.

The nervous system can elicit an external response only by acting on **effectors**, which are either muscles or glands. The response is either **movement** or **secretion**. Obviously, muscle contraction can have various expressions, from communication through speech, facial expression, and bodily posture to walking and running, respiratory movements, and changes of blood pressure. But one should bear in mind that the nervous system can only act on muscles and glands to express its "will." Conversely, if we are to judge the activity going on in the brain of another being, we have only the expressions produced by muscle contraction and secretion to go by.

On an anatomic basis we can divide the nervous system into the **central nervous system** (CNS), consisting of the brain and the spinal cord, and the **peripheral nervous system** (PNS), which connects the CNS with the receptors and the effectors. Although without sharp transitions, the PNS and the CNS can be subdivided into parts that are concerned primarily with the regulation of visceral organs and the internal milieu and parts that are concerned mainly with the more or less conscious adaptation to the external world. The first division is called the **autonomic** or **visceral nervous system**; the second is usually called the **somatic nervous system**. The second division, also called the cerebrospinal nervous system, receives information from sense organs capturing events in our surroundings (vision, hearing, receptors in the skin) and controls the activity of voluntary muscles (made up of cross-striated skeletal muscle cells). In contrast, the autonomic nervous system controls the activity of involuntary muscles (smooth-muscle and heart muscle cells) and gland cells. The autonomic system may be further subdivided into the **sympathetic system**, which is mainly concerned with mobilizing the resources of the body when demands are increased (as in emergencies), and the **parasympathetic system**, which is devoted more to the daily maintenance of the body.

The **behavior** of a vertebrate with a small and—comparatively speaking—simple brain (such as a frog) is dominated by fairly fixed relationships between a stimulus and its response. Thus, a stimulus, produced for example by a small object in the visual field, elicits a stereotyped pattern of goal-directed movements. Few neurons are intercalated between the sense organ and the effector, with correspondingly limited scope of response adaptation. Much of the behavior of the animal is therefore instinctive and automatic, and not subject to significant change by learning. In mammals with relatively small brains compared with their body weights (such as rodents), a large part of their brain is devoted to fairly direct sensorimotor transformations. In primates, the relative brain weight has increased dramatically during some million years of evolution. This increase is most marked in humans with relative brain weight double that of the chimpanzee. In humans, there are few fixed relationships between sensations and behavior (apart from a number of vital reflexes). Thus, a certain stimulus may cause different responses depending on its context and the antecedents. Consequently, we often can choose among several responses, and the response can be changed on the basis of experience. Such flexibility requires, however, increased "computational power" in terms of number of neurons available for specific tasks. The more an animal organizes its activities on the basis of previous experience, and the more it is freed from the dominance of immediate sensations, the more complex the processes that are required of the central nervous system. The behavior of humans cannot be understood merely on the basis of what happened immediately before. The British neuropsychologist Larry Weiskrantz (1992) puts it this way: "We are controlled by predicted consequences of our behavior as much as by the immediate antecedents. We are goal-directed creatures" (p. 8).

The higher processes of integration and association—that is, what we call **mental processes**—are first and foremost functions of the **cerebral cortex**. The vast number of neurons in this part of the brain primarily explains the unique adaptability and learning capacity of human beings. Indeed, the human brain not only permits adaptation to extremely varied environments; it also enables us to change our environment to suit our needs. This entails enormous possibilities but also dangers, because we produce changes that are favorable in the short run but in the long run might threaten the existence of our species.

STUDYING THE STRUCTURE AND FUNCTION OF THE NERVOUS SYSTEM

Some of the many methods used for the study of the nervous system are described in the following chapters—that is, in conjunction with discussion of results produced by the methods. Here we limit ourselves to some general features of neurobiological research.

Many approaches have been used to study the structure and function of the nervous system, from straightforward observations of its macroscopic appearance to determination of the function of single molecules. In recent years we have witnessed a tremendous development of methods, so that today problems can be approached that were formerly only a matter of speculation. The number of neuroscientists has also increased almost exponentially, and they are engaged in problems ranging from molecular genetics to behavior. Although the mass of knowledge in the field of neurobiology has increased accordingly, more important, the understanding of how our brains work has improved considerably. Nevertheless, the steadily expanding amount of information makes it difficult for the scientist to have a fair knowledge outside his or her specialty. It follows that the scientist may not be able to put findings into the proper context, with the danger of drawing erroneous conclusions

Traditionally, methods used for neurobiological research were grouped into those dealing with **structure** (neuroanatomy) and those aiming at disclosing the **function** of the structures (neurophysiology, neuropsychology). The borders are far from sharp, however, and it is typical of modern neuroscience that anatomic, physiologic, biochemical, pharmacological, psychological, and other methods are combined. Cell biological methods especially are being applied with great success. Furthermore, the introduction of modern computer-based imaging techniques has opened exciting possibilities for studying the relation between structure and function in the living human brain. More and more of the methods originally developed in cell biology and immunology are being applied to the nervous system, and we now realize that neurons are not so different from other cells as was once assumed.

Animal Experiments Are Crucial for Progress

Only a minor part of our present knowledge of the nervous system is based on observations in humans; most has been obtained in experimental animals. In humans we are usually limited to a comparison of symptoms that are caused by naturally occurring diseases, with the findings made at postmortem examination of the brain. Two cases are seldom identical, and the structural derangement of the brain is often too extensive to enable unequivocal conclusions.

In animals, however, the experimental conditions can be controlled, and the experiments may be repeated, to reach reliable conclusions. The properties of the elements of neural tissue can be examined directly—for example, the activity of single neurons can be correlated with the behavior of the animal. Parts of the nervous system can also be studied in isolation—for example, by using tissue slices that can be kept viable in a dish (*in vitro*) for hours. This enables recordings and experimental manipulations, with subsequent structural analysis of the tissue. Studies in invertebrates with a simple nervous system have made it possible to discover the fundamental mechanisms that underlie synaptic function and the functioning of simple neuronal networks.

When addressing questions about functions specific to the most highly developed nervous systems, however, experiments must be performed in higher mammals, such as cats and monkeys, with a well-developed cerebral cortex. Even from such experiments, inferences about the human nervous system must be drawn with great caution. Thus, even though the nervous systems in all higher mammals show striking similarities with regard to their basic principles of organization, there are important differences in the relative development of the various parts. Such anatomic differences indicate that there are functional differences as well. Thus, results based on the study of humans, as in clinical neurology, psychiatry, and psychology, must have the final word when it comes to functions of the human brain. But because clinicians can seldom experiment, they must often build their conclusions on observations made in experimental animals and then decide whether findings from patients or normal volunteers can be explained on such a basis. If this is not possible, the clinical findings may raise new problems that require studies in experimental animals to be solved. Basically, however, the methods used to study the human brain are the same as those used in the study of experimental animals.

Ethics and Animal Experiments

Experiments on animals are often criticized from an ethical point of view. But the question of whether such experiments are acceptable cannot be entirely separated from the broader question of whether humans have the right to determine the lives of animals by using them for food, by taking over their territories, and so forth. With regard to using animals for scientific purposes, one has to realize that a better understanding of human beings as thinkers, feelers, and actors requires, among other things, further animal experiments. Even though cell cultures and computer models may replace some of them, in the foreseeable future we will still need animal experiments. Computer-based models of the neuronal interactions taking place in the cerebral cortex, for example, usually require further animal experiments to test their tenability.

Improved knowledge and understanding of the human brain is also mandatory if we want to improve the prospects for treatment of the many diseases that affect the nervous system. Until today, these diseases—most often leading to severe suffering and disability—have only occasionally been amenable to effective treatment. Modern neurobiological research nevertheless gives hope, and many promising results have appeared in the past few years. Again, this would not have been possible without animal experiments.

Yet there are obviously limits to what can be defended ethically, even when the purpose is to alleviate human suffering. Government authorities and the scientific community itself have enacted strict rules to ensure that only properly trained persons perform animal experiments and that the experiments are conducted so that discomfort and pain are kept at a minimum. Most international neuroscience journals require that the experiments they publish have been conducted in accordance with such rules.

All Methods Have Sources of Error

Even though we do not treat systematically the sources of error inherent in the various methods discussed in this book, certainly all methods have their limitations. It often requires intimate, personal experience with a method to fully realize its limitations and sources of error. Unfortunately, when scientific results are cited and interpreted by others after their first publication, limitations and uncertainties tend to disappear, ending up with general "truths" that are perpetuated by uncritical reading and citations. One source of error when conducting animal experiments is to draw premature conclusions about conditions in humans. This problem is evident in a book like this: while the aim is to describe and understand the human brain, most of the data on neurons and their circuits derive from animal experiments.

Purely anatomic methods also have their sources of error and have led to many faulty conclusions in the past about connections between neuronal groups. In turn, such errors may lead to misinterpretations of physiologic and psychological data. The study of humans also entails sources of error—for example, of a psychological nature. Thus, the answers and information given by a patient or a volunteer are not always reliable; for example, the patient may want to please the doctor and answer accordingly. Further, the context of brain scanning (confined in a narrow tube with instructions to not move) is highly artificial and obviously influences how the person feels and responds.

Reductionism and the "Mereological Fallacy"

Scientific experiments aim at isolating structures and processes so that they can be observed in isolation (e.g., taking neurons out the brain to eliminate the number of influencing factors). However necessary such a **reductionistic** approach may be, it also means that phenomena are studied out of their natural context. Conclusions with regard to how the parts function in an intact animal in conjunction with all other parts must therefore be speculative. Arguably, **disciplinary bias** (seeing only one's own topic of research) and **reductionism** pose serious obstacles to a deeper understanding of the complex phenomena related to human beings and their brains.

As a consequence of uncritical reductionism, all too often neuroscientists ascribe attributes (psychological or behavioral) to the brain or part of the brain that can logically apply only to the whole animal. This mistake is called the **mereological fallacy** by Bennett and Hacker (2003, p. 73).[1] They point out the obvious truth that although we cannot perceive (or perform) anything without a properly functioning brain, it is not our brains that see and feel—these are concepts that make sense only in relation to a person. An analogy would be that an airplane needs an engine to fly, but we say that the airplane, not its engine, takes off from the runway.

---

1. **Mereology** is the logic of the relations between parts and the whole.

Revising Scientific "Truths" from Time to Time

That our methods have sources of error and that our interpretations of data are not always tenable are witnessed by the fact that our concepts of the nervous system must be revised regularly. Reinterpretations of old data and changing concepts are often made necessary by the introduction of new methods. As in all areas of science, conclusions based on the available data should not be regarded as final truths but as more or less probable and preliminary interpretations. Natural science is basically concerned with posing questions to nature. How understandable and unequivocal the answers are depends on the precision of our questions and how relevant they are to the problem we are studying: stupid questions receive stupid answers. It is furthermore fundamental to science—although not always easy for the individual scientist to live up to—that conclusions and interpretations be made without any bias and solely on the strength of the facts and the arguments. It should be irrelevant whether the scientist is a young student or a Nobel laureate.

Neuroethics

Due mainly to technological developments, knowledge of the human brain has increased tremendously in the past decades. Neuroscientists now approach questions about human nature that formerly were the domain of philosophy and the social sciences. Furthermore, it is now possible to interfere directly with the workings of the normal brain in ways that were unthinkable some years ago, and imaging techniques promise to reveal information about a person's personality, intentions, feelings, dispositions, and so forth. Correlations are sought between brain measures (e.g., as recorded with functional magnetic resonance imaging [fMRI]) and future outcomes in education, criminality, health-related behavior, and so forth. Numerous "neuroscience-based" educational and learning programs constitute a whole industry (often with a misconceived neuroscientific background and scant empiric support).

The surge in powerful neuroscientific methods has raised concerns that their widespread use may challenge core humanistic values. Indeed, a new field—**neuroethics**—is concerned with the growing realization that neuroscientific knowledge can be misused to legitimate value-based actions and beliefs—matters in which neuroscience can provide only indirect arguments. It is a matter of concern, for example, that psychological phenomena are commonly "explained" by referring to a part of the brain or a neurotransmitter. Further, it has become a popular, although controversial,[2] notion that brain scans can reveal a person's character, intentions, truthfulness, mental aberrations, and so forth. Indeed, neuroscientific evidence is increasingly being offered in court cases; neuroeconomics is a new field of research; insurance companies show interest in neuroscientific evidence to aid their decisions; and so forth. Such use, other than the fact that it may be scientifically flawed, needs critical evaluation in a broad and long-term perspective, including ethical, social, and legal implications.

---

2. It is one thing is to find an association between a certain brain activity and a mental state (e.g., the feeling of pain) in an experimental situation but quite another to conclude that a person who shows this brain activity is in this particular mental state (this is called the **problem of reverse inference**). Indeed, we know that similar patterns of brain activity may be associated with different mental states, and a particular mental state may be associated with different patterns of activity.

PART ONE

Main Features of Structure and Function

General information about the structure and function of the nervous system forms a necessary basis for treatment of the specific systems described in subsequent parts of this book. **Chapters 1** and **2** describe the structure of nervous tissue and some basic features of how neurons are interconnected, while **Chapters 3**, **4**, and **5** deal with the functional properties of neurons as a basis for understanding communication between nerve cells. **Chapter 6** provides an overview of the macroscopic (and, to some extent, the microscopic) structure of the nervous system with brief descriptions of functions. **Chapter 7** treats the membranes covering the central nervous system, the cavities within the brain, and the cerebrospinal fluid produced in these. Finally, **Chapter 8** describes the blood supply of the brain and the spinal cord.

Figure 1.7

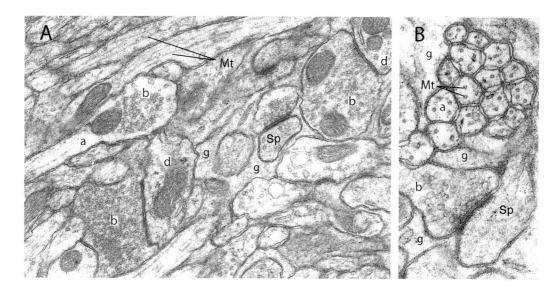

Synapses. **A, B:** Electron micrographs showing boutons (b) in synaptic contacts with dendrites (d), and dendritic spines (Sp). Note how processes of glia (g) cover the dendrites and nerve terminals except at the site of synaptic contact. Note bundle of unmyelinated axons (a) in **B**. Microtubules (Mt) are responsible for axonal transport. Magnifications, ×20,000 (**A**) and ×40,000 (**B**).

Placement of Synapses Has Functional Significance

The functional significance of a synapse depends, among other factors, on its position on the postsynaptic neuron (Fig. 1.8). In general, the closer the synapse is to the **axon hillock** (the initial part of the axon), the stronger is its effect. A synapse located far out on a dendrite has a relatively weak effect. Accordingly, many such synapses must as a rule be active simultaneously to exert a decisive influence.

Synapses formed on the cell soma are called **axosomatic**, while synapses on dendrites are called **axodendritic** (Fig. 1.8). Where dendrites are equipped with spines, one or two **axospinous** synapses are always formed with the spine head (1.7B, Figs. 1.8, and 1.9A). Interestingly, both the form and number of spines change in association with learning. Nerve terminals may also form a synapse with an axon (usually close to a terminal bouton of that axon), and such synapses are called **axoaxonic** (Fig. 1.8 and 1.9B). This enables selective control of one terminal only without influencing the other terminals of the parent axon. Axoaxonic synapses thus increase the precision of the signal transmission.

There are many more axodendritic than axosomatic synapses because the dendritic surface is so much larger. Every neuron has many thousands of synapses on its surface, and the sum of their influences determines how active the postsynaptic neuron will be at any moment.

Figure 1.8

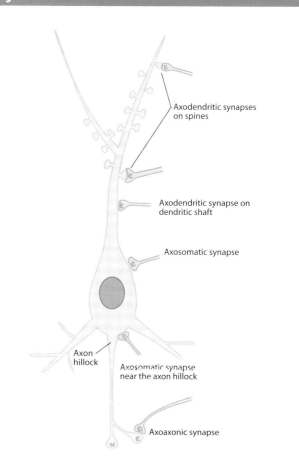

Axodendritic synapses on spines

Axodendritic synapse on dendritic shaft

Axosomatic synapse

Axon hillock

Axosomatic synapse near the axon hillock

Axoaxonic synapse

The placement of synapses. The position of a synapse determines (together with other factors) its effect on the postsynaptic neuron.

Figure 1.9

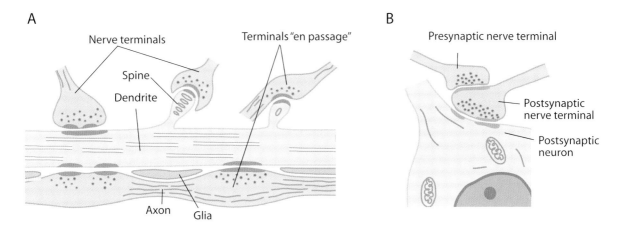

A: *Axodendritic synapses.* A nerve terminal (bouton) may form a synapse directly on the shaft of the dendrite or on a spine. The axon may also have several boutons en passage. **B:** *Axoaxonic synapse.* The presynaptic nerve terminal influences—by usually inhibiting—the release of neurotransmitter from the postsynaptic nerve terminal.

Two Main Kinds of Nerve Cell: Projection Neurons and Interneurons

Some neurons influence cells that are at a great distance, and their axons are correspondingly long (more than a meter for the longest). They are called **projection neurons**, or **Golgi type 1** (Fig. 1.10). Neurons that convey signals from the spinal cord to the muscles are examples of projection neurons; other examples are neurons in the cerebral cortex with axons that contact cells in the brain stem and the spinal cord (see Fig. 33.6). As a rule, the axons of projection neurons send out branches, or **collaterals**, in their course (Figs. 1.1 and 1.11). Thus, one projection neuron may send signals to neurons in various other parts of the nervous system.

The other main type of neuron is the **interneuron**, or **Golgi type 2** (Fig. 1.10, see also Fig. 33.7), characterized by a short axon that branches extensively in the vicinity of the cell body. Its name implies that an interneuron is intercalated between two other neurons (Fig. 1.12). Even though, strictly speaking, all neurons with axons that do not leave the CNS are thus interneurons, the term is usually restricted to neurons with short axons that do not leave one particular neuronal group. The interneurons thus mediate communication between neurons within one group. Because interneurons may be switched on and off, the possible number of interrelations among the neurons within one group

increases dramatically. The number of interneurons is particularly high in the cerebral cortex, and it is the number of interneurons that is so much higher in the human brain than in that of any other animal. The number of typical projection neurons interconnecting the various parts of the nervous system, and linking the nervous system with the rest of the body, as a rule varies more with the size of the body than with the stage of development.

The distinction between projection neurons and interneurons is not always very clear, however. Many neurons previously regarded as giving off only local branches have been shown via modern methods also to give off long axonal branches to more distant cell groups. Thus, they function as both projection neurons and interneurons. For example, many of the "classical" projection neurons in the cerebral cortex (see Fig. 33.6) give off collaterals that end within the cell group in which the cell body is located.

Tasks of Interneurons

Figure 1.12 shows how an interneuron (b) is intercalated in an impulse pathway. One might perhaps think that the simpler direct pathway shown below from neuron A to neuron C would be preferable. After all, the interneuron leads to a delay in the propagation of the signal from A to C, and this would be a disadvantage. Most important, however, is that the interneuron provides added **flexibility**. Thus, whether the signal is transmitted from a to c can be controlled by other synaptic

Figure 1.10

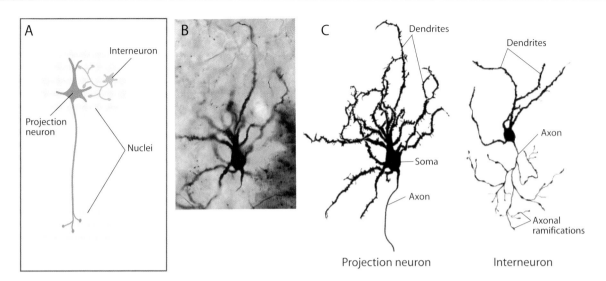

Projection neurons and interneurons. **A:** A projection neuron sends its axon to neurons in other nuclei (cell groups), often at a long distance. The axon of an interneuron ramifies and makes synaptic contacts in its vicinity (within the same nucleus). Schematic. **B:** Photomicrograph from a section treated with the Golgi method, showing a projection neuron (from the brain stem of the monkey). With this method the whole neuron is impregnated with silver salts, rendering it black. The depth of field is only a fraction of the thickness of the section (100 μm). Therefore, only part of the neuron is clearly visible in the photomicrograph. **C:** Drawing of the projection neuron shown in **B**, and an interneuron from the same material.

inputs to interneuron b. Identical synaptic inputs to neuron a may be propagated further by neuron c in one situation but not in another, depending on the state of interneuron b. This kind of arrangement may partly explain why, for example, identical stimuli may cause pain of very different intensity: interneurons along the pathways conveying sensory signals are under the influence of other parts of the brain (e.g., neurons analyzing the meaning of the sensory stimulus).

Figure 1.13 illustrates another important task performed by interneurons. Interneuron B enables neuron A to act back on itself and reduce its own firing of impulses. The arrangement acts to prevent neuron A from becoming excessively active. Thus, the negative **feedback** provided by the interneuron would stop the firing of neuron A. Such an arrangement is present, for example, among motor neurons that control striated muscle contraction (see Fig. 21.14).

Figure 1.11

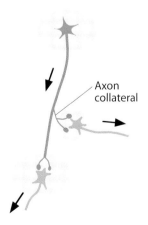

Collateral of a projection neuron. By sending off collaterals, a projection neuron may establish synapses in different cell groups (nuclei). Arrows show the direction of impulse conduction.

Figure 1.12

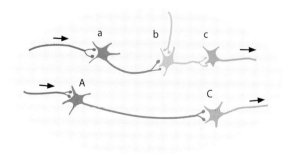

An interneuron (b) intercalated in a pathway from neuron a to neuron c. This arrangement increases the flexibility, as compared with the direct pathway from neuron A to C shown below. Arrows show the direction of impulse conduction.

Figure 1.13

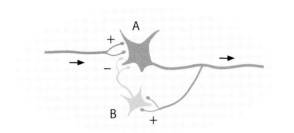

An interneuron (B) mediates negative feedback to the projection neuron (A). Arrows show the direction of impulse conduction.

Many of the tasks performed by the nervous system require very rapid conduction of signals. If unmyelinated axons were to do this, they would have to be extremely thick. Nerves bringing signals to the muscles of the hand, for example, would be impossibly thick, and the brain would also have to be much larger. Insulation is thus a very efficient way of saving space and expensive building materials. Efficient insulation of axons is, in fact, a prerequisite for the dramatic development of the nervous system that has taken place in vertebrates as compared with that in invertebrates.

Myelin and how it is formed is discussed in Chapter 2, while the conduction of nerve impulses is discussed Chapter 3.

Many Axons Are Isolated to Increase the Speed of Impulse Propagation

The velocity with which the nerve impulse travels depends on the diameter of the axon, among other factors. In addition, how well the axon is insulated is of crucial importance. Many axons have an extra layer of insulation (in addition to the axonal membrane) called a **myelin sheath**. Such axons are therefore called **myelinated**, to distinguish them from those without a myelin sheath, which are called **unmyelinated** (see Figs. 2.6 and 2.7).

White and Gray Matter

The surfaces made by cutting nervous tissue contain some areas that are whitish and others that have a gray color (Fig. 1.14). The whitish areas consist mainly of myelinated axons, and the myelin is responsible for the color; such regions are called **white matter**. The gray regions, called **gray matter**, contain mainly cell bodies and dendrites (and, of course, axons passing to and from the neurons). The neurons themselves are grayish in color. Owing to this difference in color, one can macroscopically identify regions containing cell bodies and regions that contain only nerve fibers in brain specimens.

Figure 1.14

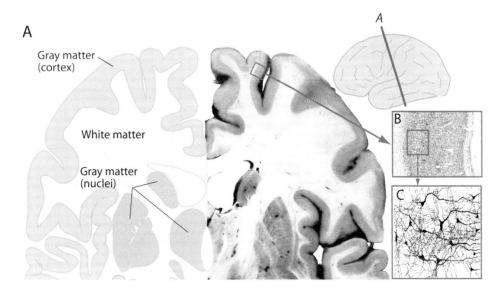

Gray and white matter. **A:** Drawing and photograph of an unstained frontal section through the human brain. The white matter consists only of axons and glial cells, whereas the gray matter contains the cell bodies, dendrites, and nerve terminals. **B:** Low-power photomicrograph of a section through the cerebral cortex (frame in **A**) stained so that only neuronal somata are visible (as small dots). **C:** Drawing of neurons in a section through the cerebral cortex (Golgi method). Only a small fraction of the neurons present in the section are shown.

Neurons Are Collected in Nuclei and Ganglia

When examining sections from the CNS under the microscope, one sees that the neuronal cell bodies are not diffusely spread out but are collected in groups. Such a group is called a **nucleus** (Figs. 1.14, 1.15, and 1.16). Neurons collected in this manner share connections with other nuclei and constitute in certain respects a **functional unit**; thus, the neurons in a nucleus receive the same kind of information and act on the same (or similar) target. In the PNS, a corresponding collection of cell bodies is called a **ganglion**.

Axons that end in a nucleus are termed **afferent**, whereas axons that leave the nucleus are **efferent**. We also use the terms afferent and efferent for axons conducting toward and away from the CNS, respectively. Thus, sensory axons conveying information from sense organs are afferent, while the motor axons innervating muscles are efferent.

Axons Form Tracts and Nerves

Axons from the neurons of one nucleus usually have common targets and therefore run together, forming bundles. Such a bundle of axons connecting one nucleus with another is called a **tract** (tractus; Figs. 1.15 and 1.16). In the PNS, a collection of axons is called a **nerve** (nervus; Fig. 1.16, see also Fig. 21.2). We also use the term **peripheral nerve** to emphasize that a nerve is part of the PNS. Tracts form white matter of the CNS, and, likewise, peripheral nerves containing myelinated axons are whitish.

Schematically, the large tracts of the nervous system are the main routes for nerve impulses—to some extent, they are comparable to highways connecting big cities. In addition, there are numerous smaller pathways often running parallel to the highways, and many smaller bundles of axons leave the big tracts to terminate in nuclei along the course. The number of smaller "footpaths" interconnecting nuclei is enormous, making possible, at least theoretically, the spread of impulses from one nucleus to almost any part of the nervous system. Normally, the spread of impulses is far from random but, rather, is highly ordered and patterned. As a rule, the larger tracts have more significant roles than the smaller ones in the main tasks of the nervous system. Consequently, diseases affecting such tracts usually produce marked symptoms that can be understood only if one has a fair knowledge of the main features of the wiring patterns of the brain.

COUPLING OF NEURONS: PATHWAYS FOR SIGNALS

In addition to the properties of synapses, which determine the transfer of signals among neurons, the function

---

Figure 1.15

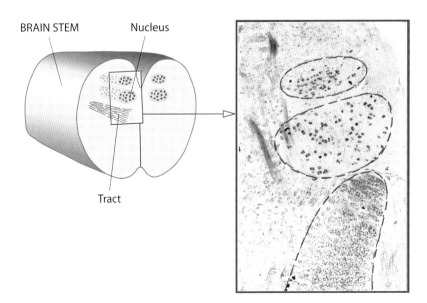

Nucleus and tract. **Left:** Schematic of part of the brain stem, showing the three-dimensional shape of two nuclei and a tract. **Right:** Photomicrograph showing the same structures in a section stained to visualize somata and myelinated axons. Magnification, ×75.

Figure 1.16

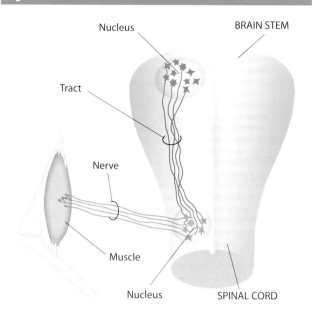

Nucleus, tract, and nerve. Three-dimensional schematic of parts of the brain stem, spinal cord, and a muscle in the upper arm. Axons from a nucleus in the brain stem form a tract destined for a nucleus in the spinal cord. The axons of the neurons in the spinal nucleus leave the CNS and form a nerve passing to the muscle.

of the nervous system depends on how the various neuronal groups (nuclei) are interconnected (often called the wiring pattern of the brain). This pattern determines the pathways that signals may take and the possibilities for cooperation among neuronal groups. Thus, although each neuron is to some extent a functional unit, it is only by

proper cooperation that neurons can fulfill their tasks. We describe here some typical examples of how neurons are interconnected, as such general knowledge is important for understanding the specific examples of connections dealt with in later chapters.

Divergence and Convergence

A fundamental feature of the CNS is that each neuron influences many—perhaps thousands—of others; that is, information from one source is spread out. This phenomenon is called **divergence** of connections. Figure 1.17 shows schematically how a sensory signal (e.g., from a fingertip) is conducted by a sensory neuron to the spinal cord and from there diverges to many spinal neurons. Each of the spinal neurons acts on many neurons at higher levels.

Another equally ubiquitous feature, **convergence** of connections, is shown schematically in Fig. 1.18. This means that each neuron receives synaptic contacts from many other neurons. The motor neuron shown in Fig. 1.18 controls the contraction of a number of striated muscle cells (but could have been almost any neuron in the CNS). The motor neuron receives synaptic contacts from many sources (peripheral sense organs, motor neurons in the cerebral cortex that initiate voluntary movements, and so forth). In this case, the motor neuron represents the **final common pathway** of all the neurons acting on it.

The nerve impulses may not necessarily follow all the available pathways shown in Figs. 1.17 and 1.18 because,

Figure 1.17

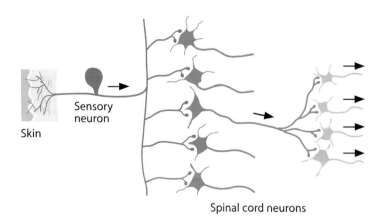

Divergence of neural connections. Highly simplified diagram. The axon collaterals of one sensory neuron contact many neurons in the spinal cord (red). Each of the spinal neurons contacts many other neurons (blue) in the cord or in the brain stem. In this way, the signal spreads from one neuron to many others. Arrows show the direction of impulse conduction.

That the two sides of the CNS cooperate extensively is witnessed by the vast number of **commissural connections**—that is, direct connections between corresponding parts in the two brain halves (Fig. 1.22B). Such connections occur at all levels of the CNS, but the most prominent one connects the two halves of the cerebral hemispheres (corpus callosum; see Figs. 6.26 and 6.27). In humans, this pathway contains approximately 200 million axons.

Single Neurons Are Parts of Neural Networks

The tasks of a neuron can be understood only in conjunction with the thousands of neurons with which it is synaptically interconnected. Further, functions of the brain are very seldom the responsibility of one neuronal group or "center" but, rather, the result of cooperation among many neuronal groups. Such cooperating groups or nuclei often lie far apart. For example, proper voluntary movements require cooperation among specific neuronal groups in the cerebral cortex, the cerebellum, and the basal ganglia deep in the cerebral hemispheres. Today we use the term **distributed system** rather than **center** when referring to the parts of the brain that are responsible for a specific function. Such a distributed system is a complicated **neural network**

of spatially separate but densely interconnected neuronal groups. Figure 1.23A gives a very simplified example of such a network that could be dedicated to, for example, the sensation of pain. Owing to the abundance of reciprocal connections, the signal traffic can take various routes within the network, and each neuronal group has connections outside the network. This means that a variety of inputs can activate the network—all presumably giving the same functional result (the sensation of pain, a specific memory, an emotion, and so forth). Nevertheless, it should not be surprising that each group, or **node**, might participate in several different, function-specific networks (Fig. 1.23B). Thus, as a rule, one neuronal group participates in several tasks.

The **anatomic connectivity** determines the possible interactions among different nodes, whereas the **functional connectivity** reflects the connections that are actively transmitting signals at any moment. Most likely, **synchronized**, **oscillatory** electrical activity is the "signature" of the operations of a network. Modern imaging techniques make it possible to study the relation between a certain behavior and the functional connectivity of specific networks.

The organization of the brain in distributed systems is particularly clear with regard to higher **mental functions**. Language is a good example: there is not one center for language but specific neuronal groups in many parts of the cerebral cortex that cooperate. Other networks are responsible for attention, spatial

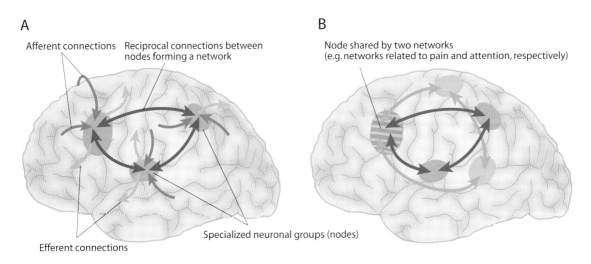

Figure 1.23

A

Afferent connections   Reciprocal connections between nodes forming a network

Efferent connections

Specialized neuronal groups (nodes)

B

Node shared by two networks (e.g. networks related to pain and attention, respectively)

Distributed neural networks. Highly simplified. **A:** Three nodes (groups of neurons) in the cerebral cortex are shown in light blue. They differ with regard to many of their afferent and efferent connections. Significantly, however, they share reciprocal connections, thus forming a network. The collective activity of the three parts of the network is responsible for its "product"—for example, the sensation of pain. **B:** Exemplifies that one node participates in more than one network.

orientation, object identification, short-term memory, and so forth. Data-based models of neural networks have provided new insight into the workings of the cerebral cortex and how symptoms arise from partial destruction of networks.

Injuries of Neural Networks

An important feature of distributed systems is that **partial damage** can degrade their performance but seldom eliminate it. Sometimes partial damage may become evident only in situations with very high demands, for example, with regard to the speed and accuracy of movements, the capacity of short-term memory, and so forth. If the number of neurons participating in the network undergoes further reduction, however, performance may deteriorate severely. In such cases, symptoms may occur rather abruptly, even though the disease process responsible for the cell loss may have been progressing slowly for years. This is typical of degenerative brain diseases such as Parkinson's disease and Alzheimer's disease.

THE CYTOSKELETON AND AXONAL TRANSPORT

The cell bodies and processes of neurons contain thin threads called **neurofibrils**, which can be observed in specially stained microscopic sections (Fig. 1.24). The neurofibrils are of different kinds but together they form the **cytoskeleton**—the name refers to its importance for development and maintenance of **neuronal shape**. The fact that neurons have very different shapes—with regard to dendrites, cell bodies, and axons—is due to cytoskeletal specializations. For example, the neurofibrils have a decisive role when axons grow for long distances (see Fig. 9.16), and the cytoskeleton serves to anchor synaptic elements at the postsynaptic density (see Fig. 4.2). The neurofibrils of the cytoskeleton are also responsible for another important cellular function: the transport of **organelles** and **particles** in the neuronal processes. Although such transport takes place in both dendrites and axons, **axonal transport** (Fig. 1.25) has been most studied (mainly because, for technical reasons, transport in dendrites is much harder to study). It is obvious that neurons need direction-specific transport mechanisms. Thus, the organelles necessary for protein synthesis and degradation of particles are present almost exclusively in the cell body. Nevertheless, dendrites contain small amounts of mRNA located at the base of dendritic spines, which may enable a limited amount of protein synthesis important for synaptic changes related to learning and memory.

Figure 1.24

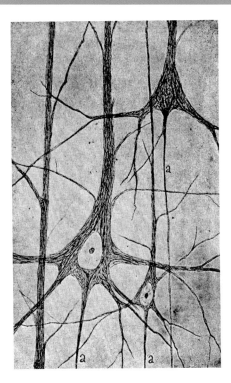

The cytoskeleton in neurons. Drawing of neurons from the cerebral cortex, as appearing in sections stained with heavy metals to visualize neurofibrils. Both dendrites and axons (a) contain numerous neurofibrils. (From Cajal 1952.)

Components of the Cytoskeleton

Electron microscopic and biochemical analyses have shown that the cytoskeleton consists of various kinds of fibrillary proteins, making threads of three main kinds:

1. **Actin filaments** (microfilaments) and associated protein molecules (approximately 5 nm thick)

2. **Microtubules** (narrow tubes) and associated proteins (approximately 20 nm thick)

3. **Intermediate filaments** or neurofilaments (approximately 10 nm thick)

Actin (microfilaments) is present in the axon, among other places. In the axon actin has an important role during development. When the axon elongates, actin together with microtubules serves to produce movements of the **growth cone** (see Fig. 9.16) at the tip of the axon (in general, actin is present in cells capable of movement, such as muscle cells). The growth cone continuously sends out thin fingerlike extensions (filopodia) in various directions. These

Glial cells are the most numerous cells in the brain and are indispensable for neuronal functioning. Glial cells are of three kinds that differ structurally and functionally. **Astrocytes** have numerous processes that contact capillaries and the lining of the cerebral ventricles. They serve important **homeostatic functions** by controlling the concentrations of ions and the osmotic pressure of the extracellular fluid (ECF), thereby helping to keep the neuronal environment optimal. Astrocytes are also involved in transmitter uptake and synapse formation and elimination. They respond to all kinds of injury and participate in **repair processes**. **Oligodendrocytes** insulate axons by producing **myelin sheaths** in the central nervous system (CNS), thus increasing the conduction velocity of the axons. **Microglial** cells seem to constantly survey the local environment of the neurons. Upon activation, they are transformed to **macrophages** that remove unwanted material. **Schwann cells** are a specialized form of glial cells that form myelin sheaths in the peripheral nervous system (PNS). Apart from these specific functions, glial cells are involved in the prenatal **development** of the nervous system, for example, by providing surfaces and scaffoldings for migrating neurons and outgrowing axons.

Although the glial cells are essential for proper neuronal functioning, **neuroinflammation** caused by activated glial cells are thought to contribute to the pathology in a number of diseases (depression, Alzheimer's disease, persistent pain, and several others).

Types of Glial Cells

It is customary to group glial cells into three categories that differ structurally and functionally: **astrocytes**, or astroglia; **oligodendrocytes**, or oligodendroglia; and **microglial cells**, or microglia. All three types have small cell bodies (compared with neurons) and send out several processes (Fig. 2.1.; see also Fig. 2.5 showing the difference in size between glial and neuronal nuclei in routinely stained sections). Astrocytes have numerous processes of various shapes (Fig. 2.1), whereas oligodendrocytes have relatively few and short processes (*oligo* means few, little). Microglial cells are—as the name implies—smaller than the other kinds. Reliable identification of the various types, however, requires immunocytochemical methods that identify specific cytoskeletal proteins. Fig. 2.2 exemplifies the identification of astrocytes by detection of **glial fibrillary acidic protein** (**GFAP**). Furthermore, differences in gene expression of receptors and signal substances help to characterize subgroups of the three main kinds of glial cell. For example, astroglia differs with regard to molecular biology in different parts of the CNS.[1]

Glial Cells Perform Many Tasks

Although they do not take part in the fast and precise information processing in the brain, glial cells are nevertheless of crucial importance to proper functioning of neurons. The name *glia* derives from the older notion that glial cells served as a kind of glue, keeping the neurons together. We now know, however, that glial cells (and astrocytes in particular) fulfill many important tasks apart from serving as a sort of scaffolding for the neurons: They serve homeostasis, regulate synaptic function, are crucial for axonal conductance, supply neurons with energy, and participate in the prenatal development of the nervous system. During infections and after trauma, glial cells are activated and carry out reparatory processes but may also contribute to tissue damage.

---

1. Such differences may help explain why **astrocytomas** (which are among the most common tumors in the CNS) arise preferentially in certain parts. Thus, astrocytes in different parts of the brain differ with regard to the expression of a tumor-suppression gene.

Figure 2.1

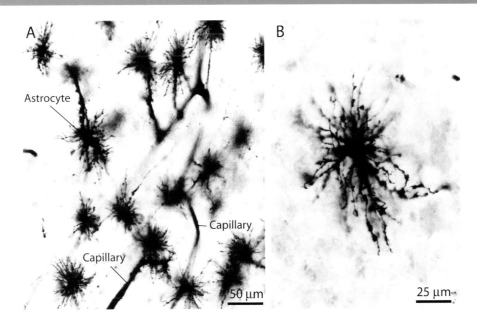

Astrocytes. Photomicrographs of Golgi-stained sections from the cerebral cortex. No neurons are visible. Note the close relationship between astrocytic processes and capillaries.

Number of Glial Cells

The number of glial cells increases during evolution and is higher than the number of neurons in humans. Thus, the ratio of glial cells to neurons in nematodes is only 0.2:1, while it is 0.4:1 in rodents and 1.4:1 in the human cerebral cortex (in other parts of the human brain the dominance of glial cells may be even greater). The absolute and relative increase in glial cells emphasize their importance for brain functioning and, more specifically, that the most complex brains are most dependent upon glial control of the neuronal local environment.

Figure 2.2

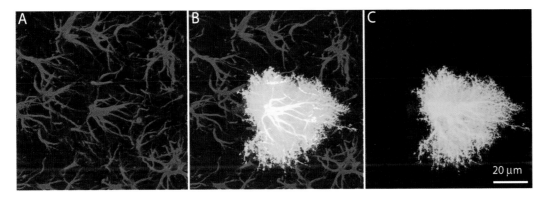

Astrocytes. **A:** Astrocytic processes visualized using an antibody against GFAP present in intermediary filaments. The antibody was labeled with a substance with red fluorescence. **B:** One of the astrocytes in A has been filled completely with intracellular injection of a substance with green fluorescence (Lucifer yellow) and reconstructed three-dimensionally. It is obvious that the astrocytic processes are much more abundant and of finer caliber than in **A. C:** View of the injected astrocyte in **B** in isolation, showing to advantage its dense and bushy halo of processes. (Reproduced with permission from Wilhelmsson et al. [2004] and *The Journal of Neuroscience*.)

to neurons, where it is metabolized aerobically. Therefore, it seems that astrocytes can deliver substrates for energy metabolism to the neurons. It is thought that this process may be important in situations with **hypoglycemia** and during periods with especially high neuronal activity.

Control of Ions

With regard to extracellular **ions**, the control of K^+ (potassium ions) is particularly important. Thus, neuronal excitability is strongly influenced even by small changes in the amount of K^+ ions extracellularly, and as neurons fire impulses, K^+ ions pass out of the cell (Fig. 2.4A). Prolonged or intense neuronal activity would therefore easily produce dangerously high extracellular levels of K^+ ions were it not for their efficient removal by glia. Further, astrocytes contribute to **extracellular pH** control by removing CO_2.

Control of Neurotransmitters

Extracellular **neurotransmitter concentration** must be tightly controlled, because proper synaptic functioning requires that their extracellular concentrations be very low, except during the brief moments of synaptic release. Most neurotransmitters are indeed removed from the ECF near the synapses by **transporter proteins** in the membranes of neurons and astrocytes. Specific transporters have been identified for several neurotransmitters (discussed further in Chapter 5). Figure 2.5 gives an impression of the abundance of a specific kind of transporter proteins (for the ubiquitous neurotransmitter glutamate, which is neurotoxic in abnormally high concentrations).

Aquaporins and Control of Water

As mentioned, astrocytes are also involved in the control of the extracellular osmotic pressure, that is, in controlling

Figure 2.5

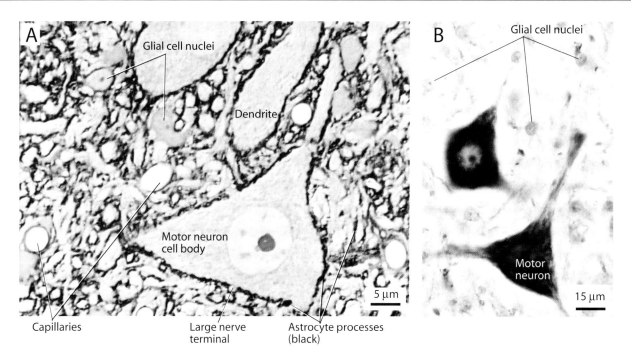

Astroglial processes in nervous tissue. **A:** Photomicrograph showing the distribution of a glutamate-transporter protein, as visualized via an immunocytochemical technique. In this 1-μm-thick section from the spinal cord, the dark spots and bands are astrocytic processes expressing glutamate transporters. They outline the somata, dendrites, and capillaries. The picture illustrates both the capacity of astroglia to take up glutamate from the ECF and the enormous astroglial surface facing neurons and capillaries. The contours of dendrites and neuronal somata are uneven because of synaptic contacts (thin arrow) breaking the otherwise continuous layer of astroglia. Capillaries are marked with asterisks. The cell body of an astroglial cell is marked with a thick arrow. (Courtesy of Drs. J. Storm-Mathisen and N.C. Danbolt, Department of Anatomy, University of Oslo.) **B:** For comparison, a photomicrograph of a thionine-stained section from the same part of the spinal cord as in **A**.

the **water balance** of the brain (Fig. 2.4A). Of particular interest in this respect are channels for transport of water—**aquaporins**—that are present in the membranes of astrocytes. Aquaporins were first described in kidney tubular systems, where they were shown to increase significantly the capacity for water passage. Interestingly, in the brain they are most abundant on the glial processes that are in close contact with capillaries and the CSF, that is, where one would expect them to be if they were involved in brain water balance (Fig. 2.4B). For example, **synaptic activity** causes rapid changes in the extracellular volume, and most likely aquaporins are instrumental in controlling such dynamic changes. Exchange by astroglial cells of small neutral molecules, such as the amino acid **taurine**, may be another mechanism to control extracellular osmolarity.

Recent research suggests that the functional role of aquaporins is not limited to regulation of the extracellular volume, although the latter has received the most attention. Thus, brain aquaporins have been implicated in tasks such as clearance of extracellular waste products, control of extracellular potassium, CSF circulation, neuroinflammation, and cell migration.

Aquaporins in Health and Disease

Two varieties of aquaporin predominate in the brain. **AQP4** is located in the astrocyte membrane and is particularly concentrated in the end-feet region close to capillaries and in glial processes bordering the CSF (Fig. 2.4B). **AQP1** is present in epithelial cells of the choroid plexus (which produces the CSF; see Chapter 7). In general, aquaporins increase water permeability of the cell membrane, thus allowing water to follow osmotic gradients and active ion transport. A function of AQP4 in the normal brain is probably to facilitate export of water. Thus, AQP4-deficient mice have increased interstitial (extracellular) fluid volume compared to normal mice. Further, in so-called **vasogenic brain edema**, wherein water accumulates extracellularly, AQP4 contributes to removal of excess water. This kind of edema arises when the brain capillaries become leaky due to, for example, traumatic brain injury. On the other hand, when water accumulates intracellularly, as typically occurs in cerebral ischemia or hypoxia (e.g., in stroke), the presence of AQP4 seems to *increase* the edema by allowing more water to enter the astrocytes. Such **cytotoxic brain edema** is caused by failure of energy-dependent ion pumping, which reduces the ability of the cells to maintain osmotic stability. Brain edema is a serious and often life-threatening complication in many brain disorders, such as stroke and traumatic brain injuries. Therefore, the discovery of a relationship between aquaporins and brain edema led to an intensive search for drugs that can modulate the activity of aquaporins. In animal experiments, inhibitors of AQP4 can reduce cytotoxic edema whereas they seem to worsen vasogenic edema. This complicates the search for the ideal drug because in human brain disorders the two kinds of brain edema usually coexist (although one may dominate depending on the specific disorder).

Oligodendrocytes and Schwann Cells

The myelin sheaths, which insulate axons, are formed by oligodendrocytes[2] in the CNS and by Schwann cells in the PNS. Although the structure and function of the myelin sheaths they produce are the same, oligodendrocytes and Schwann cells are not identical. One difference is that a single oligodendrocyte usually sends out processes to produce myelin segments for several axons (up to 40), whereas each Schwann cell forms a myelin segment for only one axon (Fig. 2.6). A particularly interesting difference concerns their differential influence on **regeneration** of damaged axons. In the PNS, a cut axon can regenerate under favorable conditions, provided that viable Schwann cells are present. In the CNS, however, such regeneration of axons does not normally occur, mainly because of inhibiting factors produced by oligodendrocytes.

In addition to forming myelin sheaths, oligodendrocytes and Schwann cells are important for **survival of the axons**. Thus, diseases affecting oligodendrocytes or Schwann cells produce axonal loss in addition to loss of myelin. In addition, oligodendrocytes and Schwann cells influence axonal thickness and **axonal transport**.

Differences between Oligodendrocytes and Schwann Cells

Even though the myelin sheaths produced by oligodendroglial cells and by Schwann cells look the same, they differ significantly in their lipid and protein composition. For example, myelin basic protein (MBP) makes up a much larger fraction of the total myelin protein in the CNS than in the PNS, whereas **peripheral myelin protein-22** (PMP-22) is absent in the CNS. Another example is **myelin-oligodendrocyte glycoprotein** (MOG), which is expressed in the CNS only. Such differences may help explain why some diseases affect only myelinated axons in the CNS (e.g., multiple sclerosis), whereas others are restricted to peripheral axons.

The Myelin Sheath

The **myelin sheath** forms an insulating cylinder around the axons (Fig. 2.6), reducing the loss of current from the axon to the surrounding tissue fluid during impulse conduction.

---

2. We do not know whether *all* oligodendrocytes form myelin. Thus, their cell bodies are often closely apposed to neuronal cell bodies, suggesting that they may have other tasks in addition to myelination.

autoimmunity) and that loss of nervous tissue was secondary. This is now being questioned, however. Thus, it seems possible that "people who develop multiple sclerosis will be shown to have a (genetically determined) diathesis [disease disposition] that does indeed predispose to neurodegeneration . . . but the exposure of that vulnerability requires an inflammatory insult without which the degenerative component does not manifest" (Compston, 2006, p. 563).

With regard to the inflammatory process, **T lymphocytes**, **microglial cells**, **brain endothelial cells**, and numerous **immune mediators** are involved, but their relative contributions are not fully understood. The role of microglia in the disease process illustrates the complexity: they may contribute both to destruction of myelin and axons and to regenerative processes (such as remyelination), presumably depending on the local situation.

Most current **therapies** aim at systemic **immune modulation** and appear to reduce significantly the frequency of disease episodes (relapses). Autologous stem cell transplantation—aiming to replace pathogenic T-cell populations—is now a promising option for patients with aggressive, relapsing MS.

Unmyelinated Axons

As mentioned, unmyelinated axons conduct much more slowly (at less than 1 m/sec) than myelinated ones, because they are thinner and lack the extra insulation provided by the myelin sheath. In the CNS, unmyelinated axons often lie in closely packed bundles without any glial cells separating them (see Fig. 1.7B). In the PNS, however, unmyelinated axons are always ensheathed in Schwann cells that do not make layers of myelin (Figs. 2.6, 2.7, and 2.8). During early development, several axons become embedded in the cytoplasm of the Schwann cells by invagination of the Schwann cell membrane. This arrangement probably serves to protect the axon from harmful substances in the interstitial fluid. Such protection may not be necessary in the CNS, as the composition of the interstitial fluid is governed by astroglia cells and by the blood–brain barrier.

Peripheral Nerves Are Built for Protection of the Axons

Fresh nervous tissue is soft, almost jellylike, with virtually no mechanical strength in itself. Protection of the CNS against external mechanical forces is afforded by its location within the skull and the vertebral canal and by its "wrapping" in membranes of connective tissue. For peripheral parts of the nervous system, the situation is different. Often located superficially, the peripheral bundles of axons and groups of nerve cells are exposed to various mechanical stresses. They are also subject to considerable stretching forces by movements of the body. Axons can be stretched only slightly

before their impulse conduction suffers, and they may even break. To prevent this, peripheral nerves contain large amounts of dense connective tissue with numerous collagen fibers arranged largely longitudinally (Fig. 2.7). The collagen fibers, specialized to resist stretching, protect the axons effectively. The presence of connective tissue in peripheral nerves is the reason that the nerves become much thicker where they leave the skull or the vertebral canal.

The connective tissue components of peripheral nerves form distinctive layers. The **epineurium** is an external thick layer of mostly longitudinally running collagen fibers. Internal to this layer, the axons are arranged into smaller bundles, or **fascicles**, which are wrapped in the perineural sheath or **perineurium** (Fig. 2.8). The collagen fibers and fibroblasts within the fascicles constitute the **endoneurium**. The perineurium is special in that it contains several layers of flattened cells. The cells, which in some respects resemble epithelial cells, interconnect through various kinds of junctions. In addition, the capillaries within the endoneurium are unusually tight and prevent passage of many substances from reaching the axons, consistent with experimental data showing that the perineurium constitutes a **blood–nerve barrier** preventing certain substances from reaching the interior of the fascicles with the axons. It is not surprising that PNS tissue also needs extra protective mechanisms to ensure that its environment is kept optimal for conducting impulses. The protection is not as efficient as in the CNS, however, and may perhaps explain why peripheral nerves are often subject to diseases that affect their conductive properties.

Diseases of Peripheral Nerves

Diseases involving peripheral nerves are called **neuropathies** and can have various causes. Whatever the cause, the symptoms are due to transitory or permanent disturbances of impulse conduction. Often there is a mixture of loss of axons and remaining axons that become hyperexcitable and spontaneously active. The latter evokes **paresthesias** (abnormal, nonpainful sensations such as tingling, pricking, vibration, coldness, and so forth) and (sometimes) persistent pain. Loss of axons produces muscle weakness and sensory loss (but can paradoxically also give persistent pain).

Axons and their myelin sheaths express membrane proteins that are specific to whether the axons are motor or sensory, thick or thin, and so forth. Thus, it may be understandable why neuropathies often affect certain nerves only or certain kinds of axons only. When motor axons are affected, the patient presents with pareses in certain muscles, while affection of sensory axons might produce loss of cutaneous sensation and joint sense. Neuropathies may also affect subgroups of sensory axons, for example, affecting only the very thin axons mediating sensations of pain and temperature but sparing axons related to touch. In other cases, only axons mediating joint sense are affected, whereas cutaneous sensation is spared (examples are

Figure 2.8

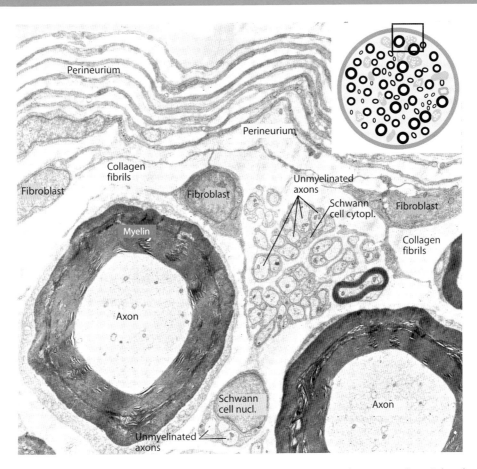

Peripheral nerve. Electron micrograph of cross section of the sciatic nerve. The picture shows a small, peripheral part of a nerve fascicle. The perineurium surrounding the fascicle is formed by several lamellae of flattened cells. Note the large difference in diameter among various myelinated axons. The thickness of the myelin sheath increases apace with the increase in axonal diameter. Between the myelinated axons are numerous unmyelinated ones. Collagen fibrils, produced by fibroblasts, fill most of the space between the axons. Magnification, ×4,000.

described in Chapter 13, under "Clinical Examples of Loss of Somatosensory Information").

Neuropathy is a well-known complication of metabolic diseases such as **diabetes** but can also be caused by toxic substances (e.g., lead). **Alcohol** abuse is a common cause of neuropathy. It is also a common side effect of **cytotoxic drugs** used for cancer treatment. Some neuropathies are due to attacks of the **immune system** on axons or myelin. This sometimes occurs after an infectious disease or in the course of cancer, probably because the immune system produces antibodies that cross-react with normal antigens expressed by axonal or Schwann cell membranes. An example is the **Guillan-Barré Syndrome** (acute inflammatory demyelinating polyradiculitis) that affects primarily the nerve roots (see Figs. 6.5 and 6.6). The disease usually starts with pareses and paresthesias in distal parts of the legs but ascends gradually to affect both extremities and sometimes the whole body.

A large group of neuropathies is **inherited**, among them, **Charcot–Marie–Tooth disease** (peroneal muscle atrophy). In most cases, the disease is inherited dominantly. The disease usually starts before the age of 20 years and leads to gradually increasing pareses and sensory loss, starting distally in the legs.

Loss of myelin and degeneration of axons cause the symptoms. Most patients with Charcot–Marie–Tooth disease have a doubling of the gene coding for the peripheral myelin protein (**PMP-22**). Animal models with overexpression of PMP-22 suggest that this defect alone can cause deficient myelination and symptoms corresponding to Charcot–Marie–Tooth disease in humans.

MICROGLIA AND REACTIONS OF THE CNS TO INJURY

Microglial Cells Monitor the Nervous Tissue

The third kind of glial cell, **microglia**, is so named because of its small size. Studies with immunocytochemical identification of specific membrane proteins show unequivocally

3 Neuronal Excitability

In Chapter 1 we considered some of the characteristic properties of neurons, such as their excitability and their ability to conduct impulses. The term **excitability** means that when a cell is sufficiently stimulated, it can react with a brief electrical discharge, called an action potential. The **action potential** (the nerve impulse) travels along the axon and is a major component in the communication among nerve cells and between nerve cells and other cells of the body. The action potential results from movement of charged particles—ions—through the cell membrane. A prerequisite for such a current across the membrane is an electric potential—the **membrane potential**—between the interior and the exterior of the cell and the presence of **ion channels** that are more or less selective for the passage of particular ions. The opening of ion channels is controlled by neurotransmitters binding to the channel (**transmitter** or **ligand-gated channels**) or by the magnitude of the membrane potential (**voltage-gated channels**). The membrane potential results from an unequal distribution of positively and negatively charged particles on either side of the membrane.[1] Energy-requiring **ion pumps** are responsible for maintaining the membrane potential. The **resting potential**, that is, the membrane potential when the neuron is not receiving any stimulation, is due mainly to unequal distribution of K^+ ions and the fact that the membrane is virtually impermeable to all ions other than K^+ in the resting state. The resting potential, with the interior of the cell negative compared with the exterior, is typically approximately −60 mV (millivolts). The **action potential** is a brief change of the membrane potential, caused by opening of channels that allow cations (especially Na^+) to enter the neuron, followed by an outward flow of K^+ ions. A net influx of cations reduces the membrane potential by making the interior less negative. This is called **depolarization**, and if it is sufficiently strong, an action potential is elicited due to opening of voltage-gated Na^+ channels.

After the brief depolarization caused by influx of Na^+ ions, the membrane potential is restored by the outward flow of K^+ ions. Restoration of the membrane potential is called **repolarization**. An increase of the membrane potential— **hyperpolarization**—makes the neuron less excitable (more depolarization is necessary to elicit an action potential). During a short period of time after an action potential, the membrane is in a **refractory state**, which means that another action potential cannot be elicited. This ensures that neurons can maintain the correct ion concentration balance.

Once an action potential is elicited, it is conducted along the axon. This is not merely a passive movement of charged particles in the fluid inside the axon. Because axons are poor conductors (compared with a metal thread), the action potential has to be renewed along the axonal membrane by cycles of depolarization and repolarization. In **unmyelinated** axons, these cycles move along the axon as a continuous wave, while in **myelinated** axons renewal of the action potential occurs only at the **nodes of Ranvier**. Because the process of depolarization–repolarization takes some time, the speed of conduction is much slower in unmyelinated axons than in myelinated ones. The action potential, when first elicited, is of the same magnitude. Neurons are nevertheless able to vary their messages because of the varying frequency and pattern of action potentials. Generally, the more synaptic inputs depolarize a neuron, the higher the frequency of axonal action potentials.

BASIS OF EXCITABILITY

The most basic property of neurons is their **excitability**— that is, their ability to respond to stimuli with an electric discharge. The discharges of billion of neurons can be recorded by placing electrodes on the head (electroencephalography [EEG]). Indeed, a "flat" EEG is used as a criterion of **brain death**, because it tells us that there are no functioning neurons left. The neuronal excitability is determined by properties of the cell membrane and active mechanisms creating and maintaining different concentrations of electrically charged particles (ions) inside and outside the cell.

---

1. Neither membrane potentials nor action potentials are properties unique to nerve cells. All cells have a membrane potential, although usually of less magnitude than that of neurons. Muscle cells and endocrine gland cells also produce action potentials in relation to contraction and secretion, respectively.

Figure 3.1

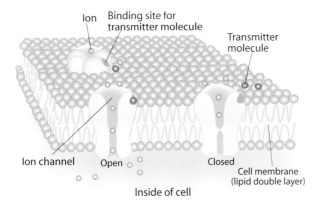

Ion channels. Schematic of a small part of the lipid bilayer of the cell membrane with interspersed ion channels. Binding of a transmitter molecule alters the opening state of the ion channel.

Cell Membrane Permeability Is Determined by Ion Channels

Ions cross the cell membrane almost exclusively through specific, water-filled channels because their electrical charges prevent them from passing through the lipid bilayer (Figs. 3.1 and 3.2). The channels are more or less **selective** for particular ions; that is, some ions pass more easily through a channel than others. Some channels are very selective, allowing passage of only one kind of ion (e.g., Na^+ ions), whereas other channels are less selective (e.g., letting through several cations such as Na^+, K^+, and Ca^{2+}). It follows that the ease with which an ion can pass through the membrane—that is, the **membrane permeability**[2] to that particular kind of ion—depends on (a) the presence of channels that let the ion through, (b) how densely these channels are distributed in the membrane, and (c) their opening state.

The current of ions through the membrane, however, does not depend solely on the density and opening of channels; an additional important factor is the **concentration gradient** across the membrane for the ion. That is, the

steeper the gradient, the greater the flow of ions from high to low concentration (provided that the membrane is not totally impermeable to the ion). Further, because ions are electrically charged particles, the **voltage gradient** across the membrane (i.e., the membrane potential) will also be important (Fig. 3.3). This means that if the interior of the cell is negative in relation to the exterior, the **cations**

Figure 3.2

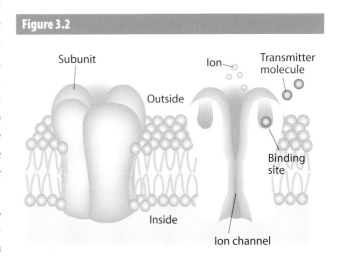

Ion channels. Five protein subunits are arranged around a central opening that can admit ions. At the outer side, the channel proteins are equipped with receptor sites for neurotransmitter molecules that regulate the opening of the channel. The figure shows the probable appearance of an acetylcholine receptor. (Based on Changeux 1993.)

2. The term **conductance** expresses the membrane permeability of a particular kind of ion more precisely. The conductance is the inverse of the membrane resistance. In an electrical circuit the current is $I = V/R$, where V is the voltage and R is the resistance (Ohm's law). This may be rewritten by using conductance (g) instead of R, as $I = g \cdot V$. In this way, one may obtain quantitative measures of membrane permeability under various conditions. For our purpose, however, it is sufficient to use the less precise term "permeability."

Figure 3.3

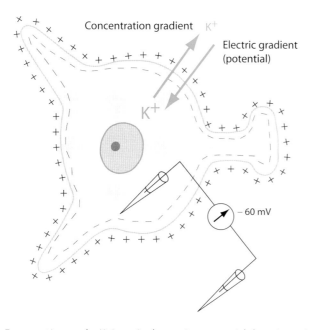

Forces acting on the K⁺ ions. At the resting potential there is equilibrium between the inward and outward forces (large arrows) acting on the K⁺ ions. One intracellular and one extracellular electrode (cones) measure the membrane potential.

Figure 3.4

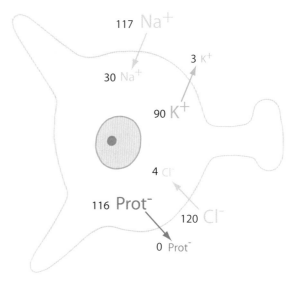

Distribution of ions of particular importance for the membrane potential. The exact concentrations depend on the resting potential (in this case –85 mV). Concentrations in mM.

(positively charged ions) on the exterior will be exposed to a force that attracts them into the cell, while the interior cations will be subjected to forces that tend to drive them out. The strength of these attractive and expulsive forces depends on the magnitude of the membrane potential. Therefore, the concentration gradient and the membrane potential together determine the flow of a particular ion through the membrane (Fig. 3.3).

The Membrane Potential and the Equilibrium Potential of Ions

In a typical nerve cell, the potential across the cell membrane is stable at approximately 60 mV in the resting state, that is, as long as the cell is not exposed to any stimuli. We therefore use the term **resting potential** in this situation (in different kinds of nerve cells, the resting potential may vary from about 45 mV to approximately 75 mV). The resting potential is due to a small surplus of negatively charged ions, **anions**, inside the cell versus the outside, and it has arbitrarily been decided to define the resting potential as negative, for example, –60 mV (Fig. 3.3).

The resting potential is caused primarily by two factors:

1. The **concentration of K⁺ ions** is about 30 times higher inside than outside the cell (Figs. 3.4 and 3.5).

2. The cell membrane is **selectively permeable** to K⁺ ions in the resting state (Fig. 3.5); that is, no other ions pass the membrane with comparable ease (the membrane is about 50 times more permeable to K⁺ than to Na⁺).

Although the concentration differs greatly inside and outside the cell for ions other than K⁺ (Fig. 3.4), the membrane is, as mentioned, almost impermeable to them (there are, e.g., very few open Na⁺ channels in the resting state). Other ions therefore influence the resting membrane potential only slightly. Therefore, to explain the membrane potential we can, for the time being, ignore ions other than K⁺. The concentration gradient will tend to drive K⁺ out of the cell, and, further, K⁺ ions can pass the membrane with relative ease through a particular kind of potassium channel that is open in the resting state. This means that positive charges are lost from the interior of the cell, making the interior negative compared to the exterior, thereby creating a membrane potential. The membrane potential reaches only a certain value, however, because it will oppose the movement of K⁺ ions out of the cell. Two opposite forces are at work: the concentration gradient tending to drive K⁺ out of the cell and the electrical gradient (the membrane

Figure 3.5

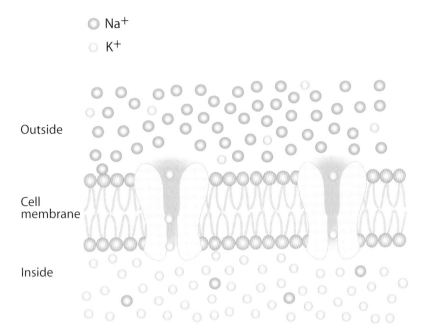

○ Na⁺
○ K⁺

Outside

Cell
membrane

Inside

The unequal distribution of K⁺ and Na⁺ ions, together with open K⁺ channels, largely explain the resting membrane potential.

potential) tending to drive K⁺ into the cell (Fig. 3.3). When the membrane potential is about −75 mV, these two forces are equally strong: that is, the flow of K⁺ into the cell equals the flow out. This is therefore called the **equilibrium potential for K⁺**, and its magnitude is determined by the concentration gradient for K⁺ ions (the concentration gradient varies somewhat among neurons).

The resting potential in most neurons, however, is lower than the equilibrium potential for K⁺ because the cell membrane is slightly permeable to Na⁺ (about 1/50th of the permeability to K⁺). Therefore, some positive charges (Na⁺) pass into the cell, driven by both the concentration gradient and the membrane potential, making the interior of the cell less negative than the equilibrium potential for K⁺. The membrane potential is consequently changed somewhat in the direction of the **equilibrium potential for Na⁺**: that is, +55 mV. In the resting state, the inflow of positive charges is equal to their outflow, and the membrane potential is therefore stable. Even though the two opposite currents of K⁺ and Na⁺ are small, over time they would eliminate the concentration gradients across the membrane. This is prevented, however, by energy-requiring "pumps" in the cell membrane that actively transport ions through the membrane against a concentration gradient. This **sodium–potassium pump** expels Na⁺ ions from the interior, in exchange for K⁺, at the same rate that the ions leak through the membrane. In

this way, the concentration gradients across the cell membrane are maintained.

Recording of Single-Cell Activity

Microelectrodes, with tips less than 1 μm thick, can be used to record the activity of single neurons and their processes (single units) intracellularly. Among other benefits, this has made it possible to study in detail the electrical events at the synapses and how they are influenced by various experimental manipulations. The effects of different concentrations of intra- and extracellular ions have been studied, as have the synaptic effects of various transmitter candidates and drugs. The **voltage clamp** technique, which permits manipulation of the membrane potential, has been instrumental to our understanding of the properties of synapses and the basic mechanisms underlying their operations. Likewise, great progress has been made with the **patch clamp technique**, making possible measurements of ion currents limited to even a single ion channel. The study of the properties of ion channels and membrane receptors is today highly interdisciplinary. **Implanted extracellular electrodes** can be used to record the activity of single neurons in relation to specific stimuli or behavioral tasks. This method has, for example, provided new insight into functional specializations within various areas of the cerebral cortex. By combining anatomic and physiologic techniques, it has been possible to determine the functional properties of structurally defined cell types. After an intracellular recording has been made from a neuronal cell body or its axon, it can be filled with a tracer substance through the same pipette. Afterward, the neuron with all its processes can be visualized in sections.

Anions Are Also Unevenly Distributed

For simplicity, we have so far dealt with only two cations, K^+ and Na^+, because they are the most important ones for the membrane potential and also for the action potential (discussed later in this chapter). Nevertheless, there are as many anions as cations. Chloride ions (Cl^-) and negatively charged protein molecules ($Prot^-$) are the major anions (Fig. 3.4). These ions are also unevenly distributed across the cell membrane: the concentration of Cl^- is 20 to 30 times higher outside than inside the cell, whereas the opposite situation exists for $Prot^-$. Therefore, **chloride** is the major extracellular anion, whereas **proteins** are the major intracellular ones. The proteins are so large that they cannot pass through the membrane; the membrane is impermeable to protein molecules. The membrane is somewhat permeable to Cl^-, however. The concentration gradient tends to drive chloride into the cell, whereas the membrane potential tends to drive it out, making the net flow of Cl^- small. In fact, the **equilibrium potential for Cl^-**, −65 mV, is close to the resting potential of most nerve cells. Therefore, no active mechanism for pumping of chloride is needed.

The Sodium–Potassium Pump and Osmotic Equilibrium

All cells depend on the sodium–potassium pump to maintain the membrane potential and osmotic equilibrium between the intracellular and extracellular fluid compartments. Particular to neurons is their need for increased pumping in association with the firing of action potentials, which arise because of a current of Na^+ into the cell and of K^+ out of it. The speed of pumping increases with increasing intracellular Na^+ concentration. A significant part of our energy in the form of ATP is spent on driving the sodium–potassium pump. In the resting state of nerve cells, this may constitute approximately one-third of the total energy requirement, whereas after high-frequency trains of action potentials it may increase to two-thirds.

The unequal distribution of ions is of fundamental importance also for the ability of neurons to maintain **osmotic equilibrium**. The distribution of ions must be such that the total concentrations of water-dissolved particles are equal inside and outside the cell. In other words, osmotic equilibrium means that the **water concentration** is equal inside and outside the cell (osmosis is the movement of water molecules from sites of high water concentration to sites of low water concentration). In case of osmotic imbalance, the cell will either swell or shrink (depending on whether the water concentration is lower inside or outside, respectively). An essential condition for osmotic balance is the low resting membrane permeability to Na^+, as both the concentration gradient and the membrane potential tend to drive Na^+ into the cell. This situation changes dramatically when the cells fire action potentials, because the membrane then becomes highly permeable to Na^+. Long trains of high-frequency action potentials may threaten the osmotic balance because more Na^+ ions enter the cell than can be pumped out.

Fortunately, neurons have properties that limit their maximal firing rate and the duration of active periods. Under pathological conditions, however, these safeguards may fail. In severe **epileptic seizures**, for example, neurons fire with abnormal frequency for long periods, and this probably contributes to cell damage by causing osmotic imbalance. Further, in situations with insufficient blood supply (ischemia), for example, after a **stroke**, ATP production suffers, resulting in slowing of the sodium–potassium pump. This, in turn, leads to osmotic imbalance and swelling of neurons. Such swelling is dangerous because neurons may be injured directly but also because swelling of the brain inside the skull (**brain edema**) reduces the blood supply.

Transmitter-Gated Ion Channels

Neurotransmitters control neuronal excitability by changing the opening state of ion channels (Figs. 3.1 and 3.2). A channel that is controlled by neurotransmitters (or other chemical substances) is called **transmitter-gated** or **ligand-gated** (the term "transmitter-activated" is also used). A large number of ion channels are now characterized that differ with regard to ion selectivity and transmitter specificity, that is, the ions that can pass a channel and the transmitter that controls it. The transmitter can either bind **directly** to the channel proteins or act **indirectly** via chemical intermediates (this is treated further in Chapter 4, under "Transmitters Act on Ionotropic and Metabotropic Receptors"). In most known cases, the transmitter opens the channel to increase the permeability of the relevant ions. We consider here only the effects of directly acting neurotransmitters (indirect effects are discussed later in this chapter). Binding of a transmitter molecule to a specific **receptor site** at the external face of a channel polypeptide may change the form of the polypeptides, thereby changing the diameter of the channel (Figs. 3.1 and 3.2). Usually, the channel is open only briefly after the binding of a transmitter molecule, allowing a brief current of ions to pass through the membrane. In this way, a chemical signal from a presynaptic neuron—the neurotransmitter—elicits an electric current through the postsynaptic membrane.

As mentioned, ion channels are more or less **selectively permeable**; that is, they let certain kinds of ions pass through more easily than others. Some channels are highly selective, allowing the passage of one kind only (such as Ca^{2+} ions), whereas others are less selective and will allow passage of, for example, most cations. Channels that are permeable for anions in general are usually termed chloride (Cl^-) channels because Cl^- is the only abundant anion that can pass through the membrane. Size and charge of the ion influence its permeability. For example, the Na$^+$ ions are more hydrated (bind more water molecules) than the K$^+$ ion and therefore are larger (Fig. 3.5). This may explain some of their differences in permeability. By regulating the channel opening, the transmitter controls the flow of ions through the postsynaptic membrane. However, the transmitter alters only the **probability** of the channel being in an open state; it does not induce a permanent open or closed state.

Voltage-Gated Ion Channels

Many channels are not controlled primarily by chemical substances but by the magnitude of the membrane potential and are therefore called **voltage-gated**. Voltage-gated Na$^+$ and K$^+$ channels, for example, are responsible for the action potential and therefore also for the propagation of impulses in the axons. There are also several kinds of voltage-gated Ca^{2+} channels, which control many important neuronal processes, for example, the release of neurotransmitters (see Fig. 4.1).

Voltage-gated channels are responsible for the activation of nerves and muscles by external **electrical stimulation**. Electrical stimulation of a peripheral nerve may produce muscle twitches by activating motor nerve fibers, as well as sensations due to activation of sensory nerve fibers. For some channels, their opening state is controlled by neurotransmitters and the magnitude of the membrane potential—that is, they are both ligand and voltage gated. An example is the so-called **NMDA receptor** (N-methyl-D-aspartate), which is part of a Ca^{2+} channel. Binding of glutamate opens the channel but only when the membrane potential is reduced (depolarized) compared with the resting potential (the NMDA receptor is discussed in Chapter 5).

The Structure of Ion Channels

The **ligand-gated** ion channels consist of five polypeptide subunits arranged around a central pore. The subunits span the membrane and extend to the external and internal faces of the membrane (Fig. 3.2). Therefore, signal molecules inside the cell may also influence the opening of ion channels. Three families of ligand-gated channels have been identified: the **nicotinic receptor superfamily** (GABA$_A$, glycine, serotonin, and nicotinic acetylcholine receptors), the **glutamate receptor family**, and the **ionotropic ATP receptors**. As an example, members of the nicotinic

receptor family consist of five equal subunits (Fig. 3.2), all contributing to the wall of the channel. The subunits are large polypeptides with molecular masses of approximately 300,000. The transmitter binds extracellularly at the transition between two subunits, but it is still unknown how the rapid binding (in less than 1 msec) produces conformational change in parts of the channel located, relatively speaking, far away. Most likely, the binding of the transmitter elicits a wave of conformational change in specific parts of the channel polypeptides. The actual opening of the channel may be caused by conformational change of just one specific amino acid.

Voltage-gated channels resemble ligand-gated ones: they consist of four subunits arranged around a central pore. The amino-acid sequence has been determined for several of the subunits, although lack of three-dimensional data has prevented clarification of the mechanisms that control their opening and ion selectivity. Presumably, subtle differences between the subunits forming the channel explain their high selectivity to particular ions.

Inherited Channelopathies

Many different genes code for channel proteins. Because ion channels determine the excitability of neurons, it is not surprising that **mutations** of such genes are associated with dysfunctions of neurons and muscle cells. Common to many such **channelopathies** is that the symptoms occur in bouts. Of particular clinical interest is that many of the channelopathies affecting neurons are associated with **epilepsy** and **migraine**. For example, mutations associated with epilepsy affect ligand-gated channels that are receptors for the neurotransmitters γ-aminobutyric acid (GABA) and acetylcholine and voltage-gated Na$^+$ and Ca^{2+} channels. Although channelopathies may not be the primary cause in the majority of patients with epilepsy, they may increase the susceptibility to other factors.

Mutations affecting channels gated by **glycine** (an inhibitory transmitter) are associated with abnormal **startle reactions**. This may be related to the fact that glycine is preferentially involved in inhibition of motor neurons.

Mutations of genes coding for a particular **voltage gated Ca^{2+} channel** (Ca$_v$2.1) are associated with several rare neurological diseases with disturbed synaptic transmission (the channel is necessary for synaptic transmitter release). Ca$_v$2.1 channel diseases include a certain kind of headache—**familial hemiplegic migraine**. Other mutations of the same gene are associated with **cerebellar ataxia** (jerky, uncoordinated movements) and a kind of epilepsy with **absences** (short episodes of disturbed consciousness).

Mutations of a kind of **voltage-gated potassium channel** (K$_v$α1.1)—expressed in highest density around the initial segment of axons—produce abnormal repolarization of motor axons and lead to repetitive discharges. This may explain the **muscle cramps** of such patients. Mutations of **voltage-gated sodium channels** cause bursts of intense **pain** (see also Chapter 13, under

"Nociceptors, Voltage-Gated Sodium and Potassium Channels, and Inherited Channelopathies"). A number of mutations affect channels in **striated muscle** membranes, many of them associated with **myotonia** (inability to relax after a voluntary muscle contraction).

Different mutations of one gene can give different **phenotypes**, such as reduced density of channels or reduced opening probability. It is noteworthy, however, that the same mutation can produce different symptoms in different individuals, even within the same family. This strongly suggests that the genes coding for the proteins of a channel do not alone determine its final properties. Additional factors, such as the products of other genes and environmental factors, must also contribute.

Many features of channelopathies are still unexplained—that they tend to occur episodically, that the symptoms often start at a certain age (in spite of the defect being present from birth), and that some forms remit spontaneously.

Alteration of the Membrane Potential: Depolarization and Hyperpolarization

As previously mentioned, in the resting state the membrane permeability for Na^+ is low. If for some reason Na^+ channels are opened so that the permeability is increased, Na^+ ions will flow into the cell and thereby reduce the magnitude of the membrane potential. Such a reduction of the membrane potential is called **depolarization**. The membrane potential is made less negative by depolarization. Correspondingly, one may predict that when the membrane permeability for K^+ is increased, more positive charges will leave the cell and the membrane potential will become more negative than the resting potential. This is called **hyperpolarization**. The same would be achieved by opening channels for chloride ions, enabling negative charges (Cl^-) to flow into the cell, provided that the membrane potential is more negative than the resting potential of Cl^-.

In conclusion, the membrane potential is determined by the **relative permeability** of the various ions that can pass through the membrane. At rest, the membrane is permeable primarily to K^+, and the resting potential is therefore close to the equilibrium potential of K^+. Synaptic influences can change this situation by opening Na^+ channels, thereby making the permeability to Na^+ dominant. This changes the membrane potential toward the equilibrium potential of Na^+ (at 55 mV). As shown in the following discussion, the action potential is caused by a further, sudden increase in the Na^+ permeability.

Markers of Neuronal Activity

Several methods can be used to visualize the activity of neurons. One method involves intracellular injection of a **voltage-sensitive fluorescent dye**. The intensity of fluorescence (as recorded with fluorescence microscopy and advanced computer technology) gives an impression of neuronal activity at a given time. Thus, this (indirect) measure of activity can be correlated with experimental manipulation of a specific transmitter, the execution of specific tasks, and so forth.

Another method takes advantage of the fact that **optic properties** of nervous tissue change with the degree of neuronal activity. This enables the recording of slow as well as rapid changes in neuronal activity in relation to experimental influences (it has been applied, e.g., in conscious persons during neurosurgery that necessitates exposure of the cerebral cortex). Other methods enable mapping of variations in neuronal activity at the time of death in experimental animals. Cells take up intravenously injected radiolabeled **deoxyglucose** in the same way as glucose. It is not broken down, however, and therefore accumulates in the cells. Because glucose is the substrate for oxidative metabolism in the neurons, its uptake correlates with degree of neuronal activity. After exposing an animal to certain kinds of stimulation or eliciting certain behaviors, one can afterward determine with autoradiography which neuronal groups were particularly active during stimulation or at the time of certain actions.

Another method utilizes the fact that a few minutes with excitatory synaptic input induces expression of so-called **immediate early-genes** in many neurons. Most studied among such genes is **c-*fos***. Without extra stimulation, C-*fos* mRNA and its protein product are present in only minute amounts in most neurons. Detection of increased levels of c-*fos* mRNA in tissue sections is therefore used as a marker of neurons that were particularly active in a certain experimental situation. This method is also used to determine where in the brain a drug exerts its effect. The method has its limitations, however. Thus, c-*fos* expression may be caused by nonspecific influences, and not all neurons express c-*fos* even when properly activated.

THE ACTION POTENTIAL

Voltage-Gated Sodium Channels Are Instrumental in Evoking an Action Potential

The basis of the action potential is found in the presence of **voltage-gated Na^+ channels**, which are opened by depolarization of the membrane (Fig. 3.6). Depolarization may be induced in several ways; for example, under artificial conditions by direct electrical stimulation. Normally, however, it is caused by neurotransmitters acting on transmitter-gated channels. The opening of transmitter-gated Na^+ channels often starts depolarization. Opening of the voltage-gated channels requires that the membrane be depolarized to a certain **threshold** value, that is, the threshold for producing an action potential (Fig. 3.6). When voltage-gated channels are opened, the permeability to Na^+ is increased beyond what was achieved by the opening of transmitter-gated channels, and Na^+ flows into the cell driven by both the concentration

Figure 3.6

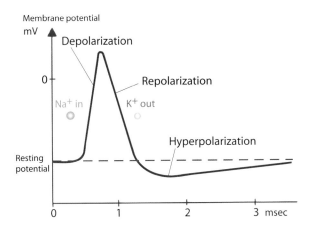

The action potential.

Figure 3.7

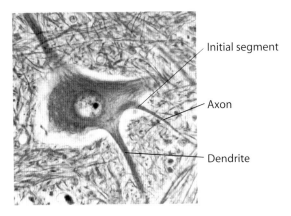

The initial segment of the axon is where the action potential usually arises. Photomicrograph of a motoneuron from the spinal cord stained with a silver-impregnation method.

gradient and the membrane potential. The membrane becomes more depolarized; in turn, this opens more voltage-gated channels and so on. In this way, as soon as the membrane is depolarized to the threshold value, the permeability to Na⁺ increases in an explosive manner. Even with all sodium channels fully open, however, the inward current of Na⁺ ions stops when the membrane is depolarized to +55 mV; at that value the inward concentration force is equal to the outward electrical force (the membrane potential). As mentioned, +55 mV is the equilibrium potential of Na⁺. Figure 3.6 shows how, during an action potential, the membrane potential quickly changes to positive values and then returns almost as rapidly to approximately the resting value. This occurs because the membrane again becomes impermeable to Na⁺; the Na⁺ channels are closed or **inactivated**.[3] Therefore, at the peak of the action potential and for a short time afterward, no Na⁺ can pass through the membrane. In this situation with a positive membrane potential, K⁺ is driven out by both the concentration gradient and the membrane potential (electrical force). Because no Na⁺ can enter the cell, there is a net outward flow of positive charges, again making the interior of the cell negative. We say that the membrane is **repolarized**. The speed of repolarization is increased by the presence of **voltage-gated K⁺ channels**, which open when the membrane is sufficiently depolarized. The opening of the voltage-gated K⁺ channels is somewhat delayed compared with the Na⁺ channels, but whereas the Na⁺ channels inactivate after about 1 msec, the K⁺ channels stay open for several milliseconds.

In sum, the action potential is caused by a brief inward current of Na⁺ ions, followed by an outward current of K⁺ ions. The whole sequence of depolarization–repolarization is generally completed in 1 to 2 msec. If the threshold is reached, an action potential of a certain magnitude arises, regardless of the strength of the stimulus that produced the depolarization.

Where Does the Action Potential Arise?

The action potential usually arises in the first part of the axon, the **initial segment** (Fig. 3.7; see also Fig. 2.6), where the density of voltage-gated Na⁺ channels is higher than in the membrane of the dendrites and the cell soma. The current spreads electrotonically (passively) from dendritic and somatic synapses toward the initial segment. If the depolarization is sufficiently strong (reaches threshold), voltage-gated Na⁺ and K⁺ channels open and produce an action potential that is propagated along the axon. Although action potentials can be elicited in dendrites, their threshold is usually much higher than in the initial segment owing to lower density of voltage-gated channels.

The Action Potential and Changes of Ion Concentrations

One might think that an action potential would cause significant changes in the concentrations of Na⁺ and K⁺ on the two sides of the membrane, but this is not the case. The number of ions actually passing through the membrane during an action potential is extremely small compared with the total number inside the cell and in its immediate surroundings. Even in an axon with a diameter of about 1 μm, with a very small intracellular volume compared to the membrane surface area, only 1 of 3,000 K⁺ ions moves out during the action potential. In addition,

3. **Inactivation** and **closure** involve different parts of the voltage-gated Na⁺ channel. This is indicated by, among other findings, that whereas closure of the channel lasts as long as the membrane potential remains below threshold, inactivation is transitory and lasts only some milliseconds.

active pumping (the sodium–potassium pump) ensures that Na$^+$ is moved out and K$^+$ is moved in between each action potential and during periods of rest. Even when the sodium–potassium pump is blocked experimentally, a nerve cell can produce several thousand action potentials before concentration gradients are reduced so much that the cell loses its excitability.

The Refractory Period

After an action potential, some time must elapse before the neuron can again produce an action potential in response to a stimulus. The cell is said to be in a **refractory state**. This ensures at least a minimal rest for the cell between each action potential and thereby puts an upper limit on the frequency with which the cell can fire. The length of the refractory period, and therefore also the maximal frequency of firing, varies considerably among different kinds of nerve cells.

Two conditions are responsible for the refractory period. One is the aforementioned inactivation of the voltage-gated Na$^+$ channels, and the other is the fact that the membrane is hyperpolarized immediately after the action potential (Fig. 3.6). The inactivation of Na$^+$ channels means that they cannot be opened, regardless of the strength of the stimulus and the ensuing depolarization. Hyperpolarization occurs because the K$^+$ channels remain open longer than required just to bring the membrane potential back to resting value. These two different mechanisms can account for why the refractory period consists of two phases. During the first phase, the **absolute refractory period**, the cell cannot be made to discharge, however strong the stimulus may be; during the **relative refractory period**, stronger depolarization than normal is needed to produce an action potential.

Calcium and Neuronal Excitability

A cation other than Na$^+$—namely, Ca^{2+}—may also contribute to the rising phase of the action potential. For Ca^{2+}, as for Na$^+$, the extracellular concentration is much higher than the intracellular one, and there are voltage-gated calcium channels in the membrane. Cellular influx of calcium can be visualized after intracellular injection of a substance that fluoresces when Ca^{2+} binds to it. During the action potential, calcium enters the cell—partly through Na$^+$ channels and partly through voltage-gated calcium channels, which have a more prolonged opening–closing phase than the sodium channels. There are also transmitter-gated calcium channels. In most neurons, the contribution of Ca^{2+} to the action potential is nevertheless small compared with that of Na$^+$. In certain other cells such as heart muscle, however, calcium is the ion largely responsible for the action potential. Because the calcium channels open and close more slowly than the Na$^+$

channels, an action potential produced by calcium currents lasts longer than one produced by flow of Na$^+$.

Another aspect of the functional role of calcium is that the extracellular calcium concentration influences the membrane excitability, which is most likely mediated through effects on the Na$^+$ and K$^+$ channels. Reducing the calcium concentration in the blood and interstitial fluid—**hypocalcemia**—lowers the threshold for evoking action potentials in neurons and muscle cells, whereas increasing the concentration—**hypercalcemia**—has the opposite effect. A typical symptom of hypocalcemia is muscle spasms—**tetany**—due to hyperexcitability of nerves and muscles. Severe hypercalcemia can cause drowsiness, nausea, and anorexia.

Neuronal Homeostasis and Control of Extracellular Potassium

Normally, the extracellular K$^+$ concentration is under tight control, as discussed in Chapter 2 ("Astroglia and the Control of Neuronal Environment"). Such control is necessary because even small alterations influence the excitability of neurons significantly. When the neurons produce action potentials, K$^+$ ions move out, increasing the extracellular concentration. This increases the excitability of the neurons in the immediate vicinity, and for each new action potential the extracellular K$^+$ concentration rises a little more. If not counteracted, this positive feedback situation would cause uncontrolled firing of neurons. Even if it initially would affect only a few neurons, the activity would spread in networks connected with the hyperexcitable neurons. This is the situation with **epileptic seizures** (see Chapter 22, under "Epileptic Seizures Starting in MI").

Under normal conditions, however, **negative feedback** mechanisms prevent the loss of homeostatic control. First the permeability (conductance) of a special kind of K$^+$ channel increases in situations with high-frequency firing. This brings the resting potential closer to the equilibrium potential of K$^+$—that is, the membrane becomes less depolarized.[4] Furthermore, **astroglia** contributes by removing excess K$^+$ from the extracellular fluid. The **refractory period** represents another homeostatic mechanism by limiting the maximal firing frequency. Although these mechanisms are effective in the short run, in the long run the

---

4. Presumably, the large repertoire of selective K$^+$ channels reflects the importance of stabilization of membrane polarization. Some channels are ligand gated; others are voltage gated (K$_v$ channels). A particular kind is **inwardly rectifying** K$^+$ **channels** (Kir), which means that the channel preferentially let K$^+$ ions *into* the cell (unlike the K$^+$ channel responsible for the repolarization phase of the action potential, Fig. 3.6). Ca^{2+} plays an important role in regulation of several K$^+$ channels.

sodium-potassium pump is all-important for control of K⁺ concentrations. Finally, **inhibitory synapses** are instrumental in controlling neuronal excitability.

Electrical Properties of Axons

We now consider how the action potential moves along the axon. The ability of the axon to conduct electrical current depends on several conditions, some of which are given by the physical properties of axons, which are very different from, for example, those of copper wire. In addition, some conditions vary among axons of different kinds. An axon is a poor conductor compared with electrical conductors made of metal because the axoplasm through which the current has to pass consists of a weak solution of electrolytes (i.e., low concentrations of charged particles in water). In addition, the diameter of an axon is small (from <1 to 20 μm) with a correspondingly enormous **internal resistance** to the current in the axoplasm. Further, the axonal membrane is not a perfect insulator, so charged particles are lost from the interior of the axon as the current passes along its length. The amount of current lost is determined by the degree of **membrane resistance** (i.e., the resistance of the membrane to charged particles trying to pass). Finally, the axonal membrane (like all cell membranes) has an **electrical capacity**; that is, it can store a certain number of charged particles in the same way a battery does. This further contributes to the rapid attenuation of a current that is conducted along an axon: the membrane has to be charged before the current can move on.

The Action Potential Is Regenerated as It Moves Along the Axon

From the foregoing it can be concluded that how well the current is conducted in an axon depends on its internal resistance (its diameter), the membrane resistance (how well insulated it is), and the capacity of the axonal membrane. If the propagation of the action potential along the axon occurred only by passive, electrotonic movement of charged particles, the internal resistance and loss of charges to the exterior would cause the action potential to move only a short distance before it "died out." The solution to this problem is that the action potential is **regenerated** as

it moves along the axon. Therefore, it is propagated with undiminished strength all the way from the cell body to the nerve terminals. As discussed, the strength of the action potential—that is, the magnitude of the changes of the membrane potential taking place—is the same regardless of the strength of the stimulus that produced it (as long as the stimulus depolarizes the membrane to threshold). Thus, increasing the strength of the stimulus increases the frequency of action potentials, whereas the magnitude of each action potential remains constant.

When the cell membrane at the initial segment (Fig. 3.7) is depolarized to threshold, an action potential is produced and is conducted passively a short distance along the axon. From then on, what occurs differs somewhat in myelinated and unmyelinated axons (Figs. 3.8 and 3.9).

Impulse Conduction in Unmyelinated Axons

The action potential is produced by positive charges penetrating to the interior of the axon, which at that point becomes positive relative to more distal parts along its

Figure 3.8

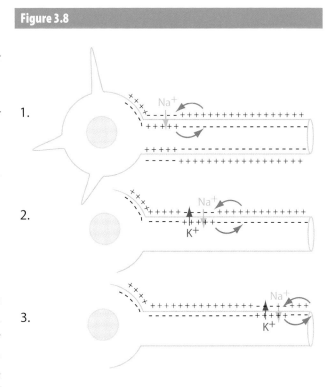

Impulse conduction in unmyelinated axons. Arrows show direction of movement of charged particles. The action potential is renewed continuously along the axonal membrane by a wave of depolarization–repolarization.

Figure 3.9

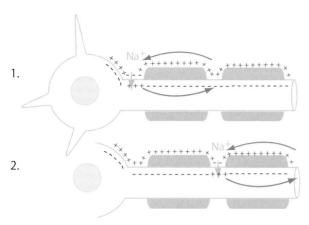

1.

2.

Impulse conduction in myelinated axons. Arrows show direction of movement of charged particles. The current moves electrotonically in the myelinated part of the axons, and the action potential is renewed only at the node of Ranvier, causing a small delay in impulse propagation.

length (Fig. 3.8). Positive charges then start moving in the distal direction (along the electrical gradient that has been set up). Outside the axon, a corresponding current of positive charges moves in the opposite direction, so that an **electrical circuit** is established. Movement of positive charges in the distal direction inside the axon means that the membrane is depolarized as the charges move along. This depolarization leads to the opening of enough voltage-gated Na⁺ and K⁺ channels to produce a "new" action potential. In this manner, the action potential moves along the axon at a speed that depends on the speed with which the charged particles (i.e., ions) move inside the axon and on the time needed for full opening of the ion channels. The membrane capacity represents a further factor slowing the propagation because the membrane has to be charged before there can be a net flow of charges through it.

In essence, the action potential is propagated as a wave of depolarization, followed closely by a corresponding wave of repolarization. When the membrane has just completed this cycle, it is in the refractory state for some milliseconds. This delay prevents the action potential from spreading "backward" toward the cell body (**antidromic** impulse conduction) and ensures that under normal conditions the impulse conduction is unidirectional. If, however, the axon is artificially stimulated (e.g., electrically) at some distance from the cell body, the action potential spreads toward both the cell body and the end ramifications (**orthodromic**

impulse conduction). Antidromic impulse conduction may occur in branches of peripheral sensory axons on natural stimulation and may play a part in certain disease symptoms (see Chapter 29, "Antidromic Impulses and the Axonal Reflex").

Impulse Conduction in Myelinated Axons

In myelinated axons, the action potential is also regenerated along the axon (Fig. 3.9). However, in contrast to that in unmyelinated axons, the action potential is regenerated only at each **node of Ranvier**—that is, where the axon membrane lacks a myelin covering and is in direct contact with the extracellular fluid (see Fig. 2.6). As in unmyelinated axons, the action potential arises in the initial segment of the axon. The current then spreads passively (electrotonically) to the first node of Ranvier. Here, the depolarization of the membrane leads to opening of voltage-gated channels and a "new" action potential. The density of voltage-gated sodium channels is particularly high in the axonal membrane at the node of Ranvier. The current can flow electrotonically as far as the first node of Ranvier (and probably sometimes farther) because the axon is so well insulated by myelin, preventing loss of charges from the interior of the axon. (Myelin dramatically increases the resistance across the membrane and also reduces the membrane capacity.) In addition, the axonal diameter is larger in myelinated than in unmyelinated axons, thus reducing the internal resistance.

In conclusion, in myelinated axons the action potential does not move smoothly and slowly along, as in unmyelinated axons, but instead "jumps" from one node of Ranvier to the next. This is also called **saltatory conduction**. Although the impulse propagation is very rapid between nodes, at each node there is a delay due to the time required for opening of channels and establishment of sufficient flow of current.

Conduction Velocities in Myelinated and Unmyelinated Axons

The main reason myelinated axons conduct so much more rapidly than unmyelinated ones is that the action potential must be regenerated only at certain sites. A figure for conduction velocity (expressed in meters per second) in myelinated axons is obtained by multiplying the axonal diameter (in micrometers) by 6. An axon of 20 μm (the maximal diameter) therefore conducts at approximately

120 m/sec, whereas the thinnest myelinated axons of about 3 μm conduct at 18 m/sec. In comparison, a typical unmyelinated axon of about 1 μm conducts at less than 1 m/sec.

Orthodromic, Antidromic, and Ephaptic Impulse Conduction

The normal situation in most neurons is that the action potential travels from the soma toward the nerve terminals. This is called **orthodromic** impulse conduction. Propagation of the action potential in the opposite direction is called **antidromic** impulse conduction. This is prevented, however, by the refractory state that arises just after membrane depolarization. (In peripheral sensory neurons, orthodromic conduction is from the terminals toward the cell body [see Fig. 1.5], whereas antidromic conduction is from the cell body toward the nerve terminals.) When an axon is stimulated artificially (e.g., electrically) somewhere along its course, action potentials travel both orthodromically and antidromically.

Antidromic impulse conduction can occur in peripheral branches of **sensory neurons** when action potentials arise in only some of the branches. The action potentials then travel orthodromically toward the CNS but also antidromically (outward) in nonstimulated nerve fiber branches. This phenomenon is important in certain disease states because the antidromically activated terminals release substances that induce tissue **inflammation** (see Chapter 13, under "Inflammatory Diseases and Release of Neuropeptides from Peripheral Branches of Sensory Neurons," and Chapter 29, under "Antidromic Impulses and the Axonal Reflex").

Under **pathologic conditions**, especially with partial damage of nerves, action potentials can spread from one axon to a neighboring one by **ephaptic** transmission. In such cases the action potential spreads most likely in both directions—that is, centrally to the CNS and peripherally to terminal axonal branches. Ephaptic transmission occurs in certain painful **neuropathies** (see Chapter 2, under "Diseases of Peripheral Nerves"). One example is **trigeminal neuralgia**, which is a condition with bouts of intense facial pain, in most cases due to compression of the trigeminal nerve by a blood vessel. The compression causes loss of myelin and abnormal axonal excitability with ephaptic transmission that most likely explains the pain.

HOW NERVE CELLS VARY THEIR MESSAGES

So far we have treated the action potential as a unitary phenomenon. As mentioned, the strength of each action potential of a neuron does not vary: whenever depolarized to the threshold, the cell fires action potentials of constant magnitude. Therefore, the action potential is an **all-or-none** phenomenon, and one might think that each neuron would be able to tell only whether or not a stimulus occurs. We know, however, that the individual nerve cell can communicate to others about the strength of the stimulation it receives—such as the intensity of light or a sound, of

something touching the skin, and so forth. It does so by varying the **frequency** and **pattern** of action potentials.

Frequency Coding

To understand how the neuron can vary its firing frequency, we need to know that a neuron is more or less continuously influenced by impulses from many other neurons. A sustained synaptic input that is strong enough to depolarize the cell to threshold does not merely produce one action potential but rather several in succession. The stronger the depolarization, the shorter the time required for reaching the threshold after each action potential. Consequently, the firing frequency depends on the strength of depolarization (Fig. 3.10). We say that the neuron uses a **frequency code** to tell how strongly it has been stimulated. The **maximal frequency** of action potentials in some neurons is more than 100 per second (100 Hz), whereas in others it is much lower.

Pattern of Action Potentials

The average firing frequency is not the only way by which the neuron can alter its message. The **firing pattern** also carries information, and each neuronal type has its characteristic firing pattern that is caused by differences in membrane properties and synaptic inputs (see "The Refractory Period," earlier in this chapter). Two neurons may both fire

Figure 3.10

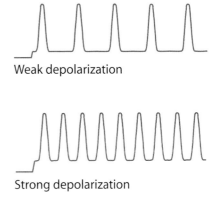

Weak depolarization

Strong depolarization

The frequency of action potentials depends on the magnitude of depolarization. Therefore, the frequency of action potentials reflects the total synaptic input to a neuron.

Figure 3.11

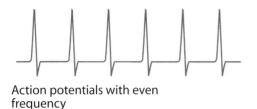

Action potentials with even
frequency

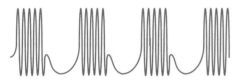

Action potentials in bursts

Different patterns of nerve impulses provide neurons with an additional means to vary the information they send to other neurons and muscle cells.

with an average frequency of, for example, 10 per second but nevertheless influence a postsynaptic cell differently. So-called **burst neurons** produce trains of action potentials with a high frequency and then pause for a while before a new train (burst) of impulses arises. Other neurons—so-called **single-spike neurons**—produce action potentials with regular intervals (Fig. 3.11).

Switching Between Regular Spikes and Bursts

Some neurons can switch between these two modes of firing. In such cases, the relationship is not linear between the strength of synaptic input and the firing frequency. The transition between the different firing patterns is evoked by a specific **neurotransmitter** (e.g., serotonin), which does not in itself produce action potentials in the postsynaptic cell but changes its reactions to other inputs. For example, the neuron may change from burst to single-spike patterns or from a high firing frequency to no firing at all.

Plateau Potentials

In some neurons, the occurrence of so-called plateau potentials causes the switch from low-frequency firing to high-frequency or bursting firing pattern. This has been shown for many neurons that control **rhythmic muscle contractions**. Plateau potentials are produced by a slow, depolarizing current, for example, by certain voltage-gated Ca^{2+} channels that are open in a limited range of membrane potentials. Such a neuron can therefore change abruptly between two entirely different behaviors. The neurotransmitter **serotonin** can evoke plateau potentials in groups of spinal motor neurons (see Chapter 21, under "Muscle Cramps and Plateau Potentials," and Chapter 22, under "Monoaminergic Pathways from the Brain Stem to the Spinal Cord"). Release of this transmitter relates to motivation and attention rather than to specific information.

In Chapter 3 we discussed the basis of nerve impulses and their conduction in axons. This chapter deals with the properties of synapses. We discuss mainly **chemical synapses**: synapses in which the signal is mediated by a neurotransmitter. Synapses with direct **electric coupling** (gap junctions) are common among glial cells but occur infrequently among neurons. The key events underlying signal transfer at chemical synapses are as follows: First, an action potential reaches the nerve terminal (bouton) and **depolarizes** it. This depolarization opens **Ca^{2+} channels**, enabling Ca^{2+} to enter the nerve terminal. Increase in intracellular Ca^{2+} concentration is a signal for release of **neurotransmitter** from vesicles by exocytosis. This produces a high concentration of neurotransmitter in the synaptic cleft. The released transmitter binds briefly to **receptors** in the **postsynaptic membrane**. After activation of the receptor, the transmitter must be **inactivated** quickly to reestablish a low background activity of the receptors, that is, to ensure a high **signal-to-noise ratio** at the synapse. Inactivation occurs partly by diffusion of the transmitter, partly by **enzymatic degradation** and partly by specific uptake mechanisms (**transporter proteins**).

There are two main kinds of transmitter receptors. **Ionotropic receptors** are parts of ion channels and therefore influence the functional state of the channel directly. Therefore, transmitter actions elicited by ionotropic receptors are fast and precise. **Metabotropic receptors** are coupled indirectly (via intracellular second messengers) to ion channels. Their effects are therefore slower to start and longer lasting than effects mediated by ionotropic receptors. We also use the term **modulatory** of the synaptic effects of metabotropic receptors, because they adjust the excitability of the postsynaptic neuron so that it responds more or less vigorously to the precise effects of ionotropic receptors (in addition, metabotropic receptors may have effects on the growth and survival of the postsynaptic neuron).

The change of the membrane potential arising as a result of synaptic influence is called a **synaptic potential**. If the synaptic influence depolarizes the postsynaptic cell, the probability that the cell will fire action potentials is increased. This synaptic effect is called an **excitatory postsynaptic potential (EPSP)**. If the synaptic potential hyperpolarizes the cell, it is called an inhibitory postsynaptic potential (IPSP) because the probability of the cell's firing is diminished. If the transmitter produces an EPSP, we use the terms **excitatory synapse** and **excitatory transmitter**. Likewise, an **inhibitory transmitter** produces an IPSP at an **inhibitory synapse**.

Because the depolarization caused by one EPSP is small, **summation** of many EPSPs is usually needed to reach a threshold for eliciting an action potential. This enables the neuron to integrate information from often many thousand synapses.

Synapses are **plastic**; that is, they can change their properties by use. This implies that certain kinds of activity can enhance or reduce the subsequent effect of a synapse on the postsynaptic neuron for a variable period (from milliseconds to years). Most likely, such **use-dependent** synaptic plasticity is the neuronal basis for **learning** and **memory**.

NEUROTRANSMITTER HANDLING AT THE SYNAPSE

The vast majority of the synapses between neurons and between neurons and muscles are chemical, and this chapter deals with this kind. Their main structural features were described in Chapter 1.

Unusual Synapses: Electrotonic and Dendrodendritic Transmission

Although it is rare, the pre- and postsynaptic elements are electrically rather than chemically coupled at some synapses. Electron microscopically, such **electrotonic (electric) synapses** differ from chemical synapses in that the synaptic cleft is only 2 nm compared to about 20 nm. This kind of cell contact is called a **nexus** or **gap junction**; it consists of channels that span the synaptic cleft. (Electrical coupling by gap junctions is much more common among **glial cells** than among neurons, and it occurs regularly among cardiac, smooth-muscle, and epithelial cells.) Through these channels ion currents can pass directly and quickly from one cell to another with no synaptic delay. In invertebrates and lower vertebrates, electrotonic synapses are formed between neurons mediating short-latency responses to stimuli (e.g., escape reactions). Electrotonic synapses may also provide electrical coupling between many neurons in a group, so that their activity may be **synchronized**. Chemical synapses may occur close to electrical ones and serve to uncouple the electrical synapse so that these apparently can be switched on and off. Even a small number of gap junctions between nerve cells—too small to produce efficient electric coupling—may be important by enabling transfer of small signal molecules, such as Ca^{2+}, cyclic AMP, and inositol triphosphate (IP_3). In this way, one neuron may alter the properties of another without ordinary synaptic contact.

There are also other unusual types of synapses. Contacts between dendrites with all the morphological characteristics of synapses have been observed in several places in the central nervous system (CNS). Such **dendrodendritic synapses** are often part of more complex synaptic arrangements. Through dendrodendritic synapses, adjacent neurons can influence each other without being connected with axons. The function of such synapses, however, is not fully understood.

Release of Neurotransmitters

We have previously described transmitter-containing synaptic vesicles, aggregated near the presynaptic membrane of boutons (Fig. 4.1; see also Figs. 1.7 and 5.9). Depolarization of the presynaptic membrane by an action potential is the normal event preceding transmitter release. The depolarization opens **voltage-gated calcium channels** and allows a flow of Ca^{2+} ions into the bouton. The rise in Ca^{2+} concentration triggers the release of transmitter by exocytosis of vesicles (Fig. 4.1). The more calcium that enters, the more transmitter is released. By exocytosis, the membrane of synaptic vesicles fuses with the presynaptic membrane. The **fusion** opens the vesicle so that its content flows quickly into the cleft (Figs. 4.1 and 4.2). It takes only 0.1 to 0.2 msec from calcium inflow to the occurrence of release, which means that only vesicles already attached to the presynaptic membrane empty their contents. Further, although voltage-gated Ca^{2+} channels are present in all parts of the nerve terminal membrane, only those situated in the presynaptic membrane can influence the fusion of the vesicle with the presynaptic membrane. This is because the fusion requires a very high concentration of Ca^{2+}, which occurs only close to the intracellular opening of the channel. In fact, there is evidence that the calcium channel constitutes a part of the protein complex that binds the vesicle to the presynaptic membrane. This ensures maximal Ca^{2+} concentration around the vesicle.

The part of the synapse where the vesicles attach to the presynaptic membrane is called the **active zone**, and it is characterized by cytoskeletal components that probably bind the vesicles to the calcium channels. The active zone is seen in electron micrographs as a **presynaptic density** (Fig. 4.2; see also Figs. 1.6B and 1.7). That fusion really occurs during release is supported by, among other data,

Figure 4.1

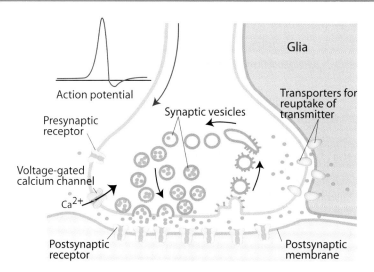

Signal transmission at the synapse. Schematic of some important features: calcium-dependent transmitter release, reuptake of transmitter by glia and neurons, and recycling of synaptic vesicles.

Figure 4.2

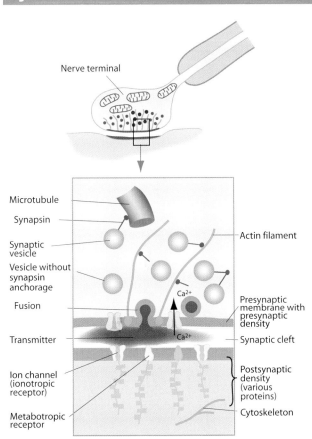

Transmitter release and some of its machinery. Calcium channels are located close to where the vesicles fuse with the presynaptic membrane. (Based on Walmsey et al. 1998.)

that are thought to help in budding of the vesicles from the membrane and in selecting their content. The recycled vesicles undergo a series of regulated steps until they are again filled with neurotransmitter (Fig. 4.1).

Several of the proteins involved in vesicle transport and fusion alter their activity in a use-dependent manner; that is, they may be involved in **synaptic plasticity** during development, recovery after brain damage, and learning in general. Some are also targets of drugs and toxins.

Mechanisms for Vesicle Transport and Fusion

Specific **transporter proteins** in the vesicle membrane fill the vesicles with neurotransmitter. After filling, the vesicles are moved toward the presynaptic membrane by a regulated process (Fig. 4.2). While some vesicles empty their contents, others move toward the presynaptic membrane and prepare for fusion. The synaptic vesicles can therefore be divided into two main groups: those situated close to the membrane that are ready for release when the Ca^{2+} concentration rises around them and those that must move to the membrane before they can release their contents. The movement of vesicles requires the presence of **actin** filaments, and **microtubules** may also play a role. A group of proteins, **synapsins**, bind the vesicles to the actin filaments (Fig. 4.2), which probably serves to assemble the vesicles in positions for further movement and is triggered by the rise in the calcium concentration. Certain **protein kinases** (phosphorylating proteins) regulate the activity of the synapsins. Phosphorylation of synapsins increases mobility of the vesicles and is most likely another way of controlling the amount of transmitter released by an action potential, for example, in response to altered use of the synapse. Several proteins take part in the **docking** of the vesicle at the presynaptic membrane, and they probably also prepare the vesicles for fusion. Vesicle-bound receptors, such as **synaptobrevin/VAMP** (vesicle-associated membrane protein), mediate attachment to receptors in the presynaptic membrane (**syntaxin** is one such receptor). These receptors interact with several others—among them, **SNAP-25** that is free in the cytoplasm—thus forming large protein complexes that anchor the vesicles to the presynaptic membrane. The fusion appears to require that the complex include **synaptotagmin**, which binds Ca^{2+} with low affinity (i.e., the concentration of Ca^{2+} must be high for bonding to occur). According to one hypothesis, synaptotagmin acts as a brake on fusion, and the binding of Ca^{2+} releases the brake. Mice lacking the gene for synaptotagmin have only reduced transmitter release, however, suggesting that other factors also play a role.

electron microscopic observations showing that the number of vesicles drops with long-term stimulation (trains of action potentials), while the number increases after a period of rest.

Exocytosis of vesicles is controlled by a large number of regulatory proteins that appear to be the same in all kinds of cells. Two features are nevertheless specific to exocytosis in neurons as compared with that in other cells: one is the speed of the process (<1 msec from arrival of the action potential to release); the other is that the release is restricted to a specific site (the synapse). This indicates that some proteins are specific to the control of exocytosis in neurons. The fusion requires specific binding of vesicle-surface receptors to receptors in the presynaptic membrane. In addition, during fusion, various proteins dissolved in the cytoplasm participate by binding to the membrane-bound receptors, thus forming large complexes.

New, empty vesicles are formed by the opposite process of exocytosis, **endocytosis**. The endocytotic vesicles are **coated** with proteins (among them **clathrin** and **dynamin**)

Neurotransmitters Are Released in Quanta

There is convincing evidence that transmitters are released in packets, or **quanta,** corresponding to the transmitter content of one vesicle. For synapses between motor nerve terminals and striated **muscle cells** (see Fig. 21.5), one vesicle contains on average 10,000 transmitter molecules. Only a few thousand molecules of each quantum are likely to bind to a receptor before they diffuse away or are removed by other means. Release of one quantum elicits a tiny excitatory postsynaptic potential (EPSP)—a **miniature EPSP**. If stimulation is increased, so that more transmitter is released, the depolarization of the muscle cell membrane increases in steps corresponding to one miniature EPSP.

In the **CNS**, each bouton probably releases from none to a few quanta for each presynaptic action potential. This means that an action potential does not necessarily elicit transmitter release; it merely increases the **probability of release**. As discussed later, many presynaptic action potentials must coincide to fire a postsynaptic neuron. The probability of release seems to be related to the **size of the active zone**, that is, to the number of vesicles that are ready for fusion. Interestingly, the size of the active zone can increase within minutes after proper use of the synapse, presumably as an expression of **use-dependent plasticity**.

Transmitters Act on Ionotropic and Metabotropic Receptors

The effects of a neurotransmitter depend primarily on the properties and localization of the receptors it can activate. There are two main kinds of transmitter receptors: ionotropic and metabotropic. **Ionotropic receptors** are parts of ion channels (Fig. 4.3A). Ionotropic receptors that are parts

of Na^+ or Ca^{2+} channels evoke fast and brief **depolarizations** of the postsynaptic membrane, thus exerting **excitatory** actions. Ionotropic receptors coupled to Cl^- channels as a rule **hyperpolarize** the postsynaptic membrane and **inhibit** the postsynaptic neuron. Synapses equipped with ionotropic receptors mediate **fast** and **precise information**—for example, about "when," "what," and "where" concerning a sensory stimulus.

The other main kind—the **metabotropic receptor**—is not coupled directly to ion channels but acts indirectly by way of **G proteins** and intracellular second messengers (Fig. 4.3B). G proteins may be regarded as universal translators, translating various kinds of extracellular signals to a cellular response (e.g., the "translation" of light and of gaseous and watery chemical substances to nerve impulses).

Most neurotransmitters act on both ionotropic and metabotropic receptors. That is, a neurotransmitter can exert both fast, direct synaptic effects and slow, indirect ones (at the same or different synapses). **Glutamate** and **GABA** (γ-aminobutyric acid) are by far the most abundant and ubiquitous transmitters acting on ionotropic receptors, although they also act on several kinds of metabotropic receptors. Several important neurotransmitters, such as **norepinephrine**, **dopamine**, and **serotonin**, exert their main actions on metabotropic receptors. We can conclude that to predict the actions of a neurotransmitter on a neuronal group, we must know the repertoire of receptors expressed by those neurons. Further, because the distribution of receptors differs,

Figure 4.3

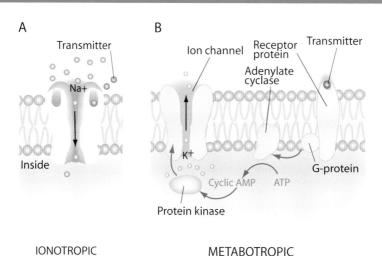

IONOTROPIC   METABOTROPIC

Two kinds of transmitter receptor. **A:** Ionotropic receptor with direct action on the ion channel. Note that the receptor is part of the channel proteins. **B:** Metabotropic receptor with indirect action on ion channels. Schematic. All indirectly coupled receptors act via G proteins, whereas other elements of the intracellular signal pathway may vary among different receptors. In this example cyclic AMP serves as the second messenger.

one transmitter may exert different actions in different parts of the brain.

Toxins Can Prevent Transmitter Release

Some of the proteins necessary for fusion are degraded by **tetanus toxin** and **botulinum toxin** (produced in certain foods if not treated properly). Both toxins are produced by anaerobic bacteria (i.e., they only grow in the absence of oxygen) and produce violent muscle spasms and paralysis, respectively. The toxins are proteases acting on the proteins that are involved in docking and fusion of synaptic vesicles. While tetanus toxin and some botulinum toxins degrade synaptobrevin, other botulinum toxins destroy SNAP-25, or syntaxin. Even extremely small amounts of the toxins produce muscle spasms (tetanus toxin) or paralysis (botulinum toxins) by preventing transmitter release. They evoke opposite effects because they act on different kinds of synapses: the botulinum toxin acts at the neuromuscular junction (see Fig. 21.5), preventing release of the excitatory transmitter acetylcholine, whereas the tetanus toxin is taken up by nerve terminals in the periphery and moved by axonal transport to the cord. There the toxin affects primarily a type of inhibitory synapse on motor neurons, making them fire action potentials with a high, uncontrolled frequency (see Chapter 5, under "Inhibitory Amino Acid Transmitters: GABA and Glycine").

Inactivation of Neurotransmitters

Synaptic signal transfer is characterized by a precisely timed start and stop. We have looked into the mechanisms responsible for precise timing of transmitter release. It is also necessary, however, that the transmitter, once released, be quickly removed from the synaptic cleft after receptor activation. Simple **diffusion** of the transmitter seems to play an important part, especially during the first few milliseconds after release. Some transmitters (acetylcholine and neuropeptides) are degraded extracellularly by specific **enzymes**. The majority of transmitters, however, are removed from the extracellular fluid by **uptake** into glial cells or neurons (see also Chapter 2, under "Astroglia and Control of the Neuronal Environment"). Specific **transporter proteins** in the cell membrane (Fig. 4.1) carry out the transmitter uptake. The transmitter transporters are driven by ion-concentration gradients across the cell membrane. There are two **families** of such transporter proteins. One is driven by the concentration gradients of Na^+ and Cl^- and transports the transmitters **GABA, glycine, dopamine, norepinephrine**, and **serotonin**. The other comprises five different transporters for **glutamate** and is driven by the concentration gradients of Na^+ and K^+ (see Chapter 5, under "Glutamate Transporters").

The task of the transporters is not to remove all traces of neurotransmitters from the extracellular fluid. Because both number and activity of the transporters are regulated, they rather serve to modulate up or down a certain baseline extracellular transmitter concentration. Even a small alteration of transporter activity can cause changes of transmitter–receptor activation. In areas with a high density of transporters (see Fig. 2.5), they also influence the ease by which neurotransmitters may activate receptors outside the synaptic cleft (on nerve terminals, dendrites, and cell bodies). In this way, the transmitter transporters participate in the control of synaptic transmission and neuronal excitability.

Because the transporter proteins have important physiologic roles, they are also interesting pharmacologically. Drugs that alter their function can be used therapeutically (such as **antidepressants** that are selective serotonin reuptake inhibitors), but some also have potential for abuse (such as **cocaine**, which inhibits the dopamine-reuptake transporter).

SYNAPTIC POTENTIALS AND TYPES OF SYNAPSES

Mechanisms of Postsynaptic Potentials (EPSPs and IPSPs)

Synaptic potentials arise when neurotransmitters activate ion channels. An **excitatory postsynaptic potential** (**EPSP**) arises at synapses where the transmitter **depolarizes** the postsynaptic membrane. An **inhibitory post-synaptic potential** (**IPSP**) arises at synapses where the transmitter **hyperpolarizes** the membrane (Fig. 4.4).

Opening of cation channels allowing Na^+ to enter and K^+ to leave the cell produces an EPSP. Because the cations outside the cell are driven inward, by both the concentration gradient and the membrane potential, whereas K^+ inside the cell is driven out only by its concentration gradient, at first the inward current is largest (see Figs. 3.3, 3.4, and 3.5). As the membrane becomes more and more depolarized, however, the outward flow of K^+ increases and counteracts further depolarization (Fig. 4.4). Transmitter-gated channel opening is not subject to self-reinforcement, unlike the voltage-gated channels that produce the action potential. This means that the synaptic potentials rise and fall gradually (Fig. 4.4 and 4.5) and last longer than the action potential. We use the term **graded potential**, as opposed to the all-or-none behavior of the action potential. The current spreads passively (electrotonically) from the synapse outward in all directions along the cell membrane. In this way,

Figure 4.4

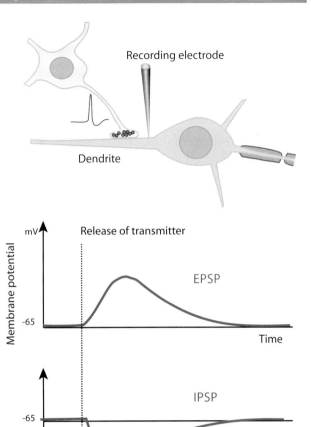

Synaptic potentials. Alterations of the membrane potential evoked by a single presynaptic action potential that releases a transmitter into the synaptic cleft. An EPSP is evoked by an excitatory transmitter (typically glutamate), while an inhibitory transmitter (typically GABA) produces an IPSP (inhibitory postsynaptic synaptic potential).

Figure 4.5

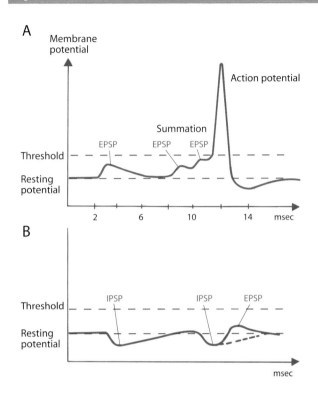

Synaptic potentials. **A:** The time course and polarity of an EPSP. In this example, one EPSP alone does not depolarize the membrane to threshold for eliciting an action potential, but if one EPSP (or more) follows shortly after the first one, the threshold is reached (summation). **B:** The time course and polarity of an IPSP and how the hyperpolarization is reduced when an EPSP is added to an IPSP.

the potential becomes gradually weaker, unlike the action potential, which is constantly regenerated. Because typical EPSPs in neurons are small (<1 mV), and the membrane has to be depolarized at about 10 mV near the initial segment to reach **threshold** for an action potential, it follows that many EPSPs must be summated to fire the neuron. We return to summation of EPSPs later.

The mechanism behind an **IPSP** is usually the opening of transmitter-gated K^+ or Cl^- channels. This results in an outward flow of K^+ or an inward flow of Cl^-. In both cases, the inside of the cell becomes more negative; that is, the membrane is hyperpolarized. This is true only if the membrane potential is less negative than the equilibrium potentials of the ions in question, however. Although this

is the normal situation for K^+ (equilibrium potential -90 mV), the equilibrium potential of Cl^- is close to the resting potential in many neurons. If the resting potential is equal to the equilibrium potential of Cl^-, there is no net flow of Cl^- ions, and, consequently, no IPSP is evoked.[1] Even in this case, however, opening of chloride channels can counteract the effects of excitatory transmitters. Thus, as long as the chloride channels remain open, even the slightest depolarization will cause Cl^- ions to flow into the cell and thereby minimize the change of the membrane potential. In this case, opening of chloride channels by an inhibitory transmitter **short-circuits** the depolarizing currents at nearby excitatory synapses.

---

1. If the resting potential is more negative than the equilibrium potential of Cl^-, the opening of chloride channels causes a net outward flow of chloride ions and the cell is depolarized. This is the case in early **embryologic development**: the transmitter GABA, which is inhibitory in the adult nervous systems, has excitatory actions in the immature brain.

Summation of Stimuli Is Necessary to Evoke an Action Potential

One or a few presynaptic action potentials leading to transmitter release do not evoke an action potential in the postsynaptic cell. As previously mentioned, the membrane has to be depolarized to a **threshold** value (Fig. 4.5A) for an action potential to be evoked. Usually, the threshold is approximately 10 mV more positive than the resting potential, and the size of an EPSP is probably in most cases less than 1 mV. As previously mentioned, to produce an action potential the current produced at synaptic sites must be strong enough to reach the initial segment and depolarize the membrane to threshold (by opening voltage-gated Na^+ channels).

A subthreshold depolarization may nevertheless be of functional significance if the synaptic potential is followed by another depolarization before the membrane potential has returned to resting value. Then the second depolarization is added to the first one so that threshold is reached. This phenomenon is called **summation** (Fig. 4.5A). The summation may be in time, as in the previous example, and is then called **temporal summation**, or it may be in space and is then called **spatial summation**. In temporal summation, impulses may follow one another in rapid succession in one terminal, whereas in spatial summation, nerve terminals at different places on the cell surface release transmitter and depolarize the cell almost simultaneously. Also, IPSPs are subject to spatial and temporal summation.

An EPSP increases the **probability** that the postsynaptic neuron will produce an action potential: for a moment, the neuron is more responsive to other inputs. Likewise, an IPSP decreases this probability.

Slow Synaptic Effects Modulate the Effect of Fast Ones

Because neurons are equipped with both ionotropic and metabotropic transmitter receptors, we may safely assume that every neuron receives both fast (direct) and slow (indirect) synaptic inputs. The slow effects modulate the effects of the fast ones, and we therefore use the term **modulatory transmitter actions**. A modulatory transmitter (when binding to an indirectly acting receptor) does not by itself evoke action potentials but alters the response of a neuron to fast, ionotropic transmitter actions. Usually, modulatory synaptic effects are mediated by altering opening states of K^+

Figure 4.6

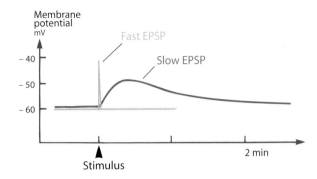

Fast and slow synaptic actions. Schematic. A fast EPSP lasts milliseconds and is caused by binding of transmitter molecules directly to channel proteins. A slow EPSP may last seconds or minutes and is due to activation of receptors indirectly coupled to ion channels.

or Ca^{2+} channels, thereby modulating both the membrane potential and the refractory period. The effects are nevertheless much more varied because there are several kinds of potassium and calcium channels, and several transmitters may influence each channel.

A brief train of impulses in axons releasing a transmitter that binds to indirectly acting receptors may keep the membrane depolarized or hyperpolarized for seconds after the train of impulses ends (slow EPSP or IPSP; Fig. 4.6). More intense stimulation may produce depolarization that lasts minutes in some neurons.

An example may make this clearer: motor neurons in the cord receive fast, excitatory synaptic input from the cerebral cortex. These signals mediate the precise, voluntary control of muscle contraction. In addition, the motor neurons receive slow, modulatory synaptic inputs from cell groups in the brain stem whose activity is related to the degree of motivation for a particular movement. The modulatory input influences the strength of the response (frequency of action potentials) to signals from the cerebral cortex, that is, how fast the movement will be. However, the modulatory input does not initiate movements on its own.

Mechanisms of Modulatory Synaptic Effects

Slow EPSPs may be mediated by transmitters closing a kind of **voltage-gated K^+ channel** that is open at the resting membrane potential. This leads to lowered K^+ permeability and reduced flow of K^+ out of the cell, which results in depolarization. Because the membrane potential is shifted toward the threshold, fast depolarization is more likely to elicit an action potential. In addition, the effect on this kind of channel makes a fast EPSP larger and longer-lasting because the fast transmitter opens the K^+ channel during the repolarization phase of the EPSP. When the modulatory transmitter counteracts the opening of the channel in this phase, the depolarization becomes stronger and the repolarization phase is prolonged. In this way the fast transmitter may produce a train of action potentials rather than just one.

Modulatory synaptic effects may not change the resting membrane potential if they are confined to channels that are not open at the resting potential. Thus, a kind of K^+ channel—closed at the resting potential—is opened by Ca^{2+} (together with Na^+) entering the cell during the action potential. This produces a relatively long-lasting hyperpolarization (the refractory period). A modulatory transmitter that reduces the opening of this K^+ channel would shorten the refractory period. As in the preceding example, a fast excitatory input might produce a train of impulses rather than only one, or the frequency of impulses during a train might be higher than without the modulatory influence.

Slow **IPSPs** are usually mediated by the indirect opening of K^+ channels. As we discuss later, the ubiquitous inhibitory transmitter GABA can act on receptors with such effect.

A Neuron Integrates Information from Many Others

We have seen that as a rule many impulses must reach a neuron almost simultaneously to make it fire, that is, to send an action potential through its axon. In other words, summation of excitatory synaptic effects is necessary. The stronger the sum of excitatory effects, the shorter the time necessary to depolarize the cell to the threshold for eliciting another action potential. This means that the frequency of action potentials, or **firing frequency**, is an expression of the **total synaptic input** to a neuron. Total synaptic input here means the sum of both excitatory and inhibitory synaptic influences. Most neurons receive thousands of synapses; for example, large neurons in the motor cortex of the monkey may receive as many as 60,000 synapses. Often a neuron is strongly influenced (many synaptic contacts) by one neuronal group and weakly influenced by many others. This means that while such a neuron primarily transmits signals from one nucleus to another, many other cell groups facilitate or inhibit the efficiency of signal transmission.

Examples of Synaptic Integration

Here we provide two examples of the integration of different synaptic inputs. The first concerns **motor neurons** of the spinal cord. Such a neuron—sending its axon to innervate hundreds of striated muscle cells in a particular muscle—is synaptically contacted by neurons in many parts of the nervous system. It may receive around 20,000 synapses, distributed over its dendrites and cell body. Some synapses inform the cell about sensory stimuli that are important for the movement produced by the muscle, others

about the posture of the body, others about how fast an intended movement should be, and so forth. The sum of all these synaptic inputs—some of them excitatory, others inhibitory—determines the frequency of action potentials sent to the muscle and by that means the force of muscle contraction (each muscle, however, is governed by many such neurons, so that their collective activity determines the behavior of the whole muscle).

The other example concerns neurons in the spinal cord that mediate information about **painful stimuli**. Although such a neuron receives its strongest synaptic input (most synapses) from sensory organs reacting to painful stimuli, it is also contacted by thousands of synapses from other sources, such as cell groups that are active when the person is anxious. This means that the final firing frequency of this sensory neuron depends not only on the actual stimuli reaching the receptors but also on the activity within the CNS itself. This correlates well with the everyday experience that the pain we feel depends not only on the strength of the peripheral painful stimulus (such as dental drilling) but also on our state of mind. Although the main task of the neuron is to convey sensory information to the brain, this information is integrated in the spinal cord with signals from other sources conveying information about the salience of the sensory information.

The Placement of Synapses Has Functional Significance

Where a synapse is located on the neuronal surface is obviously not a matter of chance (see Fig. 1.8). There are several examples of axons arising from different cell groups that end on different parts: for example, some end only on proximal dendrites, others on distal dendrites or a particular segment of the dendrite. Further, **inhibitory** synapses are often located on or near the soma of the nerve cell, whereas **excitatory** ones are most abundant on dendrites. The placement can be of functional importance, because synapses close to the **initial segment** of the axon would be expected to have a greater chance of eliciting (or preventing) an action potential than synapses far out on the dendrites. (This is due to the loss of current during electrotonic spread of the synaptic potential over long distances.) In some neurons, powerful inhibitory synapses are even located on the initial segment itself, thereby forming a very efficient "brake" on neuronal firing.

In general, a synapse far out on a dendrite would be expected to exert a weaker effect on the excitability of the neuron than one placed close to the soma, and, consequently, more summation would be needed for distal synapses than for proximal ones to fire the neuron. New findings suggest that this may not always hold true, however. Studies of pyramidal neurons (in the hippocampus) indicate that an EPSP recorded in the soma is of about equal magnitude regardless of whether it is evoked by a synapse that is proximal or distal on a dendrite. This means that a stronger depolarizing action at **distal synapses** compensates for their greater loss of current by electrotonic spread.[2]

Another important point regarding the placement of synapses is that most excitatory synapses are located on dendritic **spines** (see Fig. 1.8). A spine typically consists of a narrow neck and an expanded part called the **spine head** (see Fig. 1.9). Most of the neurons in the cerebral cortex are of the axospinous kind. Because cortical neurons constitute a large proportion of all neurons in the human brain, it is believed that about 90% of all excitatory synapses are located on spines.

Temporal Sequence of Synaptic Activation Provides Information

The temporal sequence of synaptic actions along the dendrite also seems to influence the effect of a synapse. Thus, if a sequence of synaptic activation starts distally and moves proximally, the effect at the soma is stronger than if the activation starts proximally. Whether distal or proximal synapses are activated first may depend on the direction a moving stimulus (e.g., on the skin or in the visual field). This kind of discriminative capacity was demonstrated with **two-photon microscopy** of in vitro slices of cerebral cortex, where single synapses were stimulated in a temporal and spatial sequence (Branco et al. 2010). The neuron may therefore discriminate between directions of movement and forward this information to other neurons.

Why Do We Need Inhibitory Synapses?

Inhibitory synapses are present everywhere in the CNS and are of vital importance in interrupting or **dampen excitation**, which might otherwise lead to neuronal damage. Thus, inhibition serves to maintain **homeostasis**. Figure 4.7 shows how an excitatory neuron can limit its firing by way of an **inhibitory interneuron**. Although not shown in the figure, the interneuron is influenced by many other neurons that serve to "adjust the brake," as it were. Such arrangements are common, for example, among the motor neurons that control muscle contractions (see Fig. 21.14). In general, inhibitory interneurons increase the **flexibility** of the nervous system.

---

2. Although this is shown so far only for cortical pyramidal neurons, there is reason to assume that it applies to dendrites in general. The different properties of distal and proximal dendrites relate to a higher density of NMDA receptors on distal dendrites and the fact that voltage-gated cation channels open more easily on distal than on proximal dendrites (Branco and Häusser 2011).

Figure 4.7

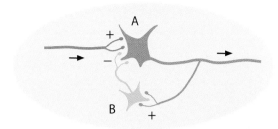

*Inhibitory interneuron (**B**) mediating negative feedback to the projection neuron (**A**). Arrows show the direction of impulse conduction.*

A salient example of the importance of inhibition is the effect of **strychnine**, which blocks inhibitory glycinergic synapses and elicits life-threatening muscle spasms. As mentioned, e**pileptic seizures** are due to uncontrolled firing of groups of neurons, and drugs reducing the tendency for seizures generally increase the effect of inhibitory transmitters. Furthermore, inhibition is necessary to suppress irrelevant **sensory information**, thereby enabling us to concentrate on certain events and leave others out. Inhibitory synapses also serve to increase the precision of sensory information by, for example, enhancing contrast between regions with different light intensity in visual images.

Inhibition is also crucial for movements by patterning and coordinating the activity of motor neurons. For example, the rhythmic pattern of muscle activation in **locomotion** depends on properly functioning inhibitory interneurons in the spinal cord.

Finally, inhibitory interneurons are instrumental in shaping the dynamic patterns of activity in distributed **cortical networks,** characterized by rhythmic **oscillations**.

Signaling by Disinhibition

In some instances, inhibitory synaptic couplings may lead to increased rather than decreased excitation. This occurs when inhibitory neurons inhibit other inhibitory neurons that in their turn act on excitatory ones (Fig. 4.8). With such an arrangement, firing of the first inhibitory interneuron (green) inhibits the next inhibitory interneuron, which thereby reduces its activity. Thus, the excitatory neuron (red) receives less inhibition and increases its firing. This is called **disinhibition**, and it plays an important role in diverse structures such as the retina and the basal ganglia (see Fig. 23.14). If an inhibitory interneuron contacts both excitatory and inhibitory neurons, it might produce both inhibition and

Figure 4.8

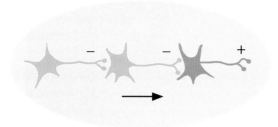

Disinhibition. Two inhibitory neurons (green) coupled in series increases the activity of an excitatory neuron (red).

Figure 4.9

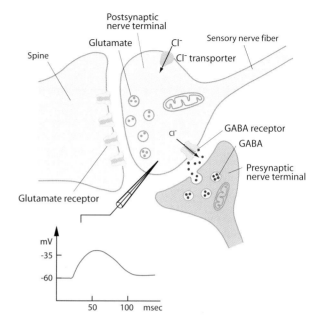

Presynaptic inhibition is mediated by axoaxonic synapses. The example is from the spinal cord where an inhibitory interneuron contacts the terminal of a sensory nerve fiber (from a spinal ganglion cell). The interneuron releases GABA that opens Cl⁻ channels and thereby depolarizes the postsynaptic nerve terminal (frame). This leads to release of less transmitter. See text for further explanations. (Based on Alvarez 1998.)

disinhibition at the same time in different neurons. By controlling the firing of such interneurons, central command centers—such as the motor cortex—can direct the signals in the desired direction. This occurs, for example, in the spinal cord where inhibitory interneurons serve to select the muscles that are best suited for a particular task.

Axoaxonic Synapses Enable Presynaptic Control of Transmitter Release

In axoaxonic synapses, the presynaptic bouton makes synaptic contact with a postsynaptic bouton, which, in turn, contacts a cell body or a dendrite (Fig. 4.9). Release of transmitter from the presynaptic bouton serves to regulate the amount of transmitter released by the postsynaptic bouton. This enables inhibition or facilitation of a subset of synaptic inputs to a neuron. The excitability of the postsynaptic neuron is unaltered, in contrast to the situation described previously with postsynaptic inhibition by IPSPs.

In the best-studied kind of axoaxonic contacts, action potentials in the presynaptic bouton lead to reduced transmitter release from the postsynaptic bouton; that is, the effect is inhibitory with regard to the neuron contacted by the postsynaptic bouton (the postsynaptic bouton usually has an excitatory action). A prerequisite for this inhibitory effect to occur, however, is that the presynaptic bouton must be depolarized (by an action potential) at the same time as or immediately before an action potential reaches the postsynaptic bouton. This phenomenon is termed **presynaptic inhibition** to distinguish it from postsynaptic inhibition. Presynaptic inhibition has been found most frequently among fiber systems that transmit sensory information; for example, sensory fibers entering the spinal cord are subject to powerful presynaptic inhibition. In this way, signals to a sensory neuron from

pain receptors can be selectively inhibited, while signals from other receptors are passed on unaltered.

Mechanisms of Presynaptic Inhibition and Facilitation

Several mechanisms may be involved in **presynaptic inhibition**. The phenomenon has been most studied in the spinal cord dorsal horn, where axoaxonic synapses are formed by inhibitory interneurons as they contact terminals of primary sensory afferents (Fig. 4.9). The transmitter released from the interneuron (usually GABA) opens chloride channels in the postsynaptic terminal (bouton). In most neurons, opening of chloride channels either hyperpolarizes or short-circuits the membrane, as described. In the sensory terminals in the cord, however, opening of chloride channels **depolarizes** the membrane, due to an unusually high intracellular chloride concentration. (To uphold this concentration gradient, these sensory neurons are equipped with a special transport mechanism for chloride coupled to the sodium–potassium pump). In this way, the equilibrium potential of Cl⁻ is more positive (−30 mV) than the resting potential (−65 mV), and, consequently, chloride ions move *out* of the nerve terminal when chloride channels open. But how can depolarization of the presynaptic terminal reduce transmitter release? The answer seems to be that depolarization reduces the amplitude of action potentials as they invade the postsynaptic terminal; in turn, this leads to opening of fewer voltage-gated calcium channels. Because the amount of transmitter released is proportional to the influx of Ca^{2+}, less transmitter will be released. It remains to be explained why depolarization of the postsynaptic terminal reduces the amplitude of the action potential. The most likely explanation is that depolarization inactivates some voltage-gated sodium channels in the postsynaptic terminal. In addition, direct influence on Ca^{2+} channels by the transmitter released from the presynaptic terminal may also contribute to presynaptic inhibition.

Presynaptic facilitation can be elicited by axoaxonic synapses by increasing CA^{2+} influx in the postsynaptic bouton. Closure of K^+ channels by the presynaptic transmitter prolongs the action potential by slowing the repolarization phase, thereby allowing more CA^{2+} to enter the postsynaptic bouton.

SYNAPTIC PLASTICITY

Basis of Learning and Memory?

There is much evidence that synapses can alter their structure and function in an **activity-dependent** or **use-dependent** manner: that is, they are **plastic**. This means that for a shorter or longer period, the postsynaptic action may be enhanced or reduced, as evidenced by altered amplitude of the postsynaptic potentials. Further, much experimental evidence supports the hypothesis that synaptic plasticity is the cellular basis of learning and memory. Martin, Grimwood, and Morris (2000, p. 650) express the hypothesis as follows: "Activity-dependent synaptic plasticity is induced at appropriate synapses during memory formation, and is both necessary and sufficient for the information storage underlying the type of memory mediated by the brain area in which that plasticity is observed." When we learn, most likely numerous synapses change their efficacy within distributed neural networks; when we later can recall what we learned, it must mean that synaptic changes have been retained. When we forget, one reason may be the decay of learning-related synaptic changes. Obviously, the most difficult part of the hypothesis to prove is a causal relationship between specific synaptic changes and memory in behavioral terms.

Under Which Conditions Do Synaptic Changes Occur?

Only a minute fraction of all the information reaching the brain is retained in memory, and, correspondingly, use of a synapse does not always change its subsequent behavior. To induce a change, the presynaptic influences must conform to certain patterns. In general, plastic changes are likely to

Figure 4.10

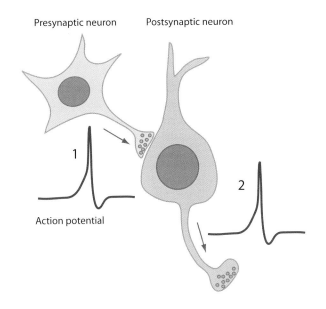

Presynaptic neuron　　　Postsynaptic neuron

1

2

Action potential

Activity-dependent synaptic plasticity. The likelihood of inducing a change of the synapse between neuron 1 and 2 is greatest if neuron 2 (postsynaptic neuron) fires an action potential immediately after receiving a synaptic input from neuron 1 (presynaptic neuron).

occur when the presynaptic activity is particularly strong and coincide in time with the postsynaptic neuron firing an action potential (Fig. 4.10).[3] This makes sense, as the immediate firing of an action potential after a synaptic input might be regarded as a sign of success. This situation is likely to arise only when several excitatory synaptic inputs reach the neuron at the same time. Looking for the functional meaning of simultaneous inputs, a crucial point may be the ability of neurons to detect **coincidences**. For example, a sensory input is significant only in a certain **context**, and only then should it be remembered. Accordingly, synaptic changes would occur only when information about the sensory event and its context coincide. However, contextual information should lead to synaptic change only if it signals that the sensory stimulus is important or unexpected. Indeed, in many situations, it appears that synaptic change depends on the coincidence of a specific input mediated by activation of ionotropic receptors and a modulatory input mediated by metabotropic receptors (Fig. 4.11). The first input provides fast and precise information—for example,

3. This was postulated by the Canadian psychologist Donald Hebb in 1949 (p. 62) in an influential attempt to explain the cellular basis of learning: "when an axon of cell A is near enough to excite a cell B and repeatedly or persistently takes part in firing it, some growth process or metabolic change takes place in one or both cells such that A's efficiency, as one of the cells firing B, is increased."

Figure 4.11

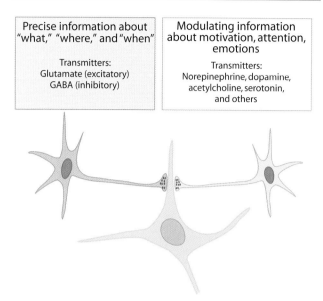

Precise information about "what," "where," and "when"	Modulating information about motivation, attention, emotions
Transmitters: Glutamate (excitatory) GABA (inhibitory)	Transmitters: Norepinephrine, dopamine, acetylcholine, serotonin, and others

Synaptic plasticity. Learning—that is, synaptic change—depends in this example on simultaneous action of a specific synaptic input and a modulatory one. The latter provides a signal about the salience of the specific stimulus

about the nature of a sensory stimulus—the other about the **salience** of the stimulus.

Mechanisms for Synaptic Plasticity

Broadly speaking, a change of synaptic efficacy may arise because

- The **presynaptic** terminal releases more or less neurotransmitter in response to an action potential.

- The **postsynaptic** neuron has increased or reduced its response to the transmitter.

We have discussed the complex cellular processes that link an action potential to transmitter release (Figs. 4.1 and 4.2), and many of the factors involved have been shown experimentally to change their activity in a use-dependent manner. For example, there may be changes in the amount and activity of intracellular second messengers and protein kinases (among other things, regulating ion channels and receptor proteins). The properties, number, and distribution of transmitter receptors are also subject to activity-dependent modifications. Nevertheless, in spite of the large number of molecular mechanisms involved in induction and maintenance of synaptic plasticity, increased

intracellular **calcium concentration** appears as a rule to **initiate** the process. The further pathways from a calcium signal to altered synaptic efficacy are multifarious and only partly known.

With regard to structural correlates of synaptic plasticity, we know that **spines** undergo changes of size and form that are correlated with altered synaptic efficacy. Further, the **formation** of new synapses (synaptogenesis) and **elimination** of old ones is very prominent during pre- and postnatal development but occur throughout adult life (Fig. 4.12).

Spines Are Crucial for Synaptic Plasticity

The functional significance of dendritic spines is still under debate. It is not simply a matter of increasing the receiving surface of the neuron because the dendritic membrane between spines may be virtually free of synapses. Since their microscopic identification more than 100 years ago, however, spines have been implicated in **learning** and **memory**, and recent animal experiments support this hypothesis. For example, the density of spines in the cerebral cortex is higher in rats that live in a challenging environment than in those that are confined to standard laboratory cages. Further, the density of spines in the cerebral cortex is markedly reduced in individuals with severe **mental retardation**. Animal experiments with electric stimulation indicate that long-term increases in synaptic efficacy (long-term potentiation [LTP]) are associated with changes of spine morphology and number. This effect is observed only among synapses affected by the increased stimulation and may be directly related to learning and memory. Improved techniques have enabled direct observation of the dynamic nature of spines. For example, using **two-photon microscopy** of genetically modified cortical neurons (made to fluoresce), the same dendrite was observed with an interval of two weeks in adult mice. It was then observed that new spines (= synapses) emerged whereas others disappeared. It was also shown that some new spines occurred while others were removed in conjunction with learning of a motor task (Fu and Zuo 2011).

An important function of spines may be to facilitate **local synaptic changes**. The narrow neck of the spines may ensure that the concentration of signal molecules responsible for LTP induction, such as Ca^{2+}, reach much higher levels in the spine head than in the dendrite. This would facilitate changes in those synapses contacting a particular spine, leaving other synapses unaffected. Spatial restriction of increased Ca^{2+} concentration may also serve a **protective role** since high intracellular Ca^{2+} concentration may damage the neuron. Indeed, experiments performed in slices of tissue from the hippocampus (a region involved in learning and memory)—enabling stimulation of single axospinous synapses—suggest that enduring changes (LTP) may be limited to the stimulated synapse. However, it seems that nearby synapses (10–20 synapses within a distance of 10 μm along the dendrite) have lowered thresholds for induction of LTP for some minutes after the stimulation. Such "crosstalk" among nearby synapses is presumably caused by dendritic spread of a diffusible substance produced in the stimulated spine.

Figure 4.12

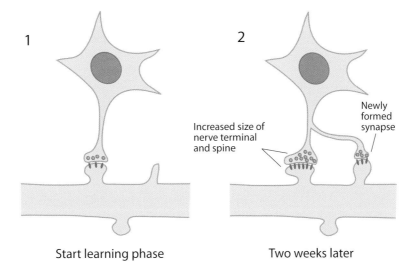

Start learning phase   **Two weeks later**

Use-dependent synaptic plasticity. Possible structural changes. Existing synapses can increase their effect by increasing the size of the nerve terminal and the spine head, thus increasing the amount of transmitter released and the number of postsynaptic receptors. In addition, sprouting of axon branches and growth of new spines can produce new synapses. Although not shown here, plasticity also comprises weakening and elimination of synapses.

Kinds of Synaptic Plasticity

Several kinds of synaptic plasticity have been described on the basis of animal experiments, and more are probably yet to be discovered. It is customary to distinguish between short-term and long-term synaptic plasticity, without a sharp transition. **Short-term plasticity** lasts from less than a second to some minutes, whereas **long-term plasticity** can last for at least several weeks. For practical reasons it is not feasible to study the phenomenon for longer periods in experimental animals. Nevertheless, if synaptic plasticity underlies memories, we know from our own experience that some synaptic changes must last for a lifetime.

The ability of synapses to express plastic changes is subject to regulation by various signal substances. This phenomenon is called **metaplasticity.** Generally, metaplasticity may serve **homeostatic** purposes, by keeping plastic changes within certain limits. However, plasticity may probably also be up- or down-regulated by environmental challenges ("enriched" environment, stress), and in neurological diseases (e.g., Alzheimer's disease, stroke, and Parkinson's disease).

Brain-Derived Neurotrophic Factor and Plasticity

Brain-derived neurotrophic factor (BDNF) is an example of a growth factor that is involved in induction of long-term synaptic plasticity. For example, alterations in BDNF expression are associated with synaptic changes induced by **stress** and also with improved learning and memory following exposure to an **enriched environment** (in rodents). The level of BDNF is generally found to be lower in conditions characterized by reduced plasticity, such as **neurodegenerative diseases** and **depression**. Interestingly, different treatments of depression (antidepressants, psychotherapy, and electroconvulsive therapy) have in common that recovery is associated with increased expression of BDNF. Presumably, recovery is facilitated by increased plasticity in mood-related brain networks.

Short-Term Plasticity

When action potentials reach the nerve terminal at relatively brief intervals, the amplitude of the ensuing postsynaptic potentials often increases gradually. This phenomenon is called **facilitation** and is due to increased transmitter release by each presynaptic action potential. The postsynaptic effect increases for each action potential until reaching a steady state after about 1 sec and then decays rapidly when stimulation stops. Further, at some synapses a series of presynaptic action potentials produce increased synaptic efficacy for minutes after the stimulation ends. This is called (synaptic) **potentiation**, and, like facilitation, it is due to increased transmitter release from the nerve terminal. Potentiation can be particularly strong and long lasting after tetanic stimulation (action potentials with maximal frequency). This is called **posttetanic potentiation**. The presynaptic terminal "remembers" that it recently received unusually intense stimulation and alters its behavior accordingly. Facilitation and posttetanic potentiation are examples of short-term plasticity that are important for the nervous system's capacity for storage of information. **Short-term depression**—that is, a weaker postsynaptic response with repeated presynaptic action potentials—is probably due to insufficient renewal of the releasable synaptic pool (Fig. 4.1).

Long-Term Plasticity: LTP and LTD

Long-term plasticity means changes of synaptic efficacy lasting for hours to weeks (years). **Long-term potentiation (LTP)** and **long-term depression (LTD)** can somewhat arbitrarily be defined as activity-dependent increases or decreases of synaptic efficacy that lasts for more than 1 hour. Presumably, LTP and LTD represent storage of information that is in some way meaningful to the individual (or interpreted as such). With these forms of long-term plasticity, cellular changes occur presynaptically and postsynaptically (not only presynaptically, as do facilitation and posttetanic potentiation). Different forms of both LTP and LTD have been described; they differ with regard to duration, the kind of activity that induces them, and molecular mechanisms. One important mechanism seems to be the **insertion of new receptors** in the postsynaptic membranes, which increases the receptor density and the effect of each quanta of transmitter released from the presynaptic terminal (see "Silent Synapses" later in this chapter). Regardless of molecular mechanisms involved in the expression of LTP and LTD, the end results are input-specific alterations of synaptic efficacy (see also Chapter 5, under "NMDA Receptors: Mediators of Both Learning and Neuronal Damage," and Chapter 32, under "Relationship between Memory and Long-Term Potentiation").

LTP and LTD are evoked by different patterns of synaptic inputs. Whereas high-frequency firing or two simultaneous inputs induces LTP, low-frequency firing or two inputs that are out of phase induces LTD. It seems reasonable that intense activity and synchronization of specific inputs strengthens connections within a network, whereas low activity or desynchronized inputs reduce strength of connectivity—the latter being interpreted as "noise" rather than meaningful information. Further, it appears that LTP is induced if a presynaptic action potential repeatedly precedes firing of the postsynaptic cell, whereas LTD occurs if the postsynaptic firing precedes

the presynaptic action potential. In this way, inputs that cause postsynaptic firing (i.e., "successful" ones) are strengthened, whereas inputs that do not contribute to postsynaptic firing are weakened.

It may seem paradoxical that the opposite phenomena—LTP and LTD—are both induced by an increase in intracellular Ca^{2+}. There is evidence, however, that intracellular responses to calcium transients can vary depending on their magnitude, time course, and site of origin.

Long-Lasting Plastic Changes Require Altered Gene Expression

Enduring changes in neurons—at either a molecular or a structural level—require altered **protein synthesis**. Proteins have a restricted lifetime, however, and it is furthermore unlikely that a synapse will remain stable for years. Indeed, animal experiments indicate that spines in the cerebral cortex are continuously removed and renewed. A logical conclusion is therefore that synaptic changes underlying stable memories must require long-term (in many instances life-long) alteration of **gene expression** that ensure continued maintenance and renewal of specific synapses. We now have much evidence that even synaptic activity lasting for minutes or less may produce altered expression of certain genes that encode for transcription factors (see Chapter 3, under "Markers of Neuronal Activity"). The experimental evidence so far mainly concerns transitory changes of gene expression; nevertheless, a number of genes have been shown to alter their expression in long-term synaptic changes. That the altered gene expression can be directed to certain synapses (those subjected to a "memorable" input) and not to others may be partially explained by the presence of mRNA and ribosomes in dendrites close to the base of the spines. Furthermore, **microRNA** may suppress the protein synthesis until a specific synaptic input (leading to plastic changes) removes the "brake."[4]

Silent Synapses

It might seem unlikely that the brain contains a large number of synapses that are not in use. Nevertheless, there is now strong evidence that some synapses do not transmit a signal, even though the nerve terminal is invaded by action potentials (this is mainly studied in the cord and the hippocampus).

---

4. MicroRNAs are short, regulatory RNA sequences that block the translation of mRNA to polypeptides.

Figure 4.13

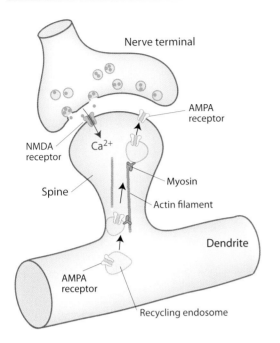

Getting silent synapses to "speak up." Activation of NMDA receptors leads to rapid influx of Ca²⁺ ions into the spine. This induces transport of so-called recycling endosomes—containing AMPA receptors—from the dendrite to the spine head. The transport depends on interaction between actin filaments and a special form of myosin molecules in the spine shaft.

This is not just a case of low release probability, because even repeated presynaptic firing is without effect (the probability that a presynaptic action potential releases the content of a synaptic vesicle varies enormously in the CNS). Further, in some areas stimulation of an axon evokes a weaker response than expected from the number of terminals. The reason for synapses being silent can be lack of either transmitter release or a postsynaptic response to the transmitter (due to lack of receptors or that the receptors are blocked). There is evidence of both mechanisms. For example, some glutamatergic synapses in the hippocampus lack the ionotropic **AMPA** (amino-methylisoxazolepropionic acid) receptors, while expressing voltage-dependent **NMDA** (*N*-methyl-D-aspartate) receptors (these are further described in Chapter 5, under "Glutamate Receptors"). Such synapses are silent because "normal" presynaptic glutamate release does not activate them. This is because the opening of NMDA receptors requires a certain magnitude of depolarization in addition to binding of glutamate. If NMDA receptors are opened by particularly strong depolarization of the postsynaptic membrane, however, this may, in turn, lead to the insertion of AMPA receptors in the postsynaptic membrane (Fig. 4.13). The receptors are transported rapidly from endosomes to the postsynaptic density, as shown with fluorescence labeling methods. Afterward, the synapse is no longer silent but "speaks up" when glutamate is released. In many instances, LTP may be caused by silent synapses being activated by insertion of AMPA receptors. The finding that silent synapses appear to be most numerous shortly after birth (in rats) supports their possible role in learning and memory.

5 Neurotransmitters and Their Receptors

OVERVIEW

Certain general properties of neurotransmitters were outlined in the preceding chapters. Recall that a signal is conveyed from one neuron to the next by release of a **neurotransmitter** (transmitter). "Conventional" or "classical" neurotransmitters are small molecules, such as amino acids and amines. Another important group of signal substances, released at synapses, are peptide molecules, called neuropeptides. Although the "typical" transmitter is released and acts at receptors in a synapse, many transmitter receptors are found **extrasynaptically**, that is, without connection to a synapse. Indeed, many transmitters act both at synapses and extrasynaptically. The latter action is called **volume transmission** and is obviously less precise than synaptic transmission. Many receptors are located presynaptically on nerve terminals. Some of them are **autoreceptors** (binding the transmitter released from the terminal), and others are **heteroreceptors** (binding other transmitters released from neurons in the vicinity). Many nerve terminals contain more than one transmitter; often a classical transmitter is **colocalized** with one or more neuropeptides.

Synthesis of a transmitter usually depends on the activity of a **key enzyme**, which controls the amount of transmitter available at a synapse. Transmitter receptors far outnumber the transmitters; thus each transmitter usually acts on several **ionotropic** and **metabotropic** receptors. The effects of a transmitter on a certain neuron therefore depend on which receptors the neuron expresses. Both the amount of transmitter available for release and the postsynaptic receptors are subject to use-dependent plasticity.

The most important **amino acid transmitters** are **glutamate** and γ-aminobutyric acid (**GABA**). Both are present in virtually all parts of the central nervous system (CNS) and are responsible for most of the fast and precise synaptic transmission by acting on ionotropic receptors. Glutamate is the dominant excitatory transmitter, whereas GABA is inhibitory. These transmitters mediate most of the spatially and temporally precise excitation and inhibition needed for perception, movements, and cognition. Glutamate binds to three families of receptors (aminomethylisoxazole propionic acid [AMPA], N-methyl-D-aspartate [NMDA], and metabotropic glutamate receptors). The **AMPA** receptors are typical ionotropic receptors with fast excitatory action, whereas the **NMDA** receptors have properties that make them especially suited to detect coincidences and induce long-term potentiation (LTP). GABA acts on ionotropic **GABA$_A$** receptors and metabotropic **GABA$_B$** receptors.

Acetylcholine is used as transmitter by a limited number of neurons in the brain stem and basal forebrain, while axonal ramifications of the neurons occur in most parts of the brain. Acetylcholine acts on ionotropic **nicotinic** receptors and metabotropic **muscarinic** receptors. The latter type dominates in the CNS, and the actions of acetylcholine are especially related to motivation, sleep–wakefulness, and memory. The group of **biogenic amines** includes the monoamines **dopamine**, **norepinephrine** (epinephrine), and **serotonin** (in addition to histamine). Like acetylcholine, these transmitters are produced in a small number of neurons but nevertheless act in most parts of the brain. They bind mostly to metabotropic receptors, with actions related to arousal, mood (emotions), and synaptic plasticity. In general, acetylcholine and the biogenic amines have **modulatory** actions that serve to regulate the excitability of neurons, thus determining the magnitude of response to fast-acting transmitters such as glutamate and GABA. **Adenosine triphosphate** (ATP) and **nitric oxide** (NO) function as signal substances with transmitter-like actions in the CNS.

A large number of **neuropeptides** have modulatory and metabolic actions in the brain, and influence a variety of processes, from basic homeostasis to complex behaviors.

How to Prove that a Substance Functions as a Neurotransmitter

Many signal substances present in the brain are small molecules, including the **amino acids** glutamate, glycine, and GABA and the **amines** norepinephrine, dopamine, serotonin, and histamine. Acetylcholine and ATP also belong to this group. These small-molecular neurotransmitters are also called **classical neurotransmitters** (presumably because they were discovered first and are best characterized functionally). Other signal substances are peptides and therefore fairly large. Such **neuropeptides** are chains of 5 to 30 amino acids. In general, the functions of the neuropeptides are far less clarified than those of the small-molecule transmitters. To prove that a substance present in a neuron actually functions as a neurotransmitter is not easy. It is not sufficient that neurons express specific **binding sites** for a substance; hormones, growth factors, and other molecules also bind to neuronal membrane receptors. Neither are there clear-cut chemical differences between neurotransmitters and other intercellular signal molecules. Indeed, the same molecule may function in several roles; for example, norepinephrine is both a neurotransmitter and a hormone. Further, some molecules—such as glutamate and glycine—are intercellular signal molecules and have a role in cellular metabolism (e.g., as building blocks for proteins).

To **prove** that a substance functions as a signal molecule, one must show the presence of corresponding receptors and that the substance is released in sufficient amounts (under physiologic conditions) to activate the receptors. Additional criteria must be met to classify such a signal substance as a neurotransmitter, however. The substance must be **produced** by neurons, it must be **stored** in nerve terminals and **released** by depolarization, and the release must be **calcium dependent**. In addition, the released substance must be directly responsible for the postsynaptic changes. Finally, there must exist mechanisms for **inactivation** of the transmitter after release. Only a few signal substances have met all of these criteria when tested experimentally. For several others, the probability that they function as transmitters is nevertheless high, and they are often described as transmitters without reservation. Strictly speaking, however, they should be termed "transmitter candidates" or "putative transmitters." Acetylcholine was the first substance to be classified with certainty as a transmitter. The excitatory action of glutamate was discovered in the 1950s, but only toward 1990 was the neurotransmitter status of this ubiquitous amino acid verified.

Determination of Neuronal Content of Neurotransmitters and Distribution of Receptors

With biochemical methods, the content of transmitters in parts of the brain and in subcellular fractions can be determined. To obtain further knowledge, however, it is also necessary to link the transmitters to specific neurons with known connections and physiologic properties. The first possibilities of studying the anatomy of neurons with known transmitters arose in the 1960s, when it was discovered that monoamine-containing neurons could be made fluorescent by a special treatment with formaldehyde. This marked the beginning of intense investigations, with other methods as well, to characterize neurons with regard to connections and at the same time with regard to their transmitters. The introduction of immunological methods, such as **immunocytochemistry**, to localize substances in nervous tissue has been of particular importance. By purifying a potentially interesting substance present in nervous tissue, **antibodies** may be raised against it. The antibodies bind antigens where they are exposed in the tissue sections, and the antibodies can be visualized subsequently with the use of secondary antibodies. The secondary antibodies may be labeled with a fluorescent molecule, or they may be identified in other ways. Such methods have been widely used to demonstrate the localization of enzymes that are critical for synthesis or degradation of certain transmitters, such as tyrosine hydroxylase, which is necessary for the synthesis of dopamine and norepinephrine (Fig. 5.1A), choline acetyltransferase (ChAT) for synthesis of acetylcholine (Fig. 5.1B), and glutamic acid decarboxylase (GAD) for GABA. Even transmitter molecules that are themselves too small to serve as antigens can be specifically identified in tissue sections via immunocytochemical methods when conjugated to tissue proteins (with glutaraldehyde). This is the case for GABA (Fig. 5.1C), glutamate, and glycine. Immunocytochemical methods can also be applied to **ultrastructural** analysis, in order to determine the transmitter accumulated at specific synapses and also whether the transmitter is localized to certain organelles, such as presynaptic vesicles (Fig. 5.2). Combination of axonal transport methods and immunocytochemical procedures makes it possible to determine the connections, as well as the transmitter candidates and other neuroactive substances of specific neuronal groups.

Even though the determination of the transmitter candidates present in a neuron is of great importance, it is not always possible to know whether the substance has been synthesized in the cell or whether it has merely been taken up. Further, the concentration of a transmitter in parts of a neuron may be so low that it cannot be reliably detected with immunocytochemical methods. The use of *in situ* **hybridization** techniques helps to overcome this kind of problem. By these methods, it is not the neuropeptides or enzymes related to transmitter metabolism that are demonstrated but the presence of the corresponding **mRNA**.

Figure 5.3

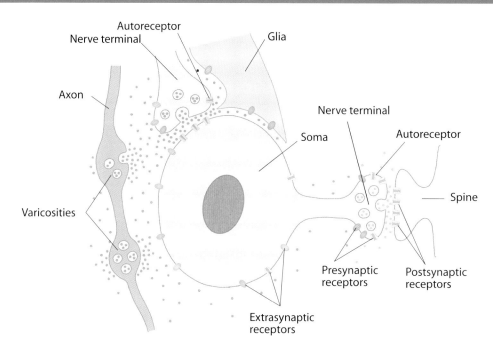

Extrasynaptic receptors and transmitter release outside synapses. Extrasynaptic receptors are localized both at the nerve terminals and on the somatic and dendritic surfaces of the neuron. Autoreceptors bind the transmitter released by the neuron itself. Note the release of transmitter from varicosities that do not form typical synaptic contacts.

TRANSMITTER RECEPTORS IN GENERAL

Binding Sites and Receptors

The many transmitters and transmitter candidates (more than 50, including the neuropeptides) have an even larger variety of receptor types to act on. More than 200 different metabotropic (G protein–coupled) receptors have been identified in the CNS. (Not all bind neurotransmitters, however; many bind hormones and a variety of growth factors.)

Several requirements must be met to conclude that a binding site for a transmitter functions as a receptor. The "final proof" requires that the amino-acid sequence of the receptor site has been determined. After cloning of the protein, one can then determine whether it binds the transmitter (and agonists and antagonists) and produces the expected physiologic effects.

Structure and Subtypes of Receptors

As discussed in Chapter 3 (under "The Structure of Ion Channels"), all the **directly** acting, **ionotropic** receptors—as

part of ion channel proteins—are similarly built, with several subunits arranged around a central pore (see Fig. 3.2). In addition, the **indirectly** acting, **metabotropic** receptors share several structural features, although they are quite different from the ionotropic receptors. The metabotropic receptors usually consist of one large protein that makes several turns through the membrane with hydrophilic (water-soluble) groups on the interior and exterior of the membrane. The receptors mediate their effects via **G proteins** (see Fig. 4.3). Several receptor types with different postsynaptic actions have been identified for each of the best-known transmitters (Table 5.1). The most abundant transmitters, such as glutamate and GABA, act on both ionotropic and metabotropic receptors.

The link between a neurotransmitter and its actions is made even more complex by the existence of **subtypes** of each main kind of receptor. Subtypes of the ionotropic (directly acting) GABA receptor (GABA$_A$) exemplify this. Each of the protein subunits forming the receptor (and the ion channel) comes in several varieties, and different combinations of them produce numerous subtypes of the GABA$_A$ receptor. These subtypes are differently distributed in the brain. This may explain why drugs acting on

Table 5.1 The Best-Known Small-Molecule (Classical) Neurotransmitters

Transmitter	Chemical	Receptor Name Mechanism, Ion Permeability*	Synaptic Action	Distribution of Receptors in the CNS†	Localization of Neurons Synthesizing the Transmitter in the CNS	Localization of Neurons in the PNS
Glutamate	Amino acid	AMPA, ionotropic, Na^+	Fast, excitation	"Everywhere"	"Everywhere"	Spinal ganglion cells
		NMDA, ionotropic, Ca^{2+}	Fast, excitation			
		MGluR1-5, metabotropic	Slow, excit. or inhib.			
GABA	Amino acid	GABA ionotropic, Cl^-	Fast, inhibition	"Everywhere"	"Everywhere"	Gut, ganglia
		$GABA_B$, metabotropic, K^+, Ca^{2+}	Slow, inhibition			
Glycine	Amino acid	Ionotropic, Cl^-	Fast, inhibition		Brain stem, spinal cord, cerebellum	
Acetylcholine	Quaternary amine	Nicotinic, ionotropic, Na^+	Fast, excitation	Cerebral cortex, spinal cord (and other places)	Motoneurons, preganglionic autonomic neurons, basal nucleus, septal nuclei, nuclei in the reticular formation of the brain stem (and other places)	
		Muscarinic, metabotropic K^+, Ca^{2+}	Slow, excitation or inhibition	Cerebral cortex, hippocampus, thalamus (and other places)		Parasympathetic ganglia
Norepinephrine Amine	α (α_1–α_2), metabotropic	Slow		"Everywhere"	Locus coeruleus and diffuse cell groups in the reticular formation	Sympathetic ganglia
	β (β_1–β_2), metabotropic	Slow				
Dopamine	Amine	D_1(D_1, D_5), metabotropic, increase cyclic AMP	Slow	"Everywhere" (especially basal ganglia and prefrontal cortex)	Mesencephalon (Substantia nigra and ventral tegmental area)	
		D_2(D_2, D_3, D_4), metabotropic, decrease cyclic AMP	Slow			
Serotonin (5-HT) Amine		$5-HT_{1A}$, metabotropic, K^+	Slow, inhibition	"Everywhere"	Raphe nuclei (brain stem)	
		$5-HT_2$, metabotropic	Slow, excitation			
		$5-HT_3$, ionotropic, Na^+	Fast, excitation			

*There are more receptor subtypes than shown here.

†The table is not complete regarding distribution of neurons and receptors.

different subtypes of the GABA$_A$ receptor have different physiologic and behavioral effects: they act on different neuronal networks.

Regulation of Receptor Density

The transmitter receptors are not static, immutable elements of the nervous system. We have discussed how changes in receptor density and activity may mediate **synaptic plasticity**. This means that learning would be expected to be associated with receptor changes. In animal experiments, for example, stressful psychological experiences leading to altered behavior also alter the activity of specific transmitter receptors. Drugs that interfere with transmitter actions often induce changes in the receptors. A drug that blocks the effect of a transmitter on a particular receptor type (antagonist) may indirectly produce increased postsynaptic receptor density. The reverse may occur with drugs that mimic the transmitter (agonist). Probably such **up- or down-regulation** of receptors represents an adaptive response: an abnormally high concentration of the transmitter (or an agonist) is counteracted by reduced receptor activity to maintain normal synaptic transmission. Down-regulation of receptors may explain many of the dramatic **withdrawal symptoms** that occur when an addicted individual abruptly discontinues a narcotic drug.

Presynaptic Transmitter Receptors

Transmitter receptors are also localized to the presynaptic membrane and can thereby modulate transmitter release (Fig. 5.3). We have discussed the axoaxonic synapses that mediate presynaptic inhibition by acting on receptors in the presynaptic membrane (see Fig. 4.9). In addition, the presynaptic membrane can express receptors for the transmitter released by the nerve terminal itself (Fig. 5.3). Here we use the term **autoreceptors**. Often, autoreceptors inhibit transmitter release as a kind of **negative feedback**. Some neurons, for example, dopaminergic ones, are equipped with autoreceptors also on the cell body and dendrites. In addition to autoreceptors, nerve terminals may express **heteroreceptors**, that is, receptors for transmitters other than those they release themselves (often released by nearby terminals).

Presynaptic Modulation Is Complex

Nerve terminals releasing **norepinephrine** can exemplify the complexity of presynaptic modulation. Such terminals can express α$_2$ adrenergic autoreceptors and muscarinic (acetylcholine), opiate, and dopamine heteroreceptors that inhibit release of norepinephrine from the terminal. In addition, the terminals also express β$_2$ adrenergic autoreceptors and nicotinic (acetylcholine) heteroreceptors that facilitate transmitter release. Thus, the amount of transmitter released by such a nerve terminal depends not only on the presynaptic activity of the neuron but also on the **local milieu** of the terminal (the concentration of various transmitters and other signal substances, as well as the presence of drugs or toxic substances). It should not come as a surprise that the functional roles of presynaptic receptors are not fully understood.

SPECIFIC NEUROTRANSMITTERS

Excitatory Amino Acid Transmitters: Glutamate and Aspartate

The amino acid group contains the ubiquitous excitatory transmitter, **glutamate** (Fig. 5.4 and table 5.1). Neurons that release glutamate at their synapses are called **glutamatergic**. The dominant effect of glutamate in the CNS is fast excitation by direct action on ion channels, although it also acts on metabotropic receptors. Glutamate is responsible for fast and precise signal transmission in the majority (perhaps all) of the large sensory and motor tracts, as well as in the numerous connections between various parts of the cerebral cortex that form the networks responsible for higher mental functions. The total concentration of glutamate in the brain is very high, although the distribution

Figure 5.4

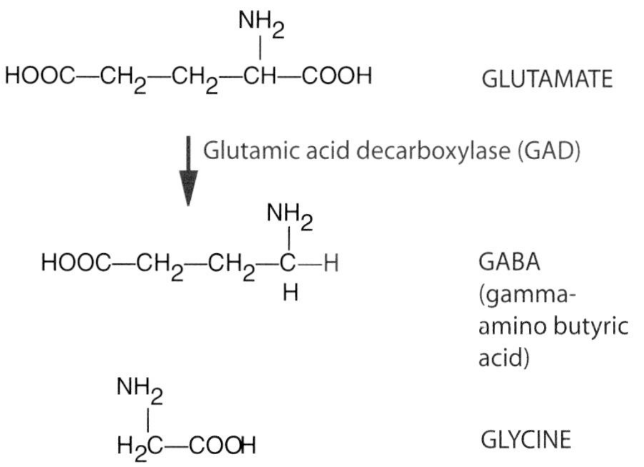

Amino acid transmitters. The enzyme glutamic acid decarboxylase (GAD) is specific for neurons that synthesize GABA.

is uneven. Notably, effective uptake mechanisms keep the extracellular concentration very low (about 1/1,000 of intracellular concentration). This is a prerequisite for glutamate's function as a neurotransmitter—acting only on specific receptors after controlled release from nerve terminals. Low extracellular concentration is also mandatory because even a small increase is toxic to the neurons. **Transporter proteins** in astroglial membranes maintain the concentration gradient (probably with a smaller contribution from transporters in neuronal membranes). In situations with poor energy supply, such as reduced blood flow or low blood sugar, glutamate leaks from the cells because the uptake mechanisms fail. The ensuing rise in extracellular glutamate concentration contributes significantly to the rapid occurrence of neuronal damage—for example, in cases of cardiac arrest (see also Chapter 11, under "Ischemic Cell Damage").

The amino acid **aspartate** is also highly concentrated in the CNS. It exerts an excitatory action by binding to glutamate receptors. Although decisive evidence is still lacking, recent studies speak in favor of aspartate being a neurotransmitter. For example, aspartate was found to be **colocalized** with glutamate in synaptic vesicles and released by exocytosis. Nevertheless, the distribution of possible aspartatergic synapses seems to be very limited in the brain. Therefore, with regard to excitatory synaptic transmission, aspartate must play a minor role compared with glutamate.

Synthesis of Glutamate

Glutamate is synthesized from two sources in the nerve terminals: **glucose** (via the Krebs cycle) and **glutamine** that is synthesized in glial cells and thereafter transported into the neurons (Fig. 5.5). Glutamine is converted in mitochondria to glutamate by the enzyme **glutaminase**. Specific transport proteins in the vesicle membrane fill the synaptic vesicles with glutamate. Glutamate is released as other transmitters by calcium-dependent exocytosis. Released glutamate is taken up by glia and converted to glutamine by the enzyme **glutamine synthetase**. Glutamine is then transported to nerve terminals, converted to glutamate, and so forth. Figure 5.5 shows the **glutamate–glutamine circuit**, which ensures reuse of the transmitter. Another advantage of the circuit is that glutamine, unlike glutamate, does not influence neuronal excitability and is not toxic in high concentrations. Therefore, its concentration need not be strictly controlled.

Figure 5.5

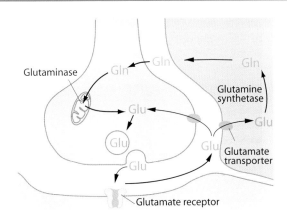

The glutamate–glutamine circuit. The enzyme glutamine synthetase converts glutamate (Glu) to glutamine (Gln) after uptake by glial cells. In contrast to glutamate, glutamine is neutral to neurons. Glutamine is transferred to nerve terminals where it is used to synthesize new glutamate that is concentrated in vesicles for release, and so forth.

Glutamate Receptors

As mentioned, the dominant action of glutamate in the CNS is fast excitation by direct binding to ionotropic receptors. In the early 1980s, however, additional kinds of glutamate receptors (**GluRs**) were found. We now recognize three groups or families of receptors that glutamate can bind to: **AMPA/ kainate receptors**, **NMDA receptors**, and **metabotropic glutamate receptors (mGluRs)**. The two first groups are glutamate-gated ion channels (ionotropic receptors). The metabotropic glutamate receptors are G protein–coupled, like other metabotropic receptors. The various glutamate receptors were discovered via use of glutamate analogs that turned out to act only on certain kinds of receptors. The receptors were named after the analog that activated them selectively (amino-methylisoxazole propionic acid [AMPA]; N-methyl-D-aspartate [NMDA]). Cloning of the receptor proteins in the early 1990s showed that AMPA, NMDA, and metabotropic receptors belonged to different protein families. To date, 10 varieties of AMPA/kainate receptors, 5 NMDA receptors, and 8 metabotropic receptors have been cloned.

AMPA receptors are ion channels admitting Na^+ (and K^+), which is typical of fast, excitatory synapses. The current view is that AMPA receptors are responsible for the majority of the fast excitatory signals in the CNS (mediating, e.g., precise sensory information and motor commands).

Kainate Receptors

Kainate receptors belong to the same family of ionotropic receptors as AMPA receptors (they seem to differ from AMPA receptors, however, by the ability to signal also through G proteins). They have been identified in many parts of the CNS and are present both pre- and postsynaptically. The concentration of kainate receptors is low in most areas, and they have not been as extensively studied as AMPA and NMDA receptors. Their total contribution to fast excitation—as compared to that of AMPA receptors—is therefore still not clarified. Kainate receptors show higher expression during brain **development** than in the adult and have been suggested to play a role in the shaping of neural networks.

Although their clinical significance remains to be elucidated, kainate receptors have been associated with a number of diseases. For example, they are expressed in spinal ganglion cells (sensory neurons), and animal experiments suggest that blockage of these receptors may alleviate persistent **pain**. Furthermore, mutations of kainate receptor coding genes have been associated with a number of brain diseases (e.g., bipolar disorders, epilepsy, and neurodegenerative diseases).

NMDA receptors have properties that distinguish them from other ionotropic receptors. They have attracted much interest due to their role in long-term potentiation (LTP) and, therefore, most likely in learning and memory. They have a much slower synaptic action than the AMPA receptors and are engaged in other tasks. One important feature of NMDA-gated ion channels is that they are much more permeable to Ca^{2+} than to Na^+ (in contrast to AMPA-gated channels). This makes possible many postsynaptic effects of glutamate binding in addition to depolarization, because Ca^{2+} can trigger a number of intracellular processes (e.g., related to synaptic plasticity). Another special feature of NMDA receptors is that they are **voltage-dependent** and remain closed at resting membrane potential. Binding of glutamate (or NMDA) to the receptor opens it only if the membrane is already depolarized—for example, by the opening of AMPA receptors in the vicinity. Depolarization removes Mg^{2+} ions that otherwise block the channel. A final characteristic feature is that when the NMDA channel is opened, the flow of Ca^{2+} through it lasts much longer than an ordinary EPSP (which is produced by opening the AMPA channels).

Metabotropic glutamate receptors (mGluRs) are located both postsynaptically and presynaptically. They fall into three groups, differing with regard to which intracellular signal pathway they activate. As to postsynaptic effects, it appears that **group I mGluRs** produce a long-lasting depolarization (slow EPSP), whereas **group II** has the opposite effect (slow IPSP). Obviously, the existence of glutamate receptors with inhibitory actions further complicates the

analysis of glutamate as a transmitter. In addition, mGluRs have metabolic effects that influence various neuronal processes—among them, the induction of LTP and LTD. As mGluRs are thought to be involved in a several brain diseases (e.g., epilepsy, schizophrenia, and stroke), drugs modulating the function mGluRs are being developed and tested in animal models of human diseases.

More about Metabotropic Glutamate Receptors

Studies with immunogold labeling indicate that metabotropic glutamate receptors (**mGluR1**) are located at the periphery of synapses, whereas AMPA receptors occupy the central region. In addition, mGluRs are found without relation to synapses (enabling extrasynaptic transmission, Fig. 5.3). Such segregation might allow the receptors to respond differentially to glutamate: the AMPA receptors would be activated by normal presynaptic stimulation (low frequency of action potentials), whereas mGluRs would be activated only by high-frequency stimulation that releases large amounts of glutamate at the synapse or by spillover of glutamate from nearby synapses.

In some GABAergic synapses, mGluRs are colocalized with GABA receptors. Presumably, some glutamate is released together with GABA, or the mGluRs are activated by glutamate diffusing from nearby synapses. While the functional significance is unknown, such observations serve to emphasize that synaptic transmission cannot be understood by considering only one transmitter and its receptors.

NMDA Receptors: Mediators of Both Learning and Neuronal Damage

Long-term potentiation (LTP) was described in Chapter 4. The transmission at an excitatory synapse can be changed for a long time when the synapse is active simultaneously with other excitatory synapses in the vicinity (associative LTP). In many areas in the CNS, the induction of LTP depends on activation of NMDA receptors, and the NMDA receptors appear to have just the right properties for this task because they require both postsynaptic depolarization and glutamate binding. (Not all LTP depends on NMDA receptors, however.) NMDA receptors have binding sites for substances other than glutamate also. The amino acid **glycine** (otherwise acting as an inhibitory transmitter) binds to the NMDA receptor, and such binding is necessary for glutamate to open the NMDA channel. Other substances that occur naturally in the brain also influence the activity of the NMDA receptors and thereby presumably determine how plastic many synapses are (**metaplasticity**). Changes in the concentrations of such substances might be relevant for learning and memory in general and for recovery after brain damage.

The NMDA receptor is also one among several candidates for mediating **cell damage** after abnormal excitatory activation (see also Chapter 11, under "Ischemic Cell Damage"). This occurs when nervous tissue receives insufficient oxygen (hypoxia), as in severely reduced blood pressure, stroke, cerebral bleeding, and so forth. Abnormally intense excitation may also occur during **epileptic seizures**. In such circumstances, extracellular glutamate concentration rises steeply, and, presumably, all kinds of glutamate receptors are activated. Activation of NMDA receptors may nevertheless be especially important because it can lead to a rapid increase of the intracellular Ca^{2+} concentration. There is evidence that increased calcium concentration is crucial for cell death, among other things by increasing depolarization and initiating a vicious cycle that activates proteolytic enzymes and induces large concentration changes of ions. Excitatory amino acid transmitters and the NMDA receptor may also be involved in the cell damage that occurs in various **neurodegenerative disorders** of the nervous system, such as amyotrophic lateral sclerosis (ALS) and Huntington's disease.

While excessive NMDA-receptor activation can harm neurons, **blockage** can also produce dramatic symptoms. This is exemplified by the drugs **ketamine** (Ketalar, used as a short-acting anesthetic) and **phencyclidine** (PCP, or "angel dust") that block NMDA receptors. Both drugs influence consciousness and disturb thought processes. Side effects of ketamine used for anesthesia are nightmares and hallucinations during awakening. The thought disturbances resemble those occurring in **schizophrenia**, and this led to the "glutamate hypothesis" for this disease. Ketamine in low doses may be effective for treating persistent **pain**, probably by blocking NMDA receptors on sensory neurons in the cord. **Alcohol** (ethanol) also influences NMDA receptors (besides many other actions in the nervous system; see "GABA Receptors Are Influenced by Drugs, Alcohol, and Anesthetics" later in this chapter).

Glutamate Receptors in Peripheral Tissues

Glutamate receptors are expressed also in peripheral tissues such as **bone** (osteoblasts and osteoclasts), in taste cells, in some ganglion cells, and in insulin-producing cells in the pancreas where they modulate **insulin** secretion. NMDA receptors (and other kinds of glutamate receptors) are expressed in the membrane of unmyelinated axons that lead from **nociceptors** (pain receptors) in the skin. The functions of glutamate receptors in peripheral tissues are less understood than those in the brain.

Glutamate Transporters

Five structurally different glutamate transporter proteins have been identified, which also differ with regard to their distribution in the brain. Two are expressed in glia and one in neurons. The quantitatively dominant transporters are concentrated in glial membranes apposing neurons, particularly around synapses (see Figs. 2.5 and 4.1). It is not unexpected that the concentration of transporters is highest in parts of the brain with a high density of glutamatergic nerve terminals. The glial transporters seem to play the major role in regulating the level of extracellular glutamate. The relatively few transporters expressed in neurons may play a more limited but fast-acting role in preventing spillover of glutamate between synapses.

The transport of glutamate into glial cells is driven by concentration gradients of Na^+ and K^+. That is, the electrochemical gradient is crucial for the activity of the transporters. Other factors also influence their activity, however. Thus, the expression of transporter proteins increases with activation of glutamate receptors, while the expression decreases after removal of glutamatergic innervation.

Glutamate Transporters and Brain Damage

Under pathologic conditions with insufficient energy supply (e.g., low blood flow or low blood glucose), the electrochemical gradient cannot be maintained. Because of the high intracellular concentration of glutamate, the transporters reverse their direction of transport so that glutamate is released into the extracellular space instead of being removed from it. In this way, the extracellular glutamate concentration can reach levels several hundred times that of the normal resting level. This leads to massive receptor activation and high flow of Na^+ and Ca^{2+} into the neurons, probably initiating a vicious cycle leading to cell death (see "NMDA Receptors: Mediators of Both Learning and Neuronal Damage" earlier in this chapter, and Chapter 11, under "Ischemic Cell Damage").

Inhibitory Amino Acid Transmitters: GABA and Glycine

GABA is the dominant inhibitory transmitter; it is present in nearly all parts of the CNS (Figs. 5.1C and 5.2). As many as 20% of all synapses in the CNS may be GABAergic. GABA is used as a transmitter mainly by **interneurons** (most projection neurons are glutamatergic). It is synthesized from glutamic acid in a single step by the enzyme **glutamic acid decarboxylase** (**GAD**, Fig. 5.4). GABA acts on ionotropic **GABA$_A$ receptors**, and metabotropic **GABA$_B$ receptors**. GABA is removed from the extracellular space by high-affinity transporters (**GAT**), which are mainly localized to neuronal membranes (differing in this respect from glutamate transporters).

GABA appears to play an important role during **development** of the nervous system and occurs very early—even before synapses are established. When synapses start to occur, GABA acts as an excitatory transmitter because it depolarizes rather than hyperpolarizes the postsynaptic neuron (by acting on GABA$_A$ receptors).[1] GABA is possibly the first excitatory transmitter to shape neuronal networks

---

1. This is probably due to high intracellular **chloride** concentration in embryonic neurons. The **equilibrium potential** for Cl^- is therefore more negative than in mature neurons, so that opening of chloride channels leads to net flow of Cl^- *out* of the neuron. The same situation appears to arise in the adult spinal cord in certain conditions with persistent **pain**, that is, GABAergic interneurons may lose their normal inhibitory action on pain transmission.

Acetylcholine Receptors (AchRs)

Acetylcholine can bind to two kinds of receptors: ionotropic **nicotinic receptors** (nAchR; see Fig. 3.2) and metabotropic **muscarinic receptors** (mAchR). The names derive from the early observations that nicotine and muscarine mimicked the effects of acetylcholine (nicotine and muscarine are plant alkaloids; muscarine is present in certain kinds of poisonous mushrooms). The nicotinic receptors produce fast, excitatory synaptic actions, whereas the muscarinic receptors mediate indirect, modulatory effects on neuronal excitability. Depending on the subtype of muscarinic receptor present, the effect may be inhibitory or excitatory. Nicotinic and muscarinic receptors are distributed differently in the nervous system, and there are several subtypes of both (which can be distinguished pharmacologically by use of different agonists and antagonists). For example, different subtypes of nicotinic receptors are expressed in striated muscle cells, in autonomic ganglia, and in the CNS.

Several **subtypes** of the **nicotinic receptor** have been identified. There are three main groups, and those include receptors in skeletal muscle, in autonomic ganglia, and in the CNS. The functional role of nicotinic receptor in the CNS is not well understood, but these receptors are present in many places and are localized mainly presynaptically. They therefore influence neuronal excitability chiefly indirectly by modulating release of other transmitters (e.g., glutamate). Much better understood are the actions of acetylcholine at the cholinergic synapses between motor neurons and **skeletal muscle** cells (see Figs. 21.4 and 21.5). Binding of acetylcholine opens the channel for cations, but the permeability is largest for Na^+. Opening of such channels elicits an action potential that spreads out in all directions to reach every part of the muscle cell membrane. This is the signal that leads to muscle contraction. (Whereas skeletal muscle cells contain only nicotinic receptors, **smooth muscle cells** are equipped only with muscarinic receptors.)

Muscarinic receptors are quantitatively the dominant acetylcholine receptors in the CNS. So far, five subtypes (**m1–m5**) have been cloned (all are blocked by **atropine**) but m1 and m2 are the quantitatively most important ones. Whereas m1 receptors are located postsynaptically, m2 receptors are found predominantly presynaptically. In the **cerebral cortex**, which receives many cholinergic nerve terminals, a major effect of acetylcholine is to reduce the permeability of a K^+ channel by acting on m1 receptors. This makes the neurons more susceptible to other excitatory inputs so that, for example, a neuron will react more easily to a specific sensory stimulus. Another kind of muscarinic receptor opens a K^+ channel, thereby producing long-lasting hyperpolarization, while a third type closes a Ca^{2+} channel.

Blockers of Acetylcholine Receptors

Curare is an antagonist (blocker) of the nicotinic receptors and was used as an arrow poison by South American natives to paralyze victims. Derivatives of curare are used to achieve muscle relaxation during surgery. **Atropine** and **scopolamine** are relatively unselective antagonists of muscarinic receptors (i.e., they block all subtypes). The snake venom α-**bungarotoxin** binds specifically to muscle nicotinic receptors and blocks the effect of acetylcholine (and kills the victim by paralyzing all skeletal muscles). The French neuroscientist Jean-Pierre Changeux and coworkers achieved the first isolation and characterization of a transmitter receptor by use of α bungarotoxin. To obtain sufficient amounts of the receptor, **electric eels** (*Torpedo*) were chosen for study because they are equipped with electric organs that produce strong electric shocks by activating nicotinic receptors.

Nicotine Addiction

Genetic variability among AchR subunits appears to be related to nicotine dependence; that is, persons with genes for a certain subunit might have an increased risk of becoming nicotine dependent. The development of addictive behavior depends, at least partly, on nicotine receptor–mediated stimulation of **dopaminergic** neurons (that release dopamine in the nucleus accumbens; see Chapter 23, under "The Ventral Striatum, Psychosis, and Drug Addiction"). However, the relation between nicotine and addictive behavior is complex, and several transmitters other than dopamine are involved (e.g., glutamate and GABA). Further, chronic nicotine consumption induces plastic changes in several neuronal groups. At the cerebral cortical level, a region called **insula** (see Chapter 34 under "The Insula") may be particularly important. For example, in one brain-imaging study, activation of neuronal groups in the insula was found to increase in relation to the person feeling an urge for a drug. Further, smokers suffering a stroke that damaged the insula were much more likely to quit smoking than were smokers suffering lesions in other parts of the brain.

Biogenic Amines

The **biogenic amines** constitute a subgroup of the small-molecule transmitters. The group includes the **monoamines** norepinephrine, epinephrine, dopamine, and serotonin (one amine group), in addition to **histamine** (two amine groups). Neurons that use monoamines as transmitters are called **monoaminergic**. The monoamines are **synthesized** by enzymatic removal of the carboxylic group from an aromatic

Figure 5.7

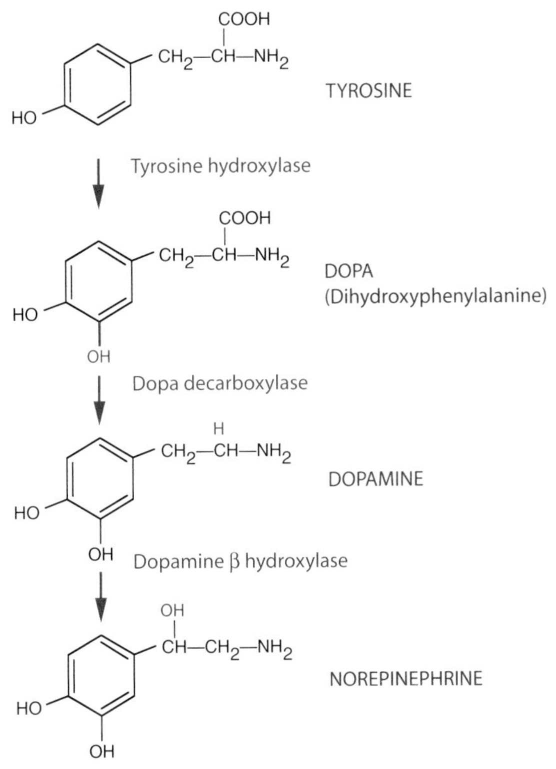

Figure 5.7

The catecholamines dopamine and norepinephrine and the key enzymes in their synthesis.

Figure 5.8

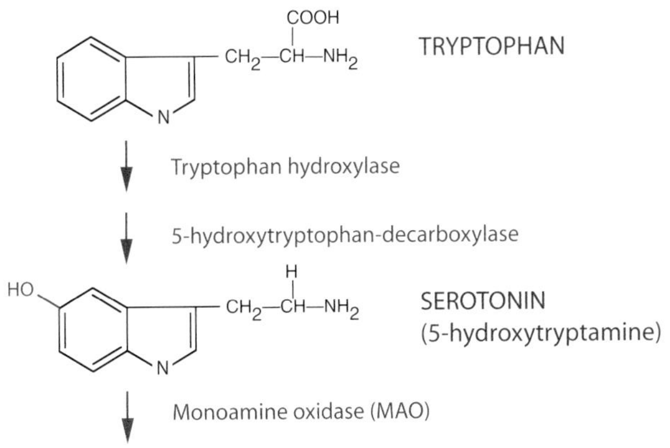

Serotonin. This neurotransmitter synthesized from tryptophan in two enzymatic steps. It is broken down by monoamine oxidase in the nerve terminals.

amino acid (Figs. 5.7 and 5.8). Norepinephrine, epinephrine, and dopamine are **catecholamines**.[6] Neurons that contain the monoamines norepinephrine, dopamine, serotonin, and histamine are said to be noradrenergic, dopaminergic, serotonergic, and histaminergic, respectively (the same terminology is used for the receptors corresponding to these transmitters).

A common feature of the biogenic amines is that they are synthesized only in a small number of neurons, which, however, have widely branching axons. In this way, these few neurons ensure that the transmitters can act in most parts of the CNS. Like acetylcholine, the biogenic amines are to a large extent released from varicosities without typical synaptic contacts (Fig. 5.3); therefore, their effects are presumably mainly mediated by **volume transmission** and binding to extrasynaptic receptors. Localization and functions of monoaminergic cell groups are discussed in Chapters 23 (dopamine) and 26 (norepinephrine and

serotonin). See also Chapter 28, under "Neurotransmitters in the Autonomic Nervous System".

Actions of the Biogenic Amines

The biogenic amines act (with one exception) on **metabotropic receptors**; that is, they exert mainly slow, **modulatory** actions. Monoaminergic (like cholinergic) neurons are therefore suited to modulate simultaneously the specific information processing mediated by glutamate and GABA in many anatomically separate neuronal groups. This is related to regulation of **attention**, **motivation**, and **mood**. In addition, the monoamines play important roles with regard to **plasticity** and **learning**. Drugs used to treat diseases such as schizophrenia, Parkinson's disease, and depression alter the functioning of monoamines.

Localization of Monoaminergic Neurons

Neurons that synthesize **catecholamines** are largely restricted to some small cell groups in the brain stem, hypothalamus, and peripheral nervous system. Most **noradrenergic neurons** in the CNS occur in somewhat diffuse cell groups in the brain stem reticular formation, the **locus coeruleus** being the largest and most distinct (see Fig. 26.7). The majority of **dopaminergic neurons** are localized to the mesencephalon in one large nucleus called the **substantia nigra** and more diffuse cells groups in the vicinity (**ventral**

6. **Catecholamines**: Compounds consisting of a catechol group (benzene ring with two hydroxyl groups) with an attached amine group.

indicate that symptoms in adult animals depend on reduced transporter activity during a short period after birth. Only animals with genetic vulnerability *plus* experience of psychological trauma in this period (such as separation from the mother) developed behavioral disturbances as adults. Therefore, it seems that normal serotonin transmission in early postnatal development is necessary for the development of neuronal networks handling emotions and stress. This assumption is further supported by other animal experiments showing that the presence of the **5-HT$_{1A}$ receptor** in early development is necessary and sufficient for normal anxiety-related behavior as an adult, regardless of whether or not the receptor is expressed in the adult animals.

Monoamine Gene Polymorphisms and Behavior: Complex Interactions

When interpreting findings of associations between certain transmitters and mental disease, one should bear in mind the complexity of the brain processes underlying human behavior. Studying the contribution of one transmitter in isolation, while necessary to obtain reliable results, is highly artificial because it leaves out numerous other factors (some known and some unknown) that interact in shaping behavior. Altered serotonin metabolism is, for example, certainly not the substrate of depression but may—together with many other transmitters—be necessary for normal signal processing in the complex networks that generate and control emotions and their behavioral expressions. Further, genetic **vulnerability** of the kind described earlier may increase the risk of developing certain mental disorders or personality traits but does not determine their development. How easily an adult person becomes mentally disturbed seems to depend on how certain brain networks developed in early childhood. This, in turn, depends on a complex interaction between inherited traits (e.g., variety of the serotonin transporter and numerous other polymorphisms) and the environment.

We should finally bear in mind that gene polymorphisms that are associated with increased disease vulnerability also might contribute positively in other aspects of human life. An example may be a COMT polymorphism that seems to provide a disadvantage in certain cognitive tasks while giving an advantage with regard to emotional processing. Also, the variant of the gene for the serotonin transporter linked to increased vulnerability to depression may, on the other hand, facilitate social adaptation.

Modulatory Transmitter "Systems"

We described some features shared by monoaminergic and cholinergic neuronal groups (with the exception of cholinergic motor neurons). First, a small number of neurons send axons to large parts of the CNS—that is, the cell bodies producing the enzymes necessary for transmitter synthesis are very restricted in distribution, whereas the transmitters and their receptors are present almost everywhere. Second, each axon ramifies extensively, and the terminal branches are equipped with numerous **varicosities** (Fig. 5.3). As mentioned, these varicosities only infrequently form typical synapses but release transmitters more diffusely (**volume transmission**), presumably by acting largely on extrasynaptic receptors. Finally, the transmitters act predominantly via **metabotropic** receptors—exerting slow, modulatory effects on neuronal excitability.

These anatomic and physiologic features imply that the monoaminergic and cholinergic cell groups do not mediate precise temporal or spatial information. They are well suited, however, to modulate the functions of specific glutamatergic and GABAergic systems, for example, by improving the **signal-to-noise** ratio. In this way, they may increase the precision of information handling in many parts of the brain—for example, in the cerebral cortex during processing of complex cognitive tasks. Their widespread connections furthermore ensure that many neuronal groups receive a similar modulatory input, as would be important for control of consciousness, awareness, different phases of sleep, emotions, motivation, and so forth. Monoamines furthermore set the level of excitability of spinal neurons to control voluntary movements and of neurons that are transmitting specific sensory information. For example, brain stem serotonergic neurons with axonal ramifications in the cord appear to both facilitate movement and inhibit sensory transmission.

Trying to bind together seemingly disparate actions, one might speculate that the modulatory transmitter "systems" ensure that sensory, motor, and cognitive processes are coordinated toward a common goal. The modulatory transmitters would do this by mediating a signal about the **value** of specific events. These speculations are supported by the well-established roles of monoamines and acetylcholine in **synaptic plasticity** (see Fig. 4.10).

In spite of their homogeneities, it is an oversimplification to regard each transmitter-specific group as a functional entity and to use terms such as "the serotonin system," "the dopamine system," and so on. First, the large number of receptors for each transmitter, with different distributions and effects in the brain, indicate that each transmitter-specific cell group has complex relations to behavior. For example, dopaminergic neurons influence neuronal networks engaged in quite different behavioral tasks. Second, even if localizations are not sharp, each transmitter-specific group contains subgroups that differ in where they send their axons and from where they receive afferents. For example, the various serotonergic raphe nuclei (see Fig. 26.6) send axons to different parts of the CNS. Third, most or all monoaminergic neurons also contain one or more neuropeptides. The effects obtained by stimulation of one of these cell groups therefore cannot be ascribed to one transmitter alone.

Adenosine Triphosphate and Adenosine

The purines adenosine triphosphate (ATP) and adenosine can exert marked effects on neuronal excitability, both in the CNS and peripherally. Only ATP, however, appears to act as a transmitter (e.g., it is concentrated in vesicles and its release is calcium dependent). The effects are mediated by purinoceptors, localized both pre- and postsynaptically. (Many other cell types besides neurons express purinoceptors—e.g., smooth muscle cells.) P_1 receptors bind adenosine, while P_2 receptors bind ATP. After release, ATP is enzymatically degraded. The transmitter role of ATP is well characterized in the **autonomic nervous system**, where it is usually **colocalized** with acetylcholine or norepinephrine. ATP and the classical transmitter are found in the same vesicles, and they are released together (see Chapter 28, under "Noncholinergic and Nonadrenergic Transmission in the Autonomic System"). As a rule, ATP excites neurons and smooth muscle cells by acting on ionotropic receptors. There are, however, examples of inhibitory effects of ATP (probably by way of metabotropic receptors) on smooth muscle cells—for example, in the longitudinal muscle layer of the large intestine. In the **inner ear**, efferent nerve fibers to the sensory cells (hair cells) release ATP together with acetylcholine and modulate the sensitivity of the sensory cells.

So far, little is known with certainty about the transmitter role of ATP in the CNS, in spite of the wide distribution of purinoceptors and possible implication in functions ranging from sensation to learning and mood. Fast purinergic transmission has been demonstrated in many parts of the brain (locus coeruleus, habenula, hippocampus, cerebral cortex, spinal cord, and other neuronal groups). ATP seems always to be **colocalized** with other transmitters (in locus coeruleus with norepinephrine, in the hippocampus with glutamate, in cortex with acetylcholine, and so forth). ATP is probably used as transmitter in a subgroup of **spinal ganglion cells**—that is, sensory

neurons conducting impulses from peripheral receptors to the spinal cord (see Chapter 13, under "Primary Sensory Neurons: Colocalization of Classical Neurotransmitters and Neuropeptides"). A population of **spinal interneurons** seems to release ATP in parts of the cord that receives signals from pain receptors (laminae I and II; see Fig. 6.10). Ionotropic P_2 receptors increase the release of glutamate and substance P from terminals of spinal ganglion cells in the dorsal horn. This may contribute to the heightened excitability of spinal neurons, which is typical of persistent pain conditions. In addition, ATP and purinoceptors mediate signals between neurons and **glial cells** and may participate in the interaction between the immune system and neurons.

As mentioned, **adenosine** has marked effects on neurons, even though it is unlikely to act as a transmitter. Injection of minute amounts of adenosine inhibits spinal cord neurons that mediate signals from **pain** receptors to the brain. Adenosine also appears to be involved—in some yet unknown way—with the **analgesic** effects of morphine and the morphine-like substances produced in the brain (opioids). Finally, adenosine influences neuronal **plasticity** and seems to be one among several substances (e.g., BDNF) that regulate plasticity (**metaplasticity**).

Purinoceptors

There are two main groups of P_2 **receptors**. One group (P_{2X}) consists of six **ionotropic** receptors with fast, excitatory action. The channels are most permeable to Ca^{2+} and have a longer opening time than, for example, AMPA receptors (but that is much shorter than for NMDA receptors). The other group (P_{2Y}) consists of seven **metabotropic** receptors. Both groups are widely distributed in the CNS, although the transmitter role of ATP is reasonably certain only in a few areas. The study of ATP as a neurotransmitter has so far been hampered by the lack of specific receptor antagonists. P_1 **receptors** are blocked by **xanthenes**, such as **caffeine** and **theophylline**. Theophylline inhibits bronchial smooth muscle cells and is used therapeutically in **asthma**.

Nitric Oxide

Nitric oxide (NO) is a gas that diffuses freely through biologic membranes. It functions as a signal molecule in many organs of the body, among them the nervous system. Its functional role in the nervous system is only partly clear, however. Even though NO often is called an "unconventional neurotransmitter," it does not meet the criteria used to define a transmitter: it is not stored in vesicles, it is not released by calcium-dependent exocytosis, and it does not bind to membrane-bound receptors.

In the **peripheral nervous system**, autonomic nerve fibers release NO that acts on smooth muscle cells. In the **CNS**, NO has a number of cellular effects and appears to take part in the control of various systems; it also influences behavior. It has quite different effects in the brain depending on its concentration, however: in low concentrations, it functions as a signal molecule that modulates neuronal behavior, whereas it is toxic in higher concentrations (which is perhaps not surprising because NO is a free radical and as such very reactive).

NO is **synthesized** from the amino acid **arginine** by specific enzymes, **NO synthases**, of which there are several different types. Synthesis of NO in nerve terminals is probably induced by the increase of intracellular Ca^{2+} concentration that is triggered by a presynaptic action potential. After synthesis, NO diffuses freely in all directions. It is not only delivered into the synaptic cleft but also enters all cells that are near the nerve terminal. Calculations from the cerebral cortex indicate that NO can diffuse more than 100 μm from its release site and reach about 2 million synapses. The most abundant **NO receptor** is a water-soluble, cytoplasmic enzyme, **guanylyl cyclase**, which controls synthesis of cyclic GMP. This is an intracellular messenger with various effects, such as activating protein kinases and acting directly on ion channels. In this way NO can modulate neuronal excitability and firing frequency.

NO synthases are present in neurons in several parts of the central and peripheral nervous system. In the cerebral cortex, they are found in GABAergic neurons, which, in addition, contain neuropeptides (substance P and somatostatin). In other parts of the brain, NO synthases occur in cholinergic and monoaminergic neurons. Although we do not know the functions of NO liberated from such neurons, there is some evidence that NO is one of numerous factors that are involved in the induction of **LTP** and therefore presumably also in neuronal **plasticity**. NO also appears to play a special role in neurons with **rhythmic** firing—such as the brain stem and thalamic neurons that regulate sleep–wakefulness and the hypothalamic neurons that control bodily functions with daily variations (**circadian rhythms**). Presumably, NO, due to its fast and wide diffusion, is particularly suited to **synchronize** the activity of many neurons.

In situations with insufficient energy supply (most often due to reduced blood flow), increased intracellular Ca^{2+} concentration leads to increased NO synthesis. This seems likely to contribute to the neuronal damage in such situations (see Fig. 11.1). On the other hand, release of NO might improve the blood supply by producing local vasodilatation.

NO and Blood Vessels

NO was first discovered in endothelial cells and named **endothelium-derived relaxing factor**. In fact, its main effect in most organs is relaxation of smooth muscle cells, causing vasodilatation and increased blood flow. NO released from autonomic (parasympathetic) nerve fibers, for example, is responsible for penile erection. **Nitroglycerin** and similar drugs give vasodilatation by inducing synthesis of NO.

NO also affects vessels in the CNS. There is evidence that NO, together with other signal molecules, mediates the increased **local blood flow** associated with increased neuronal activity. For example, the blood flow in the cortical motor area increases when the neurons increase their firing during execution of voluntary movements (see Chapter 8, under "Regional Cerebral Blood Flow and Neuronal Activity).

Neuropeptides

A large number of neuroactive peptides have so far been identified in the CNS, but many of them were first found in the peripheral nervous system and in the gut. Although there is firm evidence of a transmitter function for only a few neuropeptides, many of them have marked effects on physiologic processes and behavior when administered locally in the CNS. Several of the neuropeptides elicit slow inhibitory or excitatory synaptic potentials when administered in minute amounts close to neurons, suggesting a **modulatory** transmitter role. This assumption is supported by the identification of several G protein–coupled neuropeptide receptors. Neuropeptides can also elicit intracellular responses related to **growth** and **development**. Normally, the concentrations of neuropeptides are low in neurons. The synthesis increases, however, when the homeostasis of the nervous system is challenged (e.g., in infections, stroke, trauma). The way neuropeptides are released may perhaps fit an "**emergency**" role: it seems that neuropeptide release requires a high firing frequency or burst firing, whereas low-frequency firing suffices to release small molecule (classical) transmitters.

The duration of action appears to be longer for neuropeptides than for other neuromodulators (in spite of the presence of extracellular peptidases). Thus, the half-life after release can be very long (e.g., about 20 min for vasopressin)—giving ample time for extracellular diffusion. In addition, at least some neuropeptides are released from dendrites. Thus, it seems that the actions

Figure 5.9

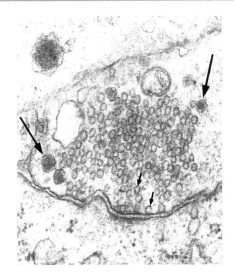

Nerve terminal containing both a "classical" transmitter and neuropeptides. Large arrows show the dense-core vesicles that contain neuropeptides with transmitter actions. Small arrows show the small, clear vesicles that contain small molecule "classical" transmitters.

of the neuropeptides are, as a rule, rather diffuse. Some of the neuropeptides may thus function more like **local hormones** than like neurotransmitters, as also suggested by a mismatch between the distribution of receptors for a neuropeptide and nerve terminals containing the neuropeptide.

A characteristic feature of neuropeptides is that they are **colocalized** in nerve terminals with small-molecule (classical) transmitters. Whereas small-molecule transmitters are stored in small, electron-lucent vesicles, neuropeptides are found in larger vesicles with an electron-dense center (**dense core vesicles**; Fig 5.9). Two or more peptides may also coexist, and there may be more than one small-molecule transmitter together with the peptides.

Several neuropeptides are mentioned in subsequent chapters in relation to various cell groups and neuronal systems.

Examples of Colocalization of Neuropeptides and Small-Molecule Transmitters

Terminals of nerve fibers innervating **salivary glands** contain both **acetylcholine** and the neuropeptide **vasoactive intestinal polypeptide** (**VIP**). Both substances are released when the nerves are stimulated, but they act on different target cells: acetylcholine elicits secretion from glandular cells, whereas VIP produces vasodilatation by relaxing smooth muscle cells, thereby increasing blood flow to the organ at the same time as its secretion is increased. Another example concerns **primary sensory neurons**

(spinal ganglion cells; see Figs. 6.9 and 13.16) mediating information from peripheral sense organs to the spinal cord. Some of these—particularly those related to painful stimuli—contain both **glutamate** and the peptides **substance P** and **calcitonin gene-related peptide** (**CGRP**). When released with glutamate, these peptides appear to have several actions: they can bind to specific postsynaptic receptors, they can act presynaptically to increase their own release and the release of glutamate, and they can sensitize the postsynaptic glutamate receptors to enhance the effect of glutamate (see also Chapter 13, under "Neuropeptides in Spinal Ganglion Cells and Nociceptors").

Spinal interneurons that receive sensory information exhibit different transmitter combinations. One group of interneurons contains **GABA** and the peptide **enkephalin**. Another group contains both **enkephalin** and **substance P** in combination with (most likely) **glutamate**. Therefore, one neuropeptide (enkephalin) may be colocalized with either an inhibitory or an excitatory transmitter with fast synaptic actions. Apparently, spinal interneurons may express a variety of transmitter combinations with correspondingly complex synaptic actions. When we also think of the variety of receptors each neuron expresses, it is easy to understand why unraveling the functional role of a single transmitter can be difficult.

In the **cerebral cortex** GABAergic interneurons express various neuropeptides, and several different morphological types of interneuron can be distinguished by their neuropeptide content (e.g., **somatostatin** (SOM), **vasoactive intestinal polypeptide** (VIP), **neuropeptide Y**, and several others).

ACTIONS OF DRUGS ON THE NERVOUS SYSTEM

Most Drugs Influence Synaptic Function

Several drugs have been mentioned in connection with discussions of synaptic function and neurotransmitters. Most drugs acting on the nervous system do so by influencing synaptic transmission directly or indirectly, regardless of whether their aim is to alleviate disorders of mood, cognition, movements, memory, or behavior. The drugs may interfere presynaptically in the synthesis, release, degradation, or reuptake of transmitters or postsynaptically in the activity, numbers, or localization of receptors. Certain drugs have one or more of these actions regarding one or several transmitters. Some drugs also seem to influence synaptic functions indirectly by changing the expression of neurotrophic factors that (among other tasks) govern synaptic plasticity.

Examples: Drugs Altering Monoamine Activity in the Brain

The most common **antipsychotic drugs** (neuroleptics) block **dopamine receptors**. Their therapeutic effects are primarily related to altering the transmitter functions of dopamine, although they also influence other transmitters (they exhibit, e.g., more or less anticholinergic and antihistaminergic effects). In addition, dopamine receptors are present in neuronal groups related to movement control and muscle tone, and this explains why motor dysfunctions are common side effects of antipsychotics. Conversely, patients with Parkinson's disease who are treated with levodopa to increase dopamine levels in the brain may develop psychotic symptoms during treatment. Nevertheless, the "dopamine hypothesis of schizophrenia," which states that the symptoms can be explained as a result of dopaminergic hyperactivity, is too simplistic. Not all symptoms can be explained in this way, and dopaminergic hyperactivity does not appear to be present in all patients. Further, psychotic symptoms can also be treated effectively with drugs that block serotonin receptors (so-called atypical antipsychotic drugs, such as **clozapine**, have higher affinity for serotonin receptors than for dopamine receptors). **MAO inhibitors** were the first drugs with significant effects on major **depressions**. Later, **tricyclic antidepressants** (TCAs) were introduced, which inhibit relatively selectively the norepinephrine transporter. The new antidepressants, such as **fluoxetine** (Prozac), inhibit rather selectively the serotonin transporter (**selective serotonin-uptake inhibitors** [**SSRIs**]). Although the clinical effects of antidepressants may appear to be caused simply by increased levels of monoamines available at the synapses, this cannot be the whole story. For example, while inhibition of the transporters occurs immediately, the clinical effect comes after days or weeks with treatment. Therefore, clinical effects were sought in compensatory processes, such as up- and down-regulation of receptors. Recent research has revealed a number of effects of antidepressants other than altering monoamine levels—for example, on expression of **neurotrophins** (notably BDNF) and neuronal **plasticity**. The fact that antidepressants, in spite of acting on different monoamine transporters, have similar clinical effects prompted the hypothesis that they act by regulating **transcription** of the same set of genes. This has received some experimental support. For example, one study identified gene transcripts that were equally regulated by treatment with different classes of antidepressants.

Cocaine inhibits the dopamine transporter very selectively; that is, its affinity to the dopamine transporter is much higher than to other monoamine transporters. The dopamine transporter has even been called a "cocaine receptor." **Amphetamine** inhibits the dopamine transporter but also other monoamine transporters, although relatively weakly compared with cocaine. In addition, amphetamine increases the release of catecholamines and has other synaptic effects as well.

Drug Effects Are Often Multifarious

Most transmitters are present in several parts of the nervous system, which differ anatomically and physiologically. Therefore, it should not be surprising that even drugs that apparently influence the actions of only one transmitter nevertheless have multifarious effects. Some of these are desired therapeutic effects, whereas others are disturbing or even dangerous side effects. Development of more specific drugs—for example, drugs acting on only one receptor subtype—may reduce the side effects but will hardly eliminate them. This is because each receptor type (even one among several subtypes for one transmitter) occurs in functionally different parts of the nervous system.

Drugs Interact with Dynamic Processes in the Brain

Another important point is that storage, release, and uptake of transmitters, as well as the expression of receptors, are **dynamic processes**. The acute perturbations caused by a drug are usually counteracted quickly by feedback loops that up- or down-regulate the transmitter release, the transporters, the receptors, and so forth. For example, when the activity of **tryptophan hydroxylase** (the rate-limiting enzyme in serotonin synthesis) is reduced, the neurons respond by increasing synthesis of the enzyme and its axonal transport to the nerve terminals.[9] Finally, we should keep in mind that alteration of one transmitter's activity as a rule leads to alterations of other transmitters as well. One mechanism behind this is the action on presynaptic receptors: a cholinergic terminal in the cerebral cortex may be equipped with serotonin receptors, so that a drug with specific action on serotonergic transmission may nevertheless also alter cholinergic transmission. Another mechanism is postsynaptic: many dopaminergic neurons receive glutamatergic synapses, so that drugs altering the action of glutamate will change dopamine release as well.

---

9. **Lithium**, used prophylactically for major bipolar disorder (manic depression), increases tryptophan uptake and initially increases serotonin synthesis (this is only one of several cellular effects of lithium). After 2 to 3 weeks with treatment, however, the tryptophan uptake is still increased, but the tryptophan hydroxylase activity is reduced so that the rate of serotonin synthesis is normal. It is possible that the therapeutic effect of lithium is due to stabilization of serotonin metabolism, which makes it less vulnerable to psychological stress or spontaneous chemical changes in the brain.

Parts of the Nervous System

OVERVIEW

In this chapter we describe the main features of the anatomy of the central nervous system (CNS), with brief mention of the functional significance of the various parts. We discuss structure and function of many of these parts in more depth in later chapters dealing with functional systems. It is assumed, however, that the reader is familiar with the names and the locations of the major cell groups and tracts of the CNS.

The CNS can be subdivided anatomically into different parts. The **spinal cord** lies in the vertebral canal, whereas the **brain** is located in the cranial cavity. The brain is further subdivided into the **brain stem**, which constitutes the upward continuation of the spinal cord, the **cerebellum** ("little brain"), and the **cerebrum** or **cerebral hemispheres**. The cerebellum and cerebrum largely cover the brain stem and constitute the major part of the brain in higher mammals and particularly in humans.

The **spinal cord** consists of a central region with gray matter surrounded by white matter. The **gray matter** contains neurons that may be subdivided based on where they send their axons. **Motor neurons** send their axons out of the cord to reach muscles and glands. **Sensory neurons** receive signals from sense organs in the body and transmit this information to the brain. The spinal **interneurons** or **propriospinal** neurons ensure communication among neurons in the spinal cord. The **white matter** contains ascending tracts carrying signals to higher levels and descending tracts enabling the brain to control spinal cord neurons (e.g., motor neurons). In addition, many propriospinal axons interconnect neurons in different parts of the cord. The cord consists of **segments**, each giving rise to a pair of **spinal nerves**. The spinal nerves and their peripheral branches transmit sensory signals from the tissues of the body and motor signals to muscles and glands. Each spinal nerve connects with the cord through a dorsal and a ventral **nerve root**. The **dorsal roots** carry only sensory nerve fibers, and the cell bodies of the sensory neurons of each root form a **spinal ganglion**, which appears as an ovoid enlargement of the dorsal root.

Functionally, the cord enables fast, automatic responses to signals from the body (e.g., withdrawal of the hand from a hot object). Nevertheless, most tasks carried out by the cord are controlled or modulated by higher levels of the CNS.

The **brain stem** is a rostral continuation of the spinal cord but has a more complex internal organization. On a purely anatomical basis, the brain stem is divided (starting caudally) into the **medulla oblongata**, the **pons**, the **mesencephalon**, and the **diencephalon** (often, however, we do not include the diencephalon). Twelve **cranial nerves** emanate from the brain stem, numbered from rostral to caudal. With some exceptions, the cranial nerves innervate structures in the head ("spinal nerves of the head") and contain sensory and motor nerve fibers. The first cranial nerve—the **olfactory nerve**—serves the sense of smell. The second—the **optic nerve**—transmit signals from the retina, while the third (**oculomotor**), fourth (**trochlear**), and sixth (**abducens**) nerves control the movements of the eyeball. The fifth nerve—the **trigeminal**—emanates from the pons and brings sensory signals from the face as well as motor signals to the masticatory muscles. The seventh nerve—the **facial**—innervates the mimic muscles of the face. The eighth nerve—the **vestibulocochlear**—carries signals from the vestibular apparatus (recording movements and positions of the head in space) and the cochlea (recording sound waves). The ninth nerve—the **glossopharyngeal**—is concerned mainly with sensations and movements of the pharynx, including taste impulses from the back of the tongue. The tenth nerve—the **vagus** nerve—participates in the innervation of the pharynx but in addition innervates the larynx and sends (autonomic) motor signals to the heart, the lungs, and the most of the gastrointestinal tract. The eleventh nerve—the **accessory**—innervates two muscles in the neck (the trapezius and the sternocleidomastoid). The twelfth nerve—the **hypoglossal**—is the motor nerve of the tongue. The cranial nerves arise in **cranial nerve nuclei**, some of which are sensory and others are motor.

Diffuse collections of neurons in between the cranial nerve nuclei are collectively termed the **reticular formation**. The reticular formation consists of neuronal groups with different tasks. Some groups are concerned with control of **circulation** and **respiration**; some regulate **sleep** and **wakefulness**, while others control **eye movements**.

The thalamus and the hypothalamus make up the bulk of the **diencephalon**. The **thalamus** is a large, egg-shaped collection of nuclei in the centre of the cerebral hemispheres. The thalamic nuclei transmit sensory information (of all kinds except smell) to the cerebral cortex. In addition, thalamic nuclei transmit information to the cerebral cortex from subcortical motor regions, notably the basal ganglia and the cerebellum. The **hypothalamus** is concerned mainly with the control of autonomic and endocrine functions that serve to maintain bodily homeostasis (e.g., circulation, digestion, and temperature control).

The **cerebral cortex** is a folded sheet of gray matter covering the cerebral hemispheres. It consists of six layers of neurons, each layer characterized by the morphology and connectivity of its neurons. In addition, the cortical mantle is divided into many **areas**, differing with regard to, among other things, their thalamic connections. Even though each area is to some extent specialized, most tasks of the cerebral cortex—whether they are motor, sensory, or cognitive—are carried out by **distributed networks** interconnecting neurons in many areas of the cerebral cortex. Among the many descending tracts from the cerebral cortex, **the pyramidal tract** targets motor neurons in the spinal cord and brain stem. The **corpus callosum**, consisting of commissural fibers, enables cooperation between the two cerebral hemispheres.

The **basal ganglia** consist of several large nuclei in the interior of the cerebral hemispheres. The **striatum** consists of **putamen** and the **caudate nucleus** and receives its main afferents from the cerebral cortex. The striatum sends efferents to the **globus pallidus** and the **substantia nigra**. From these, signals are directed to the brain stem and back to the cerebral cortex via the thalamus. By influencing motor neuronal groups in the frontal lobe of cerebral cortex (and in the brain stem), the basal ganglia contribute to the **control of movements**. Connections with other frontal areas in cerebral cortex (and certain subcortical nuclei) enable the basal ganglia to influence **cognitive functions**.

The **cerebellum**, situated dorsal to the brain stem in the posterior cranial fossa, consists of a thin sheet of highly folded gray matter and a group of centrally located **deep cerebellar nuclei**. The cerebellum is divided anatomically into a narrow middle part called the **vermis** and more bulky lateral parts called the cerebellar **hemispheres**. In addition, a deep fissure divides the cerebellum into an **anterior lobe** and a **posterior lobe**. These anatomic subdivisions correspond largely to differences with regard to connections. Thus, the vermis has reciprocal connections with the spinal cord and motor nuclei in the brain stem, whereas the cerebellar hemispheres are reciprocally connected with the cerebral cortex. These connections enable the cerebellum to play a decisive role in **coordination** of voluntary movements by acting on motor neurons in the cerebral cortex, the brain stem, and the spinal cord.

METHODS TO STUDY THE LIVING HUMAN BRAIN

Throughout this book, references are made to studies using brain-imaging techniques. Indeed, techniques for computer-based image analysis of the living human brain have revolutionized the possibilities for localizing disease processes in the brain and for studying normal structure and function. Before the computer-based imaging techniques, **electroencephalography** (EEG) was the only method available enabling studies of the activity in the living brain. EEG is usually done by placing many electrodes on the head (see Chapter 26, under "The Study of Consciousness: Electroencephalography (EEG)") and has been developed to enable study of topographic patterns of cerebral activation in relation to the performance of specific tasks. Furthermore, coherence of EEG activity in different cortical areas suggests that the areas are functionally interconnected.

Computer Tomography (CT) and Magnetic Resonance Imaging (MRI)

The first of the imaging techniques that enabled us to identify smaller parts of the living brain is **computer tomography** (CT). This method makes it possible to see X-ray pictures of thin slices through the brain. The examiner may choose the plane of sectioning. CT affords much more precise visualization of brain structures than conventional X-ray examination, which includes all tissue between the X-ray tube and the film. It also provides good visualization of the ventricular system, which previously could be visualized only by replacing the cerebrospinal fluid with air and then making an X-ray examination. CT can also visualize the distribution of a radioactive substance in the living brain, enabling the study of the distribution of neuroactive substances and also the comparison of blood flow in different parts of the brain.

Magnetic resonance imaging (**MRI**) represents a further technical development. This technique is based not on X-rays but on signals emitted by protons when they are placed in a magnetic field. Depending on the proton concentration in different tissue components, the pictures may show clearly, for example, the contrast between gray and white matter (Figs. 6.2 and 6.28). The bone of the skull gives very little or no signal and is seen as black in the pictures. With this technique, the brain can be visualized in slices with a resolution not far from that of a corresponding section through a fixed brain. Areas with changes in the tissue—for example, infarction, bleeding, or tumor—can be identified. In addition, blood vessels can be visualized (see Figs. 8.3 and 8.8). Apart from the diagnostic advantages, the MRI technique also improves the correlation of the functional disturbances with the actual damage of the brain. MRI can also be used to study dynamic processes in the brain.

Further developments of the MRI technology have added new applications. For example, with **diffusion-weighted imaging** (**DWI**) a region devoid of blood supply can be detected only minutes after **occlusion** of an artery (much earlier than with conventional MRI). Further, DWI enables study of **myelination** during normal brain development and even the visualization of major fiber tracts.

Correlation of Brain Activity with Behavior: Positron Emission Tomography (PET), Functional MRI (fMRI), Electroencephalography (EEG), and Magnetic Encephalography (MEG)

Because of the link between a change of neuronal activity and local cerebral blood flow, the flow of blood through specific parts of the brain can be correlated with certain stimuli or specific sensory, motor, or mental activities (see Chapter 8, under "Regional Cerebral Blood Flow and Neuronal Activity"). CT can be used to visualize the distribution of a radioactive substance in the living brain. This method, called **positron emission tomography** (**PET**), is based on the use of isotopes that emit positrons. Positrons fuse immediately with electrons, producing two gamma rays going in opposite directions, thus permitting the identification of their origin in the brain with the aid of a powerful computer. PET produces images that show the distribution of an inhaled or injected radioactively labeled substance at a given time. By labeling substances of biological interest, one can determine their distribution in the body. In the case of **blood flow** measurement, radioactively labeled water is injected into the bloodstream. **Functional MRI** (**fMRI**) is the other main method to visualize dynamic changes in the brain.

This method is based on the fact that the magnetic properties of hemoglobin depend on whether or not it is oxygenated, and small differences in blood oxyhemoglobin concentration can be detected with MRI. For unknown reasons, the oxygen uptake of nerve cells does not increase simultaneously with increased activity. Thus, it appears that neurons work anaerobically during a brief period of increased activity, despite a sufficient oxygen supply. The glucose uptake increases, however, and so does the blood flow. When the blood flow increases without increased oxygen uptake, more oxygen remains in the blood after passing the capillaries—that is, the **arteriovenous O_2 difference** is reduced. MRI can detect this change, and in this way the regions of increased or reduced blood flow can be visualized. An advantage over PET is that the picture of blood flow changes can be compared with the precise MRI picture of the same person's brain. This permits localization of blood flow changes to anatomic structures with a spatial resolution down to less than 2 mm.

A drawback of blood flow measurement as an indicator of neuronal activity is its low **time resolution** compared with the time scale for signal transmission in the brain. In this respect, recording the electrical activity of the brain with **electroencephalography** (**EEG**) is superior. A drawback of EEG, however, is its low spatial resolution, which means that only a crude correlation is possible between electrical activity and its origin in the brain. A more recent technique, **magnetic encephalography** (**MEG**), records the magnetic fields produced by the electric activity of the brain (while EEG reflects mainly extracellular currents, MEG is more sensitive to intracellular currents). Contrary to initial beliefs, more recent studies find that the spatial resolution is about the same for EEG and MEG. For both methods the spatial resolution becomes poorer the deeper in the brain the source of activity is located. An advantage with the MEG technique is that it can be combined with MRI. This enables precise localization of the brain areas participating in a task at the same time as the temporal aspects are analyzed (such as the sequence in which various cell groups are activated).

Methods to Study Connections in the Living Brain

Connectivity in the living brain can be studied with **transcranial magnetic stimulation** (**TMS**) and with **diffusion-weighted imaging** (**DWI**). TMS has been used to study the connections between the motor cortex and the spinal cord in healthy persons and in persons with motor dysfunction (e.g., multiple sclerosis). It can also be used to study whether parts of the brain are interconnected and, in particular, whether connectivity changes in the course of therapeutic interventions (such as rehabilitative training programs for stroke patients). DWI (and further developments of this method) enables visualization of major pathways in the brain, such as connections among various cortical areas and between the cerebral cortex and subcortical nuclei (Fig. 6.2B). The method cannot determine the polarity of connections, and the spatial resolution is limited. Provided the results are critically evaluated in conjunction with experimental tracing data from primates, the method gives important information.

*Evoking Localized Activity in the Human Brain
Can Elucidate Function*

Electric stimulation of the brain through the skull (transcranially) requires an intensity that causes pain and is therefore seldom used. With **transcranial magnetic stimulation (TMS**; also termed "magnetic brain stimulation"), however, neurons in the cerebral cortex can be activated painlessly with a short, intense magnetic pulse applied to the head. The magnetic field penetrates the skull and creates an electric current in the brain, primarily in the outer parts of the cerebral cortex. Magnetic brain stimulation also enables study of how disruption of normal activity in a specific part of the cortex affects behavior and cognitive functions.

THE SPINAL CORD

In humans, the spinal cord is a 40- to 45-cm-long cylinder of nervous tissue of approximately the same thickness as a little finger. It extends from the lower end of the brain stem (at the level of the upper end of the first cervical vertebra) down the vertebral canal (Figs. 6.1 and 6.3) to the upper margin of the second lumbar vertebra (L$_2$). Here the cord has a wedge-shaped end called the **medullary conus** (or simply "conus"). In **children**, the spinal cord extends more caudally, however, and reaches to the third lumbar vertebra in the newborn. This difference between the position of the lower end of the spinal cord in adults and infants is caused by the vertebral column growing more rapidly than the spinal cord. In early embryonic life, the neural tube and the primordium of the vertebral column are equally long (see Fig. 9.11).

Some Anatomic Terms Used in This Book

The terms **medial**, toward the midline, and **lateral**, away from the midline, are used to describe the relative position of structures in relation to a midsagittal plane of the body. The terms **cranial** (or **rostral**), toward the head or nose, and **caudal**, toward the tail, are used to describe the relative position of structures along a longitudinal axis of the body. Thus, for example, in the brain stem the mesencephalon lies cranial to the pons (Fig. 6.1). The terms **ventral** and **dorsal** are used to describe the relative position of structures in relation to the front (*venter* means belly) and the back (*dorsum*) of the body, respectively. For example, the cerebellum lies dorsal to the brain stem (Fig. 6.1). **Anterior** (front) and **posterior** (rear) are used interchangeably with ventral and dorsal, except for the human forebrain, where anterior means toward the nose and ventral means toward the base of the skull.

Furthermore, we use the term **efferent** of the direction away from something (outward) and **afferent** of the opposite direction (inward). Here we use it mostly related to fiber connections (tracts), which viewed from the CNS may be either afferent (sensory) or efferent (motor). We also use the term afferent and efferent of nuclei—for example an afferent nucleus in the brain stem receives nerve fibers from, for example, the inner ear, while an efferent nucleus sends nerve fibers to the muscles moving the tongue. Needless to say, a fiber tract is efferent when viewed from the nucleus of origin but afferent when viewed from the receiving nucleus. For example, the pyramidal tract, connecting the cerebral cortex with the spinal cord, is efferent when viewed from the motor cortex but afferent when viewed from the cord.

The spinal cord is somewhat flattened in the anteroposterior direction and is not equally thick along its length. In general, the thickness decreases caudally, but there are two marked **intumescences** (Fig. 6.3): the **cervical** and **lumbar**

Figure 6.1

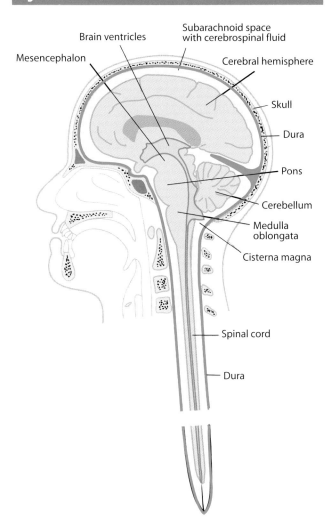

Mesencephalon
Brain ventricles
Subarachnoid space with cerebrospinal fluid
Cerebral hemisphere
Skull
Dura
Pons
Cerebellum
Medulla oblongata
Cisterna magna
Spinal cord
Dura

The central nervous system, as viewed in a midsagittal section. Compare with Fig. 6.2A.

Figure 6.2

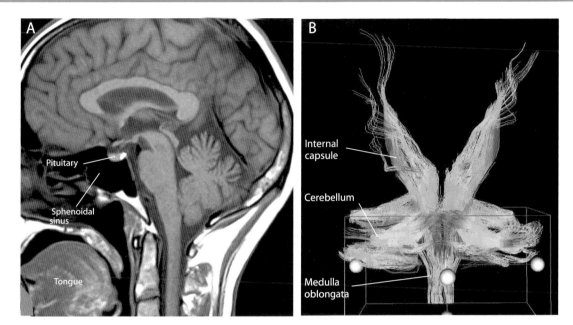

Magnetic resonance images (MRI). **A:** T1 weighted MRI at a level corresponding to the drawing in Fig. 6.1. Most of the structures seen in Fig. 6.1 can be identified in this picture. **B:** MRI tractography used to visualize major fiber bundles in the white matter of the brain stem and cerebellum. (Courtesy of Dr. S. J. Bakke, Oslo University Hospital, Oslo, Norway.)

enlargements (*intumescentia cervicalis* and *lumbalis*). The intumescences supply the extremities with sensory and motor nerves, hence the increased thickness (Fig. 6.11B).

In the midline along the anterior aspect of the cord, there is a longitudinal furrow or fissure, the **anterior (ventral) median fissure** (Fig. 6.4). Some of the vessels of the cord enter through this fissure and penetrate deeply into the substance of the cord. At the posterior aspect of the cord, there is a corresponding, but shallower, furrow in the midline—the **posterior (dorsal) median fissure**. In addition, on each side there are shallow, longitudinal sulci anteriorly and posteriorly—the **anterior** and **posterior lateral sulci**. These laterally placed sulci mark where the spinal nerves connect with the cord.

The **color** of the spinal cord is whitish because the outer part consists of axons, many of which are myelinated. The **consistency** of the cord, as of the rest of the CNS, is soft and jellylike.

Spinal Nerves Connect the Spinal Cord with the Body

Axons mediating communication between the CNS and other parts of the body make up the **peripheral nerves**.

The axons (nerve fibers) leave and enter the cord in small bundles called **rootlets** (Fig. 6.5). Several adjacent rootlets unite to a thicker strand, called a root or **nerve root**. In this manner, rows of roots are formed along the dorsal and ventral aspects of the cord: the **ventral** (anterior) **roots** and the **dorsal** (posterior) **roots**, respectively. Each dorsal root has a swelling, the **spinal ganglion**, which contains the cell bodies of the sensory axons that enter the cord through the dorsal root (Figs. 6.3 and 6.5). A dorsal and a ventral root unite to form a **spinal nerve**. The spinal ganglion lies in the **intervertebral foramen** just where the dorsal and ventral roots unite (Fig. 6.6). There is an important functional difference between the ventral and dorsal roots: the ventral roots consist of efferent (motor) fibers and the dorsal roots of afferent (sensory) fibers.

In total, 31 spinal nerves are present on each side, forming symmetrical pairs (Fig. 6.3). They all leave the vertebral canal through the intervertebral foramina on each side. As mentioned, the ventral and dorsal roots unite at the level of the intervertebral foramen to form the spinal nerves. The spinal nerves are numbered (as a general rule) in accordance with the number of vertebrae above the nerve. We therefore have 12 pairs of **thoracic nerves**, 5 pairs of **lumbar nerves**, and 5 pairs of **sacral nerves**. In humans, there is only 1 pair of coccygeal nerves. There are seven cervical vertebrae but

or **posterior funicle**. For the latter, the term **dorsal column** is used most frequently.

The Spinal Gray Matter Contains Three Main Types of Neurons

Among neurons in the gray matter of the spinal cord, there are both morphological and functional differences. Three main types may be identified according to where they send their axons (Fig. 6.7):

1. Neurons sending their axons out of the CNS

2. Neurons sending their axons to higher levels of the CNS (such as the brain stem)

3. Neurons sending their axons to other parts of the spinal cord

Often neurons of the same kind lie together in the gray matter of the cord. We next consider in some detail each of these three groups.

Efferent Fibers from the Cord Control Muscles and Glands

The cell bodies of the first kind of neuron listed previously are located in the ventral horn and at the transition between the dorsal and ventral horns. The **somatic motor neurons** or **motoneurons** have large, multipolar cell bodies and are located in the ventral horn proper (Fig. 6.8; see also Fig. 1.2). The dendrites extend for a considerable distance in the gray matter (Fig. 6.12). The axons leave the cord through the ventral root, follow the spinal nerves, and end in skeletal muscles (muscles that are controlled voluntarily). The motoneurons are discussed further in Chapter 21.

There is also another group of neurons that sends its axons out of the cord through the ventral root—the **autonomic motor neurons**. These supply smooth muscles and glands with motor signals. They belong to the autonomic nervous system, which controls the vascular smooth muscles and visceral organs throughout the body. These neurons are termed **preganglionic** because they send their axons to a ganglion (see Figs. 28.1 and 28.2). The cell bodies lie in the **lateral horn** (Fig. 6.8). Most of them form a long, slender column, the **intermediolateral cell column**.

Figure 6.7

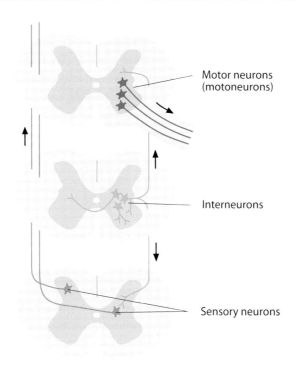

Three main types of neurons in the spinal cord. Schematic of neuronal types classified in accordance with where their axons terminate: *Motor neurons* supply skeletal muscles, smooth muscles, and glands. The *interneurons* ensure communication among neurons in the cord, and the *sensory neurons* send their axons to higher levels of the central nervous system. (See also Fig. 6.9.)

Figure 6.8

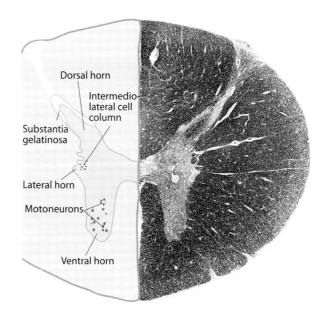

Cross section of the spinal cord at the thoracic level. Photomicrograph of a section stained so that myelinated axons appear dark. The large motoneurons in the ventral horn have also been stained (Nissl staining) and are just visible. Owing to shrinkage, a clear zone surrounds the motoneurons.

This column is present only in the thoracic and upper two lumbar segments of the cord and belongs to the sympathetic part of the autonomic nervous system. A corresponding, smaller group of neurons is present in the sacral cord (S_3–S_4) and belongs to the parasympathetic part of the autonomic nervous system.

Both the somatic and the autonomic motor neurons are under synaptic influence from higher levels of the CNS.

Sensory Neurons in the Cord Are Influenced by the Dorsal Roots and Convey Signals to the Brain

The second main type of spinal neuron sends axons to higher levels of the CNS. Their cell bodies lie mainly in the dorsal horn and in the transition zone between the dorsal and ventral horn (Figs. 6.7 and 6.9). Their job is to inform the brain of the activities of the spinal cord and especially about what is going on in the body. To fulfill the latter task, the neurons must receive signals from **sense organs**—receptors—in various parts of the body (the skin, muscles,

viscera, and so on). **Sensory**, or **afferent**, nerve fibers conducting signals from the receptors enter the spinal cord through the dorsal roots and ramify, forming terminals in the gray matter of the cord (Fig. 6.9; see also Fig. 13.12). The sensory neurons have their cell bodies in the **spinal ganglia** (Fig. 6.5; see also) and are therefore called **spinal ganglion cells** (see Fig. 13.13). These are morphologically special, as they have only one process, which divides shortly after leaving the cell body: One peripheral process connects with the sense organs, and the other extends centrally and enters the spinal cord (pseudounipolar neuron; see Fig. 1.5). In accordance with the usual definition of axons and dendrites, the peripheral process (conducting toward the cell body) should be called a dendrite, whereas the central process is an axon. Both processes are, however, morphologically and functionally axons (e.g., by conducting action potentials and by being myelinated).

The dorsal root fibers form synaptic contacts—in part directly, in part indirectly through the interneurons—with neurons in the spinal cord, sending their axons to various parts of the brain. Such axons, destined for a common target in the brain, are grouped together in the spinal white matter, forming **tracts** (Latin: *tractus*). Such tracts are named after the location of the cell bodies and after the target organ. A tract leading from the spinal cord to the cerebellum, for example, is named the "spinocerebellar tract" (*tractus spinocerebellaris*).

Interneurons Enable Cooperation between Different Cell Groups in the Spinal Cord

The axons of the third type of spinal neuron do not leave the spinal cord. Usually, the axons ramify extensively and establish synaptic contacts with many other neurons in the cord, within the segment in which the cell body is located, and in segments above and below (Fig. 6.7). Such neurons are called **spinal interneurons**, to emphasize that they are intercalated between other neurons.[1] Many spinal interneurons are found in an intermediate zone between the dorsal and ventral horns, where they receive major synaptic inputs from sensory fibers in the dorsal roots. Many of these interneurons establish synaptic contacts with motoneurons in the ventral

Figure 6.9

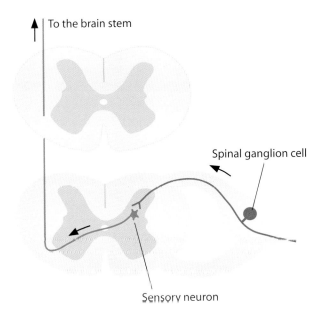

To the brain stem

Spinal ganglion cell

Sensory neuron

Sensory neuron in the gray substance of the spinal cord. The neuron, which sends its axon to the brain stem, is synaptically contacted by sensory afferents that enter the cord through the dorsal root (pseudounipolar ganglion cell). The presentation is very simplified; in reality, every sensory neuron is contacted by numerous dorsal root afferents.

horn, thus mediating motor responses to sensory stimuli. Most interneurons, however, receive additional strong inputs from other spinal interneurons and from the brain.

As mentioned, spinal interneurons also send collaterals to terminate in segments of the cord other than the one in which their cell body and local ramifications are found. Such collaterals enter the white matter, run there for some distance, and reenter the cord at another segmental level, to ramify and establish synaptic contacts in the gray matter (Fig. 6.7). Axons of this kind in the white matter are called **propriospinal fibers** (i.e., fibers "belonging" to the spinal cord itself), to distinguish them from the long ascending and descending fibers that connect the cord with the brain. **Propriospinal neuron** is, therefore, another term used for a spinal interneuron.[2]

Propriospinal fibers provide opportunities for cooperation among the spinal segments. Most of movements necessitate close coordination of the activity in many segments, each controlling different groups of muscles. Some propriospinal connections are very long and interconnect segments in the cervical and lumbar parts of the cord that control muscles in the forelimb and hind limb, respectively. Cooperation between the forelimbs and hind limbs is necessary, for example, during **walking**.

Spinal interneurons are discussed further in Chapter 13, under "Sensory Fibers Are Links in Reflex Arcs: Spinal Interneurons," and in Chapter 22, under "The Pyramidal Tract Fibers Open and Close Spinal Reflex Arcs."

The Spinal Gray Matter Can Be Divided into Zones Called Rexed's Laminae

Systematic observations with the microscope of transverse sections of the spinal cord stained to visualize cell bodies show that neurons with different sizes and shapes are also differently distributed (Fig. 6.10; see also Fig. 13.16). Essentially, neurons with common morphological features are collected into transversely oriented bands or zones. What appear as bands in the transverse plane are, three-dimensionally, longitudinal slabs or sheets. This laminar pattern is most clear-cut in the dorsal horn, whereas in the ventral horn neurons are collected into regions that form

2. It was formerly believed that propriospinal neurons—that is, spinal neurons with axons entering the white matter but not leaving the spinal cord—and interneurons represented two distinct cell groups. Recent studies have shown that spinal interneurons have local (intrasegmental) branches, as well as collaterals destined for other segments (intersegmental).

Figure 6.10

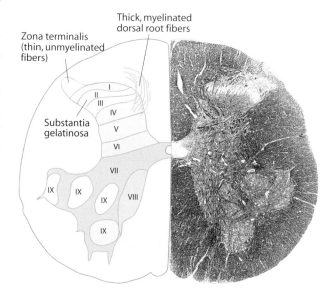

Cross section of the spinal cord at the lumbar level (*lumbar intumescence*). **Right:** Photomicrograph of section stained to show myelin and neuronal cell bodies. **Left:** The borders between Rexed's laminae. The groups of motoneurons in the ventral horn (α and γ motoneurons) constitute lamina IX; the zona terminalis (tract of Lissauer) consists primarily of thin dorsal root fibers.

longitudinal columns rather than plates (see Fig. 21.3). Nevertheless, the columns in the ventral horn, as well as the slabs in the dorsal horn, are termed **laminae**. This pattern was first described in 1952 by the Swedish neuroanatomist Bror Rexed and has since proved to be of great help for investigations of the spinal cord. Altogether, Rexed described 10 laminae; **laminae I to VI** constitute the dorsal horn, whereas **lamina IX** is made up of columns of motoneurons in the ventral horn. **Lamina II** (**substantia gelatinosa**; Figs. 6.8, 6.10, , and 6.11) is of particular importance for the control of signals from pain receptors and thus how much a painful stimulus hurts. **Lamina VII** constitutes the transition between the dorsal and ventral horns and contains mainly interneurons. **Lamina VIII**, located medially in the ventral horn, contains many neurons that send axons to the other side of the cord (commissural fibers).

Even though the cell bodies are arranged in laminae, the **dendrites** extend much wider, as shown in Fig. 6.12. Thus, a neuron belonging to a particular lamina receives synaptic inputs from nerve terminals in neighboring laminae. Nevertheless, experimental studies of the connections of the spinal cord and of the functional properties of single spinal neurons have shown that the various laminae differ in

Figure 6.11

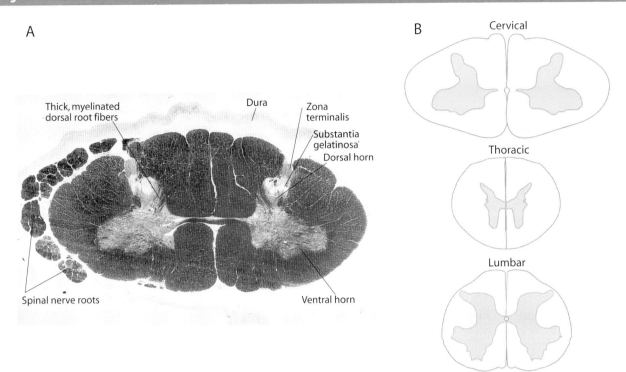

A: *Cross section of the spinal cord at the cervical level (cervical intumescence).* The broad ventral horns contain the motoneurons that supply muscles of the arm and shoulder girdle. **B:** *Comparison of cross sections of the cord at three levels.* Compared with the lumbar, the cervical cord contains more white matter in proportion to gray matter; this is because all descending and ascending fibers to and from the lower levels pass through the cervical cord. The thoracic cord, innervating the trunk, contains less gray matter than the cervical and lumbar cord.

these respects. Thus, the laminae may be regarded, at least to some extent, as the nuclei of the spinal cord. We return to Rexed's laminae when dealing with the functional organization of the spinal cord in later chapters.

The Spinal Nerves Divide into Branches

The dorsal (sensory) and ventral (motor) roots join to form spinal nerves, as described. Each spinal nerve then divides into several **branches** (**rami**) just outside the intervertebral foramen (Figs. 6.5 and 6.6). The thickest one, the **ventral ramus** (*ramus ventralis*), passes ventrally. A thinner branch, the **dorsal ramus** (*ramus dorsalis*), bends in the dorsal direction. In contrast to the spinal roots, the ventral and dorsal rami contain both sensory and motor fibers. This is caused by mixing of fibers from dorsal and ventral roots as they continue into the spinal nerves.

The **dorsal rami** innervate muscles and skin on the back, whereas the **ventral rami** innervate skin and muscles on the ventral aspect of the trunk and neck and, in

addition, the extremities. Thus, the ventral rami innervate much larger parts of the body than the dorsal ones, which explains why the ventral rami contain more nerve fibers and are considerably thicker than the dorsal rami. Some of the ventral rami join each other to form **plexuses** (see Fig. 21.2).

Each spinal nerve also sends off a small branch, the **meningeal ramus**, which passes back through the intervertebral foramen to reenter the vertebral canal (Fig. 6.5). These branches supply the meninges of the spinal cord with sensory and autonomic (sympathetic) fibers.

The Spinal Cord Consists of Subunits that Are Controlled from the Brain

Each segment of the spinal cord is to some extent a functional unit, since, as we will see in Chapter 13, a pair of spinal nerves relates to a particular "segment" of the body (see Fig. 13.14). A spinal segment may be regarded as the "local government" of a part of the body: it receives sensory

Figure 6.12

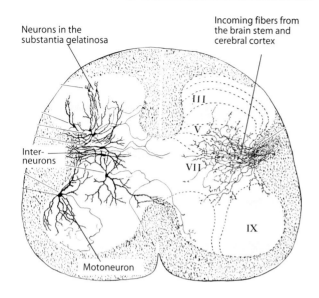

Neurons in the substantia gelatinosa

Incoming fibers from the brain stem and cerebral cortex

Inter-neurons

Motoneuron

Dendritic arborizations of spinal neurons extend beyond the laminae of their cell bodies. Composite drawing based on observations in many Golgi-impregnated transverse sections from the spinal cord of the cat. The dendrites extend far not only in the transverse plane as shown here but also longitudinally. To the right (at **A**) are the terminal ramifications of axons descending to the cord from higher levels of the CNS. (From Scheibel and Scheibel 1966.)

information from its own district, processes this information, and issues orders through motor nerves to muscles and glands to ensure adequate responses. However, just as local governing bodies in our society must take orders from higher ones (e.g., county versus national governments), the spinal segments have only limited independence. Many of the functional tasks of the spinal cord are under strict control and supervision from higher levels of the CNS. This control is mediated by fibers from the brain stem and cerebral cortex, which descend in the white matter of the cord and terminate in the gray matter of the spinal segments that are to be influenced. The brain also ensures that the activity of the various spinal segments is coordinated, so that it serves the body as a whole and not only a small part. To be able to carry out this coordination, the brain must continuously receive information about conditions in all the "local districts" of the body and in the spinal segments related to them. This information is mediated by long, ascending fibers (forming various tracts) in the white matter of the cord that terminates in the brain stem. The local cooperation among spinal segments is taken care of by the numerous propriospinal fibers coming from spinal interneurons.

THE BRAIN STEM

The brain stem represents the upward (rostral, cranial) continuation of the spinal cord (Fig. 6.1). It consists of several portions with, in part, clear-cut surface borders between them (Figs. 6.13, 6.14, and 6.15). Whereas the lowermost (caudal) part of the brain stem is structurally similar to the spinal cord, the upper parts are more complicated. The subdivisions of the brain stem are as follows (from caudal to rostral): the **medulla oblongata** (often just called medulla), the **pons** (the bridge), the **mesencephalon** (the midbrain), and the **diencephalon**. Usually, however, we use a more restricted definition including only the parts that extrude from the base of the brain: the medulla, pons, and mesencephalon.

The Brain Stem Contains the Third and Fourth Ventricles

A continuous, fluid-filled cavity varying in diameter stretches through the brain stem (Fig. 6.1). It is the upward continuation of the thin central canal of the spinal cord, and it continues rostrally into the cavities of the cerebrum (see Figs. 7.3 and 7.5). Together, these cavities constitute the ventricular system of the brain and spinal cord. The cavity in the brain stem has two dilated parts: one, the **fourth ventricle**, is at the level of the medulla and pons, whereas the **third ventricle** is situated in the diencephalon. We return to the ventricular system in Chapter 7.

The Cranial Nerves

Examination of the internal structure of the brain stem shows that it is more complicated than that of the spinal cord (compare Figs. 6.11 and 6.16). Even though gray matter is generally located centrally, surrounded by a zone of white matter in both the brain stem and the cord, the gray matter of the brain stem is subdivided into several regions separated by strands of white matter. The white matter of the brain stem consists of myelinated fibers, as in other parts of the CNS. The regions with gray matter contain various nuclei, or groups of neurons with common tasks.

Many of the nuclei belong to the **cranial nerves**. In total, there are 12 pairs of cranial nerves, which, with the exception of the first, all emerge from the brain stem (Figs. 6.13 and 6.15). They correspond to the spinal nerves but show a less regular organization. Thus, there is no clear separation

Figure 6.13

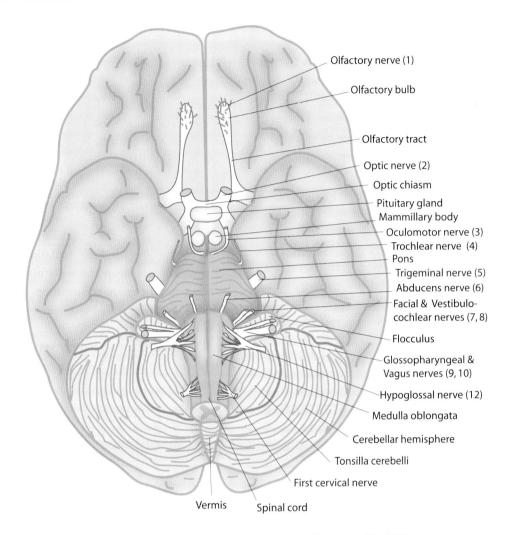

Olfactory nerve (1)
Olfactory bulb
Olfactory tract
Optic nerve (2)
Optic chiasm
Pituitary gland
Mammillary body
Oculomotor nerve (3)
Trochlear nerve (4)
Pons
Trigeminal nerve (5)
Abducens nerve (6)
Facial & Vestibulo-
cochlear nerves (7, 8)
Flocculus
Glossopharyngeal &
Vagus nerves (9, 10)
Hypoglossal nerve (12)
Medulla oblongata
Cerebellar hemisphere
Tonsilla cerebelli
First cervical nerve
Vermis   Spinal cord

The basal aspect of the brain with the cranial nerves. (The accessory nerve is not shown; see Fig. 6.15).

of sensory (dorsal) and motor (ventral) roots. The cranial nerves are numbered from rostral to caudal in accordance with where they emerge on the surface of the brain stem. Figure 8.9 shows the places on the base of the skull where the cranial nerves leave through small holes or fissures.

Many of the cranial nerves contain fibers that conduct impulses out of the brain stem; that is, the fibers are efferent, or motor. These fibers belong to neurons with their cell bodies in nuclei that are called **motor cranial nerve nuclei**. They correspond to the groups (columns) of neurons in the ventral and lateral horns of the spinal cord. The cranial nerves, like the spinal nerves, also contain sensory, afferent fibers that bring impulses from sense organs. The brain stem cell groups in which these afferent fibers terminate are, accordingly, called **sensory cranial nerve nuclei**; they correspond to the laminae of the spinal dorsal horn.

The sensory fibers entering the brain stem have their cell bodies in ganglia just outside the brain stem, **cranial nerve ganglia**, corresponding to the spinal ganglia of the spinal nerves. Most cranial nerves are mixed—that is, they contain both motor and sensory fibers—but a few are either purely sensory or purely motor.

The only cranial nerve not emerging from the brain stem is the first cranial nerve, the **olfactory nerve** (*nervus olfactorius*). This consists of short axons coming from sensory cells in the roof of the nasal cavity, which, immediately after penetrating the base of the skull, terminate in the **olfactory bulb** (*bulbus olfactorius*) (Fig. 6.13). The other cranial nerves are briefly mentioned in the next section in connection with a description of the main structural features of the brain stem. The cranial nerves and their central connections are treated more thoroughly in later chapters, particularly Chapter 27.

Figure 6.18

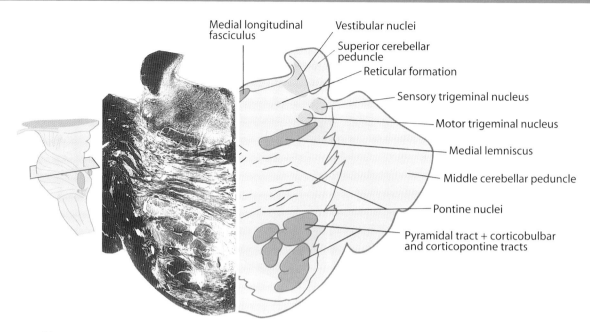

Medial longitudinal fasciculus
Vestibular nuclei
Superior cerebellar peduncle
Reticular formation
Sensory trigeminal nucleus
Motor trigeminal nucleus
Medial lemniscus
Middle cerebellar peduncle
Pontine nuclei
Pyramidal tract + corticobulbar and corticopontine tracts

Upper part of the pons. Cross section; myelin-stained.

control of voluntary movements (the pyramidal tract is discussed in Chapter 22). Close to the lower end of the medulla, on the transition to the cord, bundles of fibers can be seen to cross the midline, forming the **pyramidal decussation** (Fig. 6.15). Lateral to the pyramid is an oval protrusion (the olive), which is formed by a large nucleus, the **inferior olivary nucleus** (inferior olive), which sends its efferents to the cerebellum. Between the olive and the pyramid is a row of small bundles of nerve fibers (Fig. 6.15), which are the rootlets of the **hypoglossal nerve** (the twelfth cranial nerve, *nervus hypoglossus*). This nerve supplies the striated muscles of the tongue with motor fibers. Lateral to the olive, the rootlets of the **glossopharyngeal** and **vagus nerves** (ninth and tenth cranial nerves, *nervus glossopharyngeus* and *nervus vagus*) leave the brain stem. These two nerves supply the pharynx, the larynx, and most of the viscera with motor and sensory fibers. The **accessory nerve** (eleventh cranial nerve, *nervus accessorius*) runs cranially along the lateral aspect of the medulla. Most of its fibers come from the upper cervical spinal segments but enter the cranial cavity to leave the skull together with the glossopharyngeal and vagus nerves (see Fig. 27.8). The accessory nerve supplies two muscles in the neck with motor fibers (the trapezius and the sternoclocleidomastoid).

Figure 6.16 shows a cross section through the **lower part of the medulla**, at a level below the caudal end of the fourth ventricle. The section is stained so that regions with white matter (the myelinated fiber tracts) are dark, whereas gray matter (the nuclei) appears light. The ventrally located bundle of cross-sectioned fibers is the **pyramidal tract**, forming the pyramid (Fig. 6.15), and containing about 1 million fibers. Dorsal to the pyramid lies a highly convoluted band of gray matter, the **inferior olivary nucleus**. The **dorsal column nuclei**, the **gracile** and **cuneate** (*nucleus gracilis* and *nucleus cuneatus*), are located dorsally in the medulla. The efferent fibers from these nuclei arch ventrally and take up a position close to the midline dorsal to the pyramids, where they form a triangular area of cross-sectioned fibers. This is an important sensory tract, the **medial lemniscus** (*lemniscus medialis*), which leads from neurons in the dorsal column nuclei to nuclei in the diencephalon (see Fig. 14.1). The dorsal column nuclei receive afferent fibers that ascend in the dorsal columns (or dorsal funicles) and convey impulses from sense organs in the skin and muscles and around joints. Close to the midline, just ventral to the central canal, lies the **hypoglossal nucleus**, consisting of the cell bodies of the motor fibers that form the hypoglossal nerve. The efferent fibers of the hypoglossal nucleus pass ventrally and leave the medulla at the lateral edge of the pyramid (Fig. 6.15). Lateral to the motor cranial nerve nuclei are found several sensory cranial nerve nuclei, among them the big **sensory trigeminal nucleus** that receives sensory impulses from the face, carried in the **trigeminal nerve** (the fifth cranial nerve, *nervus trigeminus*). Note how the nuclei that are transmitting sensory impulses from the leg, arm, and face are distributed from medial to lateral in the dorsal part of the medulla (Fig. 6.16).

A cross section through the **upper part of the medulla** (Fig. 6.17) shows partly the same fiber tracts and nuclei as the section at a lower level (Fig. 6.16). In addition, we may notice the big **vestibular nuclei** situated dorsally and laterally under the floor of the fourth ventricle (these nuclei also extend cranially into the pons; see Fig. 18.7). They receive sensory signals from the vestibular apparatus in the inner ear via the **vestibular nerve** (the eighth cranial nerve, *nervus vestibulocochlearis*). One of the main efferent pathways from the vestibular nuclei forms a distinct tract, the **medial longitudinal fasciculus** (*fasciculus longitudinalis medialis*), close to the midline under the floor of the fourth ventricle (Fig. 6.18). This tract terminates in the motor nuclei of the cranial nerves supplying the eye muscles, thus conveying influences on eye movements from the receptors for equilibrium. Further, Fig. 6.17 shows the motor and sensory **nuclei of the vagus** and some of the fibers of the **vagus nerve**, which pass laterally and ventrally, to leave the medulla lateral to the olive (Fig. 6.15).

The Pons

The pons forms a bulbous protrusion at the ventral aspect of the brain stem, with clear-cut transversely running fiber bundles (Figs. 6.13 and 6.14). It is sharply delimited both caudally and cranially. The transverse fiber bundles are formed by fibers from large cell groups in the pons, the pontine nuclei, and terminate in the cerebellum. The fiber bundles join at the lateral aspect of the pons to form the **middle cerebellar peduncle** (*brachium pontis*) (Figs. 6.14 and 6.18). Several cranial nerves leave the brain stem at the ventral aspect of the pons. At the lower (caudal) edge, just lateral to the midline, a thin nerve emerges on each side. This is the **abducens nerve** (the sixth cranial nerve, *nervus abducens*) that carries motor fibers to one of the external eye muscles (rotates the eye laterally). Still at the lower edge of the pons, but more laterally, two other cranial nerves leave the brain stem. Most ventrally lies the **facial nerve** (seventh cranial nerve, *nervus facialis*), which brings motor impulses to the mimetic muscles of the face (it also contains some other kinds of fibers that are considered in Chapter 27). Closely behind the facial nerve lies the **vestibulocochlear nerve** (the eighth cranial nerve, *nervus vestibulocochlearis*), which carries sensory impulses from

the sense organs for equilibrium and hearing in the inner ear. The **trigeminal nerve** (the fifth cranial nerve, *nervus trigeminus*) leaves the brain stem laterally at middle levels of the pons. The largest portion of the nerve consists of sensory fibers from the face, whereas a smaller (medial) portion contains motor fibers destined for the masticatory muscles.

In a **cross section** through the pons, the large **pontine nuclei** can be seen easily in the ventral half of the pons (Fig. 6.18). As mentioned, the neurons of the pontine nuclei send their axons to the cerebellum. Because their main afferent connections come from the cerebral cortex, the pontine nuclei mediate information from the cerebral cortex to the cerebellum. The **medial lemniscus** borders the pontine nuclei dorsally and has turned around and moved laterally compared with its location in the medulla (Fig. 6.16). In the lower part of the pons, the nucleus of the abducens nerve, the **abducens nucleus**, is located dorsally and medially, whereas the **facial nucleus** lies more ventrally and laterally (see Fig. 27.11; this figure also shows the course taken by the efferent fibers of the abducens and facial nuclei, forming the sixth and seventh cranial nerves, respectively).

Figure 6.18 also shows the **sensory trigeminal nucleus** laterally (this nucleus extends as a slender column through the medulla, pons, and mesencephalon; Figs. 6.16, 6.17, and 6.18; see also Fig. 27.2). Medial to the sensory nucleus lies the **motor trigeminal nucleus** (the masticatory muscles), but this nucleus is present only in the pons.

The Medulla and Pons Seen from the Dorsal Side

At the dorsal side of the medulla oblongata, at caudal levels, there are two longitudinal protrusions, the **gracile** and **cuneate tubercles** (Fig. 6.19). These are formed by the **dorsal column nuclei**, mentioned earlier (they are relay stations in pathways for sensory information from the body to the cerebral cortex). The most medial of these nuclei, the **gracile nucleus**, receives signals from the leg and lower part of the trunk, whereas the laterally situated **cuneate nucleus** receives signals from the arm and upper part of the trunk. Further laterally, another oblong protrusion (*tuberculum cinereum*) is formed by the **sensory trigeminal nucleus**, the relay station for sensory impulses from the face.

Rostral to the upper end of the dorsal column nuclei, there is a flattened, diamond-shaped area, the **rhomboid**

Figure 6.19

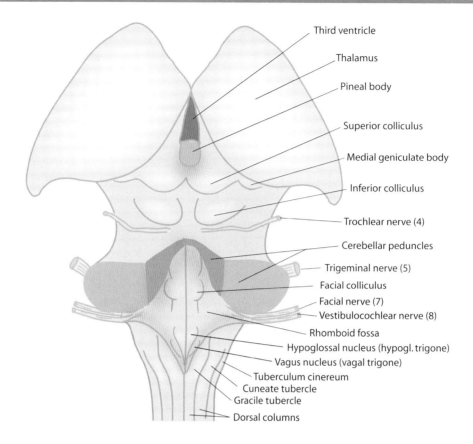

Third ventricle

Thalamus

Pineal body

Superior colliculus

Medial geniculate body

Inferior colliculus

Trochlear nerve (4)

Cerebellar peduncles

Trigeminal nerve (5)

Facial colliculus

Facial nerve (7)

Vestibulocochlear nerve (8)

Rhomboid fossa

Hypoglossal nucleus (hypogl. trigone)

Vagus nucleus (vagal trigone)

Tuberculum cinereum

Cuneate tubercle

Gracile tubercle

Dorsal columns

The brain stem. Viewed from the dorsal aspect.

fossa, extending rostrally onto the posterior face of the pons (Fig. 6.18). This constitutes the "floor" of the fourth ventricle (Fig. 6.19). Laterally and rostrally, the **cerebellar peduncles** delimit the rhomboid fossa (these have been cut in Fig. 6.19). Some of the cranial nerve nuclei and some fiber tracts form small protrusions medially at the floor of the fourth ventricle—notably the hypoglossal nucleus (hypoglossal trigone, *trigonum hypoglossi*), the vagus nucleus (vagal trigone, *trigonum vagi*) and more rostrally the root fibers of the facial nerve—the latter forming the **facial colliculus**. (Figure 27.11 explains how the facial colliculus is formed.)

The Mesencephalon (Midbrain)

The part of the brain stem rostral to the pons, the **mesencephalon**, is relatively short (Figs. 6.14 and 6.15). Ventrally, an almost half-cylindrical protrusion is present on each side of the midline—the **crus cerebri**, or **cerebral peduncle**

(Figs. 6.15 and 6.20).[3] The crus cerebri consists of nerve fibers descending from the cerebral cortex to the brain stem and spinal cord; among these fibers are those of the pyramidal tract. The fibers continue into the pons, where they spread out into several smaller bundles among the pontine nuclei (Fig. 6.18).

In the furrow between the two crura, the **oculomotor nerve** emerges (third cranial nerve, *nervus oculomotorius*) (Figs. 6.13 and 6.15). As the name implies, the nerve carries motor signals to muscles that move the eye. The oculomotor nerve innervates four of the six extraocular (striated) muscles and, in addition, two smooth internal muscles that regulate the diameter of the pupil and the curvature of the lens.

3. Strictly speaking, the term "cerebral peduncle" denotes both the crus cerebri and parts of the mesencephalon dorsal to the crus except the colliculi (the latter collectively termed the "tectum"). The region between the crus cerebri and the tectum is called the **tegmentum** and includes the periaqueductal gray, the red nucleus, and the substantia nigra. Previously, however, the crus cerebri and the cerebral peduncle were both applied to the ventralmost, fiber-rich part.

Figure 6.20

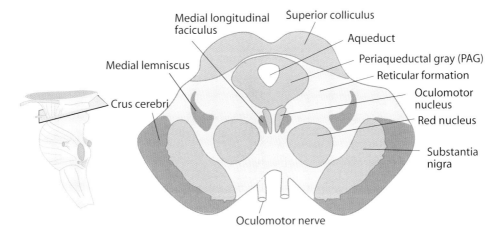

The mesencephalon. Cross section. The major nuclei are indicated in red and the major tracts are in gray.

At the **dorsal side** of the mesencephalon, there is a characteristic formation of four small, rounded protrusions, two on each side of the midline (Fig. 6.18). These are called the **colliculi** (*corpora quadrigemina*) and consist of, on each side, the **superior colliculus** and the **inferior colliculus**. The superior colliculus consists of cell groups that control reflex movements of the eyes and the head, while the inferior colliculus is a relay station in the pathways that bring auditory signals to awareness.

A thin fiber bundle, the **trochlear nerve** (fourth cranial nerve, *nervus trochlearis*), emerges on each side below the inferior colliculi (Fig. 6.19). This is the only cranial nerve that emerges on the dorsal side of the brain stem. It supplies one of the extraocular muscles with motor fibers.

In a **cross section** of the mesencephalon (Fig. 6.20), the crus cerebri can be recognized ventrally and the superior colliculus dorsally. In the midline just ventral to the colliculi there is a small hole, which is a cross section of the **aqueduct** (*aquaeductus cerebri*), a narrow canal that interconnects the third and fourth ventricles (Figs. 6.23; see also Fig. 7.5). Surrounding the aqueduct is a region of gray matter called the **periaqueductal gray substance** (*substantia grisea centralis*), which coordinates behavioral responses to stressful events and influences pain perception. Ventral to the periaqueductal gray, close to the midline, we find the **oculomotor nucleus** (or nucleus of the oculomotor nerve). Further ventrally lies the large **red nucleus** (*nucleus ruber*), so named because of its slightly reddish color. Just dorsal to the crus and ventral to the red nucleus is the **substantia nigra** (the black substance). The neurons of the substantia nigra contain a dark pigment,

making the nucleus clearly visible macroscopically. The red nucleus and the substantia nigra are both important for the control of movements.

The Diencephalon Contains the Thalamus and the Hypothalamus

Figure 6.21 shows how the diencephalon merges with the mesencephalon caudally and with the diencephalon rostrally without clear transitions (Fig. 6.13). The **optic nerve** (the second cranial nerve, *nervus opticus*) carrying afferent fibers from the retina ends in the diencephalon.

The largest part of the diencephalon is occupied by the **thalamus**, situated on each side of the third ventricle (Figs. 6.22, 6.23, 6.24, and 6.27). The thalamus consists of many smaller nuclei and is a relay station (synaptic interruption) for almost all information transmitted from the lower parts of the CNS to the cerebral cortex (notably most kinds of sensory information). Each thalamus is approximately egg-shaped with a flattened side toward the third ventricle (Fig. 6.22). Lateral to the thalamus lies a thick sheet of white matter, the **internal capsule** (*capsula interna*). It consists mainly of fiber tracts connecting the cerebral cortex with the thalamus, the brain stem, and the spinal cord, among them the pyramidal tract (Figs. 6.14, 6.24, 6.27, and 6.30). The crus cerebri is a caudal continuation of fibers of the internal capsule.

In a frontal section of the brain (Fig. 6.23) the thalamus is subdivided by narrow bands of white matter forming a Y, called the **internal medullary lamina** (Fig. 6.22). This

Figure 6.21

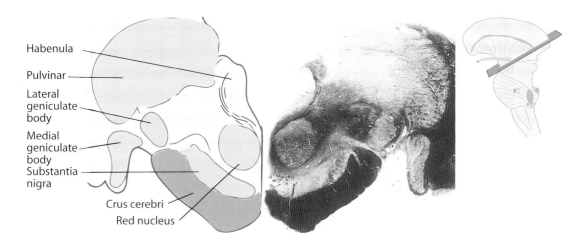

Habenula
Pulvinar
Lateral
geniculate
body
Medial
geniculate
body
Substantia
nigra
Crus cerebri
Red nucleus

Transition between the mesencephalon and the diencephalon. Oblique frontal section; myelin stained. Inset shows plane and level of the section.

divides the thalamic gray matter in three main parts: an **anterior** nuclear group (or complex), a **medial** nuclear group, and a lateral part or region made up of a **dorsal** and a **ventral** nuclear group.[4] The **pulvinar**, continuous with the lateral part, makes up most of the posterior part of the thalamus (Figs. 6.21 and 6.22). In addition, the posterior part of the thalamus includes two nuclei partly covered by the pulvinar, the **lateral geniculate body** (*corpus geniculatum laterale*) and the **medial geniculate body** (*corpus geniculatum mediale*). Each of the thalamic nuclei connects to different parts of the cerebral cortex (see Fig. 33.8). For example, the lateral and medial geniculate bodies are relay stations for visual and auditory impulses, respectively. Thus, fibers of the optic nerve end in the lateral geniculate body while fibers from the inferior colliculus end in the medial geniculate body.

The **optic nerves** from the two eyes unite just underneath the diencephalon (Figs. 6.13 and 6.15) to form the **optic chiasm** (*chiasma opticum*, or just *chiasma*), in which there is a partial crossing of the optic nerve fibers (see Fig. 16.14). In their further course from the optic chiasm to the lateral geniculate body, the fibers form the **optic tract**

(Figs. 6.15 and 6.23). The fibers from the lateral geniculate body to the visual cortex form the **optic radiation** (Fig. 16.15).

Anterior and inferior to the thalamus lies the **hypothalamus** (Fig. 6.24), which exerts central control of the autonomic nervous system—that is, with control of the visceral organs and the vessels. The hypothalamus forms the lateral wall of the anterior part of the third ventricle. The border between the thalamus and the hypothalamus is marked by the shallow **hypothalamic sulcus** (Figs. 6.23 and 6.24). The **mammillary body** (*corpus mammillare*), a special part of

Figure 6.22

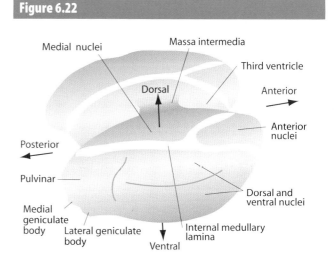

Medial nuclei
Massa intermedia
Third ventricle
Dorsal
Anterior
Anterior
nuclei
Posterior
Pulvinar
Dorsal and
ventral nuclei
Medial
geniculate
body
Lateral geniculate
body
Internal medullary
lamina
Ventral

The thalamus. Drawing of the thalami of both sides, to indicate their three-dimensional form.

4. The nomenclature of thalamic nuclear subdivisions may appear bewildering, and matters are not made easier by lack of agreement among leading investigators. For example, the nomenclature presented in the *Terminologia Anatomica* (1998) differs from that used in the scholarly book *The Human Nervous System* (Mai and Paxinos 2011). Throughout the present book, when dealing with the thalamus, we have tried to simplify matters to provide just enough anatomical detail to help the reader understand the functional organization of the thalamus.

Figure 6.23

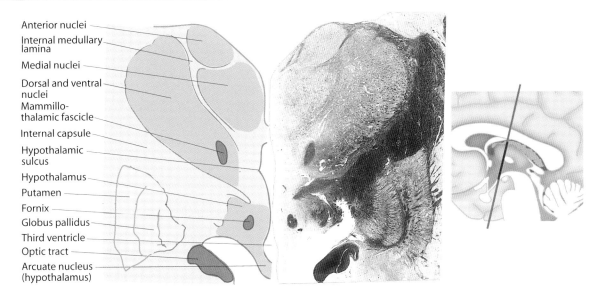

Anterior nuclei
Internal medullary lamina
Medial nuclei
Dorsal and ventral nuclei
Mammillo-thalamic fascicle
Internal capsule
Hypothalamic sulcus
Hypothalamus
Putamen
Fornix
Globus pallidus
Third ventricle
Optic tract
Arcuate nucleus (hypothalamus)

The diencephalon. Frontal section; myelin stained.

the hypothalamus, protrudes downward from its posterior part (Figs. 6.13, 6.24, and 6.29). The **fornix** is a thick, arching bundle of fibers originating in the cerebral cortex (in the so-called hippocampal region in the temporal lobe) and terminating in the mammillary bodies (see Fig. 31.2). The major efferent pathway of the mammillary body goes to the thalamus, forming a distinct fiber bundle, the **mammillothalamic tract** (*fasciculus mammillothalamicus*)

Figure 6.24

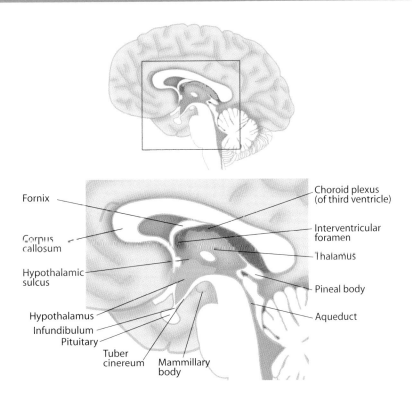

Fornix
Choroid plexus (of third ventricle)
Corpus callosum
Interventricular foramen
Hypothalamic sulcus
Thalamus
Pineal body
Hypothalamus
Infundibulum
Pituitary
Aqueduct
Tuber cinereum
Mammillary body

The hypothalamus. Drawing of midsagittal section showing the upper parts of the brain stem. The hypothalamus is indicated in green.

(Figs. 6.23 and 30.7). In front of the mammillary bodies, the floor of the third ventricle bulges downward like a funnel and forms the stalk of the pituitary gland, the **infundibulum**. The region between the mammillary bodies and the infundibulum is called the **tuber cinereum** (see Fig 30.4). It contains neuronal groups that influence the activity of the pituitary gland.

The **pituitary** (Figs. 6.13 and 6.24) consists of a **posterior lobe**, developed from the CNS, and an **anterior lobe**, developed from the epithelium in the roof of the mouth. The anterior lobe, secreting several hormones that control important bodily functions, is itself under the control of the hypothalamus. This is discussed further in Chapter 30.

The Epithalamus, the Pineal Body, and the Habenula

The diencephalon also includes a small area called the **epithalamus**, located posteriorly in the roof of the third ventricle. In addition to a small nucleus, the **habenula** (Fig. 6.21), the epithalamus contains the **pineal body** or gland (corpus pineale) (Figs. 6.19, 6.24, and 6.31). This peculiar structure lies in the midline (unpaired) and is formed by an evagination of the roof of the third ventricle. It contains glandular cells, **pinealocytes**, which produce the hormone **melatonin** (and several neuropeptides). It also contains large amounts of **serotonin**, which is a precursor of melatonin. Melatonin influences several physiologic parameters, especially those that show a cyclic variation. This is discussed more thoroughly in Chapter 30,

under "Hypothalamus and Circadian Rhythms" and under "Melatonin."

The **habenula** (Fig. 6.21) lies just underneath the pineal body (one on each side). This small nucleus (composed of several subnuclei) receives afferents from the hypothalamus and the septal nuclei, among other sources. Its main efferents go to nuclei in the mesencephalon (among them dopaminergic neurons). The pathway from the hypothalamus via habenula to the mesencephalon may be engaged in the bodily expressions of strong **emotions**—for example, rage or fear. The habenula is one among several neuronal groups that are altered in severe **depression**.

THE CEREBRUM

The cerebrum has an ovoid shape and fills most of the cranial cavity. Whereas its convexity—that is, its upper and lateral surfaces—is evenly curved, the basal surface is uneven. In the center of the basal surface, the brain stem emerges (Fig. 6.13). The cerebrum is almost completely divided in two by a vertical slit, the **longitudinal cerebral fissure** (*fissura longitudinalis cerebralis*), so that it consists of two approximate half-spheres or **cerebral hemispheres** (Figs. 6.25 and 6.26). Each of the cerebral hemispheres contains a central cavity, the **lateral ventricle** (Figs. 6.28 and 6.29). The lateral ventricles are continuous with the third ventricle through a small opening,

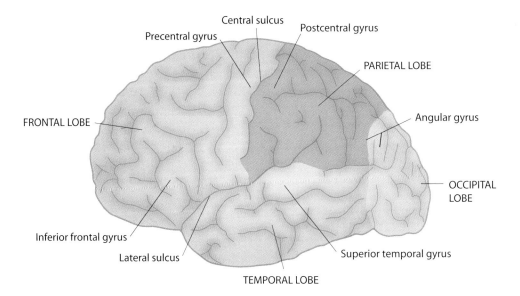

Figure 6.25

The left cerebral hemisphere. Viewed from the lateral aspect.

Figure 6.26

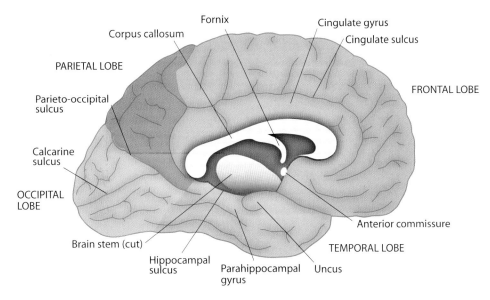

The left cerebral hemisphere. Viewed from the medial aspect. The brain stem has been cut off.

the **interventricular foramen** (Fig. 6.24). The lateral ventricles are surrounded by masses of white matter with some embedded nuclei. The surface of the hemisphere is covered everywhere by a 3- to 5-mm-thick layer of gray substance, the **cerebral cortex** (*cortex cerebri*). The structure, connections, and functions of the cerebral cortex are covered most completely in Chapters 33 and 34, but some main features are briefly described here because knowledge of them is necessary for the chapters dealing with sensory and motor systems.

The neurons of the cerebral cortex receive impulses from lower parts of the CNS, most of which are relayed through the **thalamus**. In addition, there are numerous **association fibers**—that is, fibers interconnecting neurons in various parts of the cerebral cortex of one hemisphere. Finally, a vast number of **commissural fibers** interconnect neurons in the two hemispheres. Most of the commissural fibers are collected into a thick plate of white matter, the **corpus callosum**, which joins the two hemispheres across the midline (Figs. 6.26 and 6.27). The fibers in the corpus callosum enable signals to travel from one hemisphere to the other and thus ensure that the right and left hemispheres can cooperate (see Chapter 34, under "Functions of the Commissural Connections: The Corpus Callosum"). A few commissural fibers pass in the **anterior commissure** (*commissura anterior*) (Fig. 6.26).

The Surface of the Hemisphere Is Highly Convoluted and Forms Gyri and Sulci

During embryonic development, the cerebral hemispheres fold as they grow in size (see Fig. 7.4). This leads to a great increase in their surface area and thus in the amount of cortex relative to their volume (only about one-third of the total cortical surface is exposed). The furrowed, walnut-like appearance of the cerebral hemispheres of humans and some higher mammals is highly characteristic (Figs. 6.25, 6.26, 6.27, and 6.28). The folding of the hemisphere produces deep **fissures** and more shallow **sulci**. Between the sulci, the surface of the cortex forms rounded **gyri**. Apart from the fissure that divides the two hemispheres along the midline, the longitudinal cerebral fissure, the largest fissure in each hemisphere is the **lateral cerebral sulcus** (fissure) or the Sylvian fissure (Fig. 6.25). This fissure follows a course upward and backward and extends deep into the hemisphere (Fig. 6.27). The small gyri in the bottom of the lateral sulcus form the **insula** (the island) (Figs. 6.27 and 6.30). More sulci and gyri are mentioned when dealing with the lobes of the cerebrum.

The pattern of the fissures and the larger sulci in the human brain is fairly constant. Nevertheless, variations are great enough to make it impossible to know exactly where a

Figure 6.27

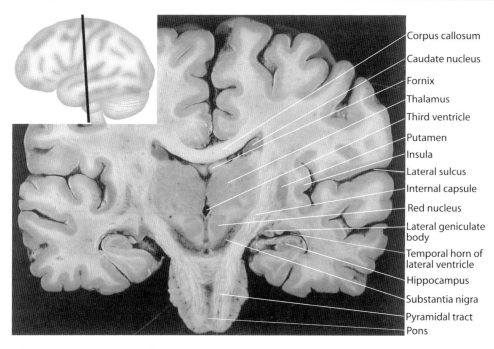

Corpus callosum
Caudate nucleus
Fornix
Thalamus
Third ventricle
Putamen
Insula
Lateral sulcus
Internal capsule
Red nucleus
Lateral geniculate body
Temporal horn of lateral ventricle
Hippocampus
Substantia nigra
Pyramidal tract
Pons

The cerebral hemispheres and upper part of the brain stem. Photograph of frontal section. Compare with Fig. 6.28.

certain sulcus is located only from landmarks on the outside of the skull. The smaller sulci and gyri are subject to considerable individual variation.

The Hemisphere Can Be Divided into Four Lobes

With more or less sharply defined borders (formed by fissures and sulci), one can distinguish four lobes of the cerebral hemispheres (Figs. 6.25 and 6.26). They are named in accordance with the bone of the skull under which they are located. The **frontal lobe** (*lobus frontalis*) lies in the anterior cranial fossa above the orbit. The frontal lobe is separated from the **parietal lobe** (*lobus parietalis*) by the **central sulcus**, which extends from the medial edge of the hemisphere laterally to the lateral sulcus. Below the lateral sulcus lies the **temporal lobe** (*lobus temporalis*). Neither the parietal nor the temporal lobe has any clearly defined border posteriorly toward the occipital lobe. The **occipital lobe** lies above the cerebellum, which is located in the posterior cranial fossa (Fig. 6.1). On the medial aspect of the hemisphere, the border between the parietal and the occipital lobe is marked

by the **parietooccipital sulcus** (*sulcus parietooccipitalis*) (Fig. 6.26).

Some Functional Subdivisions of the Cerebral Cortex

Anatomically and functionally, we divide the cerebral cortex into different regions, which do not, however, coincide with the different lobes. Here only a few points are mentioned. The gyrus in front of the central sulcus, the **precentral gyrus** (*gyrus precentralis*) (Fig. 6.25), coincides with the **motor cortex**, which is of special significance for the execution of voluntary movements. Destruction of this gyrus in one hemisphere cause pareses in the opposite side of the body. Many of the fibers in the **pyramidal tract** come from the precentral gyrus, and, as mentioned, most of these fibers cross the midline on their way to the spinal cord. The **postcentral gyrus**, situated just posterior to the central sulcus, is the major receiving region for sensory impulses from the skin, the musculoskeletal system, and the viscera. This region is called the **somatosensory cortex**. The tracts that conduct impulses from the sense organs to the cortex are

Figure 6.28

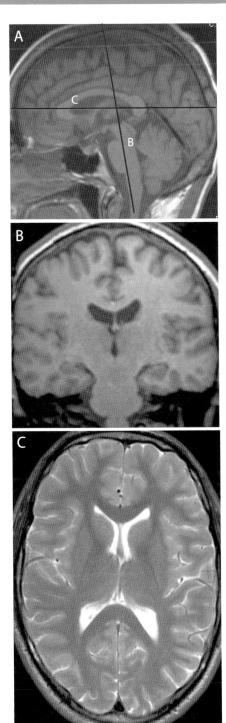

Magnetic resonance images (MRI) in the three conventional planes.
A: Midsagittal plane. **B:** frontal (coronal) plane; corresponding to
Fig. 3.27. **C:** Horizontal (transverse) plane **A** and **B** are T1 weighted
with water appearing dark. **C** is T2 weighted with water appearing
white. (Courtesy of Dr. S. J. Bakke, Oslo University Hospital, Oslo,
Norway.)

also crossed. Thus, destruction of the postcentral gyrus on one side leads to lowered sensibility (e.g., of the skin) on the opposite side of the body. We have previously mentioned the **medial lemniscus**, which is part of the pathways from the sense organs to the postcentral gyrus. The fibers of the medial lemniscus terminate in a subdivision of the **lateral thalamic nucleus** (Fig. 6.24), and the neurons there send their axons to the postcentral gyrus.

The **visual cortex**—the main cortical region receiving information from the eyes—is located in the occipital lobe around a deep sulcus (fissure), the **calcarine sulcus** (*sulcus calcarinus*) (Fig. 6.26). The impulses start in the retina and are conducted in the optic nerve and the optic tract to the **lateral geniculate body** (Figs. 6.21 and 6.22), and from there to the visual cortex (see Fig. 16.14). The visual cortex can be distinguished from the surrounding parts of the cortex in sections perpendicular to the surface: it contains a thin whitish stripe running parallel to the surface (caused by a large number of myelinated fibers). Because of the stripe, this part of the cortex was named the **striate area** by early anatomists (see Fig. 16.17).

The **auditory cortex**—the cortical region receiving impulses from the cochlea in the inner ear—is located in the superior temporal gyrus of the temporal lobe (Fig. 6.25; see also Fig. 17.11). The pathway for auditory signals is synaptically interrupted in the **medial geniculate body** (Figs. 6.21 and 6.22).

The **olfactory cortex** is a small region on the medial aspect of the hemisphere near the tip of the temporal lobe. It is part of the so-called **uncus** (Fig. 6.26) and extends somewhat onto the adjoining **parahippocampal gyrus**. The olfactory cortex receives fibers from the **olfactory bulb** (*bulbus olfactorius*) through the **olfactory tract** (*tractus olfactorius*) (Fig. 6.13). The cortex of the parahippocampal gyrus extends into the **hippocampal sulcus** (fissure), forming a longitudinal elevation, the **hippocampus** (Figs. 6.27 and 6.31; see also Fig. 32.1). The hippocampus belongs to the phylogenetically oldest parts of the cerebral cortex and has a simpler structure than the newer parts. The hippocampus and adjoining cortical regions in the medial part of the temporal lobe are of particular interest with regard to **learning** and **memory** (discussed further in Chapter 32).

The Cerebral Cortex Consists of Six Cell Layers

Examination of a microscopic section cut perpendicular to the surface of the cerebral cortex shows that the neuronal cell bodies are not randomly distributed (see Figs. 33.1 and

Figure 6.29

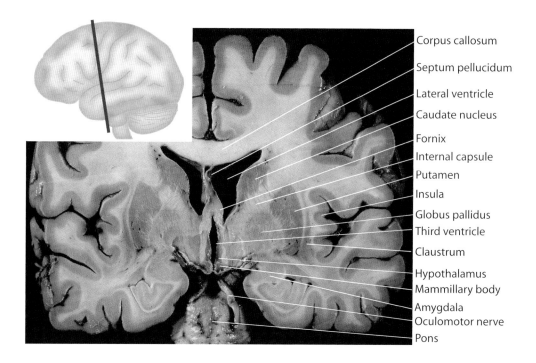

Corpus callosum
Septum pellucidum
Lateral ventricle
Caudate nucleus
Fornix
Internal capsule
Putamen
Insula
Globus pallidus
Third ventricle
Claustrum
Hypothalamus
Mammillary body
Amygdala
Oculomotor nerve
Pons

The cerebral hemispheres. Frontal section, placed more frontally than as shown in Fig. 3.27, showing the basal ganglia and amygdala.

33.2). They are arranged into **layers** or **laminae** parallel to the surface. Each layer is characterized by a certain shape, size, and packing density of the cell bodies (compare with the Rexed's laminae of the spinal cord). We number the layers from the surface inward to the white matter. **Layer 1** is cell poor and consists largely of dendrites from neurons with cell bodies in deeper layers and of axons with terminals making synapses on the dendrites. **Layers 2** and **4** are made up of predominantly small, rounded cells and are therefore called the **external** and **internal granular layer**, respectively. These two layers both have a receiving function: many of the afferent fibers to the cerebral cortex terminate and form synapses in layers 2 and 4. Fibers conveying sensory information from lower levels of the CNS end predominantly in layer 4, and consequently this layer is particularly well developed in the sensory cortical regions mentioned previously. **Layers 3** and **5** contain cells that are larger than those in layers 2 and 4, and the cell bodies tend to be of pyramidal shape, hence the name **pyramidal cells** (neurons). Many of the pyramidal cells in layer 5 send their axons to the brain stem and spinal cord, where they influence motor neurons. Layer 5 is therefore especially well developed in the motor cortex in the precentral gyrus. The pyramidal neurons in layer 3 send their axons primarily to other parts of the cerebral cortex, either in the same hemisphere (association fibers) or to cortex in

the hemisphere of the other side (commissural fibers). The cell bodies of **layer 6** are smaller and more spindle-shaped than those in layer 5. Many of the neurons send their axons to the thalamus, enabling the cerebral cortex to influence the impulse traffic from the thalamus to the cortex (feedback connections).

There are also numerous **interneurons** in the cerebral cortex, providing the opportunity for cooperation between the various layers (interneurons with "vertically" oriented axons) and between neurons in different parts of one layer (interneurons with "horizontally" oriented axons). The layers are obviously not independent units.

The Cerebral Cortex Can Be Divided into Many Areas on a Cytoarchitectonic Basis

We mentioned that some layers are particularly well developed in certain regions of the cortex—for example, layer 4 in the sensory receiving areas and layer 5 in the motor cortex. There are many more differences when all layers all over the cortex are systematically compared. Such **cytoarchitectonic** differences (i.e., differences in size, shape, and packing density of the cell bodies) form the basis of a parcellation of

Figure 6.30

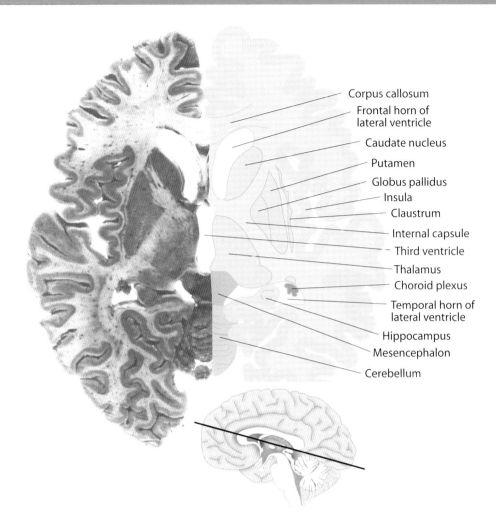

Corpus callosum
Frontal horn of
lateral ventricle
Caudate nucleus
Putamen
Globus pallidus
Insula
Claustrum
Internal capsule
Third ventricle
Thalamus
Choroid plexus
Temporal horn of
lateral ventricle
Hippocampus
Mesencephalon
Cerebellum

The internal structure of the cerebral hemisphere. The left half is a photograph of a horizontal section through the left hemisphere. Compare with Fig. 6.28C.

the cerebral cortex of each hemisphere into approximately 50 **cortical areas** (*areae*). Maps of the cerebral cortex showing the positions of the various areas were published by several investigators around year 1900 and are still in use. The German anatomist Brodmann (see Fig. 33.4) published the most widely used map. Such cytoarchitectonically defined areas have later been shown, in many cases, to differ also with regard to connections and functional properties. The numbering of the cortical areas may appear illogical. For example, the motor cortex in the precentral gyrus corresponds to area 4 of Brodmann. This borders posteriorly on area 3 but on area 6 anteriorly. Area 3 borders on area 1, which borders on area 2, and so on. It is not necessary to learn the position of more than a few of the cortical areas, however, and these are dealt with in connection with the various functional systems in Parts II to VI of this book.

The Basal Ganglia

The interior of the hemispheres contains large masses of gray substance. Largest among these are the so-called **basal ganglia**, which perform important tasks related to the control of movements and cognitive functions.[5] Here we mention only a few main points with regard to the anatomy of the basal ganglia, which are further discussed in Chapter 23. Other nuclear groups (the amygdala, the septal nuclei, and the basal nucleus) are discussed in Chapter 31. The **amygdala**, situated in the tip of the

5. The name "basal ganglia" has been retained from a time when all collections of neurons were called ganglia, regardless of whether they were located inside or outside the CNS. Today we use the term "ganglion" only for collections of neurons outside the CNS, as discussed in Chapter 1. However, the name "basal ganglia" is so well established that is not practical to exchange it.

Figure 6.31

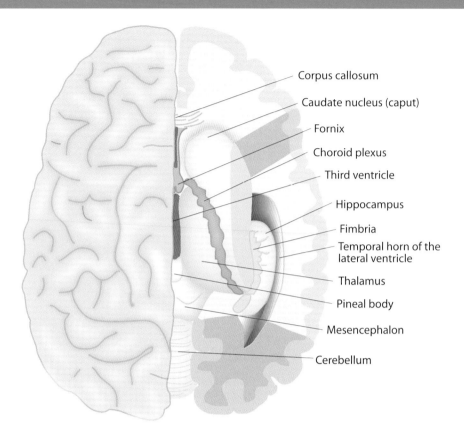

Corpus callosum

Caudate nucleus (caput)

Fornix

Choroid plexus

Third ventricle

Hippocampus

Fimbria

Temporal horn of the
lateral ventricle

Thalamus

Pineal body

Mesencephalon

Cerebellum

The internal structure of the cerebral hemispheres. The upper part of the right hemisphere has been cut away to open the lateral ventricles. In the anterior part, the caudate nucleus forms the bottom and lateral wall of the ventricle. In the temporal horn of the ventricle, the hippocampus forms the medial wall.

temporal lobe (Fig. 6.29), is of special relevance to emotions and the learning of associations between stimuli and their emotional valence.

The basal ganglia receive massive afferent connections from the cerebral cortex and acts, by way of their efferent fibers, primarily back on motor regions of the cortex. Sections through the hemispheres show that the basal ganglia consist of two main parts (Figs. 6.29 and 6.30). In a horizontal section (Fig. 6.30), one large part lies lateral to the internal capsule, and a smaller part lies medial to the internal capsule and anterior to the thalamus. The largest part is called the **lentiform nucleus** (*nucleus lentiformis*) because of its shape. It consists of two closely apposed parts: the lateral or external part is the **putamen**, and the medial or internal part is the **globus pallidus**. The part of the basal ganglia situated medial to the internal capsule is the **caudate nucleus** (*nucleus caudatus*) (Fig. 6.31). The name describes its form: a large part of the nucleus forms a long, curved "tail" (see Fig. 23.3). The

caudate nucleus consists of an anterior bulky part, the **caput** (head), and a progressively thinner **cauda** (tail). The cauda extends first backward and then down and forward into the temporal lobe, located in the wall of the lateral ventricle. Figure 7.4 shows how this peculiar form can be explained on the basis of the embryonic development of the cerebral hemispheres. The putamen and the caudate nucleus together are called the **striatum** (or neostriatum), which is the main receiving part of the basal ganglia. Globus pallidus sends efferent fibers to the thalamus, which then mediate the effects of the basal ganglia on the **motor cortical areas**. In addition, the basal ganglia have connections with the **prefrontal cortex** (areas in front of the motor areas), which are of special importance for **cognitive functions**.

The **claustrum** forms a sheet of grey matter lateral to the putamen (Figs. 6.29 and 6.30). It has reciprocal connections with most parts of the cerebral cortex. Little is known about its function or clinical significance, but based on

Figure 6.32

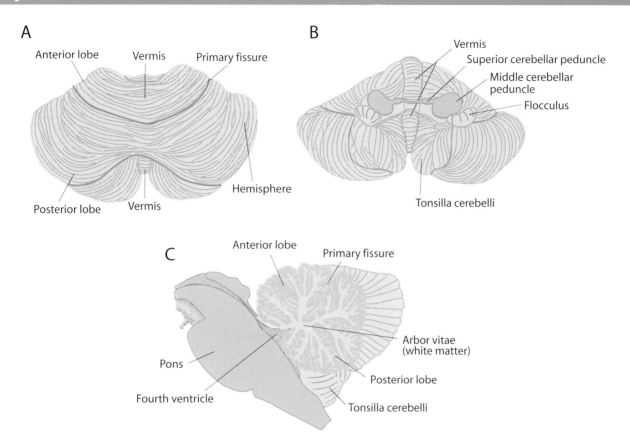

A

Anterior lobe   Vermis   Primary fissure

Posterior lobe   Vermis

Hemisphere

B

Vermis
Superior cerebellar peduncle
Middle cerebellar peduncle
Flocculus

Tonsilla cerebelli

C

Anterior lobe   Primary fissure

Pons

Fourth ventricle

Arbor vitae (white matter)

Posterior lobe

Tonsilla cerebelli

The cerebellum. **A:** Seen from the dorsal aspect. **B:** Seen from the ventral aspect (the side facing the brain stem). **C:** Midsagittal section showing the cerebellar cortex as a thin layer with white matter underneath (white matter indicated in black in the drawing).

its connections it has been suggested to deal with sensory integration. One hypothesis proposes that, by virtue of its integrative potential, claustrum may be linked with the formation of conscious percepts.

THE CEREBELLUM

The cerebellum (the "little brain") is first and foremost of importance for the execution of movements; like the basal ganglia, it belongs to the motor system. The cerebellum is located in the posterior cranial fossa, dorsal to the brain stem (Figs. 6.1 and 6.32). It is connected with the brain stem anteriorly by way of three stalks of white matter on each side: the inferior, middle, and superior cerebellar peduncles (Figs. 6.14 and 6.19). In general, the **inferior cerebellar peduncle**, or **restiform body** (*corpus restiforme*), contains fibers that carry impulses from the spinal cord to the cerebellum, whereas the **middle cerebellar**

peduncle, or **brachium pontis**, conveys information from the cerebral cortex. The **superior cerebellar peduncle**, or **brachium conjunctivum**, contains most of the fibers conveying impulses out of the cerebellum—that is, the cerebellar efferent fibers.

Like the cerebrum, the cerebellum is covered by a layer of gray substance, the **cerebellar cortex** (*cortex cerebelli*), with underlying white matter. Enclosed in the white matter are regions of gray matter, the **central (deep) cerebellar nuclei** (see Fig. 24.14). From the neurons in these nuclei come the majority of efferent fibers that convey information from the cerebellum to other parts of the CNS (the cerebral cortex, various brain stem nuclei, and the spinal cord).

The cerebellar surface is extensively folded, forming numerous narrow sheets, or **folia**, that are predominantly oriented transversely (Fig. 6.32A). The fissures and sulci between the folia are partly very deep; the deepest among them divide the cerebellum into **lobes** (Fig. 6.32A; see also Fig. 24.4). In addition, the cerebellum can be subdivided macroscopically on another basis. In the posterior part of the cerebellum, a narrow middle region is situated deeper than the much larger lateral parts (Fig. 6.32B). This middle part of the cerebellum is called the **vermis** (worm) and is present also in the anterior part of the cerebellum, although not as clearly distinguished from the lateral parts as posteriorly. The lateral parts are called the **cerebellar hemispheres**. A small bulbous part on each is connected medially with a thin stalk to the vermis. This part is called the **flocculus** (Fig. 6.32B) and lies close to the middle cerebellar peduncle, just posterior to the seventh and eighth cranial nerves (Fig 6.13). A midsagittal section through the cerebellum (Fig. 6.32C) shows clearly the deep sulci and fissures. The white substance forms a treelike structure called the **arbor vitae** (the tree of life, which is not very fitting since the cerebellum is not necessary for life). The fourth ventricle, extending into the cerebellum like the apex of a tent, is also evident in the midsagittal section.

The central nervous system (CNS) is well protected against external forces as it lies inside the skull and the vertebral canal. In addition to this bony protection, the CNS is wrapped in three membranes of connective tissue—the **meninges**—with fluid-filled spaces between the membranes. In fact, it is loosely suspended in a fluid-filled container. The innermost membrane—**pia**—is thin and adheres to the surface of the brain at all places. The outermost membrane—**dura**—is thick and fibrous and covers the inside of the skull and spinal canal. The **arachnoid** is a thin membrane attached to the inside of the dura. The **subarachnoid space** is filled with **cerebrospinal fluid** (**CSF**) and lies between the pia and the arachnoid.

The **ventricular system** consists of irregularly shaped, fluid-filled cavities inside the CNS. There are four dilatations or **ventricles**. The two lateral ventricles are the largest and are located in the cerebral hemispheres. They communicate with the third ventricle lying between the two thalami. The third ventricle, situated between the two thalami, communicates with the fourth ventricle via the narrow **cerebral aqueduct.** Vascular **choroid plexuses** in the ventricles produce about 0.5 liters of CSF per day. The CSF leaves the ventricular system through openings in the fourth ventricle and enters the subarachnoid space. Drainage of CSF occurs through small evaginations— **arachnoid villi**—of the arachnoid emptying into venous sinuses and along cranial and spinal nerve roots and then into extracranial lymphatic vessels. The CSF has a protective function; it minimizes accumulation of harmful substances in the nervous tissue, and it probably serves as a signal pathway.

The Pia Mater, the Arachnoid, and the Subarachnoid Space

The innermost one is the vascular **pia mater** (usually just called pia). It follows the surface of the brain and spinal cord closely and extends into all sulci and depressions of the surface (Figs. 7.1 and 7.2). Thin vessels pass from the pia into the substance of the brain and supply the external parts, such as the cerebral cortex, with blood (the deeper parts of the brain are supplied by vessels entering the brain at its basal surface). The next membrane, the **arachnoid**, does not follow the uneven surface of the brain but extends across depressions, fissures, and sulci. Between the pia and the arachnoid exists a narrow space, the **subarachnoid space**, which is filled with **CSF** (Figs. 7.1, and 7.5; see also Fig. 6.1). Numerous thin threads of connective tissue connect the pia with the arachnoid, thus spanning the subarachnoid space. The depth of the subarachnoid space varies from place to place because the arachnoid, as mentioned, does not follow the surface of the brain. Where it crosses larger depressions, the subarachnoid space is considerably widened, forming so-called **cisterns** filled with CSF. Several cisterns are found around the brain stem, but the largest one, the **cisterna magna**, or **cerebellomedullary cistern**, is located posterior to the medulla below the cerebellum (Fig. 7.5). The CSF enters the cisterna magna from the fourth ventricle (Fig. 7.5).

The subarachnoid space is continuous around the whole CNS. Substances released into the subarachnoid space at one place therefore quickly spread out. A **subarachnoid hemorrhage**, for example, most often caused by rupture of

Figure 7.1

A

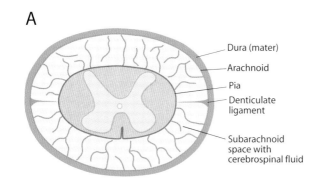

- Dura (mater)
- Arachnoid
- Pia
- Denticulate ligament
- Subarachnoid space with cerebrospinal fluid

B

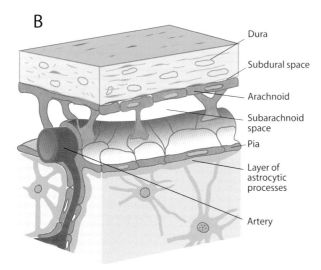

- Dura
- Subdural space
- Arachnoid
- Subarachnoid space
- Pia
- Layer of astrocytic processes
- Artery

The meninges and the subarachnoid space of the spinal cord.

a vessel at the base of the brain, quickly leads to mixing of the CSF with blood. Thus, a sample of CSF taken from the dural sac at lumbar levels will be bloody.

The Dura Mater

The outermost membrane, the **dura mater** (usually just called the dura), is thick and strong because it consists of dense connective tissue (Figs. 7.1, 7.2, and 7.5). The dura covers closely the inside of the skull, and its outermost layers constitute the periosteum. The arachnoid follows the inside of the dura closely so that there is only a very narrow space between these two meninges, the **subdural space** (Figs. 7.1 and 7.2). The dura extends down into the vertebral canal to enclose the spinal cord. It extends further down than the cord, however, forming a sac around the roots of the lower spinal nerves (the *cauda equina*). This

dural sac extends down to the level of the second-third sacral vertebra (see Fig. 6.3). Thus, below the level of the first and second lumbar vertebrae (the lower end of the cord), the dural sac contains only spinal nerve roots and CSF (see Fig. 6.3). This is a safe place to perform a **lumbar puncture**—that is, enter the subarachnoid space with a needle to take samples of the CSF, as there is no danger of harming the cord.

The dura is **innervated** by thin sensory fibers following the **trigeminal nerve** (except that fibers to the dura in the posterior fossa follow the upper cervical nerves). Sensory fibers in the dura and around the intracranial arteries contain **neuropeptides** that have been proposed to provoke neurogenic inflammation and thus cause the pain of **migraine** (see Chapter 8, under "Sensory Innervation of Brain Vessels").

Meningeal Irritation and Neck Stiffness

Electric and other kinds of stimulation (stretching, heating) of intracranial structures in humans during surgery often evoke pain. Most often the pain is felt in extracranial structures innervated by the trigeminal nerve (referred pain). Stimulation of arteries in the dura and venous sinuses and the dura at the base of the skull regularly produce intense pain, whereas stimulation of parts of the dura at a distance from the arteries and sinuses, as well as the pia and arachnoid, did not evoke pain in awake humans during surgery. It seems, however, that when inflamed by infection or irritating substances, the dura and possibly also pia and arachnoid become intensely sensitive to mechanical and chemical stimuli. Thus, infection of the meninges, **meningitis**, causes inflammation of the meninges, which also extends onto the vessels and the nerve roots in the subarachnoid space. Most likely, this **meningeal irritation** accounts for the intense pain associated with any effort to flex the back or neck (similar to the pain felt by stretching an inflamed area of the skin or a joint capsule). Straining or coughing also causes pain in patients with meningitis. Every attempt to bend the neck or the back forward evokes an immediate reflexive muscular resistance, keeping the neck stiff (**neck stiffness**). When the doctor tries to lift the patient's head off the pillow, the neck is kept straight. Forward bending (flexion) of the vertebral column elongates the spinal canal, as mentioned, and that stretches the meninges, the vessels, and the nerve roots.

However, means other than infections by bacteria and viruses can produce meningeal irritation. For example, one strong irritant is **blood** in the subarachnoid space. Thus, neck stiffness is by itself a sign only of meningeal irritation and does not indicate a specific cause. In addition to neck stiffness, meningeal irritation usually causes a strong **headache**. This occurs most dramatically with **subarachnoid hemorrhage**, in which an intense headache starts abruptly the moment the bleeding starts and blood flows into the subarachnoid space. In such instances, the cause is usually spontaneous rupture of an **aneurysm** (a sac-like dilatation) on one of the arteries at the base of the skull.

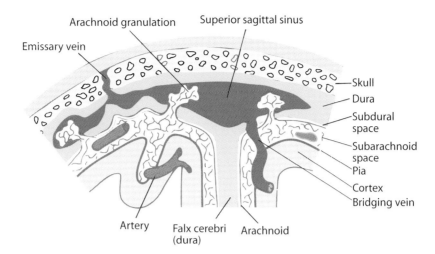

The meninges, the subarachnoid space, and the superior sagittal sinus. Schematic of a frontal section through the head, with the skull and the brain.

Anchoring of the Brain and Spinal Cord

In a few places, the dura forms strong infoldings, serving to restrict the movements of the brain within the skull. Large movements can stretch and damage vessels and nerves connecting the brain with the skull (one of the possible effects of head injuries). From the midline, the **falx cerebri** extends down between the two hemispheres (Fig. 7.2; see also Fig. 8.7). Posteriorly, the falx divides into two parts that extend laterally over the superior face of the cerebellum and attach to the temporal pyramid. These two folds meet in the midline and form the **cerebellar tentorium** (see Figs. 8.7 and 8.9). In the anterior part of the tentorium, there is an elongated opening for the brain stem. If the pressure in the skull above the tentorium increases (due to bleeding, a tumor, or brain edema), part of the temporal lobe may be pressed down or **herniate** between the tentorium and the brain stem, harming the brain stem temporarily or permanently.

The **spinal cord** is anchored to the meninges partly by the spinal nerves and partly by two thin bands, the **denticulate ligaments** (Fig. 7.1A), extending laterally from the cord to the arachnoid and dura (this is not a continuous ligament but one that forms 21 lateral extensions from the cord to the dura). The spinal cord nevertheless moves considerably up and down in the dural sac with **movements** of the vertebral column (the length of the vertebral canal varies by almost 10 cm from maximal flexion, when it is longest, to maximal extension).

THE CEREBRAL VENTRICLES AND THE CEREBROSPINAL FLUID

We have mentioned the ventricular system several times in connection with treatment of the various parts of the brain. Here we consider the ventricular system as a whole, along with the CSF.

The Location and Form of the Ventricles

The thin central canal of the cord continues upward into the brain stem. There the canal widens to form the **fourth ventricle** at the posterior aspect of the medulla and pons (Figs. 7.3 and 7.5). The ventricle has a tent-like form with the apex projecting into the cerebellum and two **lateral recesses** (*recessus lateralis*) (Fig. 7.3). The diamond-shaped **rhomboid fossa** at the dorsal aspect of the brain stem (see Fig. 6.19) forms the "floor" of the fourth ventricle, while the cerebellar peduncles form the lateral walls.

The **third ventricle** is a thin slit-like room between the two thalami (Figs. 7.3 and 7.5; see also Figs. 6.27–6.31). During embryonic development, the primordia of the hemispheres become closely apposed to the diencephalon (see Fig. 9.12). The loose masses of connective tissue between the hemispheres form an approximately horizontal plate

Figure 7.3

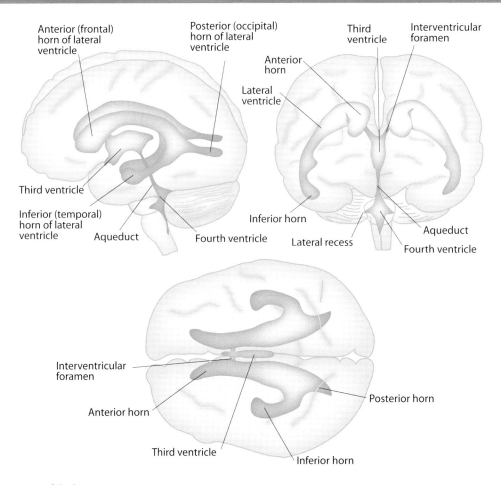

The ventricular system of the brain.

---

that constitutes the roof of the third ventricle. The choroid plexus is attached to the inside of the roof (Fig. 7.5).

The two **lateral ventricles** represent the first and second ventricles, but these terms are not used. From a central part in the parietal lobe, the lateral ventricles have processes called horns into the three other lobes: an **anterior (frontal) horn**, a **posterior (occipital) horn**, and an **inferior (temporal) horn** extending downward and anteriorly into the temporal lobe (Fig. 7.3; see also Figs. 6.27 and 6.31). The anterior horn is the largest and is bordered medially by the **septum pellucidum,**[1] (Fig. 7.5) whereas the head of the caudate nucleus bulges into it from the lateral side (see Fig. 6.29). The central part of the ventricle lies just above the thalamus (see Fig. 6.31). The inferior horn starts at the transition between the central part and the posterior horn and follows the temporal lobe almost to its tip (Fig. 7.3). Medially in the inferior horn there is an elongated elevation, the hippocampus (see Figs. 6.27 and 6.31), formed by invagination of the ventricular wall from the medial side by the **hippocampal fissure**.

The **curved form** of the lateral ventricles can be understood on the basis of the embryonic development of the cerebrum (Fig. 7.4). Both the lateral ventricles and the nervous tissue in its walls (such as the caudate nucleus and the hippocampus) eventually obtain a curved shape.

Production of the Cerebrospinal Fluid

All of the ventricles are filled with a clear, watery fluid, the **CSF.** Most of the fluid is produced by vascular tufts,

---

1. There is a thin slit between the septum pellucidum of the two sides that has nothing to do with the ventricles. In embryonic development, the slit is continuous with the room between the two hemispheres but is later closed when the corpus callosum grows across the two hemispheres. Downward, the fornices close the slit (see Fig. 6.29).

Figure 7.4

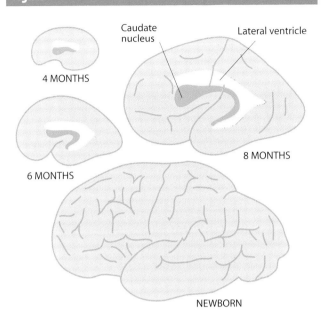

4 MONTHS

6 MONTHS

Caudate nucleus

Lateral ventricle

8 MONTHS

NEWBORN

Development of the cerebral hemispheres and the lateral ventricles. The characteristic arched shape of the ventricles can be explained by the manner in which the hemispheres fold during their growth in embryonic life. The caudate nucleus, located in the wall of the lateral ventricle, is indicated in blue. All structures in the wall of the ventricles attain the curved shape. The figure also shows the development of gyri and sulci. Compare the pattern in the newborn and in the adult (Fig. 6.25). (Based on Hamilton, Boyd, and Mossman 1972.)

the **choroid plexus**.[2] This is present in all four ventricles (Fig. 7.5), but the largest amount of choroid plexus is in the lateral ventricles (see Fig. 6.31). The plexuses arise in early embryonic life by invaginations of the innermost membrane (the pia mater) at sites where the wall of the neural tube is very thin (Fig. 7.6). An elaborate structure of thin, branching protrusions, or **villi**, arises here (Fig. 7.7). The choroid plexuses attach to the wall of the ventricles with a thin stalk (**tela choroidea**). The surface of the villi is covered by **simple cuboid epithelium** (which is continuous with the ependyma covering the inside of the ventricles). The epithelial cells have microvilli that increase their surface in contact with the CSF. The interior of the villi is composed of loose connective tissue

with numerous capillaries of the **fenestrated** type, which are rather leaky. Therefore, the **hydrostatic pressure** inside the capillaries produces a net flow of water with solutes (and a fair amount of proteins) into the interstitial space of the villi. This protein-rich fluid cannot leave the villi directly, however, because the epithelial cells covering the villi attach to each other with **tight junctions** (Fig 7.7). The transport of water through the epithelium is caused by active transport of sodium. Thus, the pumping of sodium produces an osmotic gradient so that water diffuses from the interior of the villi into the ventricles. Other ions, such as chloride and bicarbonate, follow the water passively. The epithelial cells of the choroid plexus are equipped with water channels or **aquaporins** on the apical surface (i.e., facing the CSF). Presumably, the aquaporins are important for the rapid transport of water. Indeed, the **rate of CSF secretion** by the choroid plexus (0.2 mL/min/g tissue) is much higher than in other secretory epithelia in the body.

The epithelium of the choroid plexus represents a barrier between the blood and the CSF, the **blood–CSF barrier**. Thus, many substances that can leave the capillaries of the choroid plexus cannot enter the CSF. This is obviously important, because neurons are extremely sensitive to changes in the composition of their environment. We later describe a similar but even more important barrier between the blood in the brain capillaries and the brain interstitial fluid.

Composition and Functions of the Cerebrospinal Fluid

The concentration of sodium, potassium, and several other **ions** is about the same in the CSF as in the blood (there are some minor differences, however). The concentration of **glucose** is about two-thirds that in the blood. A major difference concerns **proteins**; there is normally very little protein in the CSF (less than 0.5% of the plasma protein concentration).

Water and soluble substances are freely exchangeable between the CSF and the interstitial fluid of the nervous tissue because the **ependyma** is freely permeable to water and even small protein molecules. It is not surprising, therefore, that many neurotransmitters, peptides, and other neuroactive substances occur in the CSF, and their presence there does not by itself signify a functional role. Some substances, however—notably **peptide hormones** synthesized in the anterior pituitary—are apparently actively secreted into the

---

2. Early observations in experimental animals suggested that the choroid plexus is not solely responsible for CSF production. Thus, removal of the choroid plexus did not prevent development of hydrocephalus after blocking the CSF drainage. It is now assumed that in humans 10% to 30% of the CSF is produced by brain **interstitial fluid** passing through the ependyma.

Figure 7.5

A

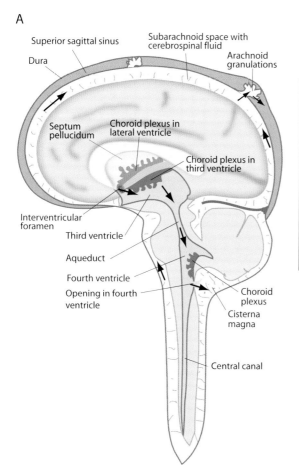

Superior sagittal sinus

Subarachnoid space with cerebrospinal fluid

Dura

Arachnoid granulations

Septum pellucidum

Choroid plexus in lateral ventricle

Choroid plexus in third ventricle

Interventricular foramen

Third ventricle

Aqueduct

Fourth ventricle

Opening in fourth ventricle

Choroid plexus

Cisterna magna

Central canal

B

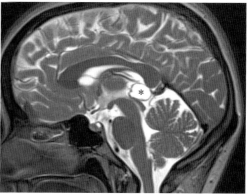

The ventricular system, the subarachnoid space, and the choroid plexus. **A:** Arrows indicate the flow of the cerebrospinal fluid. **B:** T2 weighted MRI. Water is white. Asterisk marks a cyst in the pineal body. (Courtesy of Dr. S. J. Bakke, Oslo University Hospital.)

Figure 7.6

A

B

Cerebral hemisphere

Lateral ventricle

Pia

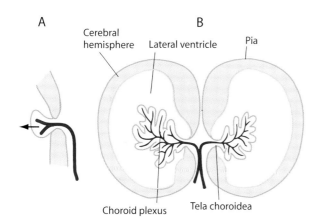

Choroid plexus

Tela choroidea

Embryonic development of the choroid plexus. Schematic of a frontal section through the cerebral hemispheres at an early (**A**) and a somewhat later (**B**) stage, showing how the choroid plexus is formed by invaginations of the pia into the ventricles.

Figure 7.7

Cuboidal epithelium with microvilli

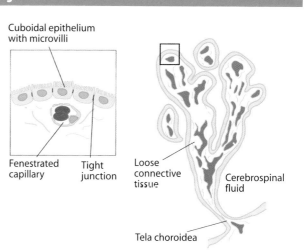

Fenestrated capillary

Tight junction

Loose connective tissue

Cerebrospinal fluid

Tela choroidea

Structure of the choroid plexus, exemplified by one villus (inset). Arrows indicate the flow of fluid from the capillaries to the ventricles.

CSF, not simply accepted by passive diffusion. Some other substances appear to use the CSF as a means to reach specific receptors close to the ventricles.

The CSF has an important **protective function** because the brain almost floats in it. Thus, theoretically **buoyancy** reduces the weight of the brain, which means less traction on vessels and nerves connected to the CNS. Further, the effect on the brain of blows to the head is dampened because water has to be pressed aside before the brain hits its hard surroundings (the skull).

Another possible functional role of the CSF can be deduced from the fact, mentioned previously, that water and solutes pass freely between it and the extracellular fluid (interstitium) of the nervous tissue. This means that diffusion into the CSF may minimize **accumulation of harmful substances** in the nervous tissue (such as potassium ions during prolonged periods of intense neuronal activity). This would be of significance, however, only for neurons that are fairly close to the ventricles, as the diffusion of molecules in the labyrinth-like brain **interstitium** is slow (much slower than in free water). Thus, after injecting representative substances in the brain, the concentration is reduced by 90% some 1 to 3 mm away from the injection site.

Regardless of the normal functions of substances in the CSF, **examination of the CSF** composition gives valuable information of the extracellular fluid of the brain. This fluid compartment is difficult to examine directly, but because the ependyma is freely permeable, one can safely assume that the composition of the CSF matches fairly well the environment of the neurons.

Cerebrospinal Fluid as a Signal Pathway

The concentration of the hormone **melatonin** (which influences sexual functions and circadian rhythms by binding to receptors in the hypothalamus) is twice as high in the third ventricle as in the lateral ventricles and 100 times higher than in cerebral arteries. This suggests that melatonin is secreted into the CSF and uses this as its main transport medium, whereas the bloodstream is of minor importance.

Some studies indicate that substances in the CSF might be of importance for **sleep**. Thus, by transferring CSF from a sleep-deprived animal, the recipient becomes sleepy. The responsible substance has not been identified but **interleukin 1β** (IL-1β) is a likely candidate. Thus, its concentration in the CSF increases by sleep deprivation and has also been shown to induce sleep. The further signal pathway of IL-1β from CSF to relevant neurons is not known, but it finally influences the neurons in the reticular formation that are responsible for regulation of sleep and wakefulness.

Several **growth factors** are synthesized and secreted by the choroid plexus. While the choroid plexus epithelium expresses receptors for such growth factors—suggesting an autocrine function—growth factors may also be expected to act on nervous tissue close to the ventricles.

Movement of the Cerebrospinal Fluid

About **one-half liter** of CSF is produced each day, yet the total volume of fluid in the ventricles and the subarachnoid space is only 130 to 140 mL (approximately 20 mL is in the ventricles). In addition, approximately 75 mL surrounds the spinal cord. Thus, the total amount is renewed several times a day. This means that effective means of drainage must exist.

Volume of the Ventricular System

The total volume of the ventricles has been determined mainly by use of plastic casts in fixed brains. The average total volume is probably some less than 20 cm³. The **individual variations** are surprisingly large, however (the normal range is probably from 7 to 30 cm³). Most studies have examined only the lateral ventricles, finding an average volume of about 7 cm³ for each. The volumes of the third and fourth ventricles appear to be some less than 1 cm³ for each. Even though the ventricular size increases somewhat with age, this can explain only a small fraction of the individual variations. In the same individual, however, the two lateral ventricles are quite similar in volume.

The **shape** and **size** of the ventricles can be determined noninvasively in living subjects by use of computer tomography and magnetic resonance imaging (see Fig. 6.28). Atrophy of the nervous tissue of the brain—for example, atrophy of the cerebral cortex, which occurs in dementia—leads to dilatation of the ventricles, whereas expansive, space-occupying processes like hemorrhages and tumors may distort and compress the ventricles.

The fluid produced in the lateral ventricles flows into the third ventricle through the **interventricular foramen** (of **Monro**) (Fig. 7.5; see Fig. 6.24). From there the fluid flows through the narrow **cerebral aqueduct** to the fourth ventricle. The choroid plexuses in the third and fourth ventricles add more fluid. The fluid leaves the ventricular system and enters the subarachnoid space (more specifically, the cisterna magna) through three openings in the fourth ventricle: one in the midline posteriorly (the **foramen of Magendie**) and two laterally (the lateral recesses or **foramina of Luschka**) (Fig. 7.5). The fluid then spreads out over the entire surface of the brain and spinal cord.

Of all cell types in the body, neurons are the most sensitive to interruption of their supply of oxygen (anoxia). Only a few minutes' stop in the blood flow may cause neuronal death. The **oxygen consumption** of the brain is high even at rest. Therefore, the blood supply of the central nervous system (CNS) is ample, and the brain receives about 15% of the cardiac output at rest. **Regulatory mechanisms** ensure that the brain gets what it needs—if necessary, at the expense of all other organs. The arteries of the brain lie within the cranial cavity and are mostly devoid of anastomoses (connections) with arteries outside the skull. Therefore, other arteries cannot take over if the intracranial ones are narrowed or occluded.

The cerebral blood flow is largely controlled by the local conditions in the nervous tissue; that is, there is a high degree of **autoregulation**. Local changes in the concentrations of ions, oxygen, carbon dioxide, and various signal substances determine the resistance offered by the arterioles. Brain vessels receive sensory innervation from the trigeminal nerve.

In most organs, small-molecule substances pass the capillary wall, and their concentration is therefore similar in the blood plasma and in the interstitial fluid. In contrast, the CNS exerts strict control of what is let in. The **blood–brain barrier** (a similar barrier exists between the blood and the cerebrospinal fluid [CSF]) is due mainly to special, selective properties of the brain capillaries.

In a few small regions adjoining the ventricles, the capillaries are fenestrated and hence let substances from the blood pass through easily. At such places, neurons are exposed to substances of the blood that do not enter other parts of the brain. These regions are called the **circumventricular organs**.

Broadly speaking, the **internal carotid artery** supplies most of the cerebral hemispheres, whereas the **vertebral artery** supplies the brain stem and the cerebellum. **Communicating arteries** at the base of the skull establish anastomoses between the posterior (vertebral) and the anterior (internal carotid) cerebral circulations. The venous blood is first collected in veins at the surface of the brain and then drained into wide, venous sinuses situated close to the inside of the skull.

The brain has a very high density of capillaries, and neurons are seldom more than 10 μm from the nearest capillary. The total length of all capillaries in the brain are said to be 400 miles and their total surface area more than 20 m^2. To understand the normal properties and the responses to disease of brain capillaries, however, they cannot be studied in isolation. The term **neurovascular unit** serves to emphasize the close structural and functional relationship between neurons, glial cells, associated capillary-endothelial cells, basal lamina, and pericytes (Fig. 8.1).

Regulation of Cerebral Circulation

Regulation of the blood flow is one among several factors governing the composition of the brain's extracellular milieu—that is, the concentration of ions, neuroactive substances, nutrients, and water (osmolarity). Control of the properties of astrocytes and the blood–brain barrier are other important factors (see Chapter 2, under "Astroglia and Homeostasis").

The cerebral circulation exhibits a high degree of **autoregulation**—that is, conditions in the brain itself determine the blood flow. If the blood pressure falls, the arteries dilate. This reduces vascular resistance so that the blood flow is upheld. If the blood pressure rises, the opposite happens: the arteries constrict. This is an important control mechanism, since increased capillary hydrostatic pressure may cause brain edema. The brain maintains almost constant blood flow as long as the systolic pressure is between 60 and 160 mm Hg. If the pressure falls below 60 mm, however, the flow falls steeply and the person becomes unconscious.

Figure 8.1

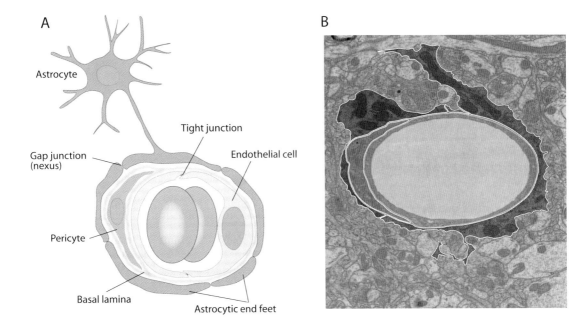

The blood–brain barrier/neurovascular unit. **A:** Schematic drawing showing the main features. Important elements are tight junctions between the endothelial cells and a continuous layer of astrocytic end feet. Gap junctions establish low-resistance connections between the astrocytes. The basal lamina also contributes to the barrier properties of the neurovascular unit. Not shown in the figure, although included in the term "neurovascular unit," are neurons that are in contact with processes of the astrocyte (see Figs. 2.3 and 2.5). **B:** Electron micrograph showing a brain capillary (hippocampus) and its relationship to processes of three astrocytes (the processes are marked with different colors). The electron micrograph is one among many in a true series of ultrathin sections, used for three-dimensional reconstruction of the astrocytic processes. This makes it possible to decide that the marked processes belong to different astrocytes. (Courtesy of Drs. Thomas Misje Mathiisen and Ole Petter Ottersen, Department of Anatomy, Institute of Basic Medical Sciences, University of Oslo, Norway.)

Among the many factors that control cerebral blood flow, local changes in the immediate surroundings of the neurons have an important role. These are changes in concentrations of ions (among them H^+ ions), CO_2 and O_2. **Hypoxia** (abnormally low concentration of O_2) and **hypercapnia** (above-normal concentration of CO_2) both cause marked vasodilatation and increased cerebral blood flow. Furthermore, increased local blood flow is closely coupled to increased neuronal activity, and this phenomenon is utilized in studies of correlations between changes in brain activity and behavior (see "Regional Cerebral Blood Flow and Neuronal Activity" later in this chapter).

Autonomic circulatory control seems to play a minor part in the brain (in contrast to in most other organs), even though **sympathetic fibers** innervate brain vessels. Such fibers release norepinephrine, neuropeptide Y (NPY), and possibly ATP, and stimulation causes **vasoconstriction**. Nevertheless, under normal conditions, activity of sympathetic fibers appears to have only marginal effects on blood flow. Thus, although sympathetic activity can constrict large brain arteries, peripheral small vessels dilate (probably because of local control). However, the sympathetic innervation may play a **protective** role during sudden increases in arterial blood pressure by preventing arterial dilatation. This would be important because passive (this is necessary because the neurons depend almost solely on glucose as a source of energy). The **glucose transporter GLUT1** is specific to brain capillaries.[2]

7. **Macromolecules**, such as some growth factors and cytokines, are to a limited extent carried from blood plasma into the brain, probably by receptor-mediated transport.

Drug Delivery and the Blood–Brain Barrier

The properties of the blood–brain barrier affect whether a **drug** may gain access to the brain; as a rule, only lipid-soluble drugs can reach therapeutic concentrations in the brain. Certain drugs such as **barbiturates** used for induction of anesthesia are highly lipid-soluble and act rapidly. Other drugs, such as penicillin, have low lipid solubility and pass the blood–brain barrier only with difficulty. In serious infections of the CNS, **penicillin** (or another drug with low lipid solubility) must be injected directly into the CSF, usually in the cisterna magna (see Fig. 7.5). The drug then easily enters the brain tissue because there is no barrier between the CSF and the brain interstitial fluid.

The need to deliver drugs noninvasively into the CNS has led to intense research activity. Many approaches have been tried (e.g., nanoparticles, peptide conjugates, viruses, and antibodies) with promising results in animal experiments but so far with limited success in treating human brain diseases. One promising approach targets the **transferrin receptor** (TfR), which mediates transport of macromolecules in vesicles through polarized cells (such as endothelial cells). TfR antibodies are linked to a therapeutic substance, which may be a drug or an antibody directed to a disease-provoking substance in the brain. For example, antibodies to the peptide **beta amyloid** (Aβ) have been successfully delivered to brain tissue across the blood–brain barrier in a mouse model of **Alzheimer's disease**. Notably, the treatment reduced the size of plaques containing beta amyloid.

Induction and Maintenance of the Blood–Brain Barrier

The special structural and functional properties of brain capillaries depend primarily on influences from surrounding elements. If peripheral tissue is transplanted into the brain, the in-growing capillaries attain the properties characteristic of the peripheral tissue: that is, no blood–brain barrier forms. The opposite happens if brain tissue is transplanted into another organ. The **astrocytic processes** that surround all brain capillaries in the adult (Fig. 8.1; see also Figs. 2.3 and 2.5), are certainly important for maintaining several features of the blood–brain barrier. Their exact

roles are not clear, however, partly due to conflicting data. For example, experiments show that astrocytes can induce tight junctions in brain endothelial cells. Nevertheless, other cell types (probably neuronal progenitor cells) appear to be responsible for the first formation of tight junctions in embryonic development, as it occurs before the appearance of astrocytes.[3] Indeed, there is good evidence that the blood–brain barrier is established and functioning in early embryonic life (Saunders et al. 2014).

Modulation of the Blood–Brain Barrier in Health and Disease

In cell cultures, a number of physiologic and pharmacological substances affect the properties of tight junctions. Normally, for example, a limited number of **lymphocytes** are allowed to enter the brain to "patrol" the tissue for foreign molecules. This requires specific receptor-mediated mechanisms that (most likely) transiently open tight junctions to let in lymphocytes. Unfortunately, some **metastatic cancer cells** also pass the blood–brain barrier. **Malnutrition** alters the blood–brain barrier, and substances like **histamine** and **bradykinin** make brain capillaries leaky (just as they do in other organs). According to animal experiments, even conditions with **inflammatory pain** (due to injection of irritants in the paw) can alter the permeability of the blood–brain barrier, presumably by circulating cytokines acting on tight junction proteins. **Stress** can increase the permeability of the blood–brain barrier to drugs, according to animal experiments. Presumably, this is so also in humans. For example, **pyridostigmine** (an acetylcholine-esterase inhibitor used to treat myasthenia gravis) normally acts only in peripheral tissues. During the first Gulf War (1990–1991) soldiers that were given prophylactic pyridostigmine (in case of nerve gas exposure) exhibited many more central side effects than are observed when the drug is given to soldiers in peacetime.

In several different, unrelated neurological diseases, the blood–brain barrier becomes less effective, mainly due to disturbed interactions between glia and endothelial cells. At the ultrastructural level, the neurovascular unit undergoes changes, such as loss of endothelial-cell tight junctions and changes of the astrocytes. In **multiple sclerosis**, for example, the blood–brain barrier is partly opened during exacerbations of the disease. Furthermore, the neurovascular unit is altered in **neurodegenerative diseases** (such as Alzheimer's disease and Parkinson's disease), in **infections** of the CNS (such as meningitis and septicemia), and in **ischemia** (due to stroke or traumatic brain injury). In the latter case, the disruption of the blood–brain barrier contributes to brain edema.

---

2. Mutations of the human *GLUT1* gene cause a syndrome with infantile seizures, delayed development, and microcephaly.

3. Growth factors of the **Wnt** family (Wnt7 and Wnt8) are secreted by the neuroepithelial cells in the earliest phases of nervous system development. Binding of Wnts to specific receptors in endothelial cells induce vessels to grow into the nervous tissue and develop their characteristic properties, such as the expression of the glucose transporter GLUT1. Mice lacking the genes for Wnt7 and Wnt8 show abnormal vascular growth, impaired blood–brain barrier properties, and lack of GLUT1 expression. (Wnt signaling also influences a number of other developmental processes in the brain.)

Figure 8.2

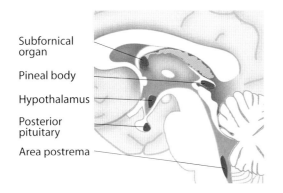

Subfornical organ

Pineal body

Hypothalamus

Posterior pituitary

Area postrema

Regions of the brain devoid of blood–brain barrier.

It is not clear, however, whether alterations of the neurovascular unit are causal to the diseases or are merely responses to the disease processes (which may nevertheless contribute to the disease manifestations).

Some Parts of the Brain Lack a Blood–Brain Barrier

In a few small regions adjoining the ventricles, the capillaries are fenestrated and hence let substances from the blood pass through easily. At such places, neurons are exposed to substances of the blood that do not enter other parts of the brain. These regions are called the **circumventricular organs** (Fig. 8.2). Among these, the **area postrema** is found in the lower end of the fourth ventricle, whereas the **subfornical organ** lies in the roof of the third ventricle just underneath the fornix close to the interventricular foramen. Both the area postrema and the subfornical organ contain many neurons that send their axons to other parts of the CNS and can thus mediate various specific influences on the nervous system. Neurons in the area postrema are involved in the **vomiting reflex** when this is elicited by toxic substances in the blood (see also Chapter 27, under "The Vomiting Reflex"). Neurons in the subfornical organ monitor the **salt concentration** of the blood. They send signals to the hypothalamus that can initiate responses necessary to maintain the fluid balance of the body. Further, neurons in the subfornical organ respond to circulating peptides involved in regulating **energy balance** (see Chapter 30, under "Control of Digestion and Feeding"). The subfornical organ and other parts of the circumventricular organs are also targets of

substances in the blood that induce **fever** and other symptoms of infections (see Chapter 30, under "Fever").

The **median eminence** (*eminentia mediana*) in the hypothalamus (Fig. 8.2) also lacks a blood–brain barrier. This region does not contain neuronal cell bodies but receives nerve fibers from other parts of the hypothalamus (see Fig. 30.8C). Hormones released from nerve terminals in the median eminence are transported by the bloodstream to the anterior pituitary (see Chapter 30, under "Influence of the Hypothalamus on the Anterior Pituitary: The Hypophyseal Portal System").

The two endocrine glands that are developed from the brain, the **posterior pituitary** and the **pineal body**, also lack a blood–brain barrier (Fig. 8.2). As with the median eminence, this is related to their release of hormones directly into the bloodstream.

ARTERIAL SYSTEM

The Brain Receives Arterial Blood from the Internal Carotid and the Vertebral Arteries

Broadly speaking, the internal carotid artery supplies most of the cerebral hemispheres, whereas the vertebral artery supplies the brain stem and the cerebellum.

The **internal carotid artery** (*arteria carotis interna*) enters the cranial cavity through a canal at the base of the skull (the carotid canal in the temporal bone) and then divides into three branches (Fig. 8.3):

1. The **ophthalmic artery** passes to the orbit through the optic canal and thus does not supply the brain itself (although, strictly speaking, the retina is part of the CNS). The **central retinal artery** (*a. centralis retinae*) enters the eye through the optic nerve and supplies the retina (see Fig. 16.1).

2. The **anterior cerebral artery** runs forward over the optic nerve and along the medial aspect of the hemisphere (Figs. 8.3 and 8.4). It supplies most of the cortex on the medial aspect of the hemisphere (except the most posterior parts and the inferior aspect of the temporal lobe). Its branches reach only a short distance onto the convexity of the hemispheres, supplying the leg representations of the motor and somatosensory areas. Shortly after its origin, the anterior cerebral artery gives off thin branches that penetrate the base of the hemisphere

Figure 8.5

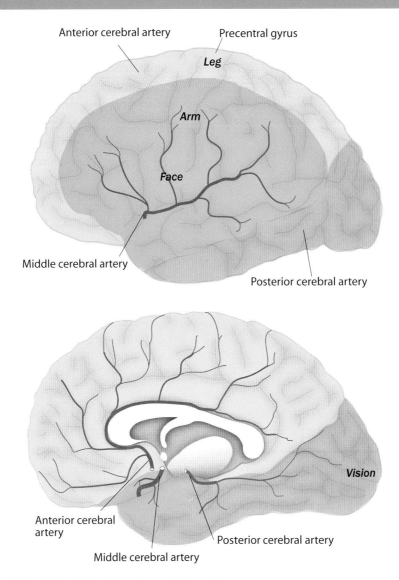

Anterior cerebral artery

Precentral gyrus

Leg

Arm

Face

Middle cerebral artery

Posterior cerebral artery

Vision

Anterior cerebral
artery

Posterior cerebral artery

Middle cerebral artery

The parts of the brain supplied with blood from the main arterial branches.

especially when the occlusion of the internal carotid artery develops slowly over the years, presumably allowing gradual compensatory widening of the communicating arteries.

The Spinal Cord Receives Arteries at Many Levels

In general, the arteries of the cord are arranged with one artery running in the midline anteriorly, the **anterior spinal artery**, and one on each side running along the rows of posterior roots, the **posterior spinal arteries** (Fig. 8.6). All three arteries begin cranially as branches of the vertebral arteries but receive contributions from the small arteries that enter the vertebral canal along with the spinal nerves.

Figure 8.6

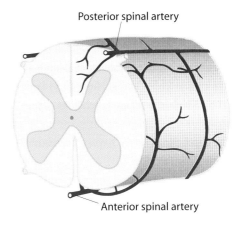

Posterior spinal artery

Anterior spinal artery

The arterial supply of the spinal cord.

Individual Variations in Size and Distribution of Cerebral Arteries Have Clinical Significance

The **symptoms** produced by occlusion of one arterial branch are variable because of individual differences in the size and exact distribution of the arterial branches. Thus, if one artery is small, another supplying a neighboring territory is usually large. The anterior and posterior inferior cerebellar arteries are examples of this phenomenon: sometimes one of them supplies the total territory normally supplied by both. Even the two vertebral arteries often differ markedly in size in one person, explaining why symptoms caused by occlusion of the artery may vary from minimal to life-threatening.

Less than 50% of the population appears to have a "typical" **circle of Willis**; that is, the communicating arteries are symmetrical and with a certain cross-sectional diameter. In some persons the anterior communicating artery is very thin or missing; in others this may concern the posterior communicating artery on one or both sides. Therefore, the ability of the carotid artery of one side to compensate for the loss of the corresponding artery of the other side would be expected to vary considerably among individuals. Similar individual variations exist with regard to the ability of the anterior (carotid) and posterior (vertebral) circulations to compensate each other.

VENOUS SYSTEM

The Venous Blood Is Collected in Sinuses

The cerebral veins can be divided into **deep** and **superficial** types. The latter partly accompany the arteries on the surface of the brain. All of the veins empty into large **venous sinuses** that are formed by folds of the dura (Figs. 8.7, 8.8, and 8.9).

The **superficial veins** at the dorsal parts of the hemispheres run upward and medially and empty into the large **superior sagittal sinus** in the upper margin of the falx cerebri. Where the falx cerebri meets the tentorium cerebelli, the superior sagittal sinus divides into two parts, the **transverse sinuses**, so named because they follow a transverse course laterally along where the tentorium is attached to the occipital bone. The **sigmoid sinus**—forming the direct continuation of the transverse sinus—empties into the **internal jugular vein** at the jugular foramen. The internal jugular vein leaves the skull and continues downward into the neck.

Most of the blood in the **deep cerebral veins** collects into the **great cerebral vein of Galen** (*vena cerebri magna*; Figs. 8.7 and 8.9). This comes out from the inferior side of the posterior end of the corpus callosum and empties into the **straight sinus** (*sinus rectus*) in the midline of the tentorium. The straight sinus drains into the superior sagittal sinus at the **confluence region**, from which the transverse sinus originates. Unlike the arteries, the cerebral veins have numerous **anastomoses**. At some locations, there are also **emissary veins** that form connections between intracranial and extracranial veins (see Fig. 7.2).

Figure 8.7

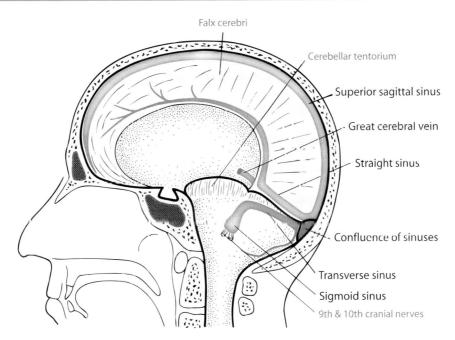

Falx cerebri

Cerebellar tentorium

Superior sagittal sinus

Great cerebral vein

Straight sinus

Confluence of sinuses

Transverse sinus

Sigmoid sinus

9th & 10th cranial nerves

Folds of the dura and the venous sinuses. The folds minimize the movements of the brain and contain venous sinuses (in blue).

PART TWO

Development, Aging, and Plasticity

The fully developed nervous system consists of incredibly complex networks of connections. There are billions of neurons in the human brain, and each one is probably, on average, connected with several thousand others. The number of possible combinations of synaptic contacts is therefore astronomic. Indeed, a section of nervous tissue stained to reveal all neuronal processes might appear as a chaotic jungle. Nevertheless, we have ample evidence that this is very far from the case: order exists everywhere, and the mutual connections between neuronal groups are far from random. This leads to a number of questions, such as: How do the thousands of individual cell groups find their highly specific positions in the brain? How do the complicated and precisely organized networks arise during development of the individual? What roles do genetic and environmental factors play in the final structure and performance of the brain? Such questions are dealt with in **Chapter 9**. In **Chapter 10**, we discuss the changes taking place in the aging brain and their consequences for function. A common theme in Chapters 9 and 10 is nervous system plasticity—that is, its ability to adapt structurally and functionally to altered demands. In **Chapter 11**, we discuss plastic changes in the nervous system as the basis for recovery of function after damage to the central nervous system. We argue that a common theme in all rehabilitative efforts is to facilitate learning.

development, precursor cells are triggered to **differentiate**—first to neurons and glial cells and then to numerous specialized subtypes of each. This occurs by modifications of the cell's chromatin, for example, by **methylation** of specific sites of the DNA, thereby modifying the expression of certain genes (without altering the DNA itself). Largely, our genome possesses the instructions that determine the final size of neurons, the shape of their dendritic trees, and the types of neurotransmitters expressed, as evidenced by growth of neurons in culture. Nevertheless, the full functional development of the brain depends critically on proper **use** of the neurons and their interconnections (discussed later in this chapter). Consequently, the normal development and performance of the nervous system depend on interactions of genetic and environmental factors.

The Central Nervous System Develops as a Long Tube

By a few days after fertilization of the egg, differentiation of the cells of the embryo to the main kinds of tissue has started. Transforming from a round lump of cells, after about a week the embryo resembles an elongated disc. In the second week the disc is covered on the upper or dorsal side and along the edges by primitive epithelium, the **ecto-derm**, whereas the under or ventral side is covered by an epithelium—the **endoderm**—which later forms the intestinal tract and its glands. Between these two epithelial layers the **mesoderm** develops, which later differentiates into the musculoskeletal system. In the third week (after 18 days), the development of the nervous system begins, with formation of a thickening, the **neural plate**, in the prospective cranial end of the disc (Figs. 9.1 and 9.2). The thickening is due to growth of the ectodermal cells so that they form a tall, simple, columnar **neuroepithelium**. Diffusible substances—called **morphogens**—from the underlying mesodermal cells induce formation of the neural plate (see also "Neuromeres and Hox Genes" later in this chapter). The differentiation of ectodermal cells to neuroepithelium proceeds in a cranial-to-caudal direction. A longitudinal infolding of the ectoderm occurs by the end of the third week (Fig. 9.1). This neural groove is subsequently closed in the fourth week; the closing starts in the middle part (Fig. 9.2) and forms the neural tube, which is soon covered by the ectoderm dorsally (Figs. 9.1 and 9.2) The wall of the tube is formed by primitive neuroepithelial cells, which proliferate enormously and develop into neurons and glial cells. The lateral edge of the neural plate forms a distinct cell group,

Figure 9.1

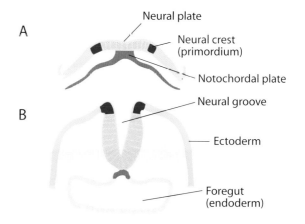

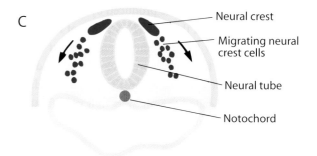

Formation of the neural tube and the neural crest. Schematic cross sections through embryos at different stages of development. **A:** The formation of the neural tube is induced by substances diffusing from the underlying mesoderm (notochordal plate). Approximately 17 days. **B:** The neural tube is formed by growth and folding of the neural plate. Approximately 21 days **C:** The neural crest gives origin to spinal ganglion cells and autonomic ganglion cells (and some other cell types). The neural crest cells migrate into the body to form ganglia. Approximately 24 days.

the **neural crest**, which later forms a longitudinal column on each side of the neural tube (Fig. 9.1). The neural crest produces the neurons of the peripheral nervous system, among them spinal ganglion cells and autonomic ganglion cells. The neural crest also produces Schwann cells and satellite cells (a kind of glia) in the ganglia.

Morphogens

Morphogens are substances that spread by diffusion from a localized source and govern the embryological development and patterning of organs and body parts. Their effects depend on their concentrations—often so that high and low concentrations exert opposite effects. Among several morphogens involved in patterning of the human nervous system, the protein **sonic hedgehog** plays an important role at very early stages. For

Figure 9.2

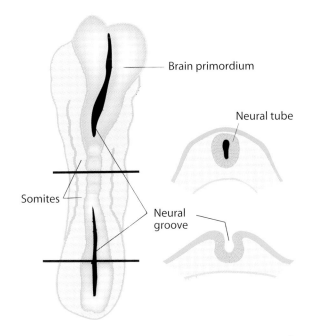

- Brain primordium
- Neural tube
- Somites
- Neural groove

The neural plate and closure of the neural groove. Drawing of a 22-day-old human embryo, approximately 1 mm long. The central nervous system is shown in pink. (Based on Hamilton, Boyd, and Mossman 1972.)

example, sonic hedgehog is expressed by the notochord when the dorsal–ventral differentiation of the neural tube begins. It also acts at later stages to guide axonal growth, attracting outgrowing axons in low concentrations and repelling them in high concentrations (as shown for retinal ganglion cell axons growing from the eye toward the brain).

The Neural Crest Produces More than Neurons and Glia

Experiments with labeling of neural crest cells before they migrate (Fig. 9.1) show that some differentiate into nonnervous structures. These include the smooth muscles of the eye (intrinsic eye muscles) and, most likely, the **pia** and the **arachnoid** (the dura mater is believed to originate from the mesoderm). Migrated neural crest cells also form the dermis and subcutis of the **face** and the cartilaginous skeleton of the **visceral arches**. Finally, neural crest cells produce endocrine cells of the **adrenal medulla**, **melanocytes** of the skin, and parts of the **septum** that divides the pulmonal artery and the aorta.

Early Development of the Cranial End of the Neural Tube

Whereas the caudal end of the neural tube—which develops into the spinal cord—retains its simple tubular form, the expanded cranial end undergoes marked changes. This occurs because different parts grow at different rates and because the tube bends, forming **flexures** (Fig. 9.3). In the fourth week three swellings or **primary vesicles** take shape (Figs. 9.3 and 9.4). The cavities inside the primary vesicles are continuous and develop into the ventricular system of the brain (see Fig. 7.3). The most cranial vesicle is called the **prosencephalon** (forebrain), the middle one the **mesencephalon** (the midbrain), and the caudal-most one the **rhombencephalon** (hindbrain). A ventrally directed bend—the **cervical flexure**—arises at the junction between the rhombencephalon and the spinal cord (Fig. 9.3). Later, a **mesencephalic flexure** arises between the rhombencephalon and the mesencephalon. A dorsally directed bend—the **pontine flexure**—later divides the rhombencephalon into two parts (Fig. 9.5).Early in the fourth week, the ventral aspect of the prospective brain exhibits shallow, transverse grooves. These are external signs of segmentation of the cranial end of the neural tube, and each segment is called a **neuromere.** The segmentation is most obvious in the rhombencephalon, and we use the term **rhombomere** in this region. Although their external signs disappear by the sixth week, the neuromeres are important because they represent the first segregation of neurons that later differentiate into the various nuclei of the brain stem. Thus, several cranial nerves and their nuclei are first laid down according to a segmental pattern, like the spinal nerves, although later development makes the cranial nerve pattern less regular.

The mesencephalon changes little during further development, in contrast to the two other primary vesicles. The **prosencephalon** develops into the diencephalon and the cerebral hemispheres, whereas the **rhombencephalon** differentiates into the medulla oblongata, the pons, and the cerebellum (Figs. 9.4 and 9.5). The rostral end of the prosencephalon produces two more vesicles (one on each side), called the **telencephalon** (Figs. 9.4 and 9.5), which later forms the cerebral cortex and basal ganglia. In addition, the **olfactory bulbs** (see Fig. 6.13) arise as evaginations from the ventral aspect of the telencephalon. The remaining caudal part of the prosencephalon forms the diencephalon, which includes the thalamus and hypothalamus. At an early stage (Fig. 9.3), cuplike

Figure 9.3

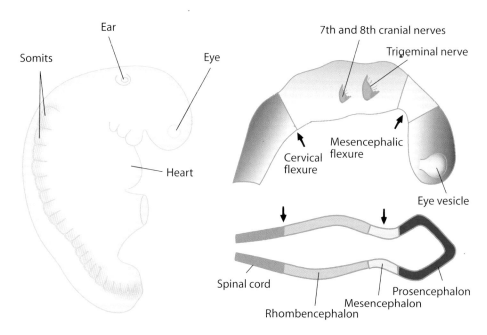

Early stages of brain development. **Left:** Drawing of a 28-day-old human embryo, approximately 3.5 mm long. **Right:** Drawings of the cranial part of the neural tube (the brain primordium) isolated and magnified compared with the drawing of the embryo. Arrows indicate the flexures of the neural tube. The lower left is cut through (seen from the dorsal aspect) to show the primary vesicles and the ventricular space. (Based on Hamilton, Boyd, and Mossman 1972.)

evaginations—the **eye vesicles**—are formed from the prosencephalon (the part later to become the diencephalon). The eye vesicles develop into the retina and the optic nerve. The rhomb-encephalon develops two parts: the **myelencephalon** forming the medulla oblongata and the **metencephalon** forming the pons and most of the cerebellum (the cerebellum also develops from the mesencephalon, as discussed next).

Figure 9.4

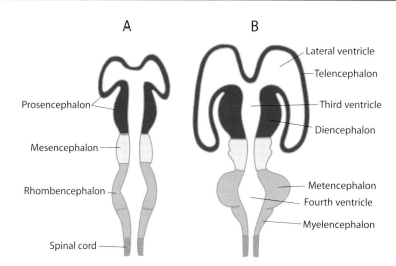

Different divisions of the brain primordium. Schematic of the cranial part of the neural tube (straightened out and cut open horizontally). **A:** Approximately the same stage as in Fig. 9.3. **B:** The same stage as in Fig. 9.13A. Note the development of the telencephalon (the hemispheres) that gradually covers the diencephalon.

Figure 9.5

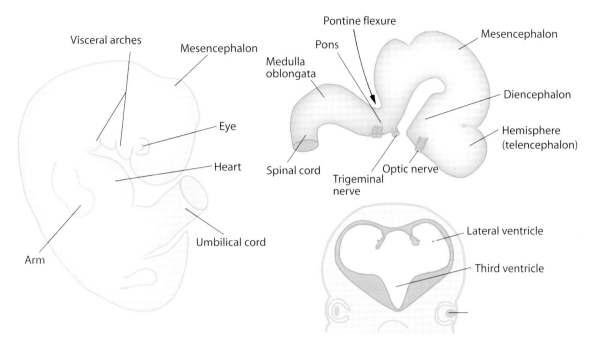

Early development of the brain. **Left:** Drawing of a 36-day-old human embryo, approximately 11 mm long. **Right:** The cranial part of the neural tube at the same stage. (Based on Hamilton, Boyd, and Mossman 1972.)

Neuromeres

We mentioned that the rostral part of the neural tube shows transient, external signs of segmentation—each segment constituting a **neuromere**. Although this phenomenon was observed in the nineteenth century, modern cell biological methods were necessary for closer study. Neuromeres are most convincingly shown in the rhombencephalon, where they are called **rhombomeres**. It is assumed that the mesencephalon consists of two neuromeres, whereas the prosencephalon probably consists of six. The great interest in neuromeres and other external signs of segmentation arose because they provide information about the mechanisms that control the early development from the undifferentiated neural tube to the adult nervous system.

Each rhombomere represents a unit of neurons that do not mix with neurons of other rhombomeres during subsequent development. This neuronal specification takes place just when the rhombomere boundaries arise. The rhombomeres arise when adjoining groups of neurons begin to express different surface markers. The neurons of one rhombomere, among other things, have a specified future peripheral target (the neurons of the neural crest in the head region are also specified with regard to their peripheral target before they start to migrate peripherally). The motor **trigeminal nucleus**, for example, is formed in rhombomeres r2 and r3, whereas the motor **facial nucleus** develops in r4 and r5. The motor and sensory cranial nerve axons already have a specified target when they start growing out from the neural tube (Fig. 9.7). Thus, when a rhombomere is transplanted to another place in the chicken embryonic brain,

it develops as if it were still in its original place and not corresponding to its new location. Such specification must be caused by the switching on of certain genes—which start to express themselves by production of mRNA—while probably other genes are switched off.

Early Phases in the Development of the Neuroepithelium

Initially, the wall of the neural tube consists of only one layer of cylindrical neuroepithelial cells (Figs. 9.1 and 9.2), bounded externally by the **external limiting membrane** (covered by the pia) and internally toward the cavity by the **internal limiting membrane**. These are basal membranes built of extracellular material, which always develop with surface epithelia. Intense **proliferation** of neuroepithelial cells soon leads to several layers of nuclei. The epithelium does not become truly stratified, however, because all cells retain a thin process reaching the internal limiting membrane (pseudostratified epithelium; Fig. 9.6). The outermost cells move toward the cavity of the neural tube (the future ventricles and central canal). The innermost layer, the **ventricular zone**, borders the cavity. In the ventricular zone, the cells divide mitotically (Figs. 9.6 and 9.13A). The future neurons, the **neuroblasts**,

Figure 9.6

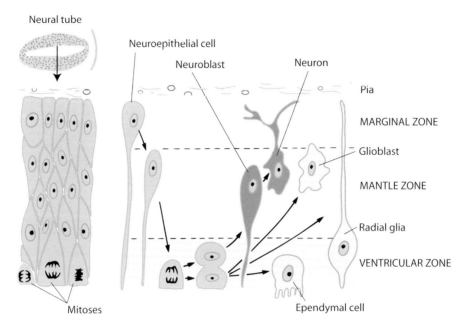

Differentiation of the neuroepithelium. **Left:** Drawing of a section through the wall of the neural tube at an early stage (cf. Fig. 9.7A). **Right:** Arrows show how the neuroepithelial cells move while they differentiate into different cell types.

afterward migrate outward to form the **mantle zone** that later becomes the gray matter. A layer without neurons, the **marginal zone**, forms external to the mantle zone and becomes the white matter. The neurons of the mantle zone send axons into the marginal zone. These axons loop back to the mantle zone, however, to synapse on neurons there (these are the first association connections to arise). Other axons leave the neural tube as motor fibers growing peripherally to contact muscle cells and glands (Fig. 9.7). After neuroblast production ends, various types of glial cells are produced by mitosis of neuroepithelial cells that remain in the ventricular zone. The last to be produced are the **ependymal cells**. These retain their internal position and cover the ventricular face of the neural tube (Fig. 9.6). The cavity is filled with cerebrospinal fluid produced by tufts invaginated from the wall into the cavity (see Fig. 7.6). These tufts—the future **choroid plexus**—are covered by ependymal cells.

The simple layering of the neural tube, with the mantle zone (gray matter) inside and the marginal zone (white matter) outside, is retained with minor changes in the spinal cord. In the cranial part of the neural tube (the future brain), however, major alterations in the mutual positions of gray and white matter occur. In the developing cerebellar and cerebral cortices, for example, neurons migrate from the mantle zone through the marginal zone and form a layered sheet of gray matter externally, just under the pia.

Hox Genes

Many so-called **Hox genes** have been identified that are expressed in a pattern corresponding to neuromeric boundaries in vertebrates. Most of these genes code for proteins that act as **transcription factors.** These bind to DNA of other genes and regulate their transcription. Typically, transcription factors are expressed temporarily during specific phases of development. (*Hox* genes not only control regional development of the nervous system but also act in pattern formation in other parts of the body.) When a certain *Hox* gene is switched on, a cascade of changes in the expression of other genes is initiated, producing signal molecules that give the neuronal groups their identity—for example, regarding location and connections. A crucial question is, of course, what controls the regionalized expression of *Hox* genes giving rise to the rhombomeres? One important factor is **retinoic acid (vitamin A)**, which normally occurs with an anteroposterior (rostrocaudal) concentration gradient in the embryo (highest concentration posteriorly or caudally). The retinoic acid seems to stem from the mesoderm adjacent to the neural tube. In low concentrations, retinoic acid acts on *Hox* genes that specify anterior parts of the neural tube, while in high concentrations it induces differentiation of posterior parts. This explains why adequate dietary levels of vitamin A are necessary for the normal development of the CNS but also why too much also may cause malformations (as may occur in women treated for acne with retinoic acid in early pregnancy).

Neuromeric borders, identified with genetic markers, are more reliable indicators of future borders between anatomically and functionally different areas than are borders between brain vesicles. For example, the **cerebellum**, traditionally regarded as arising only from the metencephalon, is also formed by neurons

Figure 9.7

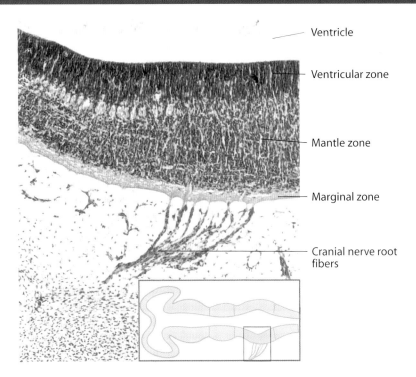

Ventricle

Ventricular zone

Mantle zone

Marginal zone

Cranial nerve root fibers

Outgrowth of cranial nerves from the rhombencephalon. Photomicrograph of a horizontal section through a chicken embryo at about the same stage as in Figure 9.3. Thin bundles of axons leave the marginal zone and penetrate the connective tissue that surrounds the brain primordium.

in the adjoining part of the mesencephalon. The rostral border of neurons forming the cerebellum coincides with a border for the expression of the *engrailed 2* gene.

Further Development of the Spinal Cord and the Brain Stem

In the fourth week, the proliferation of neuroblasts in the mantle zone produces a large ventral thickening and a smaller dorsal one on each side of the neural tube. These thickenings are called the **basal plates** and the **alar plates**, respectively (Figs. 9.8, 9.9, and 9.10). A shallow furrow, the **sulcus limitans**, marks the border between them. This remains visible in the lower part of the brain stem in the adult (see Fig. 6.17), while it disappears early in the spinal cord. The basal plate contains neuroblasts that later become motor neurons, whereas many alar plate neuroblasts become sensory neurons. This corresponds to the functional division between the ventral and dorsal horns of the cord. In the adult brain stem, the sulcus limitans marks the border between the motor and the sensory cranial nerve nuclei (Fig. 9.11). In the open part of the rhombencephalon—later

to become parts of the medulla and the pons—the motor nuclei lie medially and the sensory nuclei laterally (see Figs. 27.2 and 27.3). This is caused by lateral bending of the alar plates—away from each other—so that the roof of the rhombencephalon becomes only a thin membrane (Figs. 9.9 and 9.10). At a later stage, the **cerebellum** develops from the margins of the alar plates (the **rhombic lip**).

At an early stage, several neuronal groups in the brain stem **migrate** from their "birthplace" in the alar or basal plates. In the pons, neuroblasts move from the rhombic lip in a ventral direction and form the pontine nuclei (see Fig. 6.18). Similarly, in the medulla the inferior olive (another nucleus projecting to the cerebellum; see Fig. 6.17) is formed by neuroblasts moving ventrally from the rhombic lip. Another example is the **motor cranial nerve nuclei** that innervate visceral (branchial) arch muscles (Fig. 9.10). These neurons move in a ventral direction during early development after they have started to send out axons. The course of the root fibers in the brain stem therefore shows the path followed by the migrating neurons (see Fig. 27.11).

Until the eighth to ninth week, the **spinal cord** extends the full length of the spinal canal of the embryo. After that, however, the vertebral column and the coverings of the cord grow

(Figs. 9.3 and 9.5). The **first visceral arch**—producing the upper and lower jaw with attached masticatory muscles, along with the hammer and the anvil of the middle ear—is innervated by the **fifth cranial nerve** (the trigeminal). The **second visceral arch**—forming, among other things, the upper part of the hyoid bone, the stirrup of the middle ear, and the facial muscles—is innervated by the **seventh cranial nerve** (the facial). The **third visceral arch**—forming most of the hyoid bone and the posterior part of the tongue—is innervated by the **ninth cranial nerve** (the glossopharyngeal). The **fourth, fifth,** and **sixth visceral arches** form the cartilaginous skeleton of the larynx and the muscles of the larynx and the pharynx. These structures are innervated for the most part by the **tenth cranial nerve** (the vagus).

Cranial nerves 3, 4, 6, and 12 (the oculomotor, trochlear, abducens, and hypoglossal; see Fig. 6.14) innervate structures that most likely develop from segmentally arranged **somites** (somites are paired cubical masses giving rise to muscles, the axial skeleton, and the dermis of the skin). These nerves are homologous to spinal ventral roots. Regarding the **eleventh cranial nerve** (the accessory), it has not been determined whether the two muscles it innervates (the sternocleidomastoid and trapezius) develop from somites or from visceral arches. The latter hypothesis is supported by the fact that the accessory nerve root fibers, coming from the upper cervical segments, exit the cord more dorsally than the spinal ventral roots (corresponding to the level where visceral arch nerves leave the brain stem; see Figs. 27.1 and 27.8).

Further Development of the Diencephalon

The diencephalon represents the caudal part of the original prosencephalic vesicle (Figs. 9.4 and 9.5). The lateral wall in this part becomes thicker at an early stage and develops into the **thalamus** (Fig. 9.12A). The floor plate forms the **hypothalamus** and the **posterior pituitary** (see Figs. 6.23 and 6.24). The latter arise as an evagination of the floor plate. The furrow (**hypothalamic sulcus**; see Fig. 6.23) marking the border between the thalamus and the hypothalamus might be a continuation of the sulcus limitans (Fig. 9.10). It is not settled, however, whether the arrangement with basal and alar plates continues rostrally into the diencephalon. The thin roof plate of the diencephalon forms by invagination the **choroid plexus** of the third ventricle (see Fig. 7.6). Further, the roof plate produces the **pineal body** by evagination (see Fig. 6.24). The **eye vesicles** occur at an earlier stage (before the further differentiation of the prosencephalon; Fig. 9.3) but retain connection with the diencephalon by the future optic nerve (Fig. 9.5).

Further Development of the Telencephalon

In the fifth week, development of the **cerebral hemispheres** starts with the appearance of one vesicle on each side of the prosencephalon (Figs. 9.4 and 9.5). These are called the **telencephalic (cerebral) vesicles**. Their cavities form the lateral ventricles, which initially have wide openings to the third ventricle (interventricular foramen, Fig. 9.12A). The mantle zone of the basal part of the telencephalic vesicle thickens rapidly to form the corpus striatum of the **basal ganglia** (Fig. 9.12A). The thinner overlying part, called the **pallium**, becomes the cerebral cortex. The pallium grows dorsally, rostrally, and caudally in relation to the diencephalon (Fig. 9.4). The caudal and ventral parts of the hemispheres later fuse with the diencephalon (Fig. 9.12B).

The basal ganglia primordium is later divided into two parts—the lateral and medial **corpus striatum**—by descending axons from the cerebral cortex. These descending axons form the **internal capsule** (Fig. 9.12B). As development proceeds, the caudate nucleus and the thalamus come to lie medial to the internal capsule whereas the lentiform nucleus (the putamen and the globus pallidus) lies laterally (see Fig. 23.2).

In the medial wall of the pallium, just above the attachment of the choroid plexus, a thickening arises that bulges into the lateral ventricle (Fig. 9.12A). This is the beginning of the **hippocampus**, which is partly separated from the rest of the pallium by the hippocampal sulcus. As the hemispheres grow, their shape changes so that the temporal lobes come to lie ventrally. This produces the characteristic curved shape of the lateral ventricles and the structures in their wall, such as the hippocampus and the caudate nucleus (see Figs. 7.4 and 31.2). The hippocampus thus moves from the position in Fig. 4.12A to that in Fig. 4.12B (see also Fig. 6.31).

The **choroid plexus** of the lateral ventricles is formed by invagination of the thin part of the pallium (together with the pia) close to the dorsal aspect of the diencephalon (Fig. 9.12B; see also Fig. 7.6).

Development of the Cerebral Cortex

At first, the telencephalic vesicle consists of only one layer of neuroepithelial cells. These proliferate, however, producing rapid growth of the prospective cerebral hemisphere. At a later stage, we can differentiate a ventricular zone, mantle zone, and marginal zone, just as in other parts of the neural tube (Fig. 9.13A). At the beginning of the **eighth week**, neuroblasts from the mantle zone **migrate** into the marginal zone and start establishing the **cortical plate** (Fig. 9.13B), which in due course will develop into the mature cerebral cortex by waves of cells migrating toward the cortical

Figure 9.12

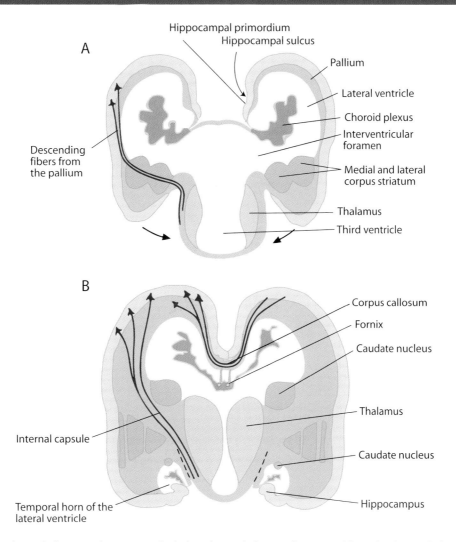

A

Hippocampal primordium
Hippocampal sulcus
Pallium
Lateral ventricle
Choroid plexus
Interventricular foramen
Descending fibers from the pallium
Medial and lateral corpus striatum
Thalamus
Third ventricle

B

Corpus callosum
Fornix
Caudate nucleus
Thalamus
Internal capsule
Caudate nucleus
Temporal horn of the lateral ventricle
Hippocampus

Development of the telencephalon. **A:** Early stage, in which the telencephalon is still separated from the diencephalon. Descending fibers have started their growth from the pallium (primordium of the cerebral cortex) to the brain stem and the spinal cord. **B:** The telencephalon is now attached to the diencephalon laterally, and the medial and lateral striatum have been separated by the internal capsule. The hippocampus has changed its position, due to the growth of the hemispheres. (Based on Hamilton, Boyd, and Mossman 1972.)

surface. The peak of migratory activity probably occurs between the third and fifth months, while migration ends in the third trimester. By the end of the seventh month (28 weeks), the cortex has developed six layers, as in the mature cortex (see Figs. 33.1 and 33.2). Synapses begin to occur in the fourth month (earliest in the prospective somatosensory cortex).

The deepest cortical layers are established first; thus, neurons destined for superficial layers have to pass through the deep layers. Neuroepithelial cells in the ventricular zone that have ceased dividing are termed **postmitotic**. The exact time a neuron becomes postmitotic—its **birth date**—appears to decide which cortical layer it will join.

Radially oriented glial cells, **radial glia** (Fig. 9.6), with processes extending from the ependyma to the pia, guide the migration of postmitotic neurons toward the cortex. The **phenotype** of postmitotic neurons—for example, whether they will develop into interneurons or projection neurons—appears to be specified at the time they start migrating toward their final destination.

Shortly after the establishment of the cortical plate, **thalamocortical fibers** start to invade the telencephalic wall, although they must "wait" several weeks below the cortical plate before they find their final destination in the developing cortex. The earliest afferent fibers to arrive, however, are **monoaminergic** (at about 7 weeks).

Figure 9.13

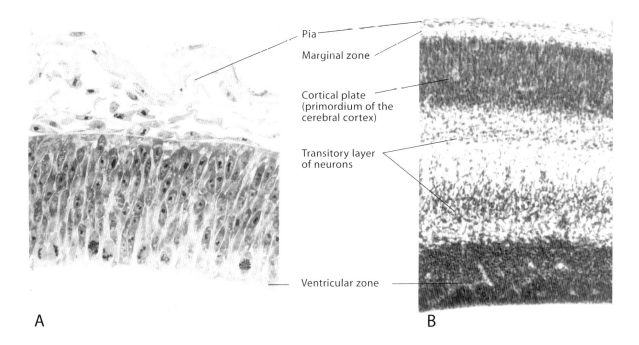

Pia
Marginal zone
Cortical plate
(primordium of the
cerebral cortex)
Transitory layer
of neurons
Ventricular zone

A   B

Differentiation of the prosencephalic neuroepithelium to the cerebral cortex. **A:** Photomicrograph of a cross section through the neural tube (prosencephalic part) at an early stage (chicken embryo, corresponding to early fourth week gestation in humans). Mitotic activity occurs in the ventricular zone. **B:** Photomicrograph of a section through the telencephalon (rat) at a much later stage than in **A**, corresponding approximately to the fourth to fifth month in human development. The ventricular zone is densely packed with neuroblasts that will soon migrate toward the cortical plate. In further development, the cortical plate develops into the adult six-layered cortex.

While probably all progenitors of projection neurons arise in the ventricular zone and migrate radially to their final destination, many prospective cortical **interneurons** arise from subcortical sites in the ventral forebrain. They then migrate tangentially along the cortical plate for varying distances before they change course and migrate perpendicularly into the cortex.[1]

Specification of Cortical Cytoarchitectonic Areas

The adult cerebral cortex consists of many areas that differ structurally and functionally (see Fig. 33.4). The differentiation of the cortical plate into distinct areas (see Fig. 33.4)—a process called **arealization**—depends on both genetic factors intrinsic to the developing cortical progenitor cells

and extrinsic influences. In the beginning, local patterning centers in the periphery of the ventricular zone produces gradients of **morphogens** that define four main, overlapping domains in the cortical plate. The morphogens in turn initiate more discrete expressions of transcription factors in cortical progenitor cells. These transcription factors are involved in the further differentiation of the cortical plate into areas with sharp borders. For example, the arealization of the frontal cortex seems to be initiated by two **fibroblast growth factors** (called Fgf8 and Fgf17).

Among **extrinsic influences**, thalamocortical afferents appear to be of particular importance for the mature **cytoarchitectonic** characteristics of an area. For example, the characteristic cytoarchitectonic differences between the primary sensory areas (compare Figs. 33.2 and 33.5) depend on from which specific thalamic nucleus the areas receive their afferents. For example, transplanting a piece of visual cortex to the somatosensory cortex makes the transplanted tissue acquire the cytoarchitectonic features that are typical of the somatosensory cortex. Further, immature **projection neurons** transplanted from one area to another develop axonal ramifications appropriate for the area to which they

---

1. All cortical interneurons are **GABAergic** but fall into different groups structurally and with regard to whether they co-express the neuropeptide **somatostatin**, **parvalbumin**, or **calretinin**). The three main groups of GABAergic interneurons seem to be specified at the time they migrate from the so-called **ventricular** (ganglionic) **eminences**.

are transplanted. Thus, the local environment contributes significantly to the neuronal phenotype.

In addition to the genetically determined development described here, proper use of cortical areas is critical for the realization of their functional specialization. This involves **use-dependent** plastic processes, stabilizing useful synaptic connections, and eliminating those that prove to be superfluous or maladaptive.

Migration and Migration Disorders

We know some of the factors governing neuronal migration, such as recognition molecules, adhesion molecules, cytoskeletal components, and others. There is a complex interplay among them, and the different factors must be present in the proper concentration at the proper time and place. For example, the early presence of certain neurotransmitters influences neuronal motility by acting on ion channels that increase the intracellular Ca²⁺ concentration. The glycoprotein **reelin** (among other factors) governs the final positioning of migrating neurons in the cortex. Because reelin is produced by **Cajal-Retzius cells** in the marginal zone (Fig. 9.6), it would seem logical that a concentration gradient of reelin between the marginal and ventricular layers is critical for normal development. The mechanisms behind the effects of reelin appear to be more complex, however. Nevertheless, mice with a mutated gene for reelin exhibit characteristic malformations of layered structures; in the cerebral cortex, the late-arriving neurons do not migrate past those that arrived first to occupy the outer layers. Although the neurons survive and establish apparently normal connections, the brain does not function normally. Another mutation, shown in some humans, affects the migration *before* the neurons enter the cortical plate and is associated with a smooth cortex lacking the normal six-layered structure (**Miller-Dieker lissencephaly**). This is just one example of a large and varied group of malformations in humans—**migration disorders**—caused by delayed or deficient migration of postmitotic neurons.

Migration disorders affect primarily the cerebral cortex and the cerebellum. Many are inherited recessively, although ischemia, radiation, and other influences can cause migration disorders (as shown in animal experiments). In the cerebral cortex, migration disorders typically are associated with defective development of the gyri (Fig. 9.14), which may be lacking (**lissencephaly**), be too small (**polymicrogyria**), or show other abnormalities. Usually, such a cortex is called **dysplastic**, and some use the term "dysplastic cortex" as synonymous with migration disorders.

Migration disorders cause a number of syndromes characterized by **cognitive** and behavioral defects (mental retardation is common). Typical of many such syndromes is **epilepsy** (which is often difficult to treat pharmacologically). This is compatible with the fact that migration disorders also are associated with molecular abnormalities of cortical neurons. Thus, animal experiments suggest that epilepsy can arise in dysplastic cortex because of an imbalance between the expression of excitatory and inhibitory receptors (up-regulation of aminomethylisoxazole propionic acid [AMPA] receptors and down-regulation of GABA_A receptors).

Figure 9.14

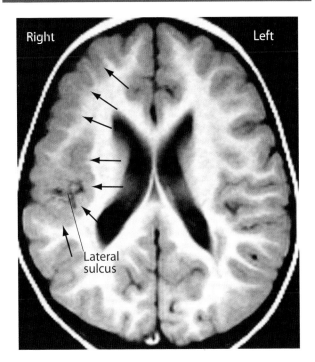

Neuronal migration disorder. Horizontal T1-weighted MRI. The right frontal cortex is dysplastic: it is thicker than normal with obliteration of normal sulci (polymicrogyria). Similar alterations occur around the lateral sulcus. (Courtesy of Dr. S.J. Bakke, Oslo University Hospital, Oslo, Norway.)

Programmed Cell Death and Competition for Trophic Factors

As previously mentioned, many more neurons are formed during the proliferation phase than are found in the mature nervous system. Cell death usually coincides in time with the period during which the neurons establish synaptic contacts. For the most intensively studied neuronal groups, such as spinal motoneurons and retinal ganglion cells, the amount of elimination depends on **target size**. If the target (e.g., striated muscle cells) is experimentally expanded, more motoneurons survive, whereas reducing the target size increases elimination. This can be explained by the neurons needing a sufficient supply of a growth-promoting substance—a **trophic factor**—to survive. The target cells produce limited amounts of this trophic factor; that is, there is not enough to keep all neurons alive. The neurons innervating the target **compete** for the trophic factor, and only the "winners" survive. Because a limited number of synapses can be formed on each neuron, the axons arriving first have an advantage. The trophic factor is taken up by the nerve terminals at the synaptic sites and transported retrogradely to the cell body. The elimination of surplus neurons appears to occur rapidly, perhaps during a few days in some systems. Overall, this kind of cell death is believed to ensure optimal numerical relationships between, for example, motoneurons and muscle cells. Cell death probably also serves to eliminate incorrect synaptic connections.

Programmed cell death is not uniform throughout the nervous system. In the primordial **cerebral cortex** probably about 90% of the neurons die, whereas in the **spinal cord** few interneurons die. About 50% of motoneurons die, and a similar rate holds for a type of interneuron in the **retina** (amacrine cells). We do not know the reasons for such differences, and many questions remain unanswered concerning programmed cell death. For example, the number of cells that die is not always related to the size of the target.

Apoptosis in the CNS

Cell death as a normal developmental process is termed **apoptosis** (in contrast to necrosis, which means cell death caused by abnormal, nonphysiologic influences). Apoptosis is characterized by the breakdown of DNA to smaller fragments and the subsequent dissolution of the cell. What triggers this process? When certain nerve cells die without the presence of a growth factor, does it happen because the cell needs the factor for vital metabolic processes or because the factor inactivates genes that trigger apoptosis? There is much evidence in favor of the latter explanation—that is, the existence of a genetic death program in each cell. In invertebrates such genes have been identified, and mutations prevent apoptosis that normally would have occurred at a certain stage of development. In vertebrates cell death due to lack of growth factors can be prevented by inhibition of mRNA and protein synthesis—indicating that gene expression is necessary for programmed cell death.

Neurotrophins and Other Growth Factors

The Italian Nobel Prize winner Rita Levi-Montalcini discovered around 1950 a substance that stimulates axonal growth in the peripheral nervous system. This substance—termed **nerve growth factor** (NGF)—is a protein produced by the cells of the target organ. Antibodies against NGF inhibit the growth of axons from autonomic ganglion cells and sensory cells derived from the neural crest. In cell cultures, axons grow into an area containing NGF and retract from areas without it. NGF binds to specific membrane receptors. It is transported retrogradely to the cell body, enabling effects on gene expressions. After the discovery of NGF, several related neuronal growth factors were

identified. Together they form the **neurotrophin family**, consisting of NGF, **brain-derived neurotrophic factor** (BDNF), and several others (neurotrophin NT-3, NT-4, and so forth). Apart from regulating many aspects of neuronal growth and differentiation during prenatal development, they are involved in synaptic plasticity and neuronal survival in the adult nervous system. The neurotrophins bind to specific **tyrosine-kinase receptors** (Trk) and to an unrelated receptor, **p75NTR** (p75 neurotrophin receptor).[2] The two kinds of receptor may help to explain further why the effects of neurotrophins are highly complex and not fully understood. Among other differences, the effects mediated via Trk and p75NTR receptors tend to be opposite. Thus, nerve growth factor prevents programmed cell death by binding to TrkA receptors, whereas binding to p75NTR promotes it. Thus, the effects of a neurotrophin on a certain neuronal population depend on the local expression of neurotrophin receptors (e.g., the balance between expression of Trk and p75 receptors). The expression of the neurotrophins and their receptors appear to be dynamically regulated by a complex interaction among intrinsic and extrinsic factors.[3] Thus, neurotrophin effects would differ among neuronal populations and on the same population at different points of time.

Among other growth factors acting in the brain are the **fibroblast growth factors** (FGFs), which influence differentiation and survival of several kinds of neurons. Several other growth factors that were initially discovered in the peripheral tissues are also expressed in the brain.

Neurotrophins, Plasticity, and Disease

As mentioned, neurotrophins play a role not only during normal development but also in the adult brain. The finding that expression of neurotrophins can be use dependent has attracted special interest in their role in **synaptic plasticity.** BDNF, for example, is involved in the induction of LTP. In the visual cortex, the expression of the receptor TrkB parallels the **sensitive period** in development, and the synthesis increases with increased use of the visual system. Beneficial effects of **physical activity** on

---

2. The Trk receptors constitute a family of three—TrkA, TrkB, and TrkC—each of which can be activated by one or more of the neurotrophins NGF, BDNF, NT-3, and NT-4. Overall, NGF seems to exert its main effects via TrkA receptors, while BDNF acts mainly via TrkB. The p75NTR belongs to the **tumor necrosis factor** receptor family (tumor necrosis factor is an inflammatory cytokine released from leukocytes, inducing apoptosis via its receptors).

3. For example, while the expression of p75NTR in normal adult brain is minimal, it increases after injury. At the same time, Trk receptor expression may be reduced. This would tend to push the effect of neurotrophin receptor activation from supporting cell survival to inducing cell death.

cognitive functions and neurogenesis appear at least in part to be mediated by increased expression of BDNF (and perhaps NGF).

Neurotrophins are also intensely investigated for their possible beneficial effects after **brain injury**. For example, administration of growth factors at the site of injured neurons might help them survive. In animal experiments, injection of NGF into the ventricular system prevented delayed cell death in the hippocampus after a period without blood supply. The role of neurotrophins in **neurodegenerative diseases** has also attracted interest. One theory proposes that the senile plaques in the brain of Alzheimer patients down-regulate FGF in their environment, thus causing neuronal death. In Parkinson's disease and Huntington's disease as well, the level of FGF is apparently reduced. The connection between such changes and the disease process is not clear, however.

Prolonged **stress** can cause neuronal death in experimental animals. Decreased production of neurotrophins—BDNF in particular—may mediate the effect of stress. Alterations of growth factors also occur in patients with severe **depression**, and both antidepressant drugs and electroconvulsive therapy have been reported to increase expression of BDNF (among other effects).

Myelination Is Required for Neuronal Connections to Function Optimally

Myelination of axons starts in the **fourth month** of gestation and is largely completed 2 to 3 years after birth. Although many axons in the CNS remain unmyelinated, the process of myelination is clearly related to functional maturation of neuronal interconnections. Full functional capacity cannot be expected before myelination is completed. As for the individual neuron, myelination starts at the soma and proceeds distally. Different tracts are myelinated at different times. Overall, tracts concerned with basic tasks, necessary for life, are the first to be myelinated (such as sucking, swallowing, retraction from harmful stimuli, emptying of bowel and bladder, and so forth). Such connections are also phylogenetically the oldest.

In the **spinal cord**, myelination starts in the cervical region and proceeds in the caudal direction. First to be myelinated are the propriospinal fibers (interconnecting various spinal segments). Ventral root motor fibers are myelinated earlier than the dorsal root sensory fibers. Myelination of ascending spinal tracts starts in the sixth fetal month, and tracts descending from the brain stem follow (reticulospinal and vestibulospinal tracts). These tracts need to be functioning at birth. In contrast, the **pyramidal tract**, which controls the most precise voluntary movements, is fully myelinated only about 2 years after birth. Connections from the cerebral cortex to the **cerebellum** (see Fig. 24.7) are myelinated at the same time as the pyramidal tract, which seems logical because these connections are important for coordination of voluntary movements.

Myelination of the **cranial nerves** starts in the sixth fetal month, except for the optic nerve (which is a central tract and not a peripheral nerve). Myelination starts shortly before birth in the optic nerve.

In the **cerebral cortex,** myelination begins shortly before birth, first in motor and sensory areas. The association areas are mainly myelinated during the first 4 months after birth, although myelination continues after that period. The last regions to become fully myelinated are the association areas in the frontal lobe (prefrontal cortex).

White Matter Increases until Adulthood

Although myelination largely occurs according to the pattern described earlier, longitudinal magnetic resonance imaging (MRI) studies indicate that the relative proportion of white matter in the brain increases (although slightly) until adult age. For example, the cross section of the corpus callosum increases from 5 to 18 years of age. Presumably, after the age of 2 to 3 years the increase in white matter is caused by increased myelin-sheath thickness of already myelinated axons. Concomitant with increased white matter, the grey matter is reduced.

Malformations of the Nervous System

We discussed migration disorders as a cause of malformations, especially of the cerebral cortex. These malformations are special since the development of the cerebral cortex is so protracted, ending late in the prenatal period. Here we consider other kinds of malformations that occur before the gross shape of the CNS has been established.

Malformations of the nervous system, as in other organs of the body, may be caused by genes or environmental factors (or by both). External agents, such as viruses and drugs, are most likely to cause serious malformations or maldevelopment if they act in the period of maximal differentiation—that is, from the **third to eighth week** after fertilization (most organs are formed during the embryonic period from the fourth to eighth week). Harmful influences before this stage usually lead to early death of the embryo.

Among the most common malformations is **defective closure** of the neural tube, which may be caused by various genetic and environmental factors. Normally, the closure is completed by the end of the fourth week. Lack of closure may affect the whole length of the neural tube but is most often restricted to either the cranial or the caudal end. When the neural tube does not develop normally, neither do overlying structures such as the skull, parts of the vertebral column, and the skin. Their normal development depends on induction by diffusible substances (morphogens) from the nervous tissue. With defective closure of the cranial end, the brain does not develop, and the remainder of the neural plate degenerates. This condition is termed **anencephaly**. Such fetuses may sometimes live until birth but always die shortly after. A defective closure of the spinal cord (most often in the lumbosacral part) is termed **spina bifida** because the vertebral arch and soft tissue dorsal to the cord do not develop normally. This condition may vary in severity. In the most serious cases the vertebral arches, muscles, and skin are absent and there is herniation of the coverings of the cord that contain degenerated nervous tissue (**meningomyelocele**). Less severe cases may involve herniation of the coverings but keep the spinal cord intact, whereas the least affected have only partial lack of the vertebral arch (**spina bifida occulta**). In the most serious cases, the cord does not develop normally, leading to pareses and sensory disturbances of the legs. When the nervous supply is deficient, the muscles do not develop to their normal size and strength.

MECHANISMS FOR ESTABLISHMENT OF SPECIFIC CONNECTIONS

The main morphologic features of the nervous system—such as its macroscopic form, the positions of major nuclei, and their interconnections—arise before birth and shortly after. In a sense, this represents the **hard wiring** of the brain. In this section, we discuss mechanisms important for forming the brain's "wiring diagrams." The growth of axons is often surprisingly goal-directed, indicating the existence of guiding mechanisms. We discuss some mechanisms that can aid axons in selecting their target. The number of known interacting players at the cellular and molecular levels is enormous, and many more are probably yet to be identified. It should therefore not come as a surprise that we cannot fully explain how the amazing connectional specificity of the mature nervous system arises.

Trial and Error

Although trial and error cannot explain the overall development of orderly connections in the nervous system, it nevertheless plays a role at the local level. Indeed, modern imagining methods permitting in vivo observation of growing neurons show that growth and retraction of neuronal processes are highly dynamic processes. Thus, at the same time that growth cones randomly explore their immediate environment and new spines bud from dendrites, errors are corrected continuously by retraction of unsuccessful growth cones and spines. The development of neuronal networks is therefore a very complex interplay of simultaneous building up and tearing down, resembling the work of a sculptor who adds an excess of clay to be able to carve out the fine details.

Distances Are Small in the Early Embryo

Knowing the complexity of the mature nervous system, one might think that most of the human genome must be devoted to specification of neuronal connections. This is not the case, of course. We should bear in mind that the whole embryo is only a few millimeters to a couple of centimeters long during the stages of most intense axonal outgrowths. Thus, the distances that axons have to grow to reach their targets are usually very short. Further, the topography of the nervous system at these early stages is also much simpler than later, as not all nuclear groups develop simultaneously. Our present knowledge suggests that combined actions of several mechanisms, each of them relatively simple, can explain how the specificity of the nervous system arises.

Time of Neuronal "Birth"

The genetically programmed time of neuronal birth can explain the development of specific connections in many cases (Fig. 9.15). If at the time of axonal outgrowth from one neuronal group only certain neurons are present in the direction of growth, the axons will hit their correct target without specific recognition molecules. In addition, programming of neurons for maximal synapse formation during a limited period ensures that synapses are established upon arrival of the proper axons. The time during which neurons readily produce synapses is usually limited. Axons encountering a particular neuronal group at a later stage cannot establish synapses, and therefore they either retract or grow past to other targets.

Trophic Factors

Timing of neuronal birth and maturation cannot explain all aspects of specificity, however. For example, what decides the direction of **axonal outgrowths**? For some neurons, such as pyramidal cells in the cerebral cortex, the initial growth direction is genetically determined. After that, however, signals in the environment of the axons determine the growth direction. Thus, cortical pyramidal cells are occasionally "inverted" with their apical dendrite pointing toward the white matter instead of toward the cortical surface. In such cases, the axons start growing toward the pial surface but soon reverse direction and grow toward the white matter, as do normal pyramidal cells (see Fig. 33.6). Such findings are best explained by the target

Figure 9.15

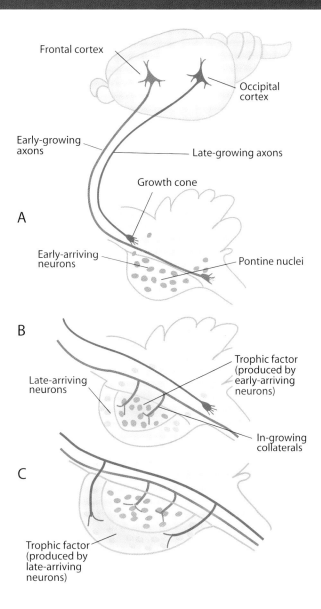

Development of topographically organized connections: example from the corticopontine projection (cf. Fig. 24.11). **A:** Because the axons from the frontal lobe start growing earlier than axons from the occipital lobe, they have reached further down in the brain stem. At this stage, neurons migrate into the ventral pons to form the pontine nuclei. **B:** At a later stage, the early-arriving pontine neurons produce a trophic substance that attracts collaterals from the descending axons. However, only the axons from the frontal lobe are sufficiently mature to emit collaterals at this stage (2 days elapse from the time the axons arrive in the pons until they can form collaterals). Immature neurons continue to invade the ventral pons and form a shell around the early-arriving neurons. **C:** Late-arriving pontine neurons are now sufficiently mature to produce the trophic factor, whereas the early-arriving ones have stopped their production. At this later stage, only the axons from the occipital lobe can emit collaterals. Thus, axons from different parts of the cerebral cortex end in different parts of the pontine nuclei, forming the orderly topographic arrangement seen in the adult (see Fig. 24.8). In this example, the topographic arrangement can be explained by genetically programmed differences in the time of birth for neurons in various parts of the cerebral cortex and the pontine nuclei. Other mechanisms may operate as well. (Based on experimental studies in the rat by Leergaard, Lakke, and Bjaalie 1995.)

organs producing growth-promoting substances—**trophic factors**—that diffuse in the tissue. Axons then grow in the direction of increasing concentration of the factor, which binds to specific receptors, so that only axons expressing the receptor are attracted. This may explain why axons from a neuronal group in some cases grow toward their correct target even if the neuronal group has been moved to another site before axonal outgrowth.

Cell-Adhesion Molecules and Fasciculation

In other instances, neurons or glia along the route apparently express specific molecules that function as "**signposts**." When the first **pioneer axons** have reached their target, the rest of the axons can get there simply by following the pioneers. (The pioneers may have a relatively simple task because, as mentioned, the distances they grow are very short and the "landscape" is simple.) Axons with a common target can express at their surface **neuronal-cell adhesion molecules** (N-CAMs) that make them sticky (N-CAMs are proteins related to the immunoglobulins). Axons expressing a particular kind of N-CAM are then kept together, whereas others are repelled or inhibited in their growth. In this way axons with common targets form bundles, or fascicles, and the phenomenon is termed **fasciculation.** The well-defined tracts of the nervous system arise in this way.

Growth Cones and Their Interactions with N-CAMs and Other Molecules

The many trophic factors, signpost molecules, recognition molecules, and N-CAMs governing the establishment of specific connections mostly act on the axonal **growth cone**. The growth cone is an expanded part of the tip of a growing axon (Fig. 9.16). It continuously sends out small extensions, or **filopodia**, as if exploring its immediate surroundings. Filopodia encountering the proper molecules in the tissue are stabilized, and this determines the direction of further growth, while other filopodia retract. The stabilization depends on increased number of **actin** molecules in the filopodia and of **microtubules** in the axon. Several N-CAMS influence the growth of the axon when they are present near the growth cone. These N-CAMs can be expressed at the surface of both the growth cone and the nearby cells. Binding of the N-CAM molecules to each other causes stickiness. In other instances, N-CAMs bind to specific receptors in the growth cone membrane and thus activate intracellular second messengers (by influx of Ca^{2+} ions). There are also **extracellular molecules** with actions on the growth cone, such as **laminin**, which is bound to the basal lamina. Laminin binds to receptors in the growth cone membrane. Laminin can occur transiently along the path of growing axons in the peripheral nervous system, guiding the growth toward the target organ. Although the action of laminin is not by itself specific, its time-specific expression ensures that only axons present at the proper time will grow.

Figure 9.16

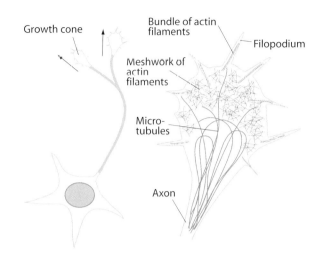

The axonal growth cone. A growth cone contains a central and stable bundle of microtubules. In addition, dynamic microtubules extend toward the filopodia and work together with actin filaments. The filopodia contain bundles of actin filaments providing motility. The filopodia extend or retract depending on the specific molecules they meet in their immediate environment. (Based on Kalil and Dent 2005.)

This is another example of the importance of **timing**—in this case of axonal outgrowth—during development.

Examples of Axonal Pathfinding

The "inverted" pyramidal cells, previously mentioned, exemplify that gradients of substances in the environment of the axon govern growth direction. Another example concerns the development of descending connections from the cerebral cortex—that is, the outgrowth of axons from **projection neurons** in the cerebral cortex. Many such axons reach the spinal cord and, in addition, emit collaterals to nuclei in the brain stem. Initially, the axons grow toward the cord without sending out collaterals (Fig. 9.15A). After a certain interval or waiting time, however, collaterals grow out and innervate the **pontine nuclei** (Fig. 9.15B). The collaterals to the pontine nuclei arise just when the pontine neurons have reached a certain stage of maturation (postmitotic age). Most likely, the pontine neurons at this stage produce a trophic factor that "attracts" growing axons. Such a mechanism, depending on diffusion, can operate only over short distances. Thus, it is less likely that trophic factors produced in the spinal cord are responsible for the goal-directed growth of corticospinal axons.

When the distance to the target is too long for trophic factors alone to guide axonal growth, we assume that there are **signpost** molecules along the route. One example illustrating this is the growth of axons from the retina through the **optic chiasm**. Figure 16.14 shows the arrangement of the axons from various parts of the retina as they pass through the optic chiasm in the adult. Axons from the nasal retina cross to the other side, whereas axons from the temporal retina pass ipsilaterally—that is, without crossing. In the adult, crossing and ipsilateral axons are segregated as they approach the optic chiasm. During the first outgrowth, however, axons from the nasal and temporal parts of the retina are mixed. Nevertheless, they take the correct path when they reach the region of the chiasm, even when this requires that some have to bend 90 degrees and that some axons must cross each other. Interaction between axons from the two eyes is not necessary, either. Thus, even if one of the eye primordia is removed before the axons have reached the optic chiasm, the axons from the remaining eye still find their way through. Neither can trophic factors from the target organ of the axons (a thalamic nucleus) play a decisive role because this nucleus is not yet established at the time the axons grow through the optic chiasm. Therefore, local clues in the region of the optic chiasm must guide the axons—at least during the first pioneering phase. In the next few weeks—when thousands of axons follow the pioneers through the chiasm—cell adhesion molecules and fasciculation are important.

Another example of the importance of local signpost cues for axonal pathfinding is the development of skeletal muscle nerve supply by **spinal motoneurons**. Even after removal of the primordial muscle, the axons that would normally supply it still find their way to the site of the (removed) muscle.

Elimination of Axon Collaterals and Synapses

As mentioned, the terminal area of a group of axons is often more extensive initially than after maturation, forming a surplus of synapses. Newborn monkeys, for example, have higher numbers of synapses on each neuron in many parts of the brain than adult monkeys (Fig. 9.17). Thus, many collaterals and synapses are eliminated during further development. When it occurs in early phases of development (prenatally), elimination is probably due mainly to programmed cell death. Later on, competition for growth factors may be more important. In this way, the axonal ramifications of each neuron are pruned, thereby increasing the spatial precision of connections. In other instances, neurons initially send axon collaterals to two (or more) nuclei, but only one collateral survives while the other disappears during further development.

Elimination of axon collaterals is exemplified by the development of descending connections from the **visual cortex**. Initially, the axons grow down to the spinal cord, sending off collaterals to the pontine nuclei (among other areas) on their way (Fig. 9.15). After the pontine collaterals are established, those to the cord disappear (in adult animals there are no connections from the visual cortex to the cord). We do not know how this happens; perhaps trophic factors from the cord or medulla "trick" the axons to grow beyond their real targets. We may further assume that, once in the cord, the axons are not able to establish synapses, perhaps because they lack specific recognition molecules or simply because the spinal neurons are not receptive at the time the axons arrive.

A further example concerns descending axons from the forelimb region of the **motor cortex** (of rodents). Initially, such axons reach both the cervical and the lumbar parts of the cord (innervating the forelimb and the hind limb, respectively). Collaterals enter the spinal gray matter only in the cervical region, however, and the branch to the lumbar cord disappears without having established synapses.

Formation and Elimination of Synapses from Newborn to Adult

While the number of neurons in the human cerebral cortex appears to be fairly constant after the twenty-eighth gestational week, the **synaptic densities** undergo marked changes until the end of puberty. In general, the synaptic density in the cerebral cortex increases steeply from before birth to late in the first postnatal year. Thereafter, the density declines slowly—presumably due to elimination of synapses—until reaching adult values between age 10 and 15. There appears to be large variations among cortical areas, with earlier maximum density and a shorter period of synapse elimination in primary sensory areas than in association areas. In the visual cortex, synaptic density at birth is about 10% of that at 4 to 8 months after birth, when the number of synapses per neuron is estimated to be 15,000. Thereafter, the number

---

Figure 9.17

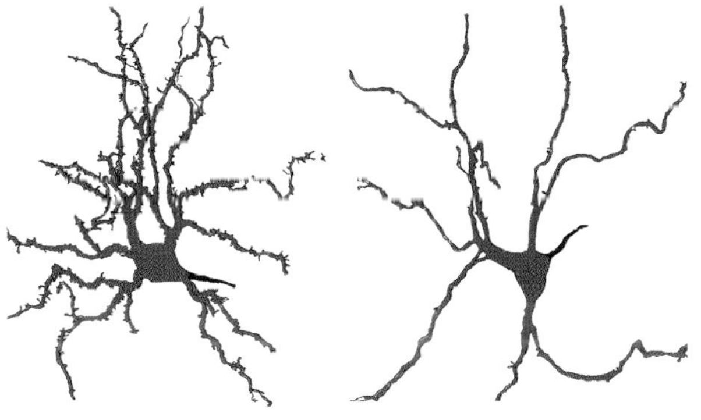

Elimination of dendritic branches and dendritic spines during postnatal development. Drawing of Golgi-impregnated neurons from the monkey pontine nuclei.

1 month   Adult

Figure 9.18

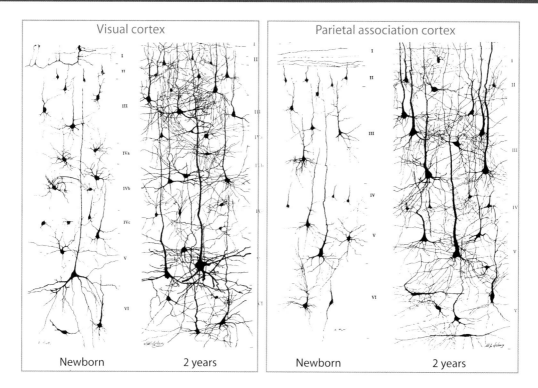

Visual cortex		Parietal association cortex	
Newborn	2 years	Newborn	2 years

Postnatal development of the human cerebral cortex. Drawings based on Golgi sections from the visual cortex showing the increase in dendritic arborizations from birth and until the age of 2 years. The increase in dendritic arborization is most likely related to the increase in the number of synapses per neuron. (From Conel 1939.)

Strong arguments for lack of specification of cortical connections at birth come from observations of infants in whom the left hemisphere has been damaged or removed. Surprisingly, such children can develop virtually normal language. This must mean that networks in the right hemisphere, which would not normally be devoted to language, can take over the task. Further, studies that correlate brain activity and language development suggest that the relevant networks undergo considerable development during the first years of life. Thus, the child's first attempts at verbal communication are associated with widespread activation in both hemispheres, whereas at 2 years the cortical activation has changed toward the adult pattern with activation of specific regions in the left hemisphere.

"Enriched Environments" and Synaptic Plasticity

Numerous animal experiments have shown robust effects of environmental conditions on brain structure and biochemistry, as well as on behavior. Early experiments showed, for example, that dendritic arborizations were more extensive in the cerebral cortex of rats raised in an **enriched environment** (a simulated natural environment with ample space and access to toys) than in rats raised in standard laboratory cages.[7] Brains of wild and tame animals represent a naturally occurring analog of experiments with enriched environments. Indeed, **wild animals** have somewhat larger brains than tame animals of the same species. The responsible influence must occur quite early, because animals born in the wild and later tamed have the same brain size as wild animals. The difference is not genetic, however, because individuals of the first generation born in captivity have smaller brains than their wild relatives. Experimental enrichment in the early postnatal period of rats induced increased synaptic density in the **hippocampus** and improved performance in certain learning and

---

7. It should be emphasized that so-called enriched environments are enriched only as compared with standard laboratory conditions. The latter is a situation of **deprivation** rather than of normality. Both the standard and the enriched conditions are therefore highly artificial. Nevertheless, when interpreted with caution, experiments with enriched environments give robust evidence of the role of environmental factors in brain development and function.

memory tasks. Results from experiments on the **motor system** further support the association between synaptic plasticity and learning: among young adult rats doing different motor tasks, some developed more synapses per neuron in the **cerebellar cortex** than others. The decisive factor was not the amount of motor activity but that the activity implied learning of new motor behaviors. Other experiments show that learning of specific skills is associated with synaptic changes in cortical areas involved in the task. For example, as monkeys gradually improved their performance in distinguishing tones of different frequencies, the part of the **auditory cortex** representing the particular frequencies increased in size. Similar changes occur in the **motor cortex** during learning of motor skills.

The preceding examples strongly suggest that formation and modification of synapses are closely linked with **learning**. It is plausible, for example, that life in the wild (or in an artificially enriched environment) requires the acquisition of a broader repertoire of adaptive behaviors than life in the cage or the bin. In general, there is good reason to assert that task-specific networks become operational during childhood because of learning processes driven by active interactions between the individual and his or her environment.

Information Must Be Meaningful

Nerve impulses are not by themselves sufficient for normal development, as shown in many animal experiments. For example, in goldfish exposed only to diffuse light (devoid of information) at the time retinal axons form synapses in the **optic tectum**, the normal ordered map of the visual environment does not develop properly. Another example concerns the development of connections from the retina to the **visual cortex**. At first, neurons in the visual cortex are influenced with equal strength from each eye. Soon after birth, however, neurons in the cortex segregate into groups, with a dominant input from one eye and a weaker input from the other. This phenomenon is called **eye dominance**. When all impulse traffic from the retina is blocked in kittens, eye dominance does not develop: each neuron continues to respond equally well to signals from either eye. Artificial electric stimulation of the optic nerve can nevertheless induce eye dominance even though the animal is blind, but only if the signals from the two eyes arrive with a minute time difference (corresponding to what occurs under natural conditions with light falling on the two retinas). With natural use of the system during development, axon terminals conveying signals from the

two eyes compete for the available synaptic sites on each neuron.

Both of the aforementioned examples from the visual system show that, in order to induce the normal synaptic pattern and connectivity, nerve impulses must convey **meaningful information**—that is, information that helps the animal adapt to its environment. (See also Chapter 4, under "Under Which Conditions Do Synaptic Changes Occur?".)

Early Social Experience Alters Brain Structure and Function

Human experiences and animal experiments strongly suggest that social conditions in early childhood can influence adult emotional and cognitive behavior and that this is associated with alterations of brain structure. Such lasting effects are caused by **epigenetic** mechanisms, by which experiences induce altered gene expressions. For example, rat pups of mothers spending much time **licking** and **grooming** them develop higher synaptic density in the **hippocampus** than do pups with mothers who pay less attention to them. In agreement with alterations of the hippocampus, the pups of "high-licking" mothers also show enhanced spatial learning and memory. Further, as adults, the offspring of high-licking mothers show a different response to stress than offspring of low-licking mothers.[8] Another example concerns the effects of exposing rat pups to **traumatic emotional experiences**, for example by separating them from their mothers. Such pups show synaptic alterations in the **anterior cingulate gyrus**, a region that is involved in emotional processing. Further, separation was associated with altered development of neural networks that control emotional responses mediated by the **autonomic nervous system.** Early life-stress in humans—for example as experienced by children in low **socioeconomic** conditions—is associated with increased risk of diseases in later life (e.g., type 2 diabetes, cardiovascular diseases, and cancer). One important cause appears to be elevated levels of inflammation as a result of

---

8. This influence appears to be mediated by (at least) two intracellular pathways. First, a **high licking** mother, as compared with a **low-licking** one, induces higher levels of serotonin in the pup's brain. This in turn leads to increased NGF expression in the hippocampus. In addition, the glucocorticoid receptor gene in the hippocampus is demethylated. This makes the gene permanently more accessible to activation by NGF, resulting in permanent high levels of glucocorticoid receptors in the hippocampus. The level of glucocorticoid receptors relates to behavioral and endocrine responses to stress in the adult animal.

The main reason for the problems encountered by this boy (and others in his situation) is most likely that he had not established the cortical networks needed for integrating visual information with other sensory modalities. Thus, his brain was not capable of using the wealth of information provided by his eyes. In contrast, if the visual system has been used normally during the sensitive period in infancy and early childhood, even many years of temporary blindness would had have no serious effects on visual capacities.

Another example concerns children who are born **deaf** and later receive a **cochlear implant** that supplies the brain with information about sounds of different frequencies. Experience shows that such children can develop useful language and hearing behavior if the implant is provided early—that is, during the first 2 to 3 years of life. As with vision, access to auditory information during the sensitive period is necessary for proper development of the hearing system. To use sounds as a basis for development of language, for example, numerous specific connections must be formed in the brain between the auditory cortex and other areas of the cerebral cortex. Such connections cannot be properly formed after the sensitive period. At least in part, this is due to other systems taking over the parts of the cerebral cortex that are normally engaged in auditory functions. Thus, deaf children activate the auditory cortex when using sign language (this is called **cross-modal plasticity**). Cochlear implants in such children do not restore sound activation of the auditory cortex.

The Nervous System and Aging

Many presumably harmful changes occur in the brain as we grow older. There are, for example, reductions of average brain **weight**, **synaptic numbers**, and **neurotransmitters**. There is also a loss of myelinated nerve fibers, and together all these changes would be expected to cause less efficient communication in neuronal networks. Age-related changes appear to affect especially networks of the **prefrontal cortex** and the **medial temporal lobe**—regions critically involved in memory and other cognitive functions. Nevertheless, most healthy elderly persons function remarkably well in spite of biologic alterations—with only a minor reduction of recent memory and some slowing of movements and mental processes. This is believed to result from compensatory, use-dependent plasticity initiated in response to the biologic changes. Thus, elderly individuals seem to activate larger parts of the brain when solving mental tasks (often both hemispheres are activated in contrast to strictly unilateral activation in younger people). Aging also entails a fairly marked loss of **peripheral receptors**, which may compromise vision, hearing, and balance. Such loss of peripheral receptors is often more bothersome than the changes occurring in the brain.

In **neurodegenerative diseases**, loss of neurons and their processes usually proceeds for many years before symptoms occur. This is at least partly due to compensatory processes going on in parallel with neuronal loss. The emerging symptoms depend mainly on which parts of the brain are subject to the neuronal loss. In spite of being caused by different mutations, **misfolding** of intracellular proteins occurs in many neurodegenerative diseases. Misfolding appears to initiate cytotoxicity. Neurodegenerative diseases with massive loss of neurons in the cerebral cortex lead to **dementia**, with Alzheimer's disease (AD) as the most common. This disease is characterized by—in addition to cortical neuronal loss—degeneration of the cholinergic **basal nucleus** (of Meynert) and marked loss of **acetylcholine** in the cortex.

AGE-RELATED CHANGES IN THE NORMAL BRAIN AND THEIR CONSEQUENCES

Biologic Changes and Their Interpretations

Comparisons of the brains of young and old persons have revealed several biologic differences. These include a reduction of average brain **weight**, enlargement of ventricles (indicative of tissue atrophy), the appearance of **degenerative patches**, and **neuronal shrinkage** (which occurs primarily in very old people). **Dendritic trees** and **synaptic numbers** appear to be reduced in the cerebral cortex. Reduced **blood flow** of the whole brain or certain regions has been found in several studies. Several other changes, particularly in **neurotransmitters** and their **receptors**, have been reported. With imaging techniques, several alterations have been reported, notably change of both **gray** and **white matter**.

The relationship between biologic changes and impairments of brain performance is still debated, however. This is partly because of conflicting evidence on several important points and uncertain interpretations of findings. Interpretations are hampered, for example, because the biologic differences usually represent small group averages, while the individual differences within each age group may be much larger. Because detailed information of a person's behavioral and cognitive performance is seldom available when examining the brain after death, correlations must be tentative. In animal experiments, formal testing can be performed before examining the brain, enabling more affirmative conclusions regarding the correlation between behavior and age-related brain alterations. Unfortunately, some biologic alterations that are well documented in aged rats and monkeys are controversial in humans.

Memory Impairment in the Elderly

Solid evidence links age-dependent memory loss to changes in specific areas of the brain. Studies of aged rats indicate that their memory impairments are due to anatomic and physiologic changes in the **hippocampal region**. The hippocampus and surrounding parts of the temporal lobe are necessary for the storage and retrieval of events, faces, names, and so forth (see Chapter 32). The changes occurring in the hippocampus are quite specific and affect only certain kinds of neurons and synapses. Some changes are presumably caused by compensatory mechanisms. For example, one kind of neuron receives fewer synapses, but each nerve terminal releases more transmitter. Long-term potentiation is more difficult to produce and does not last as long in aged rats as in young ones. The memory impairment in aged monkeys has the same characteristics as in young monkeys after removal of the medial temporal lobe. Thus, it seems likely that age-dependent loss of recent memory is caused primarily by specific changes in the hippocampus and surrounding parts of the medial temporal lobe. In addition, changes of the dorsolateral parts of the prefrontal cortex are associated with reduced working memory (the ability to hold a number of items temporarily in memory).

Loss of Peripheral Sensory Receptors with Age

For everyday problems of the elderly, changes in the central nervous system (CNS) may be less important than loss of sensory cells and neurons of the peripheral sensory organs. These losses are of sight and hearing in particular, but joint sense and sense of equilibrium also deteriorate with advancing age. For example, animal experiments show that the muscle spindles lose dynamic sensitivity. This might result in slower reflex responses to unexpected, sudden movements of the limbs. In general, thick myelinated, fast-conducting fibers are more vulnerable during aging than thin fibers. Especially, impaired **proprioception** and cutaneous sensation in the lower extremities may contribute to increased **risk of falling** among the elderly.

Transmission of sensory signals at lower levels of the CNS is serial—that is, the different links in the chain are coupled one after another (see Fig. 14.1). This contrasts with the high degree of parallel processing taking place at higher levels, particularly in the cerebral cortex. If one link in a sensory pathway is broken, all transmission stops, and the brain can compensate for the loss of sensory information only by learning to utilize alternative sources. This usually requires intense training to induce plastic changes in relevant brain networks. Unfortunately, elderly persons experiencing impaired balance tend to become less active, thus increasing the balance problem.

Balance and Loss of Vestibular Receptors

Studies of eye movements show that the **vestibulo-ocular reflex (VOR)** is less accurate in persons older than 75 than in younger persons. This reflex ensures that the gaze is kept fixed at one point in the environment when the head rotates (to keep the retinal image stable). Further, **optokinetic eye movements** become more sluggish in old age. Such eye movements are elicited when the environment moves—for example, when looking out of a car—so that the gaze is kept fixed. Suppression of the VOR, which is necessary when the head rotates in the same direction as the visual scene, is also impaired in many elderly persons. All these changes may cause difficulties with vision and orientation while moving, especially if the movement is rapid. This may be an important factor in the impaired balance and dizziness that bothers many elderly people. At the cellular level, a major cause of impaired equilibrium and eye movements may be loss of sensory cells in the vestibular apparatus. A 40% loss has been reported in persons 75 years of age.

Use-Dependent Plasticity May Compensate for Age-Dependent Losses

As we grow older, potentially harmful changes occur in the brain, as discussed in the preceding text. Yet, most elderly people manage remarkably well and show only minor functional deficits, which often become apparent only in situations with high demands. As noted by Denise Park and Patricia Reuter-Lorenz (2008, p. 183): "The puzzle for cognitive neuroscientists is not so much in explaining age-related decline, but rather in understanding the high level of cognitive success that can be maintained by older adults in the face of such significant neurobiological changes." There is now much evidence that this seeming paradox arises because the nervous system remains plastic throughout life (even though the plasticity decreases with advancing age). Thus, even in old age we can learn and thereby uphold functions that are threatened by loss of neuronal elements. Probably this process is not principally different from what takes place at any age when the brain is challenged—be it by damage or disease, need for new skills, or novel environments.

Figure 10.1

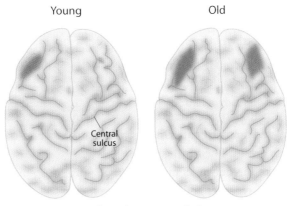

Young   Old

Central
sulcus

Prefrontal activation during
a demanding cognitive task

Altered brain activation patterns in the elderly. Comparisons with functional **MRI** of young and elderly people (older than 65 years) during execution of various cognitive tasks shows clear differences. This figure shows (in a very simplified form) that during a demanding verb-generation task, elderly persons activate the prefrontal cortex on both sides, whereas young people activate only one side (differences are apparent also in other parts of the brain). This extra activation most likely is due to compensatory (plastic) processes. It would mean that elderly people, while solving the task as well as young people, must allocate more resources to the task.

Interestingly, brain-imaging studies show that elderly and young people have different patterns of **cortical activation** during cognitive tasks, even when performance is equal. In particular, processes that are strongly lateralized in the young are more evenly divided between the two hemispheres in the elderly (Fig. 10.1). Much evidence supports that this activation pattern in the elderly is a sign of functional compensation rather than of faulty processing. For example, the tendency to use both hemispheres is associated with higher performance compared with other elderly persons using mainly one hemisphere. Elderly persons show less hippocampal activation than young people on certain **memory** tests, presumably because of age-related alterations in the hippocampal region. Among the elderly, those showing increased prefrontal activation (compared with young persons and age-matched controls) performed better on memory tests than those with less prefrontal activation. This suggests that increased prefrontal activation in the elderly compensates for reduced performance of the hippocampal region. Disrupting cortical processing by transcranial magnetic stimulation (TMS) supports that the bilateral frontal activation in the elderly is of functional significance. Thus, in the young, TMS of the left prefrontal region influenced memory performance most severely, while in older adults application to either the left or the right hemisphere reduced their performance equally. Also, for successful **motor performance**, larger parts of the cortex and the cerebellum are recruited in elderly than in young persons.

Together, these and other observations strongly suggest that plastic changes occur in the aging brain and that they counteract the detrimental effects of age-related loss of neural elements.

The Benefit of Experience

Normal aging does not affect everyday activities significantly. Indeed, it appears that all activities (motor or intellectual) that have become highly automated by long practice are quite resistant to age-dependent decline. Both speed and precision can then be maintained into advancing age. We need only think of many musicians performing with excellence after 80. Preserved superior spatial memory in old **taxi drivers** provides another example of the effect of experience. Further, a study comparing young and old **bridge** and **chess** players concluded that there was no clear age-related decline in performance, with prior experience being more important than the player's age. A generally reduced short term memory in the older players is presumably compensated by superior card recognition and specific memory for cards. Thus, old experienced players remembered more eventually in neuronal death. Although many factors are implied, **glutamate** and glutamate receptors are under particularly strong suspicion as the main villains in this drama. Thus, ischemia leads to excessive release of glutamate (see Chapter 5, under "NMDA Receptors: Mediators of Both Learning and Neuronal Damage"). In an ischemic region, whether it is due to edema, bleeding (e.g., after head injuries), or vascular occlusion, there is usually a central zone where the ischemia is so severe that all neurons die. Outside this region, however, there is a zone—the **penumbra** (from Latin *paene* [almost] and *umbra* [shadow])—characterized by neurons that are nonfunctional (unexcitable) but still viable.[1]

Inflammation is a ubiquitous result of tissue injury and seems to add to the cell damage in the ischemic region. Proinflammatory molecules are quickly released from resident astroglia and microglial cells. In addition, the **blood–brain barrier** becomes leaky some hours after the start of an ischemic injury, allowing entry of neutrophils and monocytes from the bloodstream. Cytokines such as **tumor necrosis factor** (TNFα) and **interleukin 1** (IL-1α/β) increase infarct volume in animal experiments. The relative contribution of inflammation in the total picture of ischemic cell death is not clear, however. Thus, some aspects of inflammation may increase cell damage while others promote recovery by clearing debris, remodeling, and so forth.

Vulnerability to Ischemia Differs among Regions

After global ischemia, cell death is not diffusely distributed. Especially **vulnerable** are the neurons in the CA1 field of the hippocampus (see Fig. 32.5). Regional differences in glutamate release or glutamate receptors are probably not the reason. More likely explanations concern differences among regions regarding the presence and regulation of **neurotrophic factors**.

The Search for Neuroprotection

The discovery of the delay between an ischemic episode and irreversible cell damage initiated an enormous research activity to find drugs that prevent or reduce the brain damage. In cases of focal ischemia, hopes were raised to reduce the size of the brain infarct by keeping neurons in the penumbra alive until the circulation improved (improvement may occur spontaneously or by use of **thrombolytic drugs** that dissolve the vascular obstruction). Several of the links in the pathway from start of ischemia to cell death (Fig. 11.1) have been attacked, for example by glutamate

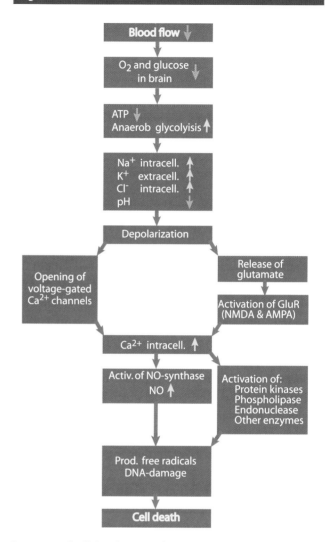

Figure 11.1

Sequence of cellular changes after focal ischemia leading to cell death (*hypothetical*). (Based on Samdani et al. 1997.)

antagonists, calcium blockers, and antioxidants. In addition, drugs that reduce the harmful effects of the inflammatory response are targeted. So far, however, the results have been disappointing in humans in spite of convincing results in animal experiments.

Among the first to be tried were **glutamate-receptor blockers** (especially of the *N*-methyl-D-aspartate [NMDA] receptor). One problem has been intolerable side effects with the doses that are necessary to obtain protection. This might not be surprising considering that glutamatergic transmission participates in virtually every neuronal network. Another reason for the failure of numerous attempts to achieve neuroprotection after stroke may be that although the activation of NMDA receptors undoubtedly is harmful in the early stages of a stroke, it may be necessary for recovery in the delayed phase. Further, it appears that the cellular events evolving in the penumbra are much more complex than assumed—with regard to both the number of substances involved and the temporal profile of cellular changes.

---

1. Cell death in the central region completely devoid of blood supply is due to necrosis, as judged from the electron microscopic appearance. There is some evidence that apoptosis may cause cell death in the penumbra.

Development of Cell Death and Edema: The Glutamate Hypothesis

According to the **glutamate hypothesis**, the sequence of events after a temporary stop of blood flow occur as follows (Fig. 11.1):

1. The loss of energy supply rapidly reduces the activity of the sodium–potassium pump, leading to (among other things)

2. Increased extracellular K^+ concentration that depolarizes the neurons so they fire bursts of action potentials, which leads to

3. Steadily worsening imbalances of ion concentrations across the cell membrane that make the neuron incapable of firing action potentials (electrically silent), while at the same time

4. The extracellular glutamate concentration rises steeply (because, among other things, the ionic imbalances reverse the pumping of glutamate by high-affinity transporters), leading to

5. Enormous activation of glutamate receptors, among them NMDA receptors[2]; this in turn is believed to induce

6. Cell damage, probably because of an uncontrolled rise in intracellular Ca^{2+} concentration. This may harm the cell in various ways, for example, by activating enzymes that degrade proteins and nucleic acids and by activating nitric oxide synthases that leads to production of free radicals. In turn this destroys other vital enzymes.

7. Before the strong inflow of calcium there is an inflow of Na^+ accompanied by Cl^- and water, which causes neurons and glia to swell, thus creating a **cytotoxic brain edema** (in contrast to the **vasogenic brain edema** caused by leaky capillaries; see Chapter 2 under "Aquaporins and Control of Water").

Neurogenesis: Production of New Neurons in the Adult Brain

In adult mammals, new neurons are produced continuously in parts of the **subventricular zone** (see Fig. 9.13) and the **dentate gyrus** of the hippocampal formation (see Fig. 32.5). The neurons produced in the subventricular zone migrate into the olfactory bulb (claims that some also populate the cerebral cortex have not been substantiated).[3] Although only a minority of the newly formed neurons appears to survive, some are incorporated into existing networks. The finding that the number of surviving neurons is use-dependent further strengthens the assumption that the new neurons are of functional significance. Neurogenesis thus seems to represent an additional but spatially restricted form of plasticity, supplementing the ubiquitous synaptic plasticity discussed earlier in this book. It remains to be determined, however, how much and in what way neurogenesis contributes to the role of hippocampus in memory formation.

Nevertheless, adult neurogenesis has attracted much interest and raised hopes that it may be induced in regions with neuronal loss due to injury or disease. Indeed, increased neurogenesis occurs in the subventricular zone after ischemic brain injury in rats, and some neurons were incorporated in adjacent parts of the striatum. Such cells are presumably diverted from their normal migratory path to the olfactory bulb. Unfortunately, the number of surviving cells in animal experiments appears to be too small for recovery of function. Much research is now directed at increasing the proliferation and survival of the newly produced neurons, with the hope that neurogenesis can be controlled in the aid of human stroke recovery.

Why Are Neurogenesis and Regeneration So Restricted in the Human Brain?

Because neurogenesis—contrary to earlier beliefs—*does* occur in adult mammals, one may ask why it is so limited in distribution. Thus, in reptiles and birds neurogenesis occurs in large parts of the nervous system. One reason may be that new neurons might be disturbing rather than beneficial if not properly integrated with existing networks and that the increasing complexity of the mammalian brain

---

2. That **NMDA receptors** are involved in ischemic cell death is indirectly supported by animal experiments involving NMDA-receptor blockers. If such drugs are given even a few hours after an ischemic episode, they reduce or prevent the cell damage. Also, blockers of AMPA receptors provide protection against ischemic cell death in such experiments.

3. A recent study found evidence that neurons produced in the subventricular zone of humans migrate to the striatum rather than to the olfactory bulb (Ernst et al. 2014). In the striatum the new neurons seemed to replace interneurons but not projection neurons.

Restitution after a Stroke Can Be Divided into Two Phases

After a person has a stroke, there is usually a **first phase** of rapid improvement lasting from days to weeks, followed by a **second phase** of slower progress lasting from months to years. Acute damage to neural tissue is usually caused by head injuries with crushing of neural tissue and bleeding or by vascular occlusion caused by thrombosis or an embolus. Secondary changes occur in the **penumbra** (the tissue surrounding the damaged area) such as edema (tissue swelling) and disturbed local circulation. If the edema subsides quickly and the circulation improves in the penumbra, neurons will regain their normal activity (compared with the transient weakness and loss of cutaneous sensation produced by pressure on a peripheral nerve).[4] This is probably why there is often a marked improvement of the patient's condition during the first week or two after the accident. For example, an arm that was totally paralyzed the day after a stroke may in a matter of days be only slightly weaker and clumsier than before the stroke. However, when the condition deteriorates rapidly after the initial insult, the reason is usually that the edema worsens and compromises the blood supply to more and more of the brain.

Certainly, plastic changes occur shortly after an injury (hours, days), as witnessed by animal experiments. Thus, there is probably no sharp distinction between the rapid and the slow phases of recovery—the nervous system starts its adaptation to the new circumstances immediately.

Studies of Recovery after a Stroke in Humans

Many stroke patients have muscular weakness (pareses) in the opposite side of the body as a dominating symptom. This is called **hemiplegia** (*hemi*, half; *plegia*, from Greek *plegé*, stroke). The symptoms are caused by destruction (due to occlusion of an artery or a bleeding) of motor pathways from the cerebral cortex to the brain stem and the cord (see Fig. 22.3). Usually, the injury occurs in the internal capsule (see Figs. 22.7 and 22.14) where the descending fibers from the cerebral cortex are collected. When such injuries cause hemiplegia, we use the term **capsular hemiplegia**. Because patients with this clinical condition are so common, and

because the site of their injury is usually well localized, they have been the subjects for many studies of restitution. Some examples elucidating mechanisms behind restitution in humans are presented here.

Regional cerebral blood flow is closely linked with neuronal activity. Thus, when we find altered blood flow—using positron emission tomography (**PET**) or functional magnetic resonance imaging (**fMRI**)—in a specific part of the brain after a stroke, it is taken as evidence of altered activity caused by the stroke. Numerous studies have compared stroke patients in varying stages of recovery with normal persons (Fig. 11.2). For example, one group of patients with capsular hemiplegia was tested 3 months after the stroke. They were then completely or substantially recovered; for example, they could all perform opposition movements with the fingers. The test was to touch the thumb

Figure 11.2

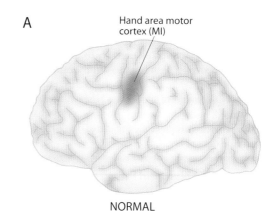

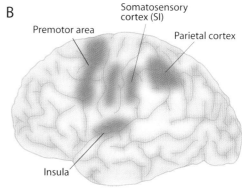

Cortical activation as associated with sequential finger movements. **A:** Normal person shows increased activity only over the motor hand area. **B:** Several areas outside the motor cortex are activated in a stroke patient with good recovery of hand function. Based on several PET and fMRI studies.

4. The often dramatic effect of **thrombolytic therapy** when given during the first few hours after stroke onset is presumably due to salvage of the neurons in the penumbra.

sequentially with the fingers, in a rhythm determined by a metronome. In normal control persons, this task is associated with increased blood flow primarily in the opposite **motor cortex** (and in subcortical motor regions like the cerebellum and the basal ganglia). This fits with the fact that the pyramidal tract, which is necessary for precise finger movements, originates in the motor cortex and is crossed. The patients differed from the controls by showing increased activity in cortical areas that are not normally activated in this kind of simple, routine movement, notably in parts of the **insula, posterior parietal cortex,** and **cingulate gyrus**. In controls, these areas showed increased activity with complex movements and problem-solving tasks that require extra attention. The regions both send association connections to the **premotor area** (see Fig. 22.10) and by this route can influence voluntary movements. Indeed, increased activity is also present in the premotor area. In addition, some of the patients differed from the controls by showing increased activity in motor cortical areas on the same (ipsilateral) side as the affected hand. Such findings suggest that functional recovery after hemiplegia is related to the patients learning to use larger parts of the cerebral cortex for control of simple finger movements than before the damage; some even used motor areas on the same side as the pareses. That some patients also involuntarily co-activated the fingers on the normal side fits with other data indicating that the undamaged hemisphere participates in the recovery.

Use of **transcranial magnetic stimulation** (TMS) in restituted stroke patients has furthermore showed that not only are cortical activation differently distributed but there is also evidence of altered connectivity, as assessed in a resting situation. Further support for **structural changes** during recovery comes from use of MRI-based morphometry, suggesting that an intense rehabilitative training program is associated with increased cortical **gray matter** in the regions most activated by movements.

The involvement of larger parts of the cerebral cortex may explain why simple, previously effortless movements require so much more **attention** and **mental energy** than before the stroke. There is evidence that descending fibers from various cortical motor areas, such as the primary motor cortex (MI), the supplementary motor area, and premotor area occupy different parts of the internal capsule. Thus, when a capsular stroke damages the most powerful and direct pathway from the cortex to the motor neurons—arising in the MI—other, parallel, descending pathways may be "trained" to activate motor neurons more powerfully than before the stroke.

The Contribution of the Undamaged Hemisphere to Recovery

As mentioned, some stroke patients activate the motor cortex of the same side as the pareses—that is, they seem to use the undamaged hemisphere for control of the paretic hand. While not all studies agree that this is beneficial, at least some observations support that use of **uncrossed motor pathways** contribute to recovery. For example, a group of patients with strokes affecting the pyramidal tract in the posterior part of the internal capsule (as verified with MRI) had initially severe paresis of the hand contralateral to the stroke, but they gradually recovered the ability to perform fractionate finger movements. In these patients, TMS of the motor cortex of the undamaged hemisphere evoked movements of both hands—not just of the contralateral hand, as in normal persons. Further, in some recovered stroke patients, involuntary movements of the unaffected fingers—**mirror movements**—accompanied voluntary movements of the paretic fingers. Finally, a peculiar experiment of nature strongly suggests that the undamaged hemisphere participates in recovery in some patients. Thus, two patients with purely motor symptoms who were in good recovery from capsular hemiplegia suffered a second stroke in the internal capsule of the other hemisphere. As expected, their previously normal side became paretic but so did the recovered side. This phenomenon is difficult to explain if we do not assume that the restitution involved the use of motor pathways from the normal hemisphere to ipsilateral muscles.

Most patients do not exhibit mirror movements, however, and several studies found no evidence of contribution of descending pathways from the undamaged hemisphere (e.g., with the use of TMS).

Animal Experiments Elucidating the Mechanisms of Recovery

Substitution implies that neuronal groups and pathways that normally participate only marginally and gradually take over the responsibility for the execution of a task. Clinical recovery after brain damage resembles a long-term learning process, involving strengthening of specific synaptic connections by repeated use.

Some redirecting of impulse traffic can occur even immediately after the damage, however. When the arm region of the **motor cortex** in monkeys doing specific wrist movements is cooled, the movements immediately become slower and weaker. This is expected because the cooling inactivates many pyramidal tract neurons. Activity in the somatosensory cortex increases simultaneously, however, as if this region were prepared to take over immediately. If the somatosensory cortex is then also cooled, the monkey becomes paralytic and is unable to do the movements at all. Cooling of the somatosensory cortex alone has almost no effect on the movements and is not accompanied by

Successful Restitution after Large Lesions of One Hemisphere

The most clear-cut examples of **successful recovery** after early brain damage concern infants with lesions—even very large ones—of one hemisphere.[5] In such cases, although the child remains hemiplegic, cognitive development may be virtually normal. The reason restitution is so successful is probably only partly that the individual neurons are more apt to send out new collaterals and remove others. Another factor could be as important: because in the young brain various regions, particularly of the cerebral cortex, are not yet fully engaged in the tasks for which they are destined, they are recruited more easily for other purposes if necessary. Furthermore, if the remaining hemisphere is undamaged, no haphazard, disturbing plastic changes are likely to occur. This may explain why the right hemisphere of the brain can take over the processing of **language** if the left hemisphere (which normally does this) is damaged at an early age. That many connections are more widespread prenatally and in infancy than later may be another contributing factor. During further development, synapses in some targets strengthen while synapses in other targets weaken or disappear. This is at least partly a use-dependent process, and, in the case of brain damage, persistence of the widespread connections probably aids restitution. As long as the damage is restricted to one hemisphere, size of the lesion does not seem to matter for success of restitution.

The most crucial negative factor in children with such lesions is the occurrence of **seizures**, which inhibits cognitive development. Presumably, ongoing epileptic activity disturbs the use-dependent development of brain networks.

Examples from Animal Experiments of Early Brain Injury

Animal experiments show that early brain injury often causes more serious symptoms than later injuries. This concerns, for example, early **cerebellar** lesions, which produce more marked behavioral deficits than later ones. Experiments with hypoxic perinatal brain damage demonstrate that an initial lesion restricted to the **hippocampus** leads to subsequent degeneration of interconnected tracts and nuclei. Thus, in some way a restricted early lesion disturbs the development of a whole system. Further, long tracts that are already established are apparently not replaced if damaged. Thus, if the left **motor cortex** (sending fibers to the right spinal cord) is removed in monkeys shortly after birth, these monkeys never learn (with their right

hand) the kinds of movements that depend on direct connections from the cerebral cortex to the cord. This is because these connections are already established at birth in monkeys (and in humans). Reports of apparent reestablishment of long fiber tracts after early injury are probably based on experiments in which the injury was inflicted before the axons from the relevant cell groups had reached their targets. In such instances, the outgrowing axons may also innervate other cell groups. This may be due to a lack of normal competition among outgrowing fiber tracts.

The Limits of Plasticity: Cerebral Palsy

Although recovery is remarkably good in some cases of early unilateral brain damage, this appears not to be the most common outcome after early brain damage. Indeed, prenatal and perinatal (at the time of birth) brain damage often causes more serious functional deficits than similar injuries acquired later in life. Thus, the child with early brain damage often presents with a mixture of symptoms, such as pareses, postural abnormalities, and involuntary movements. This is the case for children with **cerebral palsy**,[6] who suffer from the effects of lesions—such as birth-associated hypoxia, intrauterine infections, or genetic aberrations—that may have occurred at different developmental stages. Some children with cerebral palsy have additional cognitive impairments. We have discussed that during sensitive periods of development the brain is not only more plastic but also more vulnerable than later. Thus, a lesion acquired pre- or perinatally might interfere with a number of developmental processes. In addition, collateral sprouting at early stages may not necessarily be helpful. Thus, sprouts from nearby neurons may fill vacant synaptic sites, regardless of whether this is functionally meaningful. For example, in the cord sprouts from sensory fibers may innervate motor neurons that have lost their input from the cerebral cortex. Such "blind" sprouting in various parts of the brain and cord may perhaps contribute to the involuntary movements typical of many children with cerebral palsy.

Early Damage of the Corticospinal (Pyramidal) Tract in Humans

Direct connections from the cerebral cortex to the spinal cord are necessary for the acquisition and performance of most skilled movements. Although corticospinal fibers reach the cord at the seventh gestational month, the development of synaptic

---

5. The situation appears to be less favorable when the lesions affect both hemispheres (even when the lesions are relatively small).

6. Cerebral palsy is used as an umbrella term for a number of clinically different neurological disorders that appear in infancy or early childhood and are dominated by disturbances of bodily movements and posture.

connections in the cord and myelination of the corticospinal fibers go on at least until the child is 2 to 3 years old. Some connections are strengthened and others are removed during this period. Presumably, this represents a sensitive period for establishment of specific corticospinal connections. Initially, connections from each hemisphere are bilateral, but at the age of 2 the hand is controlled exclusively from the contralateral hemisphere; that is, the relevant corticospinal fibers do all cross (in the medulla). This development is at least partly use-dependent and governed by the child's efforts to learn new skills.

A frequent kind of cerebral palsy is **hemiplegia** caused by a perinatal stroke. Typically, disturbed movement control and posture in these children appear not immediately but during the first 3 years of life, and often skills acquired early are later lost. This is probably due to plastic processes that are detrimental to normal motor development. Thus, it appears that any remaining corticospinal fibers from the damaged hemisphere are prevented from establishing synaptic connections in the cord by competition from the much stronger connections of the undamaged hemisphere. Indeed, the undamaged hemisphere retains and strengthens its ipsilateral connections to the cord, rather than being weakened as would normally occur (this is shown in animal experiments and indirectly by use of TMS in human infants). Children with cerebral palsy doing **mirror movements** express this: that is, voluntary movements with one hand are always accompanied by the same movement with the other hand. Why this abnormal innervation pattern is associated with poor function is not so obvious, however. In any case, animal experiments show that stimulation of the damaged hemisphere can rescue the remaining fibers and prevent the poor functional outcome. Further, it appears that in infants with cerebral palsy early specific training (**constraint-induced movement therapy**) of the impaired arm can improve the functional outcome. Probably, in such cases use-dependent plasticity serves to prevent the gradual loss of connections from the damaged hemisphere.

PART THREE

Sensory Systems

The first chapter in this part covers the basic features that are common to all sensory receptors, or sense organs. Such knowledge will make reading the following chapters easier. The next three chapters treat various aspects of the **somatosensory system**, which is primarily concerned with sensory information from the skin, joints, and muscles. Chapter 13 deals with the peripheral parts of the somatosensory system, that is, the sense organs and their connections into the CNS. Chapter 14 deals with the central pathways and neuronal groups concerned with processing of somatosensory information, while Chapter 15 discusses pain in more depth. (Sensory information from the internal organs—visceral sensation—is dealt with mainly in Chapter 29.) In Chapter 16, we describe the **visual system**, from the peripheral receptors in the eye to the higher association areas of the cerebral cortex. Chapter 17 deals with the **auditory system** (hearing), Chapter 18 with the **vestibular system** (sense of equilibrium), and Chapter 19 with **olfaction** and **taste**.

We use the term **system** to indicate that each of these senses is mediated, at least in part, in different regions of the nervous system. In neurobiology, a system usually means a set of interconnected neuronal groups that share either one specific task or several closely related tasks. Sensory systems are designed to capture, transmit, and process information about events in the body and in the environment, such as light hitting the eye or the fullness of the bladder. We also use the term "system" for the parts of the nervous system that deal with tasks other than sensory ones. The motor system, for example, initiates appropriate movements and maintains bodily postures.

We use the term "system" rather loosely here: we do not imply that each system can be understood independently of the rest of the nervous system. Further, it is often arbitrary as to which system a particular neuronal group is said to belong. Thus, usually a cell group is used in the operations of several systems. Especially at higher levels of the brain, information from various systems converges. Cortical neuronal groups, for example, may be devoted to both sensory processing and motor preparation. **Convergence** of information from several sensory systems seems necessary for us to perceive that the different kinds of information actually concern the same phenomenon, whether it is in our own body or in the environment. How do we know, for example, that the round object with a rough surface we hold in the hand is the same as the orange we see with our eyes?

Sometimes the term "system" is misused, so that it confuses rather than clarifies; this happens when we lump structures about which we know too little, or cell groups that have such widespread connections that they do not belong to a particular system. The desire to simplify a complex reality—and the nervous system is indeed overwhelmingly complex—can sometimes become too strong.

OVERVIEW

Sensory signals from nearly all parts of the body are transmitted to the central nervous system (CNS), bringing information about conditions in the various tissues and organs and in our surroundings. The structures where sensory signals originate are called **sense organs**, or **receptors**. The receptors are formed either by the terminal branches of an axon (the skin, joints, muscles, and internal organs) or by specialized sensory cells (the retina, taste buds, and inner ear) that transmit the message to nerve terminals. We use the word "receptor" differently here than in earlier chapters where we applied it to molecules with specific binding properties. A **sensory unit** is a sensory neuron with all its ramifications in the periphery and in the CNS. The **receptive field** of the sensory neuron is the part of the body or the environment from which it samples information. These terms are applied to neurons at all levels of the sensory pathways, from the spinal ganglia to the cerebral cortex. Because of **convergence**, the receptive fields are larger at higher than at lower levels of the CNS.

Sensory receptors are built to respond preferentially to certain kinds of stimulus energy, which is called their **adequate stimulus** (mechanical, chemical, electromagnetic, and so forth). Regardless of the nature of the stimulus, it is translated into electric discharges conducted in axons—that is, the language of the nervous system. This process is called **transduction** and involves direct or indirect activation of specific cation channels. Activation produces a **receptor potential**, which is a graded depolarization of the receptor membrane (similar to a synaptic potential). We **classify** receptors by their adequate stimulus (e.g., mechanoreceptor, photoreceptor, and so forth) by their degree of adaptation and by the site from which they collect information. For example, many receptors are rapidly adapting, meaning that they respond mainly to start and stop of a stimulus. Others are slowly adapting and continue to signal a stationary stimulus. Receptors in the muscles and connective tissue are termed **proprioceptors**, while **exteroceptors** capture information from our surroundings (e.g., light, something touching the skin, and so on). **Enteroceptors** (interoceptors) inform about stimuli arising in the visceral organs. In general, contrasts and brief, unexpected stimuli are perceived much more easily than steady and familiar ones. This is partly because the majority of receptors **adapt** rapidly and partly because sensory signals are **filtered** on their way to the cerebral cortex.

SENSORY UNITS AND THEIR RECEPTIVE FIELDS

Regardless of the structure of the receptor, a sensory neuron transmits the signal to the CNS. We use the term **sensory unit** for a sensory neuron with all its ramifications in the periphery and in the CNS (Figs. 12.1 and 12.2). Such **primary sensory neurons** have their cell bodies in ganglia close to the cord or the brain stem (similar neurons are found in the retina). The **receptive field** of the sensory neuron is the part of the body or the environment from which it samples information. The receptive field of a cutaneous sensory unit is a spot on the skin (Fig. 12.1; see also Fig. 13.12). For a sensory neuron in the retina, the receptive field is a particular spot on the retina, receiving light from a corresponding part of the visual field. We can determine the receptive field of a sensory unit by recording with a thin electrode the action potentials produced in an axon or a cell body, and then we can systematically explore the area from which it can be activated.

Convergence Makes Receptive Fields Larger

We return later to the sensory unit and receptive field and exemplify them in the following chapters. Here it is important to note that these terms apply to sensory

Figure 12.1

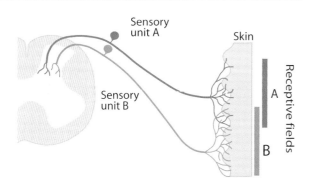

Sensory units and receptive fields. Simplified representation of two sensory units (A and B), which in this case are spinal ganglion cells. The peripheral process of each unit (fibers) ramifies in an area of the skin, which is the receptive field of this particular unit, and the receptive fields of the two units overlap. The density of terminal nerve fiber branches—endowed with receptor properties—is highest in the central part of the receptive field. Therefore, the threshold for eliciting action potentials is lower centrally than peripherally in the receptive field.

neurons at any level of the pathways that lead from the receptors to the cerebral cortex—not only of units leading into the CNS (Fig. 12.1). A neuron in the visual cortex, for example, reacts to light hitting only one particular part of the retina, which represents the receptive field of the neuron. At the cortical level the receptive field depends on **convergence** from several sensory units at lower levels (e.g., retina and thalamus). Thus, receptive fields are usually larger for cortical sensory units than for those closer to the sense organ.

Receptive Fields Are Dynamic and Context-Dependent

One might perhaps expect that the receptive field of a sensory neuron would be a constant, hard-wired property. This is not the case, however; there is ample experimental evidence that receptive fields are **dynamic.** The size of a receptive field depends on the **context** of a stimulus; for example, focused **attention** reduces the receptive fields of neurons in the visual cortex. Such rapid changes of properties are largely due to specific activation of inhibitory interneurons (see Fig. 13.4). Further, receptive fields can change because of specific **training** (learning) and of lesions that alter the sensory inputs to the CNS.

TRANSDUCTION: THE TRANSLATION OF STIMULI TO ACTION POTENTIALS

The task of the receptors is to respond to stimuli. Regardless of the nature of the stimulus, the receptor "translates" the stimulus to the language spoken by the nervous system—that is, electrical signals in the form of action potentials. We discuss in Chapter 4 how summation of many synaptic inputs evokes an action potential (depolarization to threshold) that is propagated along the axon.

Receptor Potentials

In receptors, the action potential arises near the terminal branches of the sensory neuron. This is true regardless of whether the stimulus acts directly on the terminal branches (as in the skin; Fig. 12.2A; see also Fig. 13.1) or indirectly via receptor cells as in the retina and the inner ear (Fig. 12.2B). The stimulus alters the permeability of the receptor membrane, thus depolarizing the receptor. The effect of the stimulus on ion channel openings is **graded** like a synaptic potential (see Fig. 4.4). This graded change in the membrane potential is called a **receptor potential** (Fig. 12.2A). The receptor potential that arises in the terminal branches spreads electrotonically in the proximal direction (toward the CNS, as in Fig. 12.2; see also Fig. 13.2) to the site where an action potential arises by opening voltage-gated Na^+ channels (provided the receptor potential is strong enough). The process is similar to synaptic activation of a neuron (in which the action potential usually arises where the axon leaves the cell body). In sensory cells, the stimulus does not evoke an action potential but leads to graded release of a neurotransmitter that depolarizes the terminals of the sensory cell (Fig. 12.2B).

Transduction and Transient Receptor Potential Channels

The mechanisms behind "translation," or transduction, of a stimulus to a receptor potential are only partly known. Although dozens of receptors and ion channels are involved, receptor potentials in a variety of receptors depend on activation of members of a large family of cation channels, collectively termed **transient receptor potential (TRP) channels** (mammals have more than 30 genes coding for

Figure 12.2

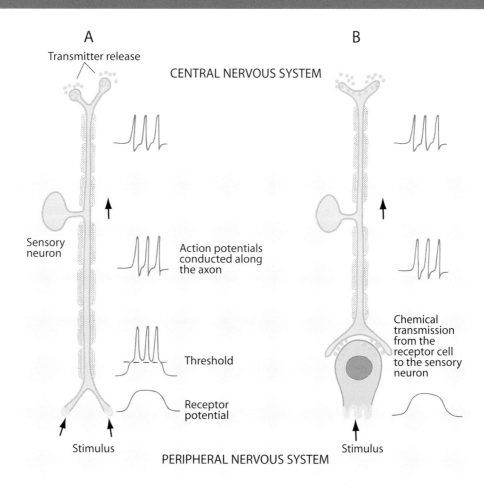

A

B

Transmitter release

CENTRAL NERVOUS SYSTEM

Sensory
neuron

Action potentials
conducted along
the axon

Chemical
transmission
from the
receptor cell
to the sensory
neuron

Threshold

Receptor
potential

Stimulus

Stimulus

PERIPHERAL NERVOUS SYSTEM

Two main kinds of sensory receptor. **A:** The most common kind, found in most parts of the body. The receptor properties are on the terminal ramifications of a sensory axon that belongs to a pseudounipolar ganglion cell. **B:** The kind of receptor found in the sense organs for taste, equilibrium, and hearing. The receptor properties are located on a sensory cell that transmits the signal to a ganglion cell. In both kinds of receptor, a stimulus produces a graded receptor potential. In the ganglion cell (A), an action potential results if the graded potential reaches the threshold. The sensory cell (B) does not produce an action potential but releases a chemical substance that depolarizes the terminals of the ganglion cell. In the CNS the signal is transmitted chemically to central sensory neurons.

TRP channels). Together, TRP channels exhibit a great variety of activation mechanisms and kinds of stimuli to which they respond.[1]

Many receptors are depolarized by binding of a specific **chemical substance** to the membrane. The chemical acts either directly on TRP channel proteins (or other channels) or indirectly via **G protein–coupled receptors**. The latter can then alter the opening state of ion channels via intracellular lipid second messengers (such as **diacylglycerol**).

Many receptors are most easily activated by **mechanical forces**. Typical examples are receptors detecting pressure on the skin or rotation of a joint. Mechanical forces can most likely evoke a receptor potential in different ways. Stretching of the cell membrane may open TRP channels directly (Fig. 12.3A). More commonly, the mechanical force transmits to membrane-receptor proteins via the rigid **cytoskeleton** (or similar structures outside the nerve terminal), which in turn either opens ion channels mechanically (Fig. 12.3B) or chemically via intracellular second messengers (Fig. 12.3C). Actions of external mechanical forces on membrane proteins have been particularly well elucidated in the sense organs for hearing and equilibrium (see Fig. 17.8).

---

1. TRP channels are not restricted to sensory neurons but are expressed in virtually all tissues of the body.

Figure 12.3

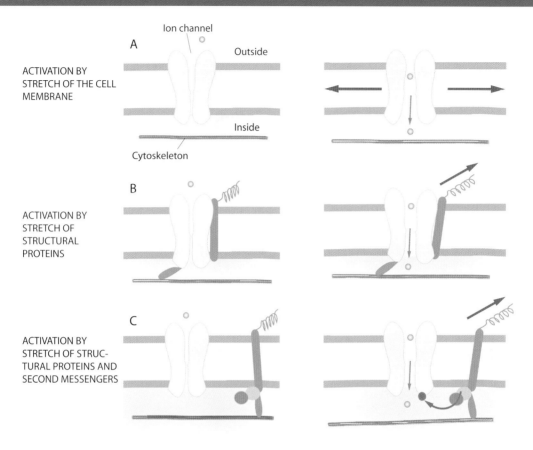

Possible means for mechanical stimuli to evoke receptor potentials via TRP ion channels. (Based on Christensen and Corey 2007).

Other receptors are particularly sensitive to the **temperature** in their surroundings. Change in temperature appears to alter the voltage sensitivity of specific subsets of TRP channels, thereby producing a receptor potential. Substances producing a cooling sensation when applied to the skin, like **menthol**, activate a TRP channel expressed in cold-sensitive receptors.

Receptors Are Often Sensitive to Several Kinds of Stimuli

Many receptors are sensitive to several kinds of stimuli; For example, many receptors evoking **pain** when activated express various kinds of TRP channels, thus combining sensitivities to mechanical, thermal, and chemical stimuli. Another example concerns some mechanoreceptors that are sensitive to **temperature**. This is most likely the explanation for why a cold object feels heavier than a warm (the "**Weber deception**" or "**silver Thaler illusion**"). Thus, some mechanosensitive skin receptors increase their firing when the temperature drops. These receptors appears to express both mechanosensitive and thermosensitive TRP channels. The biologic meaning—if any—of this dual sensitivity is unknown.

PROPERTIES AND CLASSIFICATION OF RECEPTORS

Adequate Stimulus and Specificity

Most receptors are built to respond only or preferably to one kind of stimulus energy: mechanical, chemical, thermal, and so forth. The kind of stimulus to which the receptor responds most easily—that is, with the lowest threshold—is called the **adequate stimulus** for the receptor. We also say that the receptor is **specific** for this type of stimulus, whether it is mechanical, chemical, electromagnetic (light), or thermal (warmth, cold). As we shall see, each of these broad groups of stimuli is registered by receptors with different properties.

Receptors are classified according to the nature of their adequate stimulus, that is, their stimulus specificity. A large group of receptors, the **mechanoreceptors**, responds primarily to distortion of the tissue in which they lie and thus informs the CNS about mechanical stimuli. Such receptors are numerous in the skin, in deep tissues such as muscles and joint capsules, and in internal organs. Another large group of receptors, **chemoreceptors**, responds primarily to certain chemical substances in the interstitial fluid surrounding the receptor. Many chemoreceptors respond to substances produced by or released from cells as a result of tissue damage and inflammation, regardless of the cause (mechanical trauma, burns, infection, and so forth). Other kinds of chemoreceptors are the receptors for taste and smell. Receptors in the retina responding to visible light are called **photoreceptors**. **Thermoreceptors** respond most easily to warming or cooling of the tissue in which they lie.

The **specificity** of a sensory receptor can be determined by the kind of receptor proteins and ion channels it expresses, by its position in the body, or by specialized tissue elements surrounding the nerve terminal. Thus, in some kinds of sensory receptors the nerve terminal is surrounded by cells or collagen fibers that serve as **filters**, so that only certain kinds of stimuli reach the nerve terminal (see Fig. 13.1). Furthermore, the placement in the body may ensure that the sensory receptors are subjected only to certain forms of energy (e.g., the sensory cells in the inner ear are normally influenced only by air waves).

Modality and Quality of Sensation

When a particular kind of receptor is stimulated with sufficient intensity to cause a consciously perceived sensation, we always get the same kind or **modality** of sensory experience—for example, light, touch, pressure, warmth, pain, or sound. The words "modality" and "quality" are both used to describe aspects of sensation but unfortunately somewhat differently by various authors. We use **quality** here to describe further the nature of a sensory modality; for example, pain is a sensory modality that may have a burning quality. Just because stimulation of a particular receptor always evokes a sensation of the same modality does not mean that the receptor necessarily has been subjected to its adequate stimulus. Thus, most receptors can respond to stimuli of other kinds (inadequate stimuli), although the **threshold** then is much higher for evoking a response. As an example, we can mention the perception of light upon a blow to the eye (mechanical stimulus of the photoreceptors rather than the normal light stimulus) and perception of sound upon chemical, rather than the normal mechanical, irritation of the receptors for hearing. The kind of perceived

sensation—the modality or quality of sensation—is thus characteristic for each type of receptor (**Müller's law** of specific nerve energies). Irritation of the **axon** leading from the receptor will also evoke the same sensory modality as when the receptor is stimulated by its adequate stimulus.

Threshold

Even when stimulated by their adequate stimulus, receptors vary enormously with regard to the strength of the stimulus needed to activate them; that is, they have different **thresholds** for activation. For example, in the retina, the rods are much more sensitive (have a lower threshold) to light than the cones. Another example concerns mechanoreceptors, many of which have a **low threshold** and send signals even on the slightest touch of the skin or a just barely perceptible movement of a joint. Other mechanoreceptors have a **high threshold** and require very strong stimulation to respond; we usually perceive such stimuli as painful.

Adaptation

Receptors differ in other ways too. Many receptors send action potentials only when a stimulus starts (or stops). If the stimulus is continuous, this kind of receptor ceases to respond and thus provides information about changes in stimulation only. Such receptors are called **rapidly adapting**. When after a short time we cease noticing that something touches the skin, this is partly because so many of the receptors in the skin are rapidly adapting. Other receptors, however, continue responding (and thus sending action potentials) as long as the stimulus continues. Such receptors are called **slowly adapting** (or nonadapting). Receptors responsible for the sensation of pain exemplify slowly adapting receptors. It would not be appropriate if the body were to adapt to painful stimuli because these usually signal danger and threat of tissue damage. Receptors that signal the position of the body in space and the position of our bodily parts in relation to each other must also be slowly adapting; if not, we would lose this kind of information after a few seconds if no movement took place.

That adaptation is a property of the receptors themselves can be verified by recording the action potentials from the sensory fibers supplying various kinds of receptors. For example, afferent fibers from receptors excited by warming of the skin stop sending signals if the same stimulus is maintained for some time, whereas afferent nerve fibers

the eye, for example, contains only free nerve endings but functionally there are at least four different receptors. Thus, anatomically identical receptors can differ functionally as a result of their expression of different repertoires of ion channels and receptor proteins.

Nociceptors

Receptors that on activation evoke a sensation of pain are termed nociceptors. It is characteristic that most stimuli we experience as painful are so intense that they produce tissue damage or will do so if the stimulus is continued. A more precise, physiologic **definition** would therefore be: a receptor that is activated by stimuli that produce tissue damage, or would do so if the stimulus continued. In Chapter 15, we discuss the relationship between nociceptor stimulation and the experience of pain. In the skin and, as far as we know, in all other tissues from which painful sensations can be evoked, nociceptors are **free nerve endings**. Signals from nociceptors are conducted in thin myelinated (Aδ) and unmyelinated (C) fibers.

Functionally, skin nociceptors are of three main types. One type responds to intense mechanical stimulation only (such as pinching, cutting, and stretching), and is therefore termed a **high-threshold mechanoreceptor**. The other is also activated by intense mechanical stimuli but in addition, by intense **warming** of the skin (above 45°C)[1] and by **chemical substances** that are liberated by tissue damage and inflammation. Because such receptors can be activated by different sensory modalities, they are termed **polymodal nociceptors**. In addition, recent studies indicate that many nociceptors are purely sensitive to chemical substances released in inflamed tissue. Since such receptors are unresponsive to most nociceptive stimuli used in animal experiments, they are termed **silent nociceptors**. Silent nociceptors typically require stimulation for 10 to 20 minutes to become active; thereafter, however, they may continue firing for hours and become sensitive also to mechanical stimuli. They are present in skin, muscles, and visceral organs and may constitute about one-third of all

nociceptors. They appear particularly suited to communicate about disease processes in the tissues and are probably important for communication between the **immune system** and the brain.

Many substances can excite nociceptors, and specific membrane receptors and ion channels have been identified for some. **ATP**, for example, excites nociceptors by binding to purinoceptors (Fig. 13.2). Because ATP is normally present only intracellularly, its extracellular occurrence is an unequivocal sign of cellular damage. The peptide **bradykinin**, which is produced by the release of proteolytic enzymes from damaged cells, acts on specific membrane receptors in nociceptors. Several other mediators of **inflammation**—such as cytokines, prostaglandins, histamine, serotonin, SP, and adenosine—may contribute to nociceptor activation and sensitization. H^+ **ions** (pH < 6) activate nociceptors effectively and, in addition, seem to increase their responses to inflammatory substances.

Sensitization, Hyperalgesia, and Allodynia

A characteristic feature of nociceptors is their tendency to be **sensitized** by prolonged stimulation (this is the opposite phenomenon of adaptation). Sensitization is due to upregulation of several ion channels and G-protein-coupled receptors expressed in sensory neurons, notably voltage-gated Na^+ channels and transient receptor potential (TRP) channels. Sensitization partly explains why even normally non-noxious stimuli (such as touching the skin) may be felt as painful when the tissue is inflamed. Cytokines sensitize nociceptors (Fig. 13.2) and produce a condition of **hyperalgesia,** characterized by abnormal intensity of pain compared to the strength of the stimulus. As discussed later in this chapter, hyperalgesia may also be caused by altered properties of neurons in the CNS, especially in the spinal dorsal horn. The term **allodynia** is used when innocuous stimuli, such as light touch, evoke intense pain.

Nociceptors, Voltage-Gated Sodium and Potassium Channels, and Inherited Channelopathies

Sensory neurons express a multitude of ion channels and receptors, among them several kinds of voltage-gated sodium (Na^+) and potassium (K^+) channels. Such channels are expressed in all neurons and are necessary for excitability and impulse conduction. As discussed in Chapter 3, the sodium channels are responsible for the inward current making the upstroke of the action potential, whereas the potassium channels upon opening allow an outward current that produces the down stroke of the action

---

1. Heat activates nociceptors by opening the nonselective cation channel **TRPV1** (and apparently also other varieties of the TRPV channel). Interestingly, **capsaicin**, responsible for the pungency of hot peppers, activates the heat-sensitive channel. On continued presence, however, capsaicin desensitizes the receptor, thus alleviating ongoing pain. Drugs that selectively block the TRPV1 channel have been tested in animals and found effective in alleviating inflammatory pain but also cause a rise in body temperature. Thus, the TRPV1 channel apparently contributes not only to thermal and chemical nociception but also to control of **body temperature**.

Figure 13.2

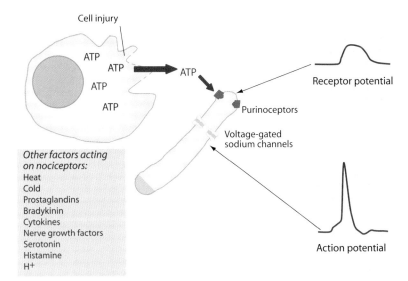

Nociceptor activation. ATP is one among many substances that activate nociceptors. Because the extracellular ATP concentration is extremely low normally, ATP is a very sensitive signal of impending cell damage. Binding of ATP to specific receptors depolarizes the nerve terminal (receptor potential). If the receptor potential reaches threshold, an action potential arises due to opening of voltage-gated sodium channels. The action potential is conducted to the CNS. Some other means of activating nociceptors are listed.

potential (Fig. 13.2). Thus, increasing the activity of nociceptor sodium channels would increase their excitability and potentially increase pain, whereas increasing the activity of the potassium channels would reduce excitability and reduce pain.

Ten voltage-gated sodium channels have been identified; they share a basic structure but have somewhat different properties and distribution. Sensory neurons express several kinds, and some of these occur primarily in small nociceptive spinal ganglion cells. Nerve injury as well as inflammation cause rapid changes in the expression of several voltage-gated sodium channels, thus rendering the ganglion cells and their free endings in the tissue hyperexcitable (as mentioned earlier in relation to hyperalgesia).

One channel—**Na$_V$1.7**—appears to be particularly important for the generation of action potentials in axons leading from nociceptors. Rare inherited diseases caused by mutations of the gene (*SCN9A*) coding for Na$_V$1.7 shed light on the function of this channel. Two gain-of-function mutations cause attacks of intense pain but with different mechanisms. Patients with **paroxysmal extreme pain disorder** suffer from attacks of pain in the eyes, jaw, and rectum, apparently caused by incomplete inactivation of the Na$_V$1.7 channel. Patients with **erythromelalgia** (primary erythermalgia) experience burning pain and redness in the hands and feet. The mutation in the latter patients causes the channel to open too easily (lowered threshold). A third variety of inherited Na$_V$1.7 channelopathy was quite recently found among members of a Pakistani family. Those afflicted show complete absence of pain sensitivity and suffer serious injuries as they grow up (**congenital analgesia**). The mutation in these patients appears to cause a loss of function of the Na$_V$1.7 channel, resulting in abolished impulse traffic from nociceptors.

Other voltage-gated sodium channels, expressed in nociceptive ganglion cells, also appear to be involved in clinical pain conditions. Great efforts are now being made to develop drugs that can block specific voltage-gated sodium channels or enhance the activity of voltage-gated potassium channels. Nonspecific sodium channel blockers, such as **lidocaine**, have long been used for local **anesthesia**.

Silent Nociceptors, the Immune System, Homeostasis, and Sickness Behavior

Since mediators released in inflamed tissues activate them, silent nociceptors most likely contribute to the pain that follows tissue damage. For example, low pH and release of prostaglandins—typically occurring together in inflammation and tissue injury—seem to be especially effective in activating silent nociceptors. It is likely that silent nociceptors play an important role in sustained inflammatory pain. In addition, silent nociceptors may play a long-term role in evaluating the status of the tissue microenvironment. Thus, they would play a role in bodily **homeostasis.** Signals from silent nociceptors may be particularly important to modulate the activity of the **immune system.** Thus, we know that the nervous system can influence the properties of the cells of the immune system, as we return to in Chapter 30. To do this, the nervous system needs information from the "battlefield" of the immune system.

Silent nociceptors seem well suited to carry out this task, as substances released from leukocytes activate them. We know, for example, that **cytokines** released in the gastric mucosa stimulate sensory nerve endings belonging to nerve fibers in the **vagus nerve**. This produces **sickness behavior**: the animal moves around less, loses its appetite, is uninterested in its surroundings, and so forth. In addition, cytokines in the bloodstream can reach neurons in certain parts of the brain, either by passing the blood–brain barrier or by acting on places devoid of a blood–brain barrier. It seems likely that signals from silent nociceptors—not only in the skin but also in deep tissues and visceral organs—contribute to "how we feel," or the feeling of the physiologic state of the body.

Thermoreceptors

Free endings of thin sensory nerve fibers are responsible for the perception of heat and cold. Although warm and cold receptors look the same, they express different kinds of TRP channels. **Cold receptors** respond with an increase of firing frequency to cooling of the skin below the normal temperature (about 32°C). They stop responding, however, at very low skin temperatures. Surprisingly, cold receptors can also be excited by skin temperatures above 45°C. This explains why a hot shower may feel cold at the beginning (until we feel pain, as mentioned previously, temperatures above 45°C excite polymodal nociceptors). This phenomenon is called **paradoxical cold** (sensation). Signals from cold receptors are conducted in thin myelinated (Aδ) fibers. **Warm receptors** respond to warming of the skin above the normal temperature up to about 45°C.

The **adequate stimulus** for thermoreceptors is the temperature of the tissue surrounding them or, rather, changes in the temperature. The receptors send action potentials with a relatively low frequency at a steady temperature, whereas a small change in the temperature elicits a marked change in the firing frequency. A heat receptor, for example, fires at constant room temperature with a low frequency, but warming the skin even slightly increases the firing rate. The response is particularly brisk if the warming happens rapidly (thus, we perceive lukewarm water as hot if the hand is cold when put into it). A change in skin temperature of 0.2°C is sufficient to cause a marked change in firing rate from a thermoreceptor. Thus, the thermoreceptors do not give an objective measure of the actual skin temperature but, rather, signal **changes** that may be significant in our adjustment to the environment (to keep the body temperature constant).

This means that they are important for the maintenance of bodily **homeostasis**.

The signals from warm receptors are conducted in **C fibers**, whereas signals from cold receptors travel much faster in thin myelinated **Aδ fibers**.

Mechanoreceptors of the Skin

The study of receptors for pain and temperature sensation is more difficult than the study of mechanoreceptors. These are particularly well studied, therefore, and among them, we know most about the low-threshold mechanoreceptors. The following account mainly deals with low-threshold mechanoreceptors of the skin. High-threshold mechanoreceptors in the skin are nociceptors and do not differ significantly from such receptors in muscles and around joints. As far as we know, they are always free nerve endings (Fig. 13.1E).

There are several kinds of **low-threshold mechanoreceptors** in the skin, ranging from free receptors to those with an elaborate capsule. Some adapt slowly or not at all; others adapt very rapidly. For example, receptors found close to the roots of **hairs** (Fig. 13.1B) are rapidly adapting. They are activated by even the slightest bending of a hair, as can easily be verified by touching the hairs on the back of one's own hand. If the hair is held in the new position, however, the sensation disappears immediately. There are also some unmyelinated afferent fibers (C fibers) from hairy skin that signal light touch (in contrast to the majority of C fibers that are either nociceptors or warm receptors). These **low-threshold C fibers** may be of special importance for mediating **emotional** aspects of touch (rather than precise, discriminative information).

Low-Threshold C Fibers

A woman with selective loss of large-diameter myelinated sensory fibers provided an opportunity to study the properties of low-threshold C fibers (Olausson et al. 2002). Light touch (stroking with a soft brush) applied to the back of the hand was felt as a very faint and diffuse but pleasant pressure (no sensation was evoked by brushing the palm of the hand, corresponding to the lack of unmyelinated low-threshold afferents from glabrous skin). Interestingly, functional magnetic resonance imaging showed activation of the **insula**—known to be related to affective aspects of sensation—but not in the primary somatosensory area (SI), which is responsible for the discriminative aspects.

Although the thick, **glabrous skin** on the palm of the hand and on the sole of the foot lacks hair, the elaborate

Table 13.1

Receptive Fields	Adaptation	
	Rapid	**Slow**
Small	*Meissner corpuscles*	*Merkel disks*
	Glabrous skin, in dermal papillae Touch: moving stimuli: Vibration < 100 Hz	Close to the epithelium Touch (judging form and surface of objects)
Large	*Pacinian corpuscles*	*Ruffini corpuscles*
	Border dermis-subcutis; Vibration > 100 Hz	Dermis, parallel to the skin surface; stretch of the skin (friction)

encapsulated receptors are particularly abundant at these locations and are obviously related to the superior sensory abilities of these parts—the fingers, in particular (Table 13.1). One such receptor is the **Meissner corpuscle**, which mediates information about touch. Meissner corpuscles are small, oval bodies located in the dermal papillae just beneath the epidermis—in fact, as close to the surface of the skin as possible without being directly exposed (Fig. 13.1A and C). Several axons approach the corpuscle and follow a tortuous course inside the capsule between the lamellae formed by connective tissue cells.[2] Meissner corpuscles respond by sending action potentials even when indenting by only a few micrometers the skin overlying the receptor. If the skin is kept indented, however, the receptor stops sending action potentials. On release of the pressure, a few action potentials are again elicited. Meissner corpuscles are thus **rapidly adapting** and obviously have a low threshold for their adequate stimulus. These corpuscles are presumably well suited to, among other things, signal **direction** and **velocity** of objects moving on the skin.

Ruffini corpuscles are also low-threshold mechanoreceptors and are **slowly adapting**. They consist of a bundle of collagen fibrils with a sensory axon branching between the fibrils (Fig. 13.1A). The collagen fibrils connect with those in the dermis, and stretching of the skin in the direction of the fibrils is the adequate stimulus for the receptor. Stretching the skin tightens the fibrils, which, in turn, leads to deformation and depolarization of the axonal ramifications, thus producing action potentials in the afferent fiber. It is therefore assumed that Ruffini corpuscles function as low-threshold **stretch receptors** of the skin, informing us about the magnitude and direction of stretch.

Another kind of **slowly adapting**, low-threshold mechanoreceptor in the skin is the **Merkel disk** (Fig. 13.1A and D), present particularly on the distal parts of the extremities, the lips, and the external genitals. An axon ends in close contact with a large epithelial cell in the basal layer of the epidermis. Even after several minutes of constant pressure on the skin overlying the Merkel disks, the receptor continues to send action potentials at about the same rate.

A final type of low-threshold mechanoreceptor, **Pacinian corpuscles** (Fig. 13.1A), is found at the junction between the dermis and the subcutaneous layer; they are also present at other locations, such as in the mesenteries, vessel walls, joint capsules, and the periosteum. Pacinian corpuscles are large (up to 4 mm long) ovoid bodies, which can be seen macroscopically at dissection. A thick axon is surrounded by numerous lamellae, which are formed by a special kind of connective tissue cell. Between the cellular lamellae there are fluid-filled spaces. Pacinian corpuscles are very **rapidly adapting**, eliciting only one or two action potentials in the afferent fiber at the onset of indentation of the skin. The adequate stimulus is therefore extremely rapid indentation of the skin. In practice, this is achieved by **vibration** with a frequency of 100 to 400 Hz. If a vibrating probe is put in contact with the skin, the frequency of action potentials in the afferent fiber follows closely the frequency of vibration. Vibration with a frequency below 100 Hz appears to be signaled by Meissner corpuscles.

Itch

Itching (pruritus) is a peculiar, unpleasant sensation evoked by stimulation—mechanical, chemical, or thermal—of free nerve endings in superficial parts of the skin and mucous membranes.

2. In addition to a thick myelinated axon, the Meissner corpuscle receives thin unmyelinated axons. The latter contain neuropeptides and express receptors typical of nociceptors. So far, however, there is no direct evidence of a contribution from Meissner corpuscles in nociceptive signaling.

The biologic meaning of itching is presumably related to its tendency to elicit scratching (scratch reflex) to remove potentially harmful objects (insects, parasites, allergens, etc.). The sensation of itch appears to be served by a specific subdivision of the neural system for pain. Thus, the signals are conducted in unmyelinated sensory (C) fibers to the spinal cord. From the cord to higher levels, the signals follow the pathways for pain, and cutting these also abolishes the sensation of itching. **Histamine** is the best-known pruritogenic substance. In the skin, it can be released from mast cells, for example cells in allergic reactions, and evoke itching. The leaves of stinging nettle (*Urtica dioica*) provoke intense itching because they contain histamine. **Microneurographic** studies in humans have identified a subgroup of peripheral sensory units (with unmyelinated fibers) that react vigorously to histamine and produce itching when stimulated. These units also respond to noxious stimuli, such as capsaicin, and inflammatory substances such as prostaglandin E and bradykinin, and therefore seem to constitute a subset of nociceptive sensory units. Nevertheless, there is evidence that this subset evokes itch when stimulated alone (by histamine or other pruritogenic substances). Accordingly, some units in the dorsal horn (lamina 1) respond primarily when histamine is applied in their receptive fields. This seems compatible with the fact that weakly painful stimuli, such as scratching the skin, suppress the sensation of itching: when noxious stimuli dominate, the evoked feeling would be pain rather than itching. Even though histamine appears to evoke activity in the same parts of the cerebral cortex as painful stimuli do, there might be subtle differences that brain scanning methods are unable to detect, explaining why we are able to discriminate the sensations of itch and pain.

Itching is a distressing symptom in several diseases (cancer, metabolic disorders, skin diseases, renal failure, and others). Histamine does not seem to be involved in such cases, however. Interestingly, interneurons in the dorsal horn producing the opioid **dynorphin** (acting on **kappa [κ] opioid receptors**) seem to be able to inhibit transmission of signals from itch receptors. Accordingly, κ-opioid receptor agonists have been found to relieve itching in animal experiments. The effect of **menthol** on itching seems to be mediated via dynorphin-containing interneurons.

Tickle

Tickling is another peculiar sensory phenomenon. It is evoked by stimulation of low-threshold mechanoreceptors, but we do not know which subgroup is involved. The sensation of tickling is strongly influenced by the **context** in which it is evoked: the same stimulus may be experienced as tickling in one situation and merely as light touch in another. For example, we know that we are unable to tickle ourselves, probably because the brain can easily distinguish sensory signals produced by our own actions and those coming from other sources. We also know that our emotional state influences whether a stimulus is felt as tickling. This example may serve to emphasize a point we return to repeatedly: the sensory messages sent from the receptors are subject to extensive processing before a conscious sensation is produced.

What Information Is Signaled by Low-Threshold Cutaneous Mechanoreceptors?

Together the four types of low-threshold mechanoreceptors described in the preceding text are thought to mediate the different qualities of our sense of touch and pressure, which are so well developed in glabrous skin (fingers, toes, and lips). One important aspect is the ability to judge the speed and direction of a moving object in contact with the skin, as well as the friction between them. Thus, we may perceive quickly that an object is slipping from our grip and judge from the friction the force needed to stop the movement. Two of the receptor types, Merkel disks and Ruffini corpuscles, are slowly adapting and, as long as the stimulus lasts, continue to provide information about slight pressure and stretching of the skin, respectively (Table 13.1). The other two, Meissner and Pacinian corpuscles, are rapidly adapting and signal only the start and stop of stimuli. It seems likely that Meissner corpuscles would be particularly well suited to signal the direction and speed of a moving stimulus. It should be noted that low-threshold mechanoreceptors in the skin also contribute to joint sense (see later) and control of posture and movements (see Chapter 18, under "More About Receptor Types and Their Contribution to Postural Control," and Chapter 21, under "Cutaneous Receptors and the Precision Grip").[3]

Microneurographic Studies of Human Skin Receptors

Studies with techniques that enable **recording** from and **stimulation** of peripheral nerves in conscious human beings have provided important information with regard to the functional properties of receptors (Fig. 13.3). The Swedish neurophysiologists Hagbarth and Vallbo pioneered this technique around 1970. With the use of very thin needle electrodes, one records the activity of single sensory axons within a nerve, such as the median nerve at the forearm. Thus, it is possible to determine the receptive field of this particular sensory unit, along with its adequate stimulus. In glabrous skin of the fingers and palms, four types of low-threshold mechanoreceptors have been so characterized. Most likely, they correspond to the four encapsulated types described earlier (Table 13.1). Thus, there are two types of rapidly adapting sensory units: one with a small receptive field (most likely the Meissner corpuscle), and the other with a large and indistinct receptive field (Pacinian corpuscle). The two other types of sensory units are slowly adapting; again, one has a small receptive field (Merkel disk) and the other a large

---

3. Cutaneous receptors may also contribute to **enteroception** (interoception)—that is, sensations attributed to internal organs. Thus, the perception of a changing heart rhythm seems to depend on signals from low-threshold receptors in the skin on the chest (Khalsa et al. 2009), presumably by informing about pressure changes and stretching of the skin.

Figure 13.3

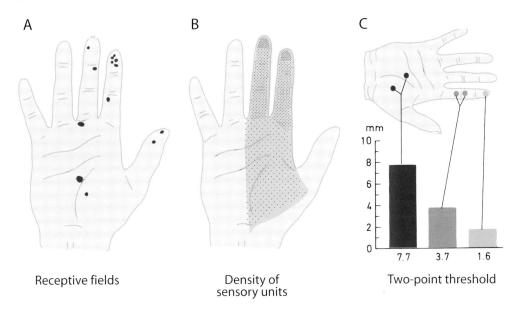

Receptive fields   Density of   Two-point threshold
                          sensory units

Receptive fields. **A:** Size and location of the receptive fields of 15 sensory units, determined by recording from the median nerve. All of these sensory units were rapidly adapting and were most likely conducting from Meissner corpuscles. Within each receptive field there are many Meissner corpuscles, all supplied by the same axon. **B:** Relative density of sensory units conducting from Meissner corpuscles (i.e., number of sensory units supplying 1 cm²). The density increases distally and is highest at the volar aspect of the fingertips. **C:** Two-point discrimination. The numbers give the shortest distance between two points touching the skin that can be identified by the experimental subject as two (reducing the distance further makes the person experience only one point touching the skin). Average of 10 subjects. (Based on microneurographic studies by Vallbo and Johansson 1978.)

but direction-specific receptive field (most likely the Ruffini corpuscle).

Stimulation of the axons of the sensory units that have been recorded enables correlations to be made between the conscious sensory experiences evoked by stimulation of only one sensory unit. Stimulation of single sensory units that most likely end in Meissner corpuscles produces a feeling of light touch, like a tap on the skin with the point of a pencil. As a rule, the person localizes the feeling to exactly the point on the skin previously found to be the receptive field of the sensory unit. Activating a sensory unit that presumably leads off from Merkel disks evokes a sensation of light, steady pressure (as long as the stimulus lasts). Stimulating axons that appear to end in Pacinian corpuscles gives a feeling of vibration.

Receptive Fields of Cutaneous Sensory Units

It has been known for a long time that cutaneous sensation is punctate, that is, there are distinct tiny spots on the skin that are sensitive to different sensory modalities. We therefore use the terms "cold," "warm," "touch," and "pain" spots. Cold spots are most easily demonstrated. Between the spots sensitive to cooling of the skin, there are others where

contact with a cold object is felt only as pressure. This is so because each sensory unit distributes all its peripheral ramifications within a limited area of the skin. Thus, the sensory unit can be activated only from this part of the skin, which constitutes its **receptive field** (Fig. 13.3; see also Fig. 12.1). Certain parts of the skin lack ramifications belonging to "cold" sensory units; consequently, sensations of cold cannot be evoked from such areas. Correspondingly, many small spots on proximal parts of the body—for example, on the abdomen and the upper arm—lack nociceptors; therefore, insertion of a sharp needle at such places is felt only as touch. The receptive fields of nociceptive sensory units are so closely spaced, however, that one has to make a thorough search to find painless spots.

The **size** of the receptive field depends on the area of the skin receiving axonal branches from the sensory neuron. In general, the **density of sensory units**—that is, the number of units innervating; for example, 1 cm² of the skin—is highest in distal parts of the body (fingers, toes, and lips), and the receptive fields are smaller distally than proximally (Fig. 13.3). This explains why the stimulus threshold is lower and the ability to localize a stimulus is more precise in the palm of the hand than at, for example, the upper arm.

Discriminative Sensation

The punctate arrangement of the cutaneous sensation is important for our ability to **localize** stimuli. Being able to determine that *two* pointed objects (such as the legs of a compass) touch the skin rather than one must mean that separate units innervate the two spots. Not surprisingly, the distance between two points on the skin that, when touched, can be identified as two is shortest where the density of sensory units is highest and the receptive fields are smallest—that is, on the fingertips (Fig. 13.3A and B). Determining this distance gives a measure of what we call **two-point discrimination** and is often used clinically. The smallest distance at which two stimuli can be discriminated is the **two-point threshold** (Fig. 13.3C). A useful test for this kind of discriminative sensation is the writing of letters or figures on the skin (with the subject's eyes closed). The figures that can be interpreted are quite small on the fingertips, somewhat larger on the palms, much larger on the upper arm, and even larger on the trunk. As one might expect, the pathways conducting the sensory signals from the spots on the skin are arranged topographically so that signals from different parts of the skin are kept separate at all levels up to the cerebral cortex.

Lateral Inhibition: Inhibitory Interneurons Improve the Discriminative Sensation

The two-point threshold (Fig. 13.3C) does not depend solely on the size and density of the cutaneous receptive fields. Inhibitory interneurons in the cord (and at higher levels) restrict the signal traffic from the periphery of a stimulated spot, thereby improving the discriminative ability compared with what might be expected from the anatomic arrangement of receptive fields (Fig. 13.4). The cutaneous sensory units (neurons) send off collaterals in the CNS that activate inhibitory interneurons that, in turn, inhibit sensory neurons in the vicinity. This phenomenon is called **lateral inhibition,** and it occurs at all levels of the sensory pathways and in all sensory systems. Figure 13.4 shows an example with a pencil pressed lightly onto the skin. The sensory units with receptive fields in the center of the stimulated spot receive the most intense stimulation. Therefore, they excite the inhibitory interneurons strongly, with consequent strong inhibition of sensory units leading from the periphery of the spot. Sensory units with receptive fields in the periphery are less strongly stimulated but receive strong inhibition.

Thus, they cannot inhibit the transmission of signals from the center of the spot. Together, the impulse traffic from the periphery of the stimulated area is reduced, and we perceive the stimulated area as smaller as and more sharply delimited than it really is. In this way, the CNS receives distorted sensory information.

PROPRIOCEPTORS: DEEP SENSATION

As mentioned, the term "proprioceptive" is used for sensations pertaining to the **musculoskeletal system**—the muscles, tendons, joint capsules, and ligaments. There are many similarities between proprioceptors and cutaneous receptors. For example, numerous free receptors (belonging to thin myelinated and unmyelinated axons) occur in the muscles, the muscle fascia, and the dense connective tissue of joint capsules and ligaments. Many of these are nociceptors as in the skin.

Here we are dealing primarily with specialized sense organs in muscles and around joints, which are of crucial importance for control of posture and goal-directed movements. These are low-threshold mechanoreceptors, and the signals from them are conducted centrally in thick, myelinated axons. The adequate stimulus of these receptors is stretching of the tissue in which they lie. Whether the receptors are located in a muscle or in a joint capsule, joint movement is the natural stimulus that leads to their activation.

We first discuss specialized sense organs in muscles—muscle spindles and tendon organs—and then receptors in joint capsules and ligaments. Chapters 18 and 21 cover the role of proprioceptors in control of movements.

Classification of Muscle Sensory Fibers

Unfortunately, other terms are used to classify sensory fibers from muscles and joints than sensory fibers from the skin (see "Classification of Sensory Nerve Fibers According to their Thickness" earlier in this chapter). Muscle afferents—that is, sensory fibers leading from muscles—are classified according to size into groups I to IV (size or thickness is closely related to conduction velocity). **Group I** muscle afferents contain fast conducting, thick myelinated fibers, while **group II** contain medium-sized myelinated fibers, and **group III** comprises the thinnest myelinated fibers. **Group IV** contains the slowly conducting unmyelinated fibers. Group I is further divided into **Ia** and **Ib** fibers, with

Figure 13.4

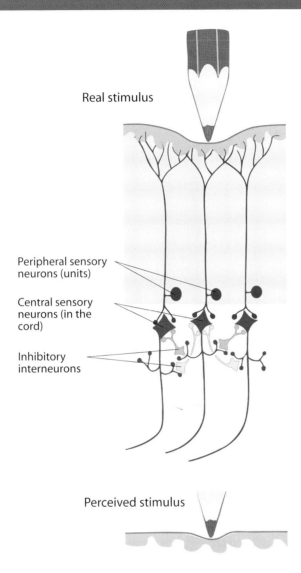

Real stimulus

Peripheral sensory
neurons (units)

Central sensory
neurons (in the
cord)

Inhibitory
interneurons

Perceived stimulus

Lateral inhibition. Simplified presentation of how inhibitory interneurons in the CNS can improve the precision of the sensory information reaching consciousness.

Ib fibers conducting slightly more slowly than Ia fibers. Signals from low-threshold mechanoreceptors in muscles that is, from muscle spindles—are conducted in group I and II fibers, while the tendon organs are supplied with Ib fibers.

Broadly, group I and II fibers correspond with regard to conduction velocity to Aα and Aβ fibers, while group III and IV correspond to Aδ and C fibers, respectively.

Nociceptors in Muscle and Tendon

As mentioned, muscles are supplied with numerous free nerve endings of thin myelinated and unmyelinated axons

(i.e., the most slowly conducting fibers). Microscopic examination of muscle nerves in experimental animals shows that almost 40% of all the axons are either thin myelinated or unmyelinated sensory fibers, terminating in tree endings (Fig. 13.5). Many—probably the majority—of the unmyelinated and thin myelinated axons lead from nociceptors in the muscle. This has been shown by recording the activity of single sensory units that innervate a muscle while systematically exploring their adequate stimuli. Such units were excited by both strong mechanical stimuli and substances liberated in inflamed tissue (such as bradykinin, known to provoke pain in humans). Inflammation also **sensitizes** the nociceptive sensory units, making them respond to normal

Figure 13.5

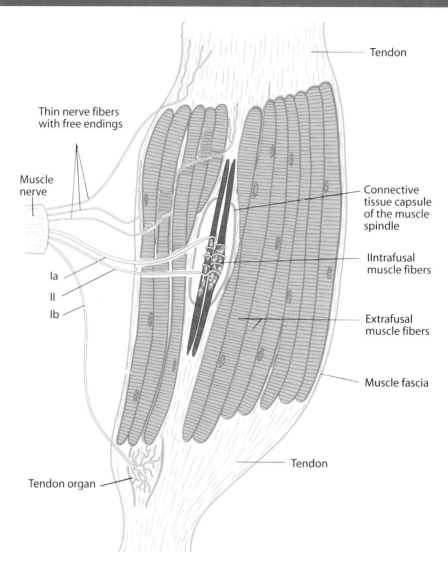

Sensory innervation of skeletal muscles. The size of the receptors relative to the muscle is exaggerated. Because the muscle spindle attaches to the tendons via connective tissue fibers, the muscle spindle is stretched whenever the whole muscle is stretched. Many of the free nerve endings are nociceptors.

movements (this may partly explain the muscle soreness after heavy exercise). Like cutaneous nociceptors, those in muscle are also sensitized by prolonged stimulation, and some sensory units are activated by **ischemia**. For example, muscle ischemia caused by a thrombotic artery, produces pain in humans.[4]

Microneurographic studies have identified sensory units in human muscle nerves that have nociceptor-like properties similar to those described in the preceding text in experimental animals. Thus, human units are slowly adapting, have a high threshold for mechanical stimuli, and can be activated by inflammatory substances. **Electrical stimulation** of small nerve fascicles in human muscle nerves produces pain as the only sensory experience. The pain is felt to be deep (not in the skin) and has a cramp-like quality. The subject localizes the pain to the muscle supplied by the nerve, not to the site of nerve stimulation that is at a distance from the muscle (recording and stimulation of single sensory fibers have confirmed these findings). If the stimulation continues, or its intensity is increased, the pain radiates to regions other than the muscle itself.

4. Animal experiments using cultured dorsal root ganglion cells indicate that the adequate stimulus for many muscle nociceptors is a combination of protons, ATP, and lactate, acting on acid sensing ion channels, purinergic type 2, and TRPV receptors, respectively. Increased levels of these metabolites would presumably mediate the pain provoked by heavy muscular exercise that causes ischemia.

A small number of axons from nociceptors in a muscle **tendon** have been investigated with microneurography. Stimulation of such a sensory unit produced a sharp pain, different from the muscle pain described earlier. The subject localized the pain to the tendon.

Ergoreceptors and Other Kinds of Free Receptors in Muscles

Not all of the thin, slowly conducting sensory fibers in a muscle nerve are nociceptors. Thus, in experimental animals, some of these fibers have a low mechanical threshold; that is, ordinary muscle contraction or gentle stretching of the muscle activates them. Their maximal firing rate is reached by stimuli much weaker than the stimuli producing pain. Such receptors may be responsible for circulatory and respiratory reflex effects known to occur at the start of muscular activity. Thus, there is a slight increase of pulse and breathing rate that occurs too early to be caused by a rise in blood CO_2 or lowered pH. Although the receptors responsible for such reflex effects have not been identified with certainty, they are called **ergoreceptors** (ergoceptors).

The Structure of the Muscle Spindle

The name "muscle spindle" is derived from the oblong shape of this sense organ. The muscle spindles are located within the muscle, among the striated muscle cells, and consist of a few (2–14) specialized muscle cells enclosed in a connective tissue capsule. The capsule is approximately 0.2 to 0.3 mm in diameter and up to 5 mm long. The muscle fibers (or

muscle cells) of the spindle are called **intrafusal** and are much thinner and shorter (7–10 mm long) than the ordinary, **extrafusal** muscle fibers. In contrast to the extrafusal muscle fibers, the intrafusal fibers show cross-striation only at their ends. This means that they are able to contract only these parts and not their middle portions. There are two main types of intrafusal fibers (Fig. 13.6). One type is called the **nuclear bag fiber** because the nuclei are all collected in the middle part of the muscle fiber. In the other type, the **nuclear chain fiber**, the nuclei are evenly distributed along the muscle fiber.

The **number** of muscle spindles varies among muscles. Although the density is generally highest in small muscles (e.g., intrinsic hand muscles), the absolute number may be much higher in large muscles (e.g., the quadriceps femoris muscle). The functional meaning of such quantitative differences is not clear but may be related to the fact that joint sense is more accurate in large proximal joints than in small distal joints.

Number and Density of Muscle Spindles: Possible Functional Significance

The number of muscle spindles has been determined in approximately 200 human muscles and varies greatly from muscle to muscle. The functional significance of such variations is not clear and has been subject to different interpretations. In large muscles such as the latissimus dorsi, the **total number** of muscle spindles is about 400, whereas the small abductor pollicis brevis contains about 80. The largest absolute number, close to 1,300, was found in the quadriceps muscle. The soleus muscle contains

Figure 13.6

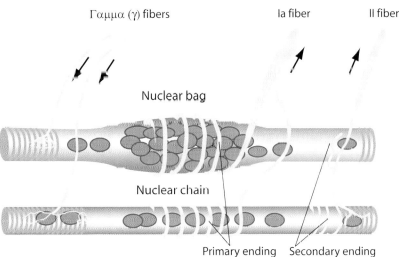

The muscle spindle. Schematic of the two kinds of intrafusal muscle fibers and their innervation. (Modified from Matthews 1964.)

Figure 13.9

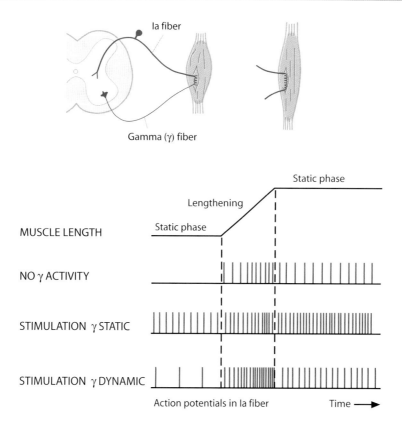

Action of γ motoneurons on the muscle spindle. The experimental setup is as in Fig. 13.8, except in addition to recording the activity of group Ia fibers in the dorsal root, γ axons are isolated in the ventral roots so they can be electrically stimulated. In this example, there is no firing of the Ia fiber at the resting length of the muscle when the γ fibers are not stimulated. Stimulation of a static γ fiber (innervating the same spindle from which the Ia fiber conducts) makes the Ia fiber fire even at the static resting length; stretching the muscle to a new static length increases the firing frequency to a new stable level. Stimulation of a dynamic γ fiber increases the firing frequency of the Ia fiber mainly during the stretching phase.

the muscle spindle is called **static sensitivity**. Because the firing rate of both group Ia and group II fibers depends on the length of the muscle, both inform the CNS about the **length of the muscle** at any time (or the static length).

During the phase in which the muscle length is changed, however, group Ia and group II afferent fibers behave differently (dynamic phase in Fig. 13.8). The firing rate of the group Ia fiber is much higher during stretching than when the length is kept stationary in the stretched position, but the group II fiber does not show this same change in firing rate. During the shortening phase, the Ia fiber becomes completely "silent." Although not shown in Fig. 13.8, the firing rate of the group Ia fiber also depends on the velocity of the length change. Thus, the Ia fiber signals that the length of the muscle is changing, as well as the **velocity** with which it is occurring. This property is called **dynamic sensitivity**.

These facts indicate that the **primary sensory ending** of the muscle spindle has both static and dynamic sensitivity: this ending is capable of informing about the actual length of the muscle (position of a joint), whether the length is constant or changing (joint movement), and the velocity of change (velocity of the movement). Because the **secondary sensory ending** almost totally lacks dynamic sensitivity, it should be able to inform primarily about the static length of the muscle.

There is much evidence to suggest that the **nuclear bag fibers** are responsible for the dynamic sensitivity of the primary sensory ending, whereas the **nuclear chain fibers** are responsible for the static sensitivity of both the primary and secondary sensory endings. That the primary and secondary sensory endings (and their afferent nerve fibers) have different properties is most likely due to differences in viscoelastic properties of the nuclear bag and nuclear chain intrafusal muscle fibers.[5]

The preceding description of the properties of the muscle spindle derives from experiments in which there was no impulse traffic in the **fusimotor γ axons** (because the ventral roots were cut before recording from the dorsal roots). As discussed in the next section, however, the properties of the muscle spindle are markedly influenced by the activity of the γ motoneurons. To understand the functioning of the muscle spindle in an intact organism, we must therefore also know the actions of the γ innervation.

Effects of Gamma (γ) Innervation on the Properties of the Muscle Spindle

As mentioned, signals in γ fibers elicit contraction of the distal, cross-striated parts of the intrafusal muscle fibers. This stretches the midportion of the intrafusal fibers with the sensory endings (Fig. 13.6). In addition, it also alters the **stiffness** of the intrafusal fibers so that their reaction to stretch is altered. In general, the γ motoneurons and their γ fibers enable the brain to control the **sensitivity** of the muscle spindle to length and changes in length.

In animal experiments, single γ fibers in the ventral roots have been stimulated while, at the same time, the activity of group Ia and group II afferent fibers in the dorsal roots were recorded. It has thus been shown that there are **two types of γ motoneurons** (Fig. 13.9). One type increases the **dynamic sensitivity** of the muscle spindle and is therefore called **gamma dynamic** (γ_D). On a fairly rapid stretch of the muscle, the firing rate of a group Ia fiber increases more when the muscle spindle receives signals from γ_D motoneurons than without such influence, but the firing rate during static length is not significantly altered (Fig. 13.9). The muscle spindle's increased sensitivity to stretch enables the CNS to react more rapidly and forcefully to any unwanted change in muscle length (imposed, e.g., by external forces that upset body balance or ongoing movements).

Signals from the other type of γ motoneurons increase the **static sensitivity** of the muscle spindle and are therefore called **gamma static** (γ_S). The activity of γ_S motoneurons increases the firing rate of muscle spindle afferent fibers

during constant length, as compared with a situation without γ activity. Although not shown in Fig. 13.9, the firing rate of both group Ia and group II afferents increases. This influence of the γ system may be important to prevent the muscle spindles from becoming "silent"—that is, sending no action potentials—during the shortening of the muscle. In other words, the **length sensitivity** of the muscle spindle increases (indeed, maximal γ firing can increase the length sensitivity tenfold). Thus, the muscle spindle may signal the length of the muscle in its entire range of movements, which is important for precise movement control and for our awareness of joint positions.[6]

Gamma Fiber Activity and Judgment of Muscle Length

We know that information from muscle spindles is crucial for judging joint position and movement (kinesthesia). In this respect, however, the γ innervation poses a problem, since the signals from muscle spindles depend not only on the absolute length of the muscle but also on the degree of γ activity. Therefore, relevant parts of the brain must be able to account for the γ activity to end up with a true measure of muscle length. In fact, as discussed in Chapter 12, this is the situation for most sensory information: the signals from one kind of receptor are seldom unambiguous and must therefore be compared with other sources to provide an optimal answer.

Muscle Spindles in Humans and α–γ Coactivation

The previous description of the properties of muscle spindles is based on experiments in animals. However, results from anesthetized animals, often with the spinal cord isolated from the rest of the brain, do not enable us to draw conclusions as to the functions of the muscle spindle in intact organisms, for example, in human voluntary movements and in proprioception. Therefore, studies in humans with **microneurographic** techniques have provided a valuable supplement to data from animals. For example, the activity of group Ia afferent fibers in the nerves of the arm and the leg has been recorded in conscious human subjects. It appears (unexpectedly based on animal experiments) that in a resting muscle there is little or no impulse traffic from the muscle spindle. Indirectly, this shows that there is no fusimotor (γ) activity either. But if the muscle contracts

---

5. In reality, the conditions are even more complex. Among other factors, there are two types of nuclear bag fibers that differ ultrastructurally and histochemically: only one of them, called **bag**$_1$, appears to be responsible for the dynamic sensitivity of the primary sensory ending. The other one, called **bag**$_2$, behaves more like a nuclear chain fiber and contributes presumably only to the static sensitivity.

6. Figure 13.7 shows that stimulation of γ_S in fact *reduces* the dynamic sensitivity of the primary sensory ending, since there is no extra increase in firing rate of the Ia fiber during the stretch phase. Thus, under the influence of γ_S, the primary sensory ending behaves more like a secondary one.

The Actions of Ib Afferents on Spinal Motoneurons

Activation of the group Ib afferents from tendon organs was shown a long time ago to inhibit (via interneurons) motoneurons of the muscle in which the tendon organs lie (**homonymous inhibition**). Although these experiments were performed on anesthetized animals and therefore should be interpreted with caution, the task of the tendon organ was said to prevent contractions from being too strong. More recent studies have shown that the effects of the Ib afferents in the cord are not limited to homonymous inhibition. In awake animals, the effect on the motoneurons depends on the locomotor phase, and the effect is reversed from inhibition to excitation when moving from the swing phase to the standing phase. Thus, tendon organs in hind limb extensors excite extensor motoneurons when the leg is in the standing phase (via excitatory interneurons). In this case the signals from the tendon organ serve to amplify the contraction of the extensor muscles that keep the upright position. This is an example of how higher motor centers (in the brain stem and cerebral cortex) can switch the impulse traffic from one route to another in the cord, depending on the motor task. Further examples of this phenomenon are provided in Chapter 21.

Perception of Muscle Force

Our conscious perception of how hard the muscles contract may depend on two sources of information. One is the total activity of neurons in the motor cortex that send commands to the muscles that contract. This requires that other parts of the brain—for example, the somatosensory cortex—receive a copy of the motor commands sent to the muscles. This is called **efference copy**, or **corollary discharge**. Based on previous experience, the somatosensory cortex (in cooperation with other cortical regions) may estimate the muscle force that corresponds to the motor command. The other source of information is the **proprioceptors** that inform about the tension in the muscles themselves and in connective tissue that is stretched by muscle contraction. As discussed, **tendon organs** are particularly suited to informing about the tension in a contracting muscle, but because muscles often insert in the joint capsule, **joint receptors** may also contribute to communication of information.

That the motor cortex output plays a part is witnessed by the fact that persons with pareses due to muscle disease judge objects to be heavier than they actually are. To compensate for the weakened muscle, the motor cortex output is presumably higher than normal while the proprioceptive feedback is correct (informing about the real muscle tension). Nevertheless, the proprioceptive information seems to be necessary also, since patients with neuropathies may experience difficulties with holding a steady force and judging the weight of objects.

Low-Threshold Mechanoreceptors around the Joints

Not only receptors in muscles and tendons but also receptors in the connective tissue around the joints provide information important for our awareness of movements and for motor control. While the relative importance of information from joint and muscle receptors is not finally settled, the prevailing view is that the contribution from joint receptors to proprioception is much less important than that of the muscle spindles.

Many sensory nerve fibers end in the joint capsules and in the ligaments around the joints (Fig. 13.11). Many are **free-ending receptors**; others are **encapsulated** endings that correspond anatomically and with regard to response properties to encapsulated receptors in glabrous skin. The encapsulated joint receptors are **low-threshold mechanoreceptors** and have been divided into four groups. The **type 1 joint receptor** resembles the Ruffini corpuscle in the dermis (Fig. 13.1A). A myelinated axon ramifies among collagen fibrils, within a thin connective tissue capsule. They are found almost exclusively in the fibrous part of the joint capsules. The **adequate stimulus** of these Ruffini-like receptors is increased tension in the part of the capsule in which they lie. The higher the capsular tension, the higher the firing rate in the afferent sensory fiber from the receptor. Like the Ruffini corpuscle in the skin, this joint receptor is **slowly adapting**. Because the tension in various parts of the capsule depends on the joint position, type 1 receptors would appear suited to signal the position of the joint. For example, receptors in the posterior part of the elbow joint capsule would be highly active in a flexed position of the joint, which stretches the capsule, and less active in an extended position, which relaxes the capsule. The receptor also has **dynamic sensitivity**, giving a stronger response (higher firing rate) to a rapid movement than to a slow one. The type 1 or Ruffini-like receptor thus seems capable of signaling static joint position, joint movements, and direction and speed of movements. As discussed later, however, the ability of the type 1 receptor to signal static joint position appears to be limited.

The **type 2 joint receptor** structurally and functionally resembles the Pacinian corpuscle but is considerably smaller

Figure 13.11

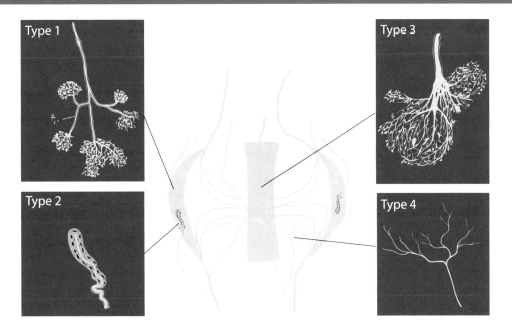

Joint innervation. Drawing of a knee joint, showing the distribution of the various kinds of joint receptors. The morphology of the four main receptor types is shown in more detail in the side panels. Type 1, 2, and 3 are low-threshold mechanoreceptors responding to small changes in joint-capsule tension. Type 4 are free nerve endings (most of them nociceptors).

(it is also called the Paciniform receptor). Type 2 receptors are present only in the fibrous part of the joint capsules. They are **rapidly adapting**, and their **adequate stimulus** is stretching of the part of the capsule in which they lie. Owing to their rapid adaptation, they can inform only of joint movements, not of static position. They appear particularly suited to signal **movement velocity** and have also been called acceleration receptors.

A third kind of encapsulated receptor (**type 3**) resembles the tendon organ and is present in **ligaments** only. It is slowly adapting (like the tendon organ), but its functional role is unknown. A protective role in signaling overstretching of joints has been proposed but has not gained experimental support.

Microneurographic studies in humans with stimulation of single afferent fibers from finger joints indicate that signals from low-threshold joint receptors can reach consciousness. Thus, when a fiber leading from a presumed type 1 receptor was stimulated, the subject reported the feeling of a movement of the relevant joint (the location and adequate stimulus of the receptor were determined before stimulation). In other instances of single-unit stimulation, the subject reported only a nonpainful, punctate feeling at the joint.

Do Low-Threshold Joint Receptors Contribute to Joint Stability?

Injury of the cruciate ligaments in the knee often leads to a feeling of lack of control and instability, even after successful surgical repair. Most likely, this is due to a proprioceptive deficit rather than a mechanical problem. In general, proprioceptive information is required for proper muscle coordination, and, more specifically, information about the tension of the cruciate ligaments may be necessary to ensure early stabilizing muscle activity. In support of this assumption, animal experiments show that stimulation of low-threshold joint receptors can increase γ-motoneuron activity (without concomitant effect on α motoneurons). In this way, muscle spindles in relevant muscles are put in a state of "alert" so they react more rapidly and strongly to knee movements.

Joint Nociceptors and Neurogenic Inflammation

The fibrous part of the joint capsule and the ligaments are richly supplied with thin myelinated and unmyelinated axons ending in free receptors. These have been termed **type 4** joint receptors. Many of these, like free endings in other tissues, are nociceptors. The joint capsules and ligaments persons become permanently dependent upon the cumbersome use of visual information to control posture and voluntary movements and to update their **body image**.

We return to proprioceptors and their central actions in Chapter 14 and discuss their relation to motor control in Chapters 18 and 21.

Clinical Examples of Loss of Somatosensory Information

In his book *The Man Who Mistook His Wife for a Hat*, neurologist Oliver Sacks gives a vivid description of a young woman, Christina, who completely lost kinesthetic sensation. A sensory neuropathy of unknown origin deprived her suddenly of virtually all kinds of proprioceptive information. Her cutaneous sensation was only slightly reduced, and motor axons were essentially spared. Nevertheless, at first she could not stand without continuously watching her feet. She could not hold anything in her hands, and they wandered around without her awareness. When stretching out to grasp an object she usually missed it—the movement stopped too soon or too late. "Something awful's happened, I can't feel my body. I feel weird—disembodied," she said, and "I may 'lose' my arms. I think they're one place and I find they're another." After having proprioception explained, she said: "This 'proprioception' is like the eyes of the body, the way the body sees itself. And if it goes, as it's gone with me, it's like the body is blind . . . so I have to watch it—be its eyes. Right?"

Another example concerns a 36-year-old man who gradually lost both cutaneous and kinesthetic sensation of the extremities due to a sensory neuropathy (described by Rothwell et al. 1982). His muscle power was hardly reduced, and he did surprisingly well on several routine tests of motor function. He performed, for example, various finger movements that require cooperation between muscles in the forearm and the hand. He could move his thumb with fair precision over three different distances and with three different velocities, and he could judge reasonably well the resistance to a movement. In spite of this, his hands were almost useless in daily life. He could not hold a cup with one hand, hold a pen and write, or button his shirt. Most likely this can be explained by lack of automatic adjustment of ongoing movements and by an inability to maintain constant muscle force for more than a few seconds (without seeing the part). The problems seemed to arise also because he was unable to do longer sequences of simple movements without constantly watching what he was doing.

THE SENSORY FIBERS AND THE DORSAL ROOTS

Afferent (sensory) fibers from the receptors follow the peripheral nerves toward the CNS. Close to the spinal cord, the sensory fibers are collected in the **dorsal roots** and enter the cord through these (Fig. 13.12). The sensory fibers of the spinal nerves have their cell bodies in the dorsal root

Figure 13.12

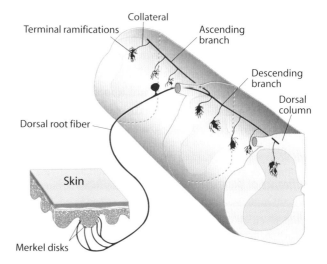

Terminal pattern of a dorsal root fiber. A dorsal root fiber (in this case conducting from Merkel disks) divides into an ascending and a descending branch after entering the cord. These branches give off several collaterals that end in the dorsal horn. The piece of the cord shown is about 1 cm long, but the axon continues beyond this in both directions. Corresponding reconstructions have been made for sensory units leading from several other kinds of receptors, and each sensory unit has a characteristic terminal pattern in the dorsal horn. (Based on Brown 1981.)

ganglia (see Figs. 6.5 and 6.9). Likewise, the sensory fibers in the cranial nerves have their cell bodies in ganglia close to the brain stem (see Fig. 27.4).

Spinal Ganglion Cells and Satellite Cells

As mentioned, the spinal ganglion cells are pseudounipolar (see Figs. 1.5 and 12.2) and send one long process peripherally, ending freely or in encapsulated sense organs. Functionally and structurally, both the peripheral and the central processes are axons. The **central process** enters the cord and then divides into an ascending and a descending branch (Fig. 13.12). These branches give off several collaterals ventrally to the gray matter of the cord. One sensory neuron, entering the cord through one dorsal root, can therefore influence spinal neurons at several segmental levels of the cord.

The dorsal root axons vary greatly in thickness, as described previously. The thick fibers belong to ganglion cells with large cell bodies, and the thin fibers belong to those with small cell bodies (Fig. 13.13). Thus, the small ganglion cells belong mostly to axons conducting from

Figure 13.13

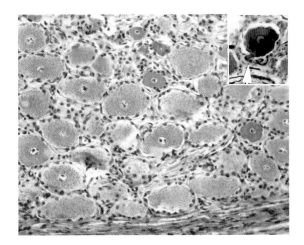

Spinal ganglion. Photomicrograph of a section from a human spinal ganglion. The cell bodies of the pseudounipolar neurons are different sizes. The cell bodies are surrounded by satellite cells. Inset: Photomicrograph of section treated with a silver impregnation method showing axons. Arrow points to the axon leaving the cell body of the ganglion cell.

nociceptors and thermoreceptors while the large ones belong to axons from low-threshold mechanoreceptors.

A layer of **satellite cells** surrounds the cell bodies of the ganglion cells and control their immediate environment (there is no blood–nerve barrier in the spinal ganglia; cf. Chapter 2 under "Peripheral Nerves Are Built for Protection of the Axons"). Satellite cells share several properties with **astroglia**. Thus, they contribute to homeostasis, are electrically coupled to their neighbors with gap junctions, and control extracellular K⁺ concentration. Activation of satellite cells may contribute to **persistent pain** by increasing ganglion cell excitability, for example after a nerve injury.

Are There Sensory Fibers in the Ventral Roots?

We now know that there are exceptions to the rule that sensory fibers enter the cord through the dorsal roots and that motor fibers enter through the ventral roots (the law of Magendie). The fact that cutting the dorsal roots—dorsal **rhizotomy**—does not always abolish pain indicates that not all sensory information passes through the dorsal roots. Electron microscopic investigations have proved the presence of many **unmyelinated fibers** in the ventral roots of several species, including humans. Many of these are efferent, preganglionic autonomic fibers, but physiologic data show that others (30% in the rat) are sensory and react to stimulation of **nociceptors**. However, few, if any, of these unmyelinated fibers have been proved actually to enter the cord through the ventral root. With retrograde

transport methods, their cell bodies have been shown to lie in the **dorsal root ganglia**. Some ventral root sensory fibers leave the ventral root to innervate the pia at the ventral aspect of the cord; others reverse direction before they enter the cord. Some of these then enter the cord through the dorsal root, whereas the further course of the others is unknown. We also do not know whether these peculiar arrangements have a special biological meaning.

Fiber Categories and Sensations

Relationships between signals conducted in sensory fibers of various thickness and sensations have been investigated primarily via graded electrical stimulation of peripheral nerves and selective blockage of axonal conduction. By electrical stimulation of peripheral nerves, the weakest stimulation evokes activity only in the thickest myelinated fibers, and with increasing intensity, the thinner fibers are recruited progressively. Thus, the thickest fibers have the lowest electrical threshold for activation. In human subjects, **pain** is evoked by such stimulation only if the stimulus is strong enough to activate **Aδ fibers**. The person then typically reports that the pain is of a sharp, pricking quality. If the stimulus strength is increased to recruit **C fibers** as well, the person experiences an intense, often burning pain that continues after the stimulus stops. These experiments are in agreement with the common experience that one usually can distinguish two phases of pain after an acute injury. The first phase, or **fast pain**, is experienced immediately after the stimulus, is well localized, and is not very intense; the second phase, or **slow pain**, occurs with a longer latency and is more unpleasant, is not well localized, and usually continues after the end of the stimulus. The slow pain is delayed because it depends on signals being conducted in C fibers with a conduction velocity of less than 1 m/sec. The difference in conduction velocity between fibers that give rise to fast and slow pain is most easily observed when something hits the foot hard enough to cause pain—for example, when a toe is bumped against a hard object. The pathway from the toe to the cerebral cortex is longer than from any other part of the body, so the time lag between the signals conducted in thick and thin fibers is greatest. In fact, the very first sensation is only that something touched the foot, due to activation of low-threshold mechanoreceptors. Almost simultaneously, the sharp and well-localized fast pain is perceived, and we then know that the pain will soon be worse—the diffuse, burning, and intensely unpleasant slow pain continuing for some time.

Blocking Conduction in Peripheral Nerves by Local Anesthetics and Pressure

Injection of **local anesthetics** around a peripheral nerve blocks the thinnest (C) fibers first and the thickest myelinated ones last. Accordingly, with local anesthetics the pain disappears first, whereas the tactile sensation remains considerably longer, and some sensations may remain throughout the period of anesthesia. When peripheral nerves are subjected to **pressure**, conduction in thick fibers is blocked first, and, accordingly, there first occurs a reduction of the ability to perceive light touch and to judge the position of joints, while pain perception is still present. For local anesthetics, which act by blocking voltage-gated Na^+ channels in the axonal membrane, access to the channels is more direct in unmyelinated fibers than in thick, myelinated ones. Pressure affects primarily thick myelinated fibers, presumably because of their high oxygen demand that make them more vulnerable than unmyelinated fibers to ischemia.

The Segmental Innervation: The Dermatomes

The **ventral branches** (rami) of the spinal nerves form plexuses supplying the arms (see Fig. 21.2) and the legs. Each nerve emerging from these plexuses contains sensory and motor fibers arising from several segments. In the peripheral distribution of the fibers, however, the segmental origin of the fibers is retained. Thus, sensory fibers of one spinal segment—that is, of one dorsal root—supply a distinct part of the skin. The area of the skin supplied with sensory fibers from one spinal segment is called a **dermatome**. In the thorax and abdomen, dermatomes form circular belts; in the extremities, however, conditions are more complicated (Figs. 13.14 and 13.15). Because the dermatomes **overlap**, each spot on the skin is innervated by sensory fibers from at least two dorsal roots.[7] Interruption of a single dorsal root therefore may not produce a clear-cut sensory deficit.

How the Dermatomes Have Been Determined

The oldest method for determining the dermatome is to follow the distribution of the nerves by dissection. To follow the course of fibers from a root through the plexuses is, of course,

far from easy. Certain diseases may affect single dorsal roots and produce changes restricted to the dermatome. **Shingles** (herpes zoster), for example, is a viral infection of the spinal ganglion cells that produces skin eruptions in the dermatome of the affected dorsal roots. Examination of many patients with this disease served as a basis for maps showing the dermatome (Head 1920). **Electrical stimulation** of dorsal roots during operations and comparison of observations during operations for herniated intervertebral disks with the information given previously by the patient of where the pain and sensory loss were localized also help determine the location of dermatomes. **Local anesthesia** of single or several dorsal roots in healthy volunteers has also been of value (Keegan and Garrett 1948). The best method is to eliminate impulse conduction in several dorsal roots on each side of one that is left intact (**method of remaining sensibility**). Sherrington (1898) did this experimentally in monkeys, but the results are not directly applicable to humans. The German neurosurgeon Foerster (1933) made more sporadic observations based on the method of remaining sensibility in patients in whom the dorsal roots were cut to relieve pain. Keegan and Garrett (1948) based their map on observations of a large number of patients with **root compressions** (usually due to a herniated intervertebral disk) and, in addition, on examination of the distribution of reduced sensation in volunteers who had been subjected to local anesthesia of dorsal roots.

Different Dermatomal Maps and Individual Variations

All dermatomal maps are composites of many single observations; no more than one or a few dermatomes have been determined in any single person. Thus, all maps showing dermatomes for the whole body are approximations because they do not take into account the considerable individual variations that exist. For example, experiments with electric stimulation of nerve roots shows that the thumb—indicated in Figure 13.14 as belonging to the C_6 dermatome—in some persons is innervated by fibers from the C_7 root. The big toe is shown in Figure 13.15 to lie mainly within the L_4 dermatome, while the L5 root supplies it in some persons. Individual variations, together with the fact that different methods have been used to explore the distribution of the dermatomes, probably explains why the maps of different authors vary so much. It should be noted, however, that the differences between the various dermatome maps are smaller in **distal parts** of the extremities than more proximally.

Because we do not know a person's exact dermatomal distribution, for the student the emphasis should be on learning the main features rather than the artificial borders between the dermatomes indicated on the maps.

---

7. Animal experiments indicate that the dermatomes are about twice as large as what appears from ordinary testing conditions, and the overlap is correspondingly larger. Inhibitory propriospinal fibers in the **tract of Lissauer** (Fig. 13.16) seem to inhibit weak sensory inputs from the peripheral parts of the dermatome, so that only signals from its central parts evoke a sensation. Under pathological conditions, however, the spinal neurons may become hyperexcitable and therefore respond to sensory inputs that normally are too weak to activate them.

Figure 13.14

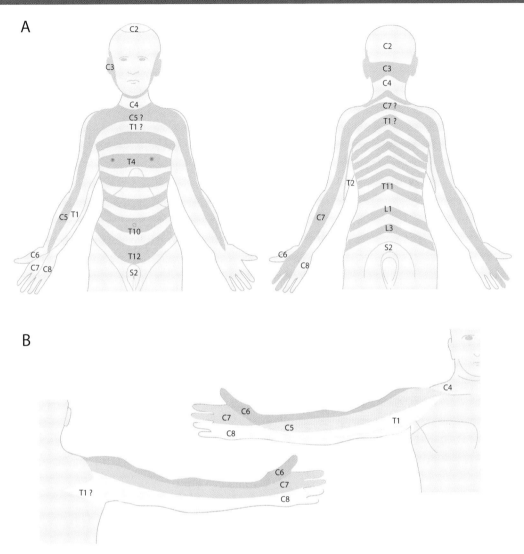

Dermatomes of the trunk and the upper extremity. Schematic. Because neighboring dermatomes overlap considerably, the map gives a false impression of the extension of the dermatomes; in reality the borders as presented in Figs. 13.14 and 13.15 are imaginary. The map presented here is based on Keegan and Garrett (1948), with modifications based on Lee et al. (2008). The main modification is that that the C_5 and T_1 dermatomes do not extend onto the trunk, in contrast to the original map published by Keegan and Garrett.

Clinical Significance of Dermatomes

Knowledge of the segmental innervation of the skin (and also of the segmental innervation of muscles and viscera, dealt with in Chapters 21 and 27) is of great practical value in clinical neurology. Due to the considerable overlap between neighboring dermatomes, **interruption** of a dorsal root produces no obvious sensory loss. Nevertheless, careful examination—especially of the distal parts of the extremities—usually shows a narrow zone (centrally in the dermatome) where the cutaneous sensation to touch is slightly reduced and that for pain may be abolished (analgesia). The usually more marked reduction in pain than in touch sensation is due to less extensive overlapping of fibers from nociceptors than of fibers from low-threshold mechanoreceptors.

When a dorsal root is subjected to **irritation**, as may occur by compression or stretching in connection with growth of an intraspinal tumor, protrusion of an intervertebral disk, or degenerative changes narrowing the intervertebral foramen, the result can be pain and other sensory phenomena (numbness, pricking, tingling, and so forth) in the vicinity of the dermatome. Often the symptoms are felt only in smaller parts of the dermatome. With a protruding (herniated) intervertebral disk in the lumbar spine, for example, most often the roots of the fifth lumbar or first sacral nerves are affected, and the pain is felt in the leg (**sciatica**). It should be emphasized that conclusions as to which root is affected must be based also on (if present) the distribution of motor symptoms (reflex changes, pareses).

Figure 13.15

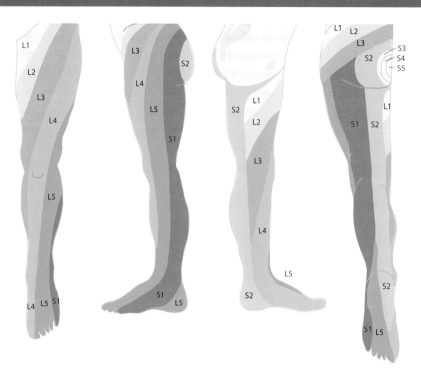

Dermatomes of the lower extremity. In contrast to the original maps of Keegan and Garrett (1948), there is now good evidence that the spinal nerves L$_4$, L$_5$, and most often S$_1$ do not send sensory fibers to the back and gluteal region. (Based on Keegan and Garrett 1948 and Lee et al. 2008).

Fibers from Different Receptors End in Different Parts of the Dorsal Horn

The thin (Aδ and C) and thick (Aα and Aβ) dorsal root fibers end almost completely separated in the cord (Fig. 13.16). This indicates that afferents from nociceptors and low-threshold mechanoreceptors make monosynaptic contacts on different neuronal populations, as confirmed by recordings from single units in the dorsal horn. Nevertheless, the extensive dendrites of spinal neurons (see Fig. 6.12) and numerous interneurons enable convergence of signals from different receptor types. Thus, in the dorsal horn, some neurons are **modality specific**, whereas others integrate signals from different kinds of receptors.

Thin **Aδ** and **C** fibers conducting signals from **nociceptors** end almost exclusively in the dorsalmost parts of the dorsal horn, in **laminae I** and **II** (**substantia gelatinosa**), but to some extent the Aδ fibers also terminate in lamina V. Low-threshold receptors around the joints send signals mainly to lamina VI. Signals from cutaneous **low-threshold mechanoreceptors** activate mostly neurons in deep parts of the dorsal horn—that is, in **laminae III** to **V**. Signals from

low-threshold mechanoreceptors and from nociceptors (and thermoreceptors) follow different routes from the dorsal horn to the cerebral cortex, as we discuss in Chapter 14.

Tracing of Single Doral Root Fibers

Combination of physiologic and anatomic techniques verified the differential terminal patterns of dorsal-root fibers. Further, such experiments made it possible to study in detail the termination of individual sensory units, as exemplified in Fig. 13.12. Single axons in the dorsal root were penetrated with thin glass microelectrodes (pipettes). After determination of the receptive field and adequate stimulus of the sensory unit, a tracer substance was injected in the axon with the same pipette. The axon and its ramifications were subsequently traced in serial sections of the spinal cord. A remarkable degree of specificity exists in the pattern of termination of fibers that belong to functionally different receptors.

Thin Sensory Fibers from Muscles, Joints, and Viscera: Nociception and Homeostasis

Whereas the thin afferent fibers (the majority from nociceptors and thermoreceptors) from the **skin** end mainly in

Figure 13.16

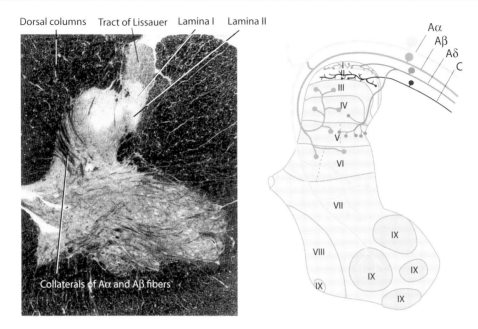

Dorsal columns   Tract of Lissauer   Lamina I   Lamina II

Collaterals of Aα and Aβ fibers

Terminal regions of the dorsal root fibers in the cord. **Left:** Photomicrograph of myelin stained transverse section through the cervical cord. **Right:** Schematic drawing. The thickest myelinated fibers (Aα, from muscle spindles and tendon organs) end in the deep parts of the dorsal horn and partly also in the ventral horn. Thick, myelinated fibers from cutaneous mechano receptors (Aβ) end in laminae III to VI. The thinnest myelinated and unmyelinated dorsal root fibers (Aδ and C)—many of them leading from nociceptors—end in laminae I, II, and parts of V. Based on experiments with axonal transport of tracer substances.

laminae I and II, corresponding fibers from the **viscera** appear to end almost exclusively in **laminae I** (and, to some extent, lamina V), thus avoiding the substantia gelatinosa. Thin **muscle** and **joint** afferents appear to terminate in the same parts of the dorsal horn as the fibers from viscera (although there are some conflicting data). Another feature of afferents from muscles and joints is their extensive **rostrocaudal distribution** in the cord. For example, afferent fibers from a single **facet joint** of the back terminate in seven to eight segments of the cord (cat). It is a common experience that pain of visceral origin has different qualities than pain evoked from the skin; visceral pain is much more diffuse and difficult to localize. In addition, pain that arises in muscles and joints is less precisely localized than cutaneous pain and radiates out from the site of the noxious stimulus. We also mentioned that muscle pain has a cramplike quality. Presumably, the anatomic arrangements in the dorsal horn may contribute to such differences.

    Lamina I of the dorsal horn has attracted interest because of its possible role in **homeostasis**. Due to the unique convergence of thin sensory fibers (especially C fibers) from virtually all tissues of the body—many of them chemoreceptors—lamina I neurons may monitor the metabolic status of the organism (such as the concentration of lactic acid and other metabolites produced in working muscles). At higher levels of the CNS, information from lamina I neurons most likely elicits appropriate autonomic and endocrine adjustments, while increasing afferent activity is perceived as discomfort and pain. The latter feelings are, of course, strong "recommendations" to the brain to change behavior (so that homeostasis is reestablished). (See also Chapter 14 under "Homeostatic Surveillance: A Task of Ascending Tracts from Lamina I?")

Primary Sensory Neurons: Colocalization of Classical Neurotransmitters and Neuropeptides

Probably all primary sensory neurons release a classical transmitter with fast synaptic actions in the spinal cord. Among other evidence, this is based on the observation that nerve terminals in the cord originating from dorsal root afferents contain small, clear vesicles, which have been shown in other parts of the nervous system to contain classical neurotransmitters. It has been estimated that at least 70% of all dorsal root fibers release an excitatory amino acid transmitter. Both ionotropic and metabotropic **glutamate receptors** are present in the dorsal horn, with the highest concentration in the dorsalmost laminae (I and especially II). *N*-methyl-D-aspartate (**NMDA**) receptors have attracted much interest because of their possible role in development of central **sensitization** in chronic pain. There is also evidence that some primary sensory fibers release **ATP** (probably together with glutamate), exerting fast, excitatory synaptic actions.

Several **neuropeptides** are present in the central and peripheral terminals and in the cell bodies of spinal ganglion cells, as shown with immunocytochemical techniques. These include **substance P** (SP), **vasoactive intestinal polypeptide** (VIP), **cholecystokinin**, **somatostatin, CGRP, galanin**, and others. Many ganglion cells contain more than one neuropeptide; for example, 80% of all SP-containing cells contain CGRP as well. The neuropeptides probably always colocalize with a classical transmitter with a fast, excitatory action. The peptides appear to mediate slow, modulatory synaptic actions in the dorsal horn, probably largely by acting on **extrasynaptic receptors** (see Fig. 5.3). When applied locally in the dorsal horn, SP and CGRP increase the release of glutamate. Further, SP receptors (neurokinin receptors) and NMDA receptors (glutamate) interact, making the NMDA receptors more sensitive to glutamate. Release of SP in the dorsal horn might therefore enhance and prolong the excitation produced by incoming signals from sensory receptors. We return in Chapter 15 to how this phenomenon may relate to increased pain sensitivity.[8]

Neuropeptides in Spinal Ganglion Cells and Nociceptors

Most of the neuropeptides are found only in **small ganglion cells** (Fig. 13.13), which have thin axons; these are probably mainly C fibers but also some Aδ fibers. Substance P, for example, is present in most of the small ganglion cells (in about 20% of all, large and small together). The **neuropeptide receptors** are concentrated in **laminae I and II** (with

the exception of CGRP receptors). These data suggest that the neuropeptides are particularly involved in transmission from **nociceptors** and **thermoreceptors**. Correspondingly, several neuropeptides and their receptors in the dorsal horn are up- or down-regulated in conjunction with **inflammation, nerve injury**, and **enduring pain**. Especially SP and its receptors (**neurokinin 1 [NK-1]**) are likely to be involved in processing of signals from nociceptors. Thus, SP is released from dorsal root fibers in the dorsal horn on nociceptor activation, and microinjection of SP in the dorsal horn make neurons more susceptible to sensory stimulation. Blocking NK-1 receptors prevents this effect.[9] The mechanism appears to be as follows: local injection of SP (and CGRP) in the dorsal horn increases the release of glutamate. Furthermore, SP and NMDA receptors interact, thereby making the NMDA receptors more sensitive to glutamate. Release of SP therefore would increase and prolong the response in the dorsal horn to signals from peripheral sensory receptors.

Inflammatory Diseases and Release of Neuropeptides from Peripheral Branches of Sensory Neurons

The function of neuropeptides present in the peripheral ramifications of primary sensory neurons is less understood than their functions in the central terminals. We do not know, for example, whether these peptides are released under normal circumstances and take part in the normal homeostatic control. We know, however, that the peptides can be released in the peripheral tissue by **noxious stimuli** and by **antidromic activation** of the axon (see Chapter 29, under "Antidromic Impulses and the Axonal Reflex"). Several of these peptides, when released in the tissues, have profound effects on vessels, as shown in the skin and mucous membranes. **SP** and **VIP** both produce vasodilation, and thereby increased blood flow and extravasation of fluid from the capillaries leading to edema. Furthermore, SP can activate cells of the **immune system**, resulting in phagocytosis and release of inflammatory mediators. AS mentioned, this phenomenon is termed **neurogenic inflammation** (see "Joint Nociceptors and Neurogenic Inflammation" earlier in this chapter).

Inhalation of irritating gases may provoke release of SP from peripheral sensory fibers in the **airways**, and the same takes place in the **skin** upon strong mechanical stimulation, such as scratching. The liberation of SP in such cases is probably due to an axonal reflex because afferent signals from the receptors are transmitted not only toward the spinal cord but also distally in branches of the sensory fibers (i.e., distally in the branches that were not stimulated).

Injury to the nerve or the innervated tissue changes the neuropeptide expression of the ganglion cells. For example,

8. A relationship seems to exist between the kind of **tissue** a neuron innervates and its neuropeptide content. For example, many more of the ganglion cells innervating viscera contain SP and CGRP than do those cells innervating the skin. About two-thirds of the ganglion cells supplying joints contain SP and CGRP. The evidence so far is too limited, however, to draw conclusions regarding relations between neuropeptides, sensory modalities, and tissue or organ specificity.

9. Although SP is clearly associated with nociception, the correlation is not absolute (as judged from studies combining physiologic and immunocytochemical characterization of single spinal ganglion cells). Thus, an SP-containing ganglion cell is not necessarily nociceptive, and many nociceptive neurons do not contain SP.

experimental arthritis leads to a marked increase of SP and CGRP in the cell bodies of the ganglion cells that innervate the affected joint (the arthritis is produced in animals by injecting the joint with a local irritant). SP enters the synovial fluid and induces release of such substances as **prostaglandins** and **collagenase** from leukocytes. Such substances may contribute to the damage of the joint cartilage in arthritis. Indeed, blocking the SP receptors (NK-1) or depleting the nerves of SP with **capsaicin** reduces the inflammatory reaction. Peripheral release of neuropeptides is now believed to play a role in several human diseases, including **rheumatoid arthritis**, **asthma**, **inflammatory bowel disease**, and **migraine**.

Sensory Fibers Are Links in Reflex Arcs: Spinal Interneurons

Sensory information reaching the spinal cord through the dorsal roots is further conveyed to higher levels of the CNS. In addition, the majority of the spinal neurons that are contacted by dorsal root fibers are not links in ascending sensory pathways but have axons that ramify within the cord—that is, they are **spinal interneurons**. The axons of these interneurons establish synaptic contacts with other spinal neurons, among them **motoneurons** and **sympathetic neurons** in the intermediolateral cell column, giving origin to efferent fibers to smooth muscles and glands. In this manner, **reflex arcs** (see Fig. 21.9) for several important somatic (skeletal muscle) and autonomic (visceral) reflexes are established. Most, if not all, spinal interneurons also establish connections between neurons at different segmental levels (propriospinal fibers). Each spinal interneuron thus establishes synaptic contacts with a large number of other neurons in the spinal cord. Signals entering the cord through one dorsal root may influence neurons at several segmental levels, by both their own ascending and descending collaterals and their influence on interneurons with propriospinal collaterals (Fig. 13.12; see also Fig. 21.10).

How far the signals from one dorsal root fiber spread from interneuron to interneuron depends on the other synaptic influences these interneurons receive. For example, **descending connections** from the brain can selectively facilitate or inhibit spinal interneurons. This enables the impulse traffic from dorsal root fibers to be directed so that certain reflex arcs are used, whereas others are "switched off," in accordance with the need of the organism as a whole. **Presynaptic inhibition** is an important mechanism in this respect (see Fig. 4.9). For example, separate groups of interneurons mediate presynaptic inhibition of group I muscle afferents, group II muscle afferents, and group Ib tendon organ afferents. Spinal reflexes are discussed in more detail in Chapter 21.

14

Central Parts of the Somatosensory System

OVERVIEW

There are two major somatosensory pathways, both consisting of **three neurons** forming a chain from the receptors to the cerebral cortex (Fig. 14.1). The first, the **primary sensory neuron**, has its cell body in a spinal ganglion or in a cranial nerve ganglion; the next, the **secondary sensory neuron**, has its cell body in the gray matter of the spinal cord or in the brain stem; and the third, the **tertiary sensory neuron**, has its cell body in the thalamus. Both somatosensory pathways are **crossed**, so that signals from one side of the body are brought to the cerebral hemisphere of the other side. The actual crossing over takes place at different levels for the two pathways, however (Fig. 14.1). Another important point is that the pathways are **somatotopically organized**, which implies that neurons that conduct signals from different parts of the body are kept separate.

Whereas axons conducting from different kinds of receptors lie intermingled in the peripheral nerves and the dorsal roots, they are grouped according to their thickness as soon as they enter the spinal cord. The thick dorsal root fibers (Aα and Aβ) pass medially, whereas the thin ones (Aδ and C) follow a more lateral course into the dorsal horn. Largely, then, neurons conveying signals related to low-threshold mechanoreceptors and nociceptors (and thermoreceptors) are kept separate in the spinal cord, as previously discussed. This segregation is maintained in the pathways that lead from the cord to higher levels.

The medially located **thick dorsal root fibers** continue without synaptic interruption rostrally in the **dorsal columns** (dorsal funiculus), without synaptic interruption in the cord. The first synaptic interruption occurs in the **dorsal column nuclei**, which contain the cell bodies of the secondary neurons in this pathway. The secondary axons cross in the medulla to end in the **thalamus** on the opposite side, forming the so-called **medial lemniscus**. From the thalamus, the tertiary neurons send their axons to the **primary somatosensory cortex** (SI) in the postcentral gyrus. Together, these three links constitute the so-called **dorsal column–medial lemniscus pathway**. From the prevalence of thick fibers conducting from low-threshold mechanoreceptors, it follows that the dorsal column–medial lemniscus pathway is important for perception of **touch**, **pressure**, **vibration**, and **kinesthesia**, but it is of primary importance for the **discriminatory aspects** of sensation—that is, the ability to distinguish differently placed and different kinds of stimuli. The pathway appears not to be necessary for the mere perception of, for example, light touch or movement of a joint.

The central pathway followed by signals conducted in the **thin dorsal root fibers** differs from that followed by the thick fibers. The thin fibers make synaptic contacts in the gray matter of the dorsal horn, where most of the secondary sensory neurons of this pathway are located. The axons of the secondary neurons cross to the other side of the spinal cord and form the **spinothalamic tract**. As the name implies, the fibers of this tract terminate in the thalamus. The spinothalamic tract is primarily important for the perception of **pain** and **temperature**, which is consistent with the observation that it transmits information mainly from Aδ and C dorsal root afferents. (There are also some other, less specialized pathways capable of transmitting somatosensory information.)

As mentioned, the sensory signals conducted in the medial lemniscus and the spinothalamic tract finally reach the **SI**. Here, the body is represented **somatotopically** with the face most laterally on the convexity and the foot on the medial side of the hemisphere. In addition, the spinothalamic tract sends signals to several other parts of the cerebral cortex (notably the anterior cingulate gyrus and the insula). Sensory information reaching the SI is subject to some processing before being forwarded to the **posterior parietal cortex** for further analysis and integration with other sensory modalities. In addition, many fibers pass from

Figure 14.1

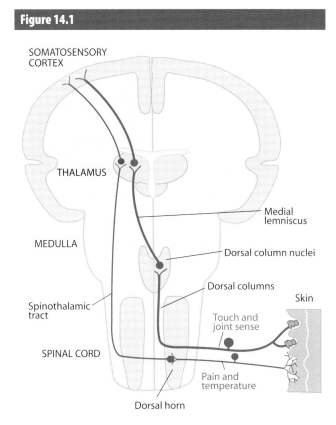

Somatosensory pathways. Highly simplified to show the main features of the two major pathways: the medial lemniscus–dorsal column pathway and the spinothalamic tract. The two pathways cross at different levels and differ in the sensory modalities they mediate.

the SI to the precentral motor cortex, contributing to control of voluntary movements.

CENTRAL SOMATOSENSORY PATHWAYS

Chapter 13 dealt with the peripheral parts of the somatosensory system—the receptors and the primary sensory neurons. We now turn to the tracts and nuclei conveying and processing somatosensory information within the central nervous system (CNS). The main pathways consist of three neurons forming a chain from the periphery to the cerebral cortex, crossing the midline in the spinal cord or brain stem (Fig. 14.1). The signals from low-threshold receptors and from nociceptors take different courses, but both pathways are synaptically interrupted in the thalamus.

The term "somatosensory pathways" is not entirely appropriate, however, because these pathways transmit signals not only from somatic structures, such as skin, muscles,

and joints, but also from internal (visceral) organs. Most signals from internal organs are not consciously perceived, and visceral sensory processes have been less intensively investigated than somatosensory ones. We discuss sensory information from the internal organs in Chapter 29.

Before we describe the somatosensory pathways in more depth, a few basic features of the thalamus need to be emphasized.

The Thalamus: Synaptic Interruption of Sensory Pathways

All pathways conducting sensory information from the receptors to the cerebral cortex (except the olfactory pathways) are synaptically interrupted in the thalamus. In addition, the thalamus has a decisive influence on the general level of neuronal activity of the cerebral cortex and thus on **consciousness** and **attention** (these aspects are discussed in Chapter 26, under "Thalamocortical Neurons Have Two States of Activity," and in Chapter 33, under "The Corticothalamic Connections" and "Higher-Order Thalamic Nuclei.")

The macroscopic appearance of the thalamus is described in Chapter 6 (see Figs. 6.22, 6.23, and 6.27). Three major subdivisions, delimited by the Y-shaped **internal medullary lamina**, can be identified macroscopically (Fig. 14.6; see also Fig. 6.23): an **anterior** nuclear group (or complex), a **medial** nuclear group, and a **lateral region** or part made up of a **dorsal** and a **ventral** nuclear group (see Fig. 6.22). Within and close to the internal medullary laminae are several less clearly defined groups of neurons, called the **intralaminar thalamic nuclei** (Fig. 14.6).[1]

Each of the three major thalamic subdivisions can be further subdivided into smaller nuclei based on cytoarchitectonic differences. These are called the **specific thalamic nuclei**, because most of them are relays in precisely organized, major pathways that reach only certain parts of the cerebral cortex. The various specific nuclei have different functional tasks, and they receive fiber connections from the somatosensory nuclei, the retina, the nuclei of the auditory pathways, the cerebellum, the basal ganglia, and some other neuronal groups. As a rule, each nucleus receives afferents from only one of these sources. The somatosensory

---

1. The intralaminar thalamic nuclei were formerly called the "unspecific thalamic nuclei" because their connections with the cerebral cortex were thought to be diffusely distributed, in contrast to the connections of the specific thalamic nuclei. More recent studies have questioned the nonspecific nature of the intralaminar nuclei, however.

pathways terminate in the ventral nuclear group, as is dealt with in more detail later in this chapter.

The Dorsal Columns and the Medial Lemniscus

The thick, myelinated fibers in the medial portion of the dorsal roots curve rostrally within the **dorsal columns** (funiculi) just after entering the cord. Many of these fibers ascend to the dorsal column nuclei in the medulla (see Figs. 6.16 and 6.19), where they terminate and establish synaptic contacts (Figs. 14.1 and 14.2). As the fibers ascend in the dorsal columns, they send off collaterals ventrally to the spinal gray matter (see Fig. 13.12). Most of these collaterals establish synaptic contact with interneurons, but some reach as far as the ventral horn and contact α motoneurons (primary afferents from muscle spindles). Therefore, the same sensory neuron influences spinal reflexes and evokes conscious sensations.

The fibers occupying the medial part of the dorsal columns—the **gracile fascicle**—conduct signals from the lower part of the trunk and the legs. These fibers end in the **gracile nucleus** (Fig. 14.2). Signals from the upper part of the trunk and the arms are conducted in the lateral part of the dorsal columns, the **cuneate fascicle**. The fibers of the cuneate fascicle terminate in the **cuneate nucleus**. Why the longest fibers of the dorsal columns lie most medially is explained by the simple fact that they enter the cord at the lowermost level, where no other long ascending fibers are present. At higher levels, fibers entering from the dorsal root occupy positions lateral to those that have entered at more caudal levels. Initially the fibers of the dorsal columns are arranged **segmentally**, but as they ascend, the fibers rearrange themselves so that they are organized **somatotopically**—that is, fibers conducting from the hand lie together, separated from those of the forearm, and so on (Fig. 14.2). Thus, fibers from different dorsal roots are mixed at higher levels of the dorsal columns.

The primary afferent fibers ascending in the dorsal columns end in a particular cytoarchitectonic subdivision—the **cluster region**—of the dorsal column nuclei. The morphology and arrangement of the neurons in the cluster regions ensure a particularly precise topographic arrangement of the afferent and efferent connections. The neurons of the cluster regions of the dorsal column nuclei send their axons rostrally to the thalamus, forming the **medial lemniscus**. The fibers first course anteriorly and cross the midline to

Figure 14.2

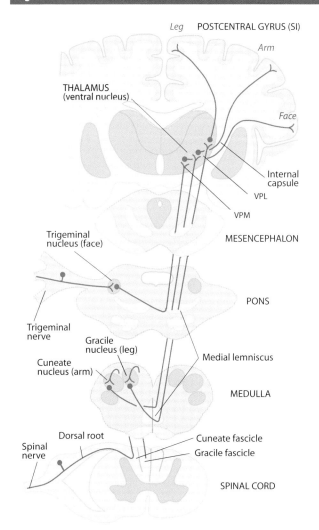

The dorsal column–medial lemniscus pathway. This is the main pathway for transmission of signals from low-threshold mechanoreceptors. Fibers leading signals from mechanoreceptors in the face join the medial lemniscus in the brain stem.

occupy a position just dorsal to the pyramid (Fig. 14.3; see also Fig. 6.17). In the pons and the mesencephalon, the medial lemniscus is placed more laterally (Fig. 14.3; see also Figs. 6.18 and 6.20).

The medial lemniscus ends in the **ventral posterolateral nucleus** (**VPL**) (Figs. 14.2 and 14.6). The fibers of the medial lemniscus are **somatotopically** organized,[2] and this pattern is maintained as the fibers terminate in the VPL.

---

2. That fibers carrying signals from the leg are located more anteriorly within the medial lemniscus than are those related to the arm (Fig. 14.3) is simply because the gracile nucleus is situated more caudally than the cuneate nucleus. When fibers from the cuneate nucleus join those from the gracile nucleus, the anterior position is already occupied.

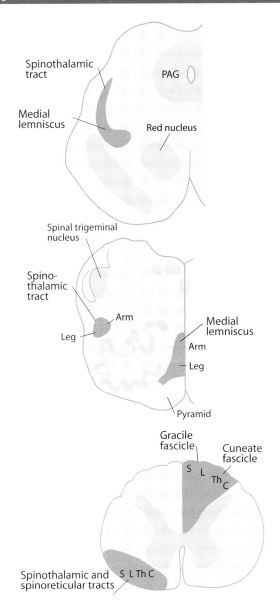

Somatosensory pathways. Position and segmental arrangement in the cord, medulla, and mesencephalon. The spinal cord is disproportionally large.

Fibers from the gracile nucleus (sensory signals from the leg) terminate most laterally, with fibers from the cuneate nucleus (arm) terminating more medially. Most medially, in a separate nucleus, the **ventral posteromedial nucleus (VPM)** ends the fibers from the sensory trigeminal nucleus (relaying signals from the face).

Neurons of the dorsal column nuclei that send their axons in the medial lemniscus most likely use **glutamate** as transmitter (like most other long, precisely organized tracts in the CNS).

The Dorsal Columns Contain More than Primary Afferent Fibers

The dorsal columns carry four kinds of nerve fibers:

1. Primary afferent fibers that reach the dorsal columns and establish synaptic contacts there; that is, the fibers forming a link in the dorsal column–medial lemniscus pathway.

2. Primary afferent fibers in the dorsal columns that do not reach the dorsal column nuclei, even though they may pass through many segments—for example, from the lumbar to the cervical levels. Such fibers constitute a large proportion of the fibers in the dorsal columns.

3. The dorsal columns contain a large number of axons from neurons located in the spinal gray matter. Most of these are **propriospinal** fibers extending just for one or a few segments to end in the cord. Others, however, end in the dorsal column nuclei and are called **postsynaptic dorsal column neurons**. These seem to play a particular role in transmission of **nociceptive** signals from the viscera (see Chapter 29, under "The Dorsal Columns Carry Signals from Visceral Nociceptors").

4. A number of axons **descend** in the dorsal columns to make synaptic contacts in the dorsal horn (especially in lamina V, containing neurons excited by signals from nociceptors). These descending fibers come from neurons in a subdivision of the dorsal column nuclei (the **reticular zone**) that receives afferents from the cerebral cortex and the reticular formation. Thus, the dorsal column nuclei are part of a neuronal network that—by way of descending connections—control the flow of sensory information from the cord (see "The Brain Controls the Transmission of Sensory Signals" later in this chapter).

Thalamocortical Pathway to the SI and SII

The neurons of the VPL and the VPM send their axons into the internal capsule (Fig. 14.2) and further through this to the **postcentral gyrus**. This part of the cortex, made up of cytoarchitectonic fields 3, 1, and 2 (after Brodmann; see Fig. 33.4), constitutes the **primary somatosensory area (SI;** Figs. 14.2 and 14.6). In addition, some fibers from the VPL and the VPM end in the **secondary somatosensory area (SII)**, situated in the upper wall of the lateral cerebral fissure (Fig. 14.6). On **electrical stimulation** of the SI or SII, conscious human subjects report sensory phenomena such as tingling, itching, numbness, and so forth. Just as the somatosensory pathways are **somatotopically** organized, this is also the case within the SI and SII (Figs. 14.2 and 14.7). Fibers conducting signals from the leg end most medially within the postcentral gyrus, then follow fibers conveying signals from the trunk, arm, and face successively in the lateral direction.

Epileptic Seizures Demonstrate the Cortical Somatotopic Pattern

On irritation of the cortex within the postcentral gyrus—for example, by a chip of bone from a skull fracture—the patient may experience fits of abnormal sensations. In the same person, the fits have the same characteristic pattern each time: The sensations are felt in one particular part of the body and then spread gradually to other parts. The spreading follows the known somatotopic pattern within the SI (see Fig. 14.8). For example, the patient may first experience a tingling sensation in the thumb; then it may move to the index finger and the other fingers and then to the forearm, upper arm, shoulder, and even further. Such epileptic seizures are called **Jacksonian fits** (after the famous British neurologist Hughlings Jackson). They signify the presence of a local disease process of the brain, and the starting point of the abnormal sensations indicates the focus of the disease. Often the sensory phenomena are followed by muscle spasms (convulsions) due to spreading of the abnormal cortical electrical activity to the motor cortex of the precentral gyrus.

Single-Unit Properties in the Dorsal Column–Medial Lemniscus System

As mentioned, the dorsal columns contain primarily fibers coming from **low-threshold mechanoreceptors** in the skin, muscles, and joints. Recording the activity of single units in the dorsal columns has confirmed this and has shown that there is a predominance of **rapidly adapting** sensory units; relatively few are slowly adapting. They have small **receptive fields**, mostly at the **distal parts** of the extremities (see Fig. 13.3). Recordings from neurons in the **cluster regions** of the dorsal column nuclei show that many neurons are activated by only one kind of receptor. Some are activated only by joint movements, others only by light touch of the skin, others only by vibration, and so forth. These neurons are called **modality specific** (because they only react to one kind of stimulus) and **place specific** (because they are activated only from one restricted part of the body).

Neurons in the **VPL** and **SI** also have the same characteristic response properties as those described for the neurons of the dorsal column nuclei. Nevertheless, there is a difference since in the VPL, and even more so in the SI, a larger fraction of the neurons are activated by more than one kind of receptor. In addition, the receptive field tends to be somewhat larger for neurons in the SI than, for example, in the dorsal column nuclei. Thus, many neurons in the thalamus, and even more in the SI, receive signals from primary afferents with different modalities and receptive fields; that is, they **integrate** various kinds of information.

Functions of the Dorsal Column–Medial Lemniscus System

Most of the axons at all levels of the dorsal column—medial lemniscus system are thick and rapidly conducting. This, together with the data from single-unit recordings mentioned earlier, enable us to conclude that the dorsal column–medial lemniscus system is particularly well suited to bring fast and precise information from the skin and musculoskeletal system about the type of stimulus, the exact site of the stimulus, and when the stimulus starts and stops. Thus, it provides information about the **sensory quality** and the **spatial and temporal characteristics** of any stimulus of low intensity (the "what," "where," and "when"). The next question is then: How does the CNS use this information? Unfortunately, on this point conclusions are largely based on the deficits observed when the system is not working. Further, because of the adaptive changes that take place after an injury, we have to distinguish between the **acute** and **long-term** functional deficits. Other problems of interpretation arise because, with incomplete lesions, functional deficits may be revealed only by tests that require full use of the system. For example, experiments in cats show that the ability to judge the roughness of surfaces is only slightly reduced even after cutting 90% of the dorsal column fibers.

The sensory deficits occurring after lesions of the dorsal columns all concern spatial and temporal comparisons of stimuli, or what we call **discriminative sensation**. Such sensory information is crucially important for the performance of many **voluntary movements**; indeed, disturbances of voluntary movements are characteristic of the lesions that affect the dorsal column–medial lemniscus system. After the acute phase, the movement deficits first concern movements that require fast and reliable feedback information from the moving parts. For example, the ability to adjust the grip when an object is slipping is clearly reduced. Delicate movements, such as writing and buttoning, are performed only with difficulty after lesions of the dorsal columns. It is not possible to throw an object accurately or to perform a precise jump, presumably because such activities require feedback information from skin receptors to judge the pressure exerted on the hand by the object or by the ground against the sole of the foot.

In conclusion, the dorsal column–medial lemniscus system is of primary importance for complex sensory tasks, such as determination (comparison) of direction and speed of moving stimuli. Further, many precise voluntary movements—especially of the hand—depend on the fast sensory feedback provided only by this system. In fact, after damage to the system, the motor deficits may be more disturbing than the purely sensory ones.

Acute and Long-Term Sensory Impairments Differ

Most studies (with some exceptions) indicate that in monkeys, as in humans, **acute damage** to the dorsal columns produces severe **ataxia** (insecure and uncoordinated movements), which recedes partly or completely within weeks to months after the damage. In some patients, the ataxia may be so severe that they cannot walk without support. Observations some time after the damage indicate, however, that the dorsal column–medial lemniscus system is not necessary for all aspects of cutaneous sensation and kinesthesia. First, temperature and pain perception are unaltered by lesioning the dorsal columns; second, light touch of the skin can easily be felt, as can passive joint movements. Two-point discrimination may not be appreciably reduced, and some reports even indicate that the ability to recognize objects by manipulation may be retained (clinical observations do not support the latter point, however). What appears to be consistently impaired is the ability to solve tasks that require spatially and, in particular, temporally very accurate sensory information. Thus, a coin pressed into the palm of the hand may perhaps be recognized, but the patient is unable to decide which is the larger of two coins. The patient may also correctly identify that something is moving on the skin but not the direction of the movement. To ask the patient to identify figures written on the skin, for example, is one sensitive test of the function of the dorsal column–medial lemniscus system. Further, some careful clinical observations indicate that the perception of joint position and movement is abnormal after lesions of the dorsal columns.

The Dorsal Columns and Kinesthesia

Observations in humans have provided conflicting results as to whether lesions of the dorsal column–medial lemniscus system give impaired kinesthesia. A thorough clinical study by Nathan and coworkers (1986, p. 1032), however, concluded that complete lesions of the dorsal columns do produce clear-cut and enduring kinesthetic deficits. But they emphasize that "routine examination of tactile sensibility does not show up these defects as well as everyday activities of living. The further one gets away from this testing situation, the easier it is to see the effects of these disturbances of sensibility." One example may illustrate this point: a patient with damage to the dorsal columns was aware of a toe being passively moved by the examiner; nevertheless, his shoe would easily slip off his foot without his noticing, and he was unable to roll over in bed because he did not realize that one leg was hanging off the bed.

In monkeys, Vierck and Cooper (1998) described deficient kinesthetic sensation of the **hands** after cutting the cuneate fasciculus, although only specific and detailed testing revealed the problems. Thus, the perception of passive finger movements was impaired only if the movements were small or slow. This is indeed what we would expect when eliminating a system devoted to very precise sensory information. It is furthermore worth noticing that the monkeys had more obvious problems with precise hand movements than with kinesthesia. In the **legs**, however, joint sense remained normal in monkeys after lesions of the dorsal columns at thoracic or cervical levels. This may be explained by the finding (in monkeys) that primary afferent fibers conveying signals from slowly adapting low-threshold mechanoreceptors in leg muscles and joints leave the gracile fasciculus at the low thoracic level. Then they enter the dorsal horn, where they synapse on second-order sensory neurons. The axons of the latter continue in the dorsal part of the lateral funiculus, not in the dorsal columns. Thus, a lesion of the dorsal columns at cervical levels would not interrupt signals from leg proprioceptors. We do not know, however, whether this arrangement pertains also to humans.

Clinical Examination of the Dorsal Column–Medial Lemniscus System

Many of the deficits that occur after damage to the dorsal column–medial lemniscus system may not show up during a routine neurological examination. Nevertheless, they may render the patient severely handicapped in daily life. We described earlier in this chapter similar symptoms occurring after loss of thick myelinated nerve fibers in the peripheral nerves. This is not surprising because many of these fibers continue into the dorsal columns. The deficits may be more severe with peripheral loss, however, because reflex effects from low-threshold mechanoreceptors (among other things) are also lost. Based on these considerations, a routine examination of kinesthesia (asking the patient to indicate the direction of movement in a joint being passively moved) would not provide definite information because such a test may be negative (i.e., normal performance) in spite of damage to the dorsal columns or the medial lemniscus. Neither is testing the sense of vibration a reliable source of information; several clinical studies show that vibration is not always reduced after damage to the dorsal columns. A routine testing of cutaneous sensation would not necessarily reveal the lesion. The most reliable information is presumably obtained by testing the ability to judge the direction of a stimulus to the skin and to examine the patient's ability to identify numbers written on the skin.

applied to alleviate intense pain that cannot be overcome in any other way. After such an operation, sensations of pain and temperature are almost totally abolished in the opposite side of the body in the parts supplied by sensory fibers from the spinal segments below the level of interruption.

Although both lamina I and lamina V contain a mixture of WDR and HT neurons, it appears that **lamina I** contains a majority of HT (nociceptive specific) neurons, whereas WDR neurons dominate in the deeper parts of the dorsal horn.

Terminations of the Spinothalamic Tract and Further Projections to the Cortex

The **thalamic** termination site of the spinothalamic tract is more extensive than that of the medial lemniscus, and the same holds for the further signal transmission to the cerebral cortex. Many of the spinothalamic fibers end in the **VPL** with a **somatotopic** pattern (Fig. 14.4) but not in

exactly the same parts as the fibers of the medial lemniscus (corresponding fibers from the spinal trigeminal nucleus end in the VPM). The terminal ramifications are also different for the two pathways, and nociceptor activation of VPL neurons requires more **summation** than activation from low-threshold mechanoreceptors. In addition, many of the spinothalamic fibers end in parts of what is now collectively referred to as the **posterior thalamus,** notably in the **ventromedial nucleus.** Spinothalamic fibers also end in parts of the **intralaminar nuclei** (e.g., the central lateral nucleus), the **mediodorsal nucleus,** and some other nuclei.

The multiple terminations of spinothalamic fibers probably explain how signals from nociceptors, by way of thalamocortical fibers, can reach several regions of the cortex in addition to the SI and SII. Recordings of single-unit activity in monkey **SI** indicate that neurons activated by high-intensity (presumably noxious) cutaneous stimuli are concentrated in a narrow zone at the transition between Brodmann's **areas 3** and **1** (Fig. 14.6). This may primarily concern signals relayed through the

Figure 14.6

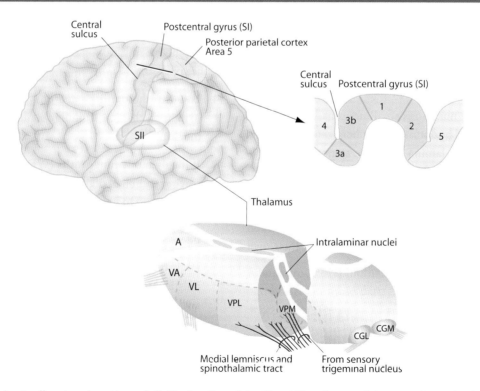

The SI and its thalamic afferent nucleus. **Upper left:** The location of the SI and SII and parts of the posterior parietal cortex in the left hemisphere. **Upper right:** The extension of the various cytoarchitectonic areas of the central region. **Below:** The VPL—supplying the SI and SII with somatosensory signals—is marked on a schematic drawing of the left thalamus. The main afferent pathways to the VPL are also indicated. A, anterior thalamic nucleus; LG, lateral geniculate body; MG, medical geniculate body; VA, ventral anterior nucleus; VL, ventral lateral nucleus; VPM, ventral posteromedial nucleus; VPL, ventral posterolateral nucleus.

VPL, whereas signals from other parts of the thalamus receiving spinothalamic fibers may directly and indirectly influence other cortical areas, such as the **anterior cingulate gyrus** and the **insula**.

Does the Spinothalamic Tract Consist of Distinct Discriminative and Affective Parts?

The spinothalamic tract has been proposed to consist of two anatomically and functionally different components. One part—ending in the lateral thalamus (mainly in the VPL and VPM) with further transmission to the SI—is responsible for the discriminative aspects of pain perception; that is, our ability to localize a painful stimulus and to judge its quality (sticking, burning, cramp-like, and so forth). The other part—consisting of fibers ending in the medial thalamus (especially in the intralaminar nuclei) and projecting on to the **insula**—is responsible for the affective, emotional aspects of pain. There is much evidence, however, that this division is at least an oversimplification. For example, many spinothalamic fibers send collaterals to both lateral and medial thalamic nuclei (and to parts of the reticular formation in the brain stem). Furthermore, some spinothalamic fibers send branches to the VPL/VPM and posterior thalamus. Accordingly, the VPL/VPM and the ventromedial nucleus both receive signals from HT and WDR sensory units (although the ventromedial nucleus may receive the majority of lamina I afferents, which are mainly of the HT kind). Thus, it seems highly unlikely that signals from spinothalamic neurons with different physiologic properties (HT, WDR, and so forth) are treated separately in the thalamus. In support of this conclusion, **microstimulation** of the lateral thalamus in humans (presumably in the ventromedial nucleus) evoked pain that could be precisely localized *and* at the same time evoked strong emotions (anxiety, discomfort).

Spinothalamic Cells Receive Signals from the Skin, Muscles, and Visceral Organs

Recording from spinothalamic cells in the spinal cord has shown that many can be activated by nociceptive stimuli applied to **visceral organs** and to the **skin**. Signals from the skin and viscera **converge** onto the same neuron, which then conveys the information to the thalamus. Nociceptive signals from **muscles** and skin can also converge onto the same spinothalamic neuron. Sensory convergence of this kind pertains to regions of the skin and deep tissues and to visceral organs that receive sensory innervation from the same segments of the cord. The primary sensory fibers can activate the spinothalamic cells monosynaptically or through one or more interneurons (polysynaptically). In addition, in some spinal ganglion cells the peripheral process divides, with one branch innervating the skin and the other a visceral organ or a muscle.

The observations of convergence on spinothalamic cells and branching of sensory fibers may help explain why pain arising from a visceral organ is often felt as if it comes from the skin. This phenomenon is called **referred pain** and is discussed further in Chapter 29.

What Tracts in the Anterolateral Funiculus Can Mediate Alone: A Case History

A woman with a knife-stab partly severing the cord at the Th$_3$ level illustrates what the anterolateral funiculus alone can mediate of somatic sensations (Danzinger et al. 1996). The lesion, which was verified during open surgery, severed the cord completely except for the anterolateral fascicle and adjoining parts of the lateral funicle on the left side. Shortly after the accident, with some difficulty, she was able to feel and localize light touch on both sides of the body below the lesion. She was able to perceive passive joint movements on the left side but not vibration. Eighteen years after the lesion her sensibility was virtually unchanged. The lesion did not abolish control of the bladder and the rectum, and she retained some voluntary control of movements of the left leg (whereas the right leg was paralytic, she was, e.g., able to lift the left leg 30° in the supine position).

Additional Pathways from Nociceptors

Pathways other than the spinothalamic tract may transmit signals from nociceptors to consciousness, even if their contribution may be minor under normal conditions. It should be emphasized that nociceptive signals reach numerous subcortical nuclei (in the rat apparently more than 20), many of which have ascending projections. Concerning transmission from **visceral nociceptors**, postsynaptic fibers in the **dorsal columns** seem to contribute in addition to the spinothalamic tract. There is also evidence that signals in the dorsal columns may contribute to persistent pain in some instances (this is further discussed in Chapter 29, under "Visceral Pain"). Further, many nociceptor-activated spinal neurons send their axons to brain stem nuclei that mediate automatic responses to noxious stimuli, such as changes of blood pressure, heart rate, sweating, breathing, muscle tone, bladder and bowel function, and so forth. Parts of the **reticular formation**, the periaqueductal gray (**PAG**), and the **parabrachial nucleus** all receive signals from nociceptors and participate in automatic behavioral responses to nociceptor activation. Among these, the parabrachial nucleus is special since it receives spinal afferents mainly from **lamina** extent, from nociceptors. Somatosensory signals also reach other cortical regions, however, such as the **motor cortex** (MI) in the precentral gyrus. Not unexpectedly, primarily signals from **proprioceptors** are conveyed to the motor cortex.

The parts of the SI receiving sensory signals from the feet, hands, and face are much larger than those receiving signals from other parts of the body (Fig. 14.8). Further, the region devoted to the thumb is larger than that devoted to the palm of the hand, which, in turn, is larger than that devoted to the forearm, and so on. This is mainly a reflection of the much higher **density of sensory units** that supply the skin at distal parts of the extremities (and parts of the face) than more proximal parts of the trunk. To use this very detailed information from the most densely innervated parts of the body, a large volume of cortical gray matter—that is, many neurons—has to be available for information processing. A **magnification factor** gives a numerical representation of the cortical representation of certain body parts. Similar over-representations exist within the visual and auditory systems.

Brain-imagining techniques have brought a wealth of information on the contribution of specific cortical areas in motor, sensory, and cognitive processes. Brief descriptions of these and some other methods were given in Chapter 6, under "Methods to Study the Living Human Brain." We refer to results from brain-imaging studies throughout this book.

The Primary Somatosensory Area (SI)

The primary somatosensory area, in particular, has been the subject of intense anatomic and physiologic investigations. The subdivision of the SI into different **cytoarchitectonic areas—3, 1,** and **2** of Brodmann (see Figs. 22.4 and 33.2)—corresponds to functional differences. These areas extend as narrow strips from the midline laterally along the postcentral gyrus: that is, perpendicular to the somatotopic arrangement (Fig. 14.6; see also Fig. 33.4). Animal experiments, particularly by the American neurophysiologist Mountcastle, show that the cytoarchitectonic subdivisions differ with regard to the kinds of receptor from which they receive information. **Area 3a**, on the transition to the MI (see Fig. 22.4), receives sensory signals from **muscle spindles** in particular.[5] Neurons in **area 3b** are mainly activated

by stimulation of **cutaneous receptors** (predominantly by low-threshold mechanoreceptors). Neurons receiving information from rapidly adapting receptors appear to be separated from those receiving from slowly adapting receptors. **Area 2** is influenced by **proprioceptors** to a larger extent than area 3b is; for example, bending of a joint most easily activates many neurons. Within each of the cytoarchitectonic subdivisions it appears that the whole body has its representation; thus there are probably three **body maps** within the SI. The map in Fig. 14.7 therefore gives a somewhat misleadingly simplified presentation.

Figure 14.8 shows the representation of body parts based on electric stimulation of the cortical surface in conscious patients (during neurosurgery for therapeutic reasons). The patient tells where she feels something when a certain cortical site is stimulated. Although later studies overall agree with the findings of Penfield and Rasmussen (1950; Fig. 14.8), an exception seems to concern the representation of the **genitals**, which most likely are represented on the convexity near the lower part of the abdomen (and not on the medial aspect of the hemisphere close to the foot, as originally indicated by Penfield and Rasmussen).[6]

Even though many neurons in the SI are activated only or most easily from one receptor type—that is, they are **modality-specific**—there are other neurons in the SI with more **complex properties**. For example, many neurons have large receptive fields, indicating that they receive convergent inputs from many primary sensory neurons. Further, movement of just one joint in one direction activates some neurons, while other neurons are activated by several joints. Still other neurons in the SI require specific combinations of receptor inputs to be activated. Thus, processing of the "raw" sensory information already begins at the first cortical stage; the SI is not merely a receiver of sensory information.

Efferent **association connections** from the SI pass posteriorly to the **posterior parietal cortex** (Fig. 14.6), which processes the sensory information (see later discussion), and anteriorly to the **MI**. The latter connections appear to be of particular importance while **learning** new movements, whereas they are not crucial for the performance of well-rehearsed movements (judging from lesion experiments in monkeys). This may be explained by an extra need for fast and precise feedback from the moving parts during

---

5. Some have argued that area 3a should be considered a part of the MI rather than of the SI. In certain respects, anatomically and physiologically, area 3a represents at least a transitional zone. Like the other subdivision of the SI, area 3a receives thalamic afferents from VPL, whereas MI (area 4) receives them from VL. The afferents from other parts of the cortex are more like those of MI than of the other parts of the SI, however.

6. Representation of the genitals on the medial aspect of the hemisphere would be in conflict with the principle of continuous representation of body parts (Fig. 14.7). Indeed, a recent study using natural peripheral stimulation and fMRI (rather than stimulation of the cortical surface) concluded that the penis is represented on the convexity in the transition zone between the lower abdomen and the thighs (Kell et al. 2005).

learning. The connections from the SI to the MI, furthermore, are necessary for motor **recovery** after cutting the connections from the cerebellum to the MI, as discussed in Chapter 11 (under "Animal Experiments Elucidating the Mechanisms of Recovery"). This may also be regarded as a learning situation.

Further Processing of Sensory Information Outside the SI

Although processing of somatic sensory information starts in the SI, clinical and experimental observations show that the cortex posterior to the SI is necessary for comprehensive utilization. The posterior parietal cortex comprises **area 5** and **area 7** (Fig. 14.6; see also Fig. 33.4) and belongs to the association areas of the cerebral cortex (further discussed in Chapters 33 and 34). Areas 5 and 7 do not receive direct sensory information from the large somatosensory pathways but via numerous association fibers from the SI and SII. They also receive numerous connections from other parts of the cortex. Broadly speaking, in areas 5 and 7 the bits of information reaching the SI are put together and compared with other inputs, such as visual information and information about the salience of a stimulus and about movement **intentions**. Neurons in area 5 often have large receptive fields and respond to complex combinations of stimuli, as shown in monkeys. Their activity depends not only on what is occurring in the periphery but also on whether the **attention** of the monkey is directed toward the stimulus. The posterior parietal cortex sends **efferent** connections to motor areas in the frontal lobe, thereby linking sensory information with **goal-directed movements**. This link is evidenced by neurons in the parietal cortex being active in conjunction with the monkey stretching its arm toward something it wants. Accordingly, electrical stimulation of the posterior parietal cortex in human subjects evoked a desire to move the contralateral arm or foot (Desmurget et al. 2009).

In addition to the posterior parietal cortex, the **SII** (Fig. 14.6) and adjoining areas in the **insula** (Fig. 14.9) also process information from the SI. The anterior part of insula integrates somatosensory information with other sensory modalities (taste, smell, and signals from vestibular receptors). Sensory units in these areas typically have large receptive fields and are activated from both sides of the body. Insula is, however, more strongly linked with processing of visceral sensory information and pain (see later in this chapter and Chapter 34 under "The Insula").

Symptoms after Lesions of the Somatosensory Areas

Lesions of the **SI** in humans entail reduced sensation in the opposite half of the body. A localized destruction of the SI, or of the fibers reaching it from the thalamus, may produce loss of sensation in a restricted area (corresponding to the somatotopic localization within the SI). Not all sensory qualities are affected equally, however. **Discriminative** cutaneous sensation and **kinesthesia** are particularly disturbed; much less reduced (if at all) is pain sensation. As is the case with lesions of the dorsal columns, the sensory deficits gradually diminish after the time of the lesion. The least improvement with time is seen in the discriminative aspects of sensation, whereas pain sensation improves considerably. This can perhaps be explained by the fact that the pathways for signals from nociceptors are to a larger extent bilateral than are the pathways from low-threshold

---

Figure 14.9

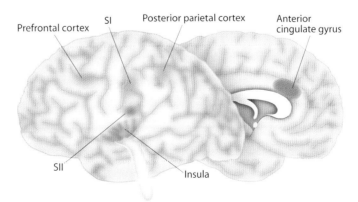

Prefrontal cortex · SI · Posterior parietal cortex · Anterior cingulate gyrus · SII · Insula

Regions of the cerebral cortex showing increased activity during pain experience. (Based on data from a meta-analysis published by Peyron et al. 2000.)

p. 54): "pain is an *opinion* on the organism's state of health rather than a mere reflexive response to an injury." Nociceptor activation is only one among many factors that determine a person's experience of pain, and, as we will see, it is not even necessary. The **meaning** we attribute to what happens to us determines to a large extent whether we will experience pain and how much suffering it will cause.

Pain Is of Vital Importance

In the clinical situation, where pain is often the main presenting complaint of patients, it is easy to forget the advantages of pain perception. Children born without the ability to feel pain have severely reduced quality of life and often die young. The following description from *Pain: The Gift Nobody Wants* (Brand and Yancey, 1993, p. 3) explains why: "Tanya, now eleven, was living a pathetic existence in an institution. She had lost both legs to amputation . . . her failure to limp or shift weight when standing (because she felt no discomfort) had eventually put intolerable pressure on her joints. Tanya had also lost most of her fingers. Her elbows were constantly dislocated. She suffered the effects of chronic sepsis from ulcers . . . Her tongue was lacerated and badly scarred from her nervous habit of chewing it." The ability to feel pain is indeed necessary for us to be able to prevent injuries from innumerable small (and occasional large) physical threats. Also, lowered pain threshold and spontaneous pain in conjunction with tissue damage are biologically meaningful, because they ensure protection and optimal conditions for healing. In a wider context, the pain system constitutes an integral part of the bodily systems for **defense** and **homeostatic control**, as discussed in Chapter 14, under "Homeostatic Surveillance: A Task of Ascending Tracts from Lamina I?"

The vital importance of the pain system might perhaps give us a clue to why it so often goes awry. In the inevitable balance between **sensitivity** and **specificity,** the system is biased heavily in favor of sensitivity: we cannot afford to miss alarms of potential life-threatening events. Thus, the specificity would be correspondingly low, leaving the system open to false alarms. Indeed, some poorly understood pain conditions, such as **fibromyalgia**, might perhaps be understood in such terms.

"Change Behavior and Remember What Happened!"

The aforementioned example of a child born without the ability to feel pain also exemplifies that the feeling of pain is

as a strong signal to **change behavior**. The lack of adaptation in the pain system—on the contrary, it easily **sensitizes**—is meaningful: it might be disastrous if we stop paying attention to a steady stream of signals from nociceptors. This is very different from the situation for other sensory systems where adaptation is a characteristic property. Further, pain is a forceful stimulus to **learning**: we quickly learn to avoid everything that previously led to tissue injury or threatened to do so. As a child—mostly through learning by doing—develops mastery and control of his or her environment, the experience of pain is a central guide. In this sense, physical pain is just one aspect of discomfort and suffering and belongs perhaps conceptually more to the category of brain systems handling **punishment** and **reward** (suffering and pleasure) than that of sensory systems. Interestingly, functional magnetic resonance imaging (fMRI) studies show overlap between brain regions that are activated when we feel pleasure and pain. Overlap also exists between the brain activity related to physical and **social pain** (e.g., when social relationships are threatened or lost). Especially the anterior **cingulate** gyrus, the **orbitofrontal cortex**, and the **insula** are sites where pain and emotions meet.

Plasticity of the Pain System

For the development of various maladaptive pain conditions, the pain system's well-developed plasticity seems to be crucial. For example, even a relatively short train of signals from nociceptors alters the properties of the receiving dorsal horn neurons. Presumably this property is necessary for proper functioning of the pain system, for example, to ensure the necessary high level of sensitivity. Nevertheless, plasticity too often seems to go awry, causing **pathologic pain**, that is, pain that cannot be explained by adequate nociceptor activation and has no protective or reparative function. In cases of pathologic pain, plastic changes occur at all levels of the pain system, from the dorsal horn to the cerebral cortex.

Nociceptors and the Perception of Pain

It is important to realize that "pain perception" and "nociceptor activity" are not synonymous terms. Thus, nociceptor activity and the feeling of pain may occur independently of each other. The usual **definition** of a **nociceptor** is purely physiologic: a receptor that is activated by stimuli that produce tissue damage or would do so if the stimulus continued. In contrast, **pain** is a feeling that is defined in psychological terms: an unpleasant sensory and emotional experience, which occurs together with actual or threatening tissue damage or is described as if it were caused by tissue damage. Usually, of course, nociceptor activation causes the pain, and when we feel pain, we automatically ascribe it to something that harms our body. Indeed, pain is always felt somewhere in our body, even if it is caused solely by abnormal activity of neurons in the brain. Thus, on the one hand, a person may suffer the most intense pain, yet there may be no evidence of nociceptor stimulation; on the other hand, there are many examples of persons exposed to massive nociceptor stimulation who feel no pain. Examples of the latter situation are seen in serious accidents in which the injured person may experience no pain immediately afterward, in spite of considerable tissue damage.[1] This is most likely explained by brain systems that can prevent nociceptive signals from reaching consciousness (discussed further later in this chapter). In certain situations, such pain suppression may be necessary to survive.

WHEN THE PAIN SYSTEM GETS OUT OF CONTROL

Acute and Persistent Pain

Many observations suggest that acute, "ordinary" pain differs from pain of longer duration (chronic) regarding central mechanisms. The former is clearly related to nociceptor activation; it ends when (or shortly after) the stimulus ends. The threshold for eliciting acute pain is high (see the preceding definition of a nociceptor). There is good correspondence between the intensity of nociceptor stimulation and the experience of pain. In such instances, pain is a homeostatic factor, serving as a signal to change behavior to avoid tissue damage. Persistent pain, in contrast, is characterized by a weak or absent correlation between stimulus and experience of pain. For example, **hyperalgesia**—the experience of pain on nociceptor stimulation—is more intense than normal—is often present.[2] Thus, the somatosensory system

is abnormally sensitive. We all experience this altered state of the somatosensory system with, for example, a sprained ankle or a local infection, that is, in situations with inflammation. Even slight movement or touching of the injured part evokes intense pain, or it may be painful also at rest. In this situation the pain can be seen as biologically meaningful, as it ensures that the injured part receives the necessary rest; moreover, the pain subsides in parallel with the inflammation as the tissue heals. Hyperalgesia is due to **sensitization** of both the nociceptors (primary hyperalgesia) and of neurons in the dorsal horn and at higher levels (secondary hyperalgesia). Experimentally, dorsal horn neurons can be made hyperexcitable by inducing inflammation in a joint or in the skin.

The Unfortunate Use of the Term "Chronic"

The indiscriminate use of the term "chronic pain" has been criticized for several reasons, and it is now customary to replace it with words like "persistent" or "enduring." One reason for criticism is because the term "chronic pain" lacks precision and encompasses a variety of conditions with different causes, courses, and prognoses. Indeed, definitions of chronic pain differ widely. Some define it as pain that persists longer than the course of natural healing; others classify it as pain that lasts longer than 3 or 6 months. Some even use as a criterion that the pain has not responded to available (drug) treatment. The International Association for the Study of Pain defines chronic pain as "pain which persists past the normal time of healing ... With non-malignant pain, three months is the most convenient point of division between acute and chronic pain, but for research purposes six months will often be preferred."

Another reason to abandon the term "chronic pain"—at least in communication with patients—is that most people perceive the word "chronic" to mean that their pain will last forever with no hope of relief. Thus, the doctor's words serve to deprive the patient of **hope** and belief in his or her own ability to influence the situation.

Allodynia and Radiating Pain

Some, but not all, patients with persistent pain have a lowered threshold, so that normal innoxious stimuli (such as touching the skin) can elicit intense and long-lasting pain. This phenomenon is called **allodynia** and appears to be caused by (abnormal) activation of nociceptive neurons in the cord by dorsal root fibers (Aβ) leading from low-threshold mechanoreceptors. Change of presynaptic inhibition is probably instrumental in causing such a switch in the signal traffic. (The normal situation is that activity in thick myelinated dorsal root fibers *inhibits* nociceptive neurons,

---

1. Of patients admitted to an emergency ward, 40% reported no pain at the time of injury, 40% reported pain that was judged (by the doctors) as stronger than expected on the basis of the injury, but only 20% reported pain that was judged as "adequate" (Hardcastle 1999).

2. The International Association for the Study of Pain has proposed that **hyperalgesia** be used as an umbrella term for all conditions of increased pain sensitivity (Loeser and Treede 2008). Allodynia would then be a special case of hyperalgesia.

as discussed under "Analgesia Can Be Produced by Nerve Stimulation and Acupuncture" later in this chapter).[3]

Another characteristic of long-lasting pain is the tendency to **radiate**—the pain spreads out from the original painful site. This is most likely due to sensitization of (among others) spinothalamic neurons in the segments above and below the dorsal roots leading from the inflamed region (the dorsal root fibers divide in an ascending and a descending branch that may pass for several segments; see Fig. 13.12).

Central Sensitization: NMDA Receptors and Glia

Hyperalgesia, allodynia, and radiating pain are at least partly due to altered synaptic transmission in the CNS: persistent pain is associated with **plastic changes** that make neurons in many parts of the somatosensory system hyperexcitable. This is best documented in the dorsal horn but occurs also at higher levels. As with plastic changes in other systems, N-methyl-D-aspartate (**NMDA**) **receptors** have a crucial role. **Substance P** increases (via binding to neurokinin receptors) the sensitivity of NMDA receptors to glutamate. Thereby, wide-dynamic range spinothalamic neurons might react more vigorously to inputs from low-threshold mechanoreceptors. Activation of NMDA receptors also leads to activation of protein kinases that alter the properties of ion channels and thereby neuronal excitability.

Glial cells seem to be implicated in development and maintenance of persistent pain. Activation of glial cells can occur in response to release of substance P and amino acid transmitters from nociceptive dorsal root fibers, either by prolonged noxious stimuli or by injury of the primary sensory neurons in the periphery. In the cord astrocytes and activated **microglia** release neuroactive substances (interleukins, tumor necrosis factor, nitric oxide, ATP, BDNF, and others). These substances may, partly via activation of NMDA receptors, increase transmitter release from central terminals of nociceptive dorsal root fibers. Further, activated glial cells can sensitize dorsal horn neurons, among them spinothalamic ones.

Memory for Pain

Intense pain of some duration may leave "memory traces" in the brain so that, later, minimal provocation may suffice to revive the pain. For example, a man who had a painful spine fracture re-experienced the pain when, many years later, he suffered a myocardial infarction. Synaptic changes in the **amygdala** may be crucial in this connection. Thus, the amygdala is one of the neuronal groups with consistently altered activity in persistent pain, and it is especially important for learning the connection between a stimulus and its valence (e.g., painful–pleasant).

Another example of plastic changes that alter pain experience is the effects of electric stimulation during brain surgery of the somatosensory **thalamus**. Thus, this part seems to become hyperexcitable in patients with persistent pain syndromes. For example, patients with panic attacks accompanied by chest pain and patients with deafferentation pain reported their usual pain on thalamic stimulation. In contrast, patients undergoing surgery for movement disorders reported no pain on stimulation at the same thalamic sites. Finally, pain relief following sudden **amnesia** in two patents (with persistent pain and opiate dependence) indicates that memory processes may in some way contribute to persistent pain (Choi et al. 2007). Conceivably, this may be related to **learning** of certain associations that enhance pain experience—for example by linking a certain stimulus, thought, or feeling to expectations of threats and danger.

Persistent Pain Is Associated with Loss of Gray Matter

A large number of studies of patients with various persistent pain conditions document alterations of **gray matter** (in most cases volume reductions). The specific cellular changes that underlie these findings are unknown but most likely involve synaptic changes related to altered connectivity. Unfortunately, the distribution of reported gray matter alterations differs considerably among studies, hampering interpretation of their functional meaning. A recent meta-analysis, however, focusing on networks rather than isolated regions, indicates that alterations of the **attention** and **salience** networks seem to be common to all persistent pain conditions. (These include nodes in prefrontal regions, the thalamus, the anterior cingulate gyrus, and the insula; see Fig. 34.2). Apart from this core of affected areas, different pain conditions seem to be associated with more specific, additional areas of gray matter changes.

Most likely, the gray matter alterations represent *reactions* to the pain condition rather than their cause. Thus, the alterations have been reported to normalize with successful therapy. For example, a study of patients with painful **coxarthrosis** showed that loss of gray matter in parts of the thalamus was normalized after successful hip replacement therapy (removing the pain). Furthermore, in patients with **complex regional pain syndrome** (CRPS), the **somatosensory-cortex** representation of the painful part seems to shrink but normalizes during successful therapy.

Pathologic Pain

Persistent pain can occur not only on increased nociceptor activity but also after loss of sensory information, either

---

3. Increased excitability of certain spinal interneurons most likely contributes to allodynia. Several mechanisms might contribute; for example, persistent inflammation may induce synthesis of substance P in Aβ fibers—in contrast to the normal situation in which substance P is restricted to nociceptive C-fibers (see Chapter 13, under "Neuropeptides in Spinal Ganglion Cells and Nociceptors").

from nociceptors or from low-threshold mechanoreceptors. It can also occur without any apparent cause, as sometimes is the case with CRPS. We use the term **pathologic pain** here rather loosely to describe conditions in which pain occurs without any nociceptor activation (or peripheral tissue pathology)—that is, pain that has no obvious biologic function (in contrast to "normal" or "physiologic" pain). Pathologic pain may have quite different causes, such as partial damage to peripheral nerves or destruction of central somatosensory pathways, for example, in the spinal cord or in the thalamus. There are several varieties of pathologic pain, among them so-called **neuropathic pain**, that is, pain associated with damage to nervous tissue. Another variety is **deafferentation pain,** which is pain that, paradoxically, occurs after loss of sensory information from a body part. A striking example of the latter is patients with **avulsion of dorsal roots** (this occurs sometimes with the roots of the brachial plexus upon a violent pull of the arm). In spite of no sensory nerves entering the cord, such patients often develop excruciating pain in the denervated arm. Pathologic pain also occurs in some patients below a **transverse lesion of the cord,** even though all ascending sensory pathways are interrupted. Pathologic pain may also be felt in an area of the skin with reduced sensibility in patients who have had shingles (**postherpetic pain**). A stroke destroying parts of the thalamus leading to reduced sensibility in a body part is sometimes associated with enduring pain (**thalamic pain**).

Neuropathic Pain

The definition of neuropathic pain has changed over time. The International Association for the Study of Pain (IASP) defined it in 1994 as "Pain initiated or caused by a primary lesion or dysfunction of the nervous system." Many found this definition too vague, and the IASP replaced it recently with the following: "Pain arising as a direct consequence of a lesion or disease of the somatosensory system" (Treede et al. 2008). This implies that some pain conditions that formerly were classified as neuropathic no longer fit the definition because the brain lesions do not affect the somatosensory system directly. Conditions like **fibromyalgia** and **complex regional pain syndrome 1** (**CRPS1**) are not included due to lack of firm evidence of neural lesions as causative (although both conditions fit the wider definition of pathologic pain).

Phantom pain, often occurring for shorter or longer periods after amputations, refers to pain felt in the missing body part. It is usually not due to abnormal activity in peripheral nerves or ascending sensory pathways. Often the pain occurs together with a vivid experience of abnormal movements or postures of the missing limb. Probably the brain misinterprets the lack of sensory information from the missing body, drawing the conclusion that something is seriously "wrong" out there. This peculiar phenomenon is associated with plastic changes in the brain, especially in the somatosensory cortex. The area in the somatosensory cortex formerly receiving signals from the amputated part is taken over by signals from adjacent body regions—for example, after amputation of the hand, the hand area receives signals from the face. In such cases the person might experience the phantom pain upon touching the face. Finally, pain together with sensory loss is common in peripheral **neuropathies**, for example diabetic neuropathy.

It is fair to say that our understanding of pathologic pain syndromes is far from satisfactory. It is particularly enigmatic why apparently identical injuries cause persistent pain in some patients but not in others (the majority). Furthermore, in patients with the same lesion or disease (e.g., postherpetic pain) the mechanism causing the pain may be different (loss of nerve fibers or hyperactive nociceptors). An association between pathologic pain syndromes and certain personality traits has not been convincingly demonstrated.

Why Do Some People Develop Pathologic Pain While the Majority Do Not after Similar Injuries?

Animal and human experiments indicate that several gene **polymorphisms** play a role in determining a person's susceptibility to pathologic pain. For example, a particular variety of a K⁺-channel subunit, which is expressed in spinal ganglion cells, is associated with pathologic pain. Similarly, polymorphisms for a voltage-gated **Na⁺-channel** ($Na_V1.7$) subunit may influence the risk of persistent pain. Other genetic differences concern a person's ability to suppress signals from nociceptors after an injury, probably because descending inhibition from the brain stem is less active (see "Descending Control of Transmission from Nociceptors" later in this chapter). Such **descending inhibition** may be necessary to prevent development of long-term plastic changes in the dorsal horn. The next question, then, is "who" determines whether to turn on the descending inhibition? Presumably, such control is exerted by higher networks that analyze and interpret tissue damage and pain in a wider context (networks including the amygdala, the insula, the cingulate gyrus, and the prefrontal cortex). Several gene polymorphisms that influence the functioning of these networks seem to influence a person's vulnerability with regard to development of persistent pain. Examples are **monoamines** and **serotonin** (cf. Chapter 5 under "Monoamine Metabolism. Implications for Personality, Cognition, and Mental Disorders") and **opioid peptides** (polymorphisms in the μ-opioid receptor gene).

Twin studies suggest that 30% or more of the variation in persistent pain among people may be due to heritable factors. Nevertheless, each of the polymorphisms that are associated with persistent pain conditions (and more are being discovered) contributes only a little to the total variance. Thus, at the individual level one would expect that whether or not pathologic

Figure 15.1

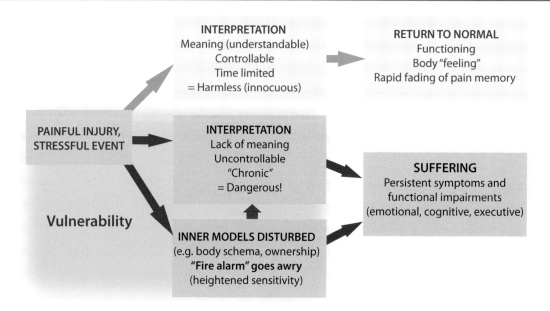

Persistent pain. Possible steps and factors that may differentiate the normal situation, in which the pain abates in pace with the healing, from situations with development of persistent pain.

pain ensues depends on the person's total setup of pain-related genes in interaction with environmental factors. Such interactions presumably occur from early childhood and determine the person's susceptibility to persistent pain (Fig. 15.1).

CRPS: A Special Kind of Pathologic Pain

In some patients pain continues in spite of complete healing of an injury (most often in the extremities). What started as a "normal," nociceptor-driven pain continues for unknown reasons as a pathologic pain (Fig. 15.1). For example, an apparently trivial fracture of the radius is sometimes followed by pain for years after the fracture has healed. Similar persistence of pain can occur after partial lesions of peripheral nerves (neuropathic pain). Usually such patients also suffer from hyperalgesia and allodynia, and even light touch may provoke excruciating pain. Often they also show signs of **autonomic dysfunction**, such as abnormal sweating and circulatory disturbances. This condition used to be called reflex sympathetic dystrophy, **reflex dystrophy**, or sympathetically mediated pain. In some cases, especially after nerve injury, the pain has a peculiar burning quality, and the name **causalgia** refers to this condition (Greek: *kausos*, heat; *algos*, pain).

It is especially unfortunate, however, that names of poorly understood diseases implicate an etiology, like "reflex" and

"sympathetic." The term **complex regional pain syndrome** (CRPS) was introduced in an attempt to avoid the many confusing terms for these kinds of pathologic pain conditions. CRPS is a purely descriptive term, reflecting that we do not know the pathophysiologic mechanisms leading to the various symptoms. It has two subgroups, with reasonably precise definitions, corresponding largely to reflex dystrophy (CRPS type I) and causalgia (CRPS type II), respectively.

CRPS and the Sympathetic System

As mentioned, patients with CPRS often show evidence of autonomic dysfunction in the painful part—mainly hyperactivity of the sympathetic system. The often-used term "reflex sympathetic dystrophy" implies that sympathetic dysfunction *causes* the syndrome. The pain relief achieved in some patients by a sympathetic block (e.g., of the stellate ganglion in case of pain in the hand) would seem to support this assumption. Nevertheless, **microneurographic** and other kinds of studies have not confirmed abnormally increased activity of sympathetic postganglionic fibers in such patients, even in those with obvious signs of sympathetic hyperactivity such as profuse sweating and extreme cutaneous vasoconstriction. This seeming paradox may perhaps be explained by the up-regulation of **adrenergic receptors** in **spinal ganglion cells** and their ramifications (Fig. 15.2). This is most likely caused by inflammatory mediators. Thus, normal levels circulating catecholamines may activate sensory neurons and contribute to persistent pain. There is furthermore evidence that in some CRPS patients neuropeptides (substance P and

Figure 15.2

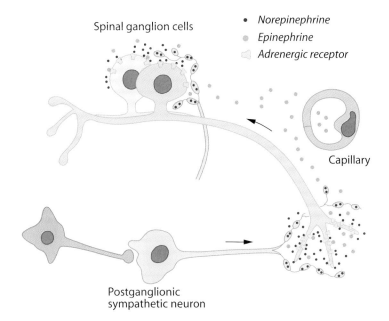

Spinal ganglion cells

- Norepinephrine
- Epinephrine
- Adrenergic receptor

Capillary

Postganglionic
sympathetic neuron

Sensory neurons (spinal ganglion cells) express adrenergic receptors in certain persistent pain conditions. Receptors are located on the cell body and the peripheral branches.

cholecystokinin [CCK] in particular) are released from sensory nerve endings in the skin of the painful parts. This causes **neurogenic inflammation,** which may produce some (but not all) of the autonomic signs in CRPS. The relationship between neurogenic inflammation and pain in CRPS is not clear, however.

CENTRAL CONTROL OF PAIN SENSATION

We now realize that a complex network—stretching from the spinal cord to the cerebral cortex—modulates transmission of signals from nociceptors and pain perception (Fig. 15.3). Although inhibition has attracted most interest, we now know that there are descending connections that facilitate transmission of nociceptive signals as well. For example, descending connections can facilitate development of central hyperalgesia secondary to inflammation and also contribute to development of neuropathic pain. As mentioned, how we conceive the meaning of a situation determines how we perceive signals from nociceptors. Indeed, the effects of the neurotransmitters used in the descending control systems are not fixed: depending on the cause of the pain and the context in which it occurs, the same transmitter may have opposite effects.

In the modulatory network, **serotonin**, **norepinephrine**, and **opioid peptides** (endorphins) seem to play crucial roles, although several other neurotransmitters also participate.

Descending Control of Transmission from Nociceptors

A dramatic observation by Reynolds (1969) was the starting point for much later research on central control of nociception. He showed that by electrical stimulation of a mesencephalic region, the **periaqueductal gray matter** (**PAG**; Fig. 15.3; see also Fig. 6.20), conscious rats could be subjected to major surgery without apparently feeling any pain (as judged from their behavior and other observations). The stimulation produced **analgesia** (no experience of pain on noxious stimuli). Subsequent research indicates that the effect of PAG stimulation can be explained, at least in part, by activation of descending connections to the dorsal horn. Although a sparse direct pathway from the PAG to the spinal cord exists, the main pathway appears to be synaptically interrupted in cell groups in the medulla, especially the **raphe magnus nucleus** (NRM) (Fig. 15.3; see also Figs 26.5 and 26.6) and other nearby cell groups in the **medullary reticular formation.** The descending fibers from these nuclei (raphespinal fibers) lie in the dorsolateral funiculus of the cord and end preferentially in the **substantia gelatinosa** (Fig. 15.4). Cutting the dorsolateral funiculus abolishes the effects of PAG stimulation almost completely. Further, electrical stimulation of NRM inhibits spinothalamic cells.

procedure is called **transcutaneous nerve stimulation**. One kind of analgesia occurs immediately and is mediated by activity of **thick myelinated fibers** in the stimulated nerves (i.e., fibers leading from low-threshold mechanoreceptors). Selective stimulation of such fibers is elicited by electrical stimulation with **high frequency** and low intensity or by natural stimuli such as vibration, light touch, or pressure. The analgesia is restricted to parts of the body innervated by the peripheral nerves, and it usually disappears when the stimulation stops. It is mediated by activity in collaterals of the thick dorsal root fibers that inhibit impulse transmission from the thin (Aδ and C) fibers in the dorsal horn, via inhibitory interneurons and presynaptic inhibition. Melzack and Wall (1965) proposed such interaction between thick and thin dorsal root fibers in their **gate-control theory**. It is presumably the basis of the everyday observation that it helps to blow at a finger that hurts, that it may help to move the part that has received an acute injury, that labor pains may be alleviated by rubbing over the lower back, and so forth.

Another kind of stimulation-induced analgesia requires that **thin sensory fibers** be activated. This can be achieved by electrical stimulation of **low frequency** with relative high intensity. Classical **acupuncture** probably obtains the same effect by rotation of thin needles in the tissue. The analgesia produced by this kind of stimulation occurs with latency but may last for hours after termination of the stimulation. Analgesia is not limited to the parts of the body that were stimulated. This kind of stimulation-induced analgesia is most likely due, at least in part, to activation of the descending connections from the brain stem. The activation may happen by way of collaterals from spinothalamic and spinoreticular cells to the PAG and adjacent parts of the reticular formation. The analgesia can be reversed or prevented by intravenous injection of **naloxone**. Further, in animal experiments it has been blocked by sectioning the dorsolateral fascicle. The results of such control experiments are in part contradictory, however, and indicate that not all aspects of stimulation-induced analgesia can be explained by liberation of endorphins.

Functional Role of Pain-Modulating Systems

A dominating view today is that modulation of pain is just one among several bodily adjustments—controlled by the nervous system—to physical and mental challenges. The person's mindset and his or her interpretation of the situation determine the choice of responses. In other words, **expectation** of what a stimulus will cause is more decisive for the response than the stimulus itself. Nevertheless, we do not fully understand the functional role of the pain-modulating systems, nor under which conditions they are activated. It is reasonable to assume, however, that **inhibiting** systems are active in situations with severe injuries and no experience of pain (as, e.g., in war and major civil accidents). In such situations, suppression of pain may enable continuation of intense physical activity, which may be of vital importance.

Markedly reduced pain sensitivity may also occur in more peaceful situations, such as sport competitions. Further, pain-suppressing systems (at several levels) appear to be active in expectation-dependent analgesia, although expectation may also increase pain perception (see the next section in this chapter, "Placebo and Nocebo"). Animal experiments indicate that **stress-induced analgesia** can occur in situations characterized by the inability to escape. However, the mental state of the animal seems to influence whether analgesia occurs. Thus, in one study analgesia occurred only if the animal was calm at the start of the period of stress, whereas anxious animals became hyperalgesic.

Anxiety together with pain may be understood as a result of how the person perceives the meaning of the pain: if the pain is thought to be caused by a serious threat and to be uncontrollable, pain intensity and anxiety will both be high. In such a situation, the descending system will presumably **facilitate** the transmission from nociceptors (Fig. 15.3). It seems biologically meaningful that the more threatening the pain is felt to be, the stronger the alarm (discomfort, distress, anxiety), and, consequently, the system should ensure that the alarm keeps going until necessary action is taken—or the threat is reinterpreted.

PLACEBO AND NOCEBO

The **placebo** effect is probably best understood as one part of a repertoire of responses to challenges that threaten our mental or physical stability (see also Chapter 30, under "The Hypothalamus and Mental Functions" and "Stress," and Chapter 31, under "Amygdala and Conditioned Fear"). Although it has attracted most attention in connection with the treatment of pain, we now know that placebo effects concern several physiologic processes. The beneficial placebo effect depends on the patient's positive expectations, but negative expectations may evoke increased pain and harmful physiologic alterations. This is called the **nocebo** effect. However, placebo (and nocebo) effects may in addition involve **conditioned responses**, for example elicited by the taste of a drug that previously was experienced as effective (e.g., a painkiller).[5] In this

---

5. In one study, patients received the immunosuppressant **cyclosporine** in association with a flavored drink. After a number of repetitions of the association, the flavored drink alone induced immunosuppression. Several other studies in experimental animals and in humans have shown similar conditioning of immune responses. The endocrine system is also subject to placebo conditioning. The conditioned immune and endocrine responses do not require conscious expectations.

respect, the placebo response is **learned,** depending on prior experience. Even the observation of another person receiving a beneficial treatment induces a placebo response in the observer.

As discussed, descending connections from the brain stem can inhibit or enhance nociceptive signal transmission, depending on the situation (Fig. 15.3). Such mechanisms are most likely involved in the placebo and nocebo effects on pain. One likely pathway goes from the amygdala to the PAG. At the cortical level, expectation of pain relief reduces the activity of the pain network (Fig. 15.5A). Further, during the expectation phase cortical regions usually involved in cognitive and evaluative processes show enhanced activity (Fig. 15.5B).

A common misconception is that the placebo effect works only with moderate pains and only in comparison to "weak" drugs. However, if the patient believes that the drug he or she receives is morphine, the placebo effect is much greater than if the patient believes it to be aspirin. Indeed, postoperative, intravenous administration of a placebo (saline) in full view of the patient had the same analgesic effect as 6 to 8 mg of morphine given covertly.

The question remains, however, how **expectancy** controls the activity in the "pain network" and pain-suppressing systems. Put more broadly: How do thoughts and feelings express themselves through the body? We discuss this theme further in Chapters 31 and 32 although, admittedly, we are far from a full understanding.

Placebo

The word "placebo" (literally: "I shall please") has been used for a long time about mock medicine—that is, drugs and procedures that the doctor knows have no effect. In clinical trials, for example, inert tablets are given as a placebo to decide whether a drug has a specific effect on a disease. Thus, it is well known that a treatment without any specific effect may influence the disease and the experience of pain. We know that the effect is present only if the patient expects the treatment to work. Further, surgery produces a larger placebo effect than drugs, and injection of a drug is more efficient than oral administration.

Figure 15.5

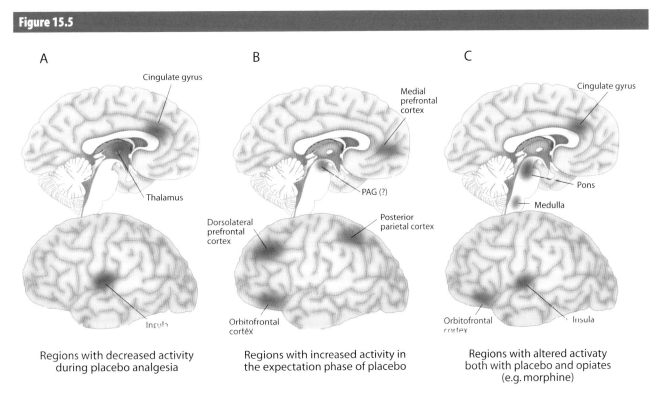

A — Regions with decreased activity during placebo analgesia

B — Regions with increased activity in the expectation phase of placebo

C — Regions with altered activaty both with placebo and opiates (e.g. morphine)

Brain regions involved in placebo analgesia. The size and position of the relevant regions are only approximations, and regions other than those shown here are involved in placebo analgesia. The regions shown in **B** are activated by cognitive and evaluative processes, as shown in other fMRI studies. (Based on fMRI data published by Petrovic et al. 2005 and Wager et al. 2004.)

iris, forming the **pupillary dilatator muscle** (*musculus dilatator pupillae*) widen the pupil when they contract.

The space inside the eye in front of the lens and the iris is called the **anterior chamber**. It is filled with a clear watery **fluid** that is produced by small processes of the ciliary body. The space behind the lens is filled with a clear jellylike substance called the **vitreous body** (*corpus vitreum*).

The eyeball is moved inside the orbit by six small striated muscles, the **extraocular muscles** (see Figs. 25.1 and 27.16). The muscles originate in the wall of the orbit, and their tendons insert in the sclera. The extraocular muscles are innervated by the **third**, **fourth**, and **sixth cranial nerves**. They cooperate very precisely to produce the movements of the eyes that ensure that the visual axes (Fig. 16.2) of the eyes are always directed toward the point of fixation (Fig. 16.3C).

The Visual Field

The visual field is the part of our surroundings from which the eyes can perceive light (without movement of the eyes or the head). Together, the two eyes cover a large area (Fig. 16.3A and B). Light from a particular point in the visual field falls on a particular point on the retina. Because of the refraction of the light when it passes the optic media of the eye, the image on the retina is upside down. For convenience, we divide the retina and the visual field vertically into two halves: the **temporal** parts—that is, lateral parts, toward the temple—and the **nasal** parts (Fig. 16.3C). The nasal halves of the retina receive light from the temporal halves of the visual field, and the temporal halves of the retina receive light from the nasal visual field. The situation is the same for the upper and lower halves of the retina and the corresponding parts of the visual field. Thus, light from the lower half of the visual field reaches the upper half of the retina. The lateral 30 degrees of the visual field is viewed by one eye only, because the nose prevents light from reaching the anterior part of the temporal retina (Fig. 16.3C), and is therefore called the **monocular zone**. Both eyes view the rest of the visual field, the **binocular zone**.

Damage to parts of the nasal retina in one eye produces a blind spot in the temporal visual field; damage in the upper half of the retina in one eye produces a blind spot in the lower visual field; and so forth. Damage that affects the binocular zone usually goes unnoticed by the person affected. Therefore, the visual field must be examined for each eye separately. This is done with the person fixating the gaze at a target straight ahead while one eye is covered. Often it suffices to test the outer borders of the visual field by moving an object (e.g., the finger of the examiner) from well outside the visual field toward its center. A systematic examination covering all parts of the visual field for each eye is called **perimetry**.

The Lens and the Far and Near Points of the Eye: Accommodation

The lens is transparent and built of cells that form long fibers. It is elastic, and, when loosened from the ciliary body to which it is attached with thin **zonular fibers** (Figs. 16.1 and 2), it becomes rounder. Contraction of the ciliary muscle reduces the diameter of the ring formed by the ciliary body. This slackens the zonular fibers and enables the lens to become rounder; that is, its curvature (convexity) and thus also the refraction of the light increase. Sharp contraction of the ciliary muscle is required to see objects that are closer to the eye than approximately 6 m. This distance is called the **far point of the eye.** In a normal—**emmetropic**—eye, the length of the eyeball is accurately adjusted to the refraction of the cornea and the lens in the relaxed state. When viewing objects at distances greater than about 6 m, the lens maintains the same convexity, and yet the image is always focused on the retina. This is because the light rays entering the eye from points at such distances are all virtually parallel and are therefore collected in the plane of the retina (like a camera focused at infinite distance). If the length of the eyeball differs from the normal (even by only a few hundred microns), the light rays are not collected in the plane of the eye and the sight is blurred. If the eyeball is too long, the light rays are collected in front of the retina. This condition is called **myopia** and is corrected by concave (−) glasses.[1] If the eyeball is too short, the light rays meet behind the retina. Convex (+) glasses correct this **hypermetropia** (in children, because of their elastic lenses, the error is easily corrected by constant accommodation).

The closer an object comes within the far point of the eye, the more the convexity of the lens must be increased by contraction of the ciliary muscle. Such adjustment of the lens for near sight is called **accommodation**. The closest distance from the eye at which we can see an object sharply is called the **near point of the eye**. One's own near point can be easily determined by fixing the eyes on an object (e.g., a finger) that is gradually moved closer to the eye until it no longer can be viewed sharply.

---

1. A correlation seems to exist between much reading (i.e., accommodating for long periods) and development of myopia in adolescents. Animal experiments confirm that how the eye is used influences the growth of the eyeball. Thus, when 3-month-old monkeys were equipped with +3 glasses, the length of the eye changed to compensate for the refraction error (Hung et al. 1995).

The far point of the eye depends on the curvature of the lens in its "relaxed" state—that is, with no contraction of the ciliary muscle—and remains stable throughout life. The near point, however, depends on the ability of the lens to increase its curvature and moves gradually away from the eye from birth until about the age of 60. This happens because the lens becomes gradually stiffer and less elastic, so that the ability to increase its convexity declines steadily. At about the age of 45 so much accommodation is lost—or, in other words, the near point is so far away—that it is difficult to read fine print. This condition, called **presbyopia**, is corrected by the use of convex (+) glasses of appropriate strength.

THE RETINA

The retina forms the innermost layer of the eye (Fig. 16.2). The outer part of the retina, which adjoins the choroid, is the **pigmented epithelium,** consisting of one layer of cuboid cells with large amounts of pigmented granules in their cytoplasm. Internal to the pigmented epithelium follows a layer with **photoreceptors** and then two further layers with neurons (Fig. 16.4). The processes of the photoreceptors contact the **bipolar cells**, which, in turn, transmit signals to the **retinal ganglion cells**. The axons of the ganglion cells leave the eye in the **optic nerve** to end in nuclei in the diencephalon and the mesencephalon. The pigmented epithelium extends forward to the edge of the pupil (Fig. 16.2), whereas the photoreceptors, bipolars, and ganglion cells are present only in the parts of the retina situated posterior to the ciliary body (*pars nervosa retinae*).

Unlike many other receptors, the photoreceptors are not of peripheral origin but belong to the central nervous system. The retina develops in embryonic life as an evagination of the diencephalon (see Fig. 9.3). Strictly speaking, the term "retinal ganglion cell" is therefore not correct, but it is nevertheless maintained.

Because the photoreceptors are located external to the two other neuronal layers, the light has to pass through the latter to reach the photoreceptors. Because there are no myelinated axons in the retina, however, the layers internal to the photoreceptors are sufficiently translucent.

In addition to the aforementioned neuronal types, the retina also contains many **interneurons: amacrine cells** and **horizontal cells** (Fig. 16.4; these neurons are treated in more detail under "Interneurons in the Retina" later in this chapter). The horizontal cells are responsible for **lateral**

Figure 16.4

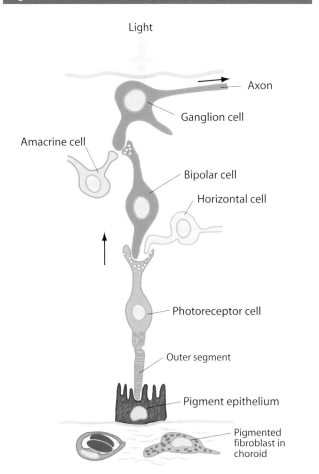

The retina. The main cell types and their interconnections (highly simplified).

inhibition (see Fig. 13.4), among other things. More processing of sensory information takes place in the retina than in any other sense organ. Thus, the visual information transmitted to higher centers of the brain from the retina is already "distorted" by enhancement of the contrast between light and darkness and by preference for signals caused by light from moving objects.

The Retina Has a Layered Structure

Under a microscope, several distinct layers of the retina can be identified in sections cut perpendicular to its surface (Figs. 16.5 and 16.12). Externally, toward the pigmented epithelium, lie the light-sensitive parts of the photoreceptors—their **external segments**. The two types of photoreceptors, the **rods** and the **cones**, can be distinguished because the external segments of the cones are thicker and usually

Figure 16.5

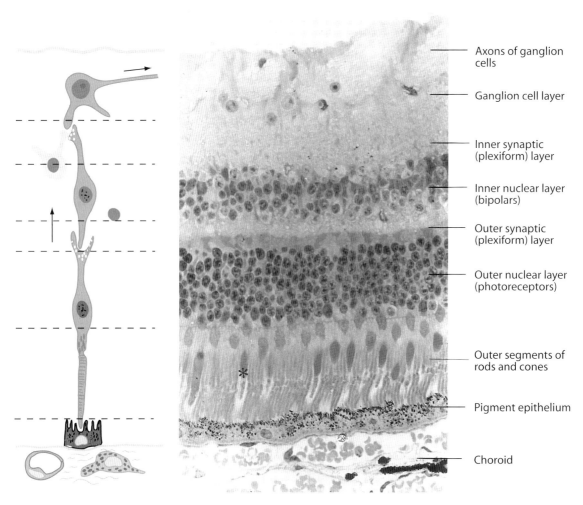

The retina. Photomicrograph of a microscopic section showing the various layers (monkey). The section is from the peripheral part of the retina (this explains the lower density of ganglion cells here than in Fig. 16.12). The outer segment of a cone is marked with an asterisk. Magnification, ×175.

somewhat shorter than those of the rods. Internal to the layer of the external segments, there are three distinct layers with cell nuclei. The **outer nuclear layer** consists of the nuclei of the photoreceptors. The nuclei of the bipolar cells (and many of the interneurons) form the **inner nuclear layer**. The innermost layer of nuclei belongs to the ganglion cells—**the ganglion cell layer.** Between the nuclear layers lie processes of the neurons and their synapses, consequently termed the **outer** and **inner synaptic layers** (or plexiform layers). In the outer synaptic layer, the processes of the bipolar cells end in depressions in the processes of the photoreceptors (Fig. 16.4). The photoreceptor processes contain synaptic vesicles close to the presynaptic membrane.

A special kind of astroglial cell—the **Müller cells**—extends through the retina from the pigmented epithelium to the vitreous body.

Photoreceptors and the Photopigment

Electron microscopy reveals that the **outer segments** of the rods and cones are packed with folded membrane, forming a large surface containing the light-sensitive **photopigment**. In the rods, the folds of membrane lie mostly intracellularly, whereas in the cones they are partly invaginations of the surface membrane. The photoreceptors constantly remove and resynthesize the membrane folds.

The rods and the cones contain different kinds of photopigment. The **rods** contain **rhodopsin**, which has been the most studied. It consists of a protein part, **opsin**, and **retinal**, which is an aldehyde of the **vitamin A** molecule. Retinal is light absorbing and is changed by light (absorption of photons). Simultaneously the opsin part is changed,

Figure 16.6

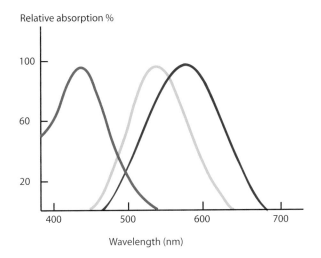

The three different kinds of visual pigment. The diagram shows the efficiency with which the three kinds of cones absorb light of different wavelengths. Note the marked overlapping of the absorption curves.

and this leads to alteration of the membrane potential of the photoreceptor (hyperpolarization by closure of Na⁺ channels). The **transduction** mechanism involves activation of G proteins and the intracellular signal molecule cyclic GMP. Structurally the photopigments resemble closely other G protein–coupled receptors (e.g., muscarinic receptors, and receptors for smell). The hyperpolarization of the photoreceptors by light stimuli affects the bipolar cells (and retinal interneurons), which then act on the ganglion cells to alter the frequency of action potentials conducted in the optic nerve to the visual centers of the brain.

The photopigment of the **cones** differs slightly from rhodopsin in the structure of the opsin molecules. Further, there are three varieties of **cone opsin** molecules, which explain why we have three kinds of cones absorbing light of different wavelengths (Fig. 16.6). The opsin of the cones is also bound to retinal, but the opsin molecule determines the wavelength sensitivity of retinal.

Dark Adaptation and Light Adaptation

When looking into the eye (e.g., through an ophthalmoscope), the color of the retina is a deep purple because of the content of rhodopsin. The reflection of light from the retina produces the red eyes of flash photography. The color bleaches quickly on illumination of the retina, but it returns slowly in the dark. The light has broken down the rhodopsin, and it takes some time to resynthesize it. We experience the time needed for this process of **dark adaptation** when entering a dark room from strong sunlight.

In the beginning, we can hardly see anything, but gradually the ability to see returns. This happens in two stages; first, there is a rapid stage of improvement of about 10 minutes and thereafter a slower stage of almost 1 hour until full light sensitivity has been restored (if the initial illumination was very intense). Because the rods are responsible for vision in dim light (scotopic vision), the dark adaptation depends on resynthesis of rhodopsin in the rods.

We experience the opposite phenomenon of dark adaptation, **light adaptation**, when moving from darkness into strong light (photopic vision). Also then, after first seeing nothing, vision gradually returns. The strong light bleaches the photopigment massively—that is, there is an intense, brief stimulation of many receptors, producing the almost painful sensation of blinding light. The rhodopsin of the rods remains bleached as long as it is exposed to strong light and the rods cannot contribute to vision under these conditions. The cones are first maximally hyperpolarized and are therefore unable to respond. This explains why we cannot discriminate forms and colors at first. However, within a few seconds the outer segments of the cones depolarize to a level where they again can respond to changes of illumination. Change of intracellular Ca²⁺ concentration is of crucial importance for this depolarization. Light adaptation, then, depends on change of the cone-membrane potential. Additional adaptations occur when passing from darkness to light, such as **constriction of the pupils** to reduce light entering the eye (anyone entering a sunlit street after having the pupils widened by atropine has experienced the importance of this adaptation).

Rods and Cones Have Different Properties

The rods are much more sensitive than the cones and react to extremely small amounts of light, whereas the cones need strong light to react. This is partly because the outer (external) segment of the rod is longer and contains more photopigment than that of the cone. The rods are thus responsible for vision when the light is dim, called **scotopic vision**, whereas the cones are responsible for vision in good light—**photopic vision**. (That vitamin A is necessary for the synthesis of rhodopsin explains why vitamin A deficiency causes night blindness.) The distribution of light sensitivity for different wavelengths of light is the same for all the rods (maximal sensitivity for wavelengths around 500 nm); hence, they cannot help us **discriminate** between light of different **wavelengths**, which is a prerequisite for color vision. The cones, in contrast, are as mentioned of three kinds, each with a particular variety of photopigment with maximal light sensitivity to different wavelengths. One kind of cone responds best to light with wavelengths in the **blue** part of the spectrum, another in the **red** part, and the other in the **green** part (considerably fewer cones react to blue than to red and to green). One kind of cone alone cannot inform about color, however. This is so because each photopigment is bleached not only by light with wavelengths to which it is maximally sensitive but also by stronger light with shorter and longer wavelengths (Fig. 16.6). Only by **comparing the degree of activation** of the different kinds of cones can the neurons receiving signals from them extract information about the distribution of wavelengths in the light falling on the retina. Together, the three kinds of cones are responsible for **color vision**. As mentioned, however, the cones are not very sensitive to light; from daily experience, we know that we need good light to perceive the color of objects. In poor light, everything appears as a variation of gray.

Dopamine and the Shift from Scotopic to Photopic Vision

Two kinds of photoreceptors with different sensitivities to light enable the visual system to give meaningful information even when exposed to extreme variations of light intensities. Release of **dopamine** from one kind of amacrines (Fig. 16.4) seems to support the change from scotopic (rods) to photopic (cones) vision. Light induces release of dopamine, which enhances the signal transmission from the cones compared with the rods. Further, dopamine uncouples electric synapses between amacrines and a certain kind of bipolars so that signals are less widely distributed horizontally in the retina. This presumably contributes to the enhanced spatial resolution with photopic vision.

Spatial Resolution Depends on the Cones

Other important differences between rods and cones concern their interconnections with other neurons in the retina. Notably, many rods connect to each bipolar cell—that is, there is a high degree of **convergence**. For the cones, on the other hand, there is typically much less convergence, with a few cones connected to one bipolar cell. This also helps us understand why less light is required to convey signals through the optic nerve from the rods than from the cones. The difference in convergence means that the cones provide information with a higher **spatial resolution** than the rods—that is, two points must be farther apart to be perceived as two when the rods are responsible for transmitting the information than when the cones are responsible. This explains our inability to perceive visual details, such as small letters, in dim light. Therefore, the cones are responsible not only for color vision but also for our ability to perceive visual details: they are responsible for precise perception of **patterns** and **form**.

What Is Color?

Light reflected from objects evokes a sensation we call "color." We can only learn the definition or meaning of the name of a color by referring to samples—the grass is green, an apple is red, and so forth. (A person who never has seen a red object cannot know what the experience of red is.) Nevertheless, as we discuss later in this chapter, how we perceive the color of an object depends not only on its physical properties but also on how the brain processes information about the wavelength composition of the light reflected from the object and from all other objects in the same visual scene.

Color Blindness

In most cases color blindness is an inheritable condition, due to either lack of one kind of cones or an error affecting one of the three cone photopigments. Green or red blindness (or weakness) are the most common forms, affecting about 3% of the male population, whereas blue blindness is very rare. Genes at the X chromosome code the photopigments of the red- and green-sensitive cones, whereas the genes for the blue-sensitive photopigment and for rhodopsin are at autosomal chromosomes. Since the condition is recessively heritable, it is understandable that almost only men are color blind.

Rarely are two kinds of cones lacking, or even all three. Finally, deficient or absent color vision can sometimes be caused by disease of the retina or a lesion of the visual cortex.

Signal Transmission in the Retina

The photoreceptors do not behave like other receptors when exposed to their adequate stimulus: they are hyperpolarized instead of depolarized. Here we briefly discuss how hyperpolarization of the receptors can elicit action potentials in the neurons conducting the signals to the brain.

One important point is that the **photoreceptors** are unusual in another respect: they are in a **depolarized** state in the dark, with a membrane potential around −30 mV. Na$^+$ channels that are open in darkness probably cause this. Like other receptors, the photoreceptors (and the bipolar cells) do not produce action potentials but only graded changes of the membrane potential. Because the distance is very short from the outer segment—where the membrane potential changes arise—to the synapses between the photoreceptors and the bipolar cells, even small membrane-potential fluctuations cause alterations of the transmitter release from the photoreceptors. (There is thus no need for the production of action potentials, which are necessary only when signals are to be propagated over long distances.) Light falling on the retina causes closure of Na$^+$ channels by degradation of the photopigment and **cyclic GMP**. Closing of Na$^+$ channels hyperpolarizes the cell. Transmitter release from the photoreceptors (as from other neurons) is caused by membrane depolarization without any definite threshold that must be exceeded. Thus, in the dark, photoreceptors release transmitter continuously, whereas the release is reduced by light (as if darkness were the adequate stimulus).

Recording from **bipolar cells** has shown that they are of two kinds: one is depolarized by light and is called **ON bipolars**, and the other is hyperpolarized and is called **OFF bipolars**. **Glutamate**—which is the transmitter released from the photoreceptors—has a depolarizing (and therefore excitatory) effect on neurons in other parts of the central nervous system. With regard to the bipolars, however, ON bipolars are hyperpolarized by glutamate, whereas OFF bipolars are depolarized (Fig. 16.7), due to the expression of different kinds of glutamate receptors.[2]

We can **summarize** the events as follows. When light hyperpolarizes the photoreceptors, the release of glutamate is reduced, as mentioned. This leads to less hyperpolarization, which is the same as depolarization, of one kind of bipolar (ON); thus, some of the bipolars are depolarized and therefore increase their own transmitter release. This is an example of **disinhibition.** The opposite happens with the other kind of bipolar cell (OFF), which is hyperpolarized (receives less depolarization) and therefore reduces its transmitter release. Thus, one kind of bipolar reacts with increased transmitter release when light is turned on and the other kind when the light is turned off (Fig. 16.7).

The bipolar cells have depolarizing (excitatory) effects on the **retinal ganglion cells** (and on amacrine cells), and we can then understand why there are also two kinds of ganglion cells: one that is excited and one that is inhibited by light hitting the photoreceptors to which they are coupled. We therefore use the terms **ON** and **OFF ganglion cells.** In contrast to the photoreceptors and the bipolars, the ganglion cells produce action potentials (conducted in the optic nerve to the higher visual centers).

Couplings from Rods and Cones Are Different

Figure 16.7 shows that there are two **parallel signal pathways** from the **cones**. The ON ganglion cells increase their firing frequency with increasing intensity of light hitting the cones

---

2. In general, OFF bipolars express ionotropic glutamate receptors (AMPA/kainate) opening cation channels, whereas ON bipolars express metabotropic glutamate receptors (mGluR6) triggering closure of cation channels. Conditions are complex, however. There are, for example, more than 10 different kinds of bipolars with somewhat different synaptic arrangements and expressions of receptors.

Figure 16.7

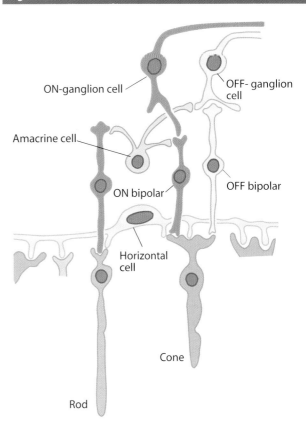

ON and OFF bipolar and ganglion cells in the retina. Simplified diagram showing the coupling of a cone to two different bipolar cells and further coupling of the bipolars to ganglion cells that increase or decrease their activity, respectively, when light falls on their receptive fields. Amacrine cells are intercalated in the coupling of rods to ganglion cells.

with which they are connected, whereas the OFF ganglion cells increase their firing frequency with increasing darkness. These two channels enable the ganglion cells to inform of a much wider range of light intensities than if there were only one channel. However, the bipolars and the ganglion cells do not inform about the absolute light intensity but the intensity in a small spot on the retina in comparison to the surroundings. This is caused by **lateral inhibition** produced by **horizontal cells** (Fig. 16.7), which are electrically coupled.

The coupling from the **rods** to the ganglion cells is more complicated than from the cones. Thus, bipolars excited by rods do not influence ganglion cells directly but via a special kind of **amacrine cells** (Fig. 16.7). These amacrines excite ON bipolars and inhibit OFF bipolars. It should be noticed that the rods and cones are coupled to the same ganglion cells. Consequently, a ganglion cell transmitting signals from cones in daylight transmits from rods in the dusk.

As mentioned, the retina contains interneurons in addition to the photoreceptors, bipolars, and ganglion cells (Fig. 16.4). The **horizontal cells** send their processes in the plane of the retina—that is, perpendicular to the orientation of the photoreceptors and the bipolars (Fig. 16.7). The horizontal cell processes establish contact with the inner segments of the photoreceptors and with the dendrites of the bipolars. They therefore regulate the transmission from the photoreceptors to the bipolars. There is good evidence that the horizontal cells are responsible for the typical receptive fields of the bipolars and ganglion cells with central excitation and peripheral inhibition (or vice versa). This involves complex and unusual synaptic mechanisms that are not fully understood. The horizontal cells are interconnected with **electric synapses**, probably enabling transmission for several millimeters in the plane of the retina. They release γ-aminobutyric acid (**GABA**) in their efferent synapses onto the inner segments of the photoreceptors. Each horizontal cell is depolarized by **glutamate** released from many photoreceptors. Thus, light hitting the photoreceptors leads to hyperpolarization of the horizontal cells; that is, they release less GABA so that the photoreceptors are disinhibited. Conversely, the horizontal cells hyperpolarize the photoreceptors in darkness.

The other kind of retinal interneuron, the **amacrine cell**, is located with its cell body in the inner nuclear layer and establishes contact with both the axons of the bipolar cells and the dendrites of the ganglion cells (Fig. 16.7). Amacrine cells are thus intercalated between bipolar cells and ganglion cells, and many bipolar cells exert their effect on ganglion cells only or mainly via amacrine cells. As mentioned, this is the rule for **rod bipolars** (bipolars connected with rods). Such amacrines (**AII**) form **electric synapses** with ON (depolarizing) bipolars and chemical **glycinergic** synapses with OFF (hyperpolarizing) bipolars. Some of the processes of the amacrine cells also extend horizontally for considerable distances. The actions of the amacrine cells are varied and complex, and there are numerous morphological varieties. They are also heterogeneous with regard to their transmitter content, and, as mentioned, some establish both chemical and electric synapses. One subgroup of amacrines contains **GABA**, for example; others contain **acetylcholine** or **dopamine**. At least seven different **neuropeptides** have been associated with amacrine cells. Twenty different kinds of amacrine cells have so far been identified, considering differences in both synaptic connectivity and transmitter content. The amacrines play an important role in influencing the activity of many ganglion cells with properties that cannot be explained by transmission directly from bipolars to ganglion cells. For example, amacrine cells appear to be partly responsible for making certain ganglion cells sensitive to light stimuli (contrasts) with a specific orientation.

Receptive Fields of Retinal Ganglion Cells

Most retinal ganglion cells are excited most effectively by shining light on small circular spots on the retina. These are the **receptive fields** of the ganglion cells and can be defined as the **area** of the retina from which a ganglion cell can

be influenced. The receptive field can of course be determined not only for ganglion cells but also for neurons at all levels of the visual pathways. The ganglion cells are typically excited from a small central circle and inhibited from a peripheral circular zone, or vice versa (Fig. 16.8A). The American neurophysiologist Stephen Kuffler first demonstrated this in the early 1950s. He introduced the terms **on-center** and **off-center** for ganglion cells that are activated and inhibited, respectively, by light hitting the central zone of the receptive field. These correspond to ON and OFF ganglion cells, described previously with reference to the center of their receptive fields (Fig. 16.7). Thus, as mentioned, illumination of a small spot on the retina can lead to increased activity in one chain of neurons—forming, as it were, a channel for signal transmission to the higher visual centers—and reduced activity in another. (The arrangement of a central excitatory field and a peripheral inhibitory zone is also found in the somatosensory system.) For receptive fields of the retinal ganglion cells, the central excitatory or inhibitory part of the receptive field can be explained by direct coupling from photoreceptors to bipolars and further to ganglion cells, whereas the peripheral zone with opposite effects must involve **horizontal cells** producing lateral inhibition (Fig. 16.7). As expected, illumination of the complete receptive field—the central and peripheral zones simultaneously—gives a much weaker response from the ganglion cells than illumination of the central zone only (Fig. 16.8).

In conclusion, each ganglion cell brings information to higher visual centers about a particular small, round area in a definite position on the retina and thus in the visual field. Together, the receptive fields of all ganglion cells cover the whole visual field with the same type of concentrically arranged receptive fields. Ganglion cells that lie side by side in the retina have overlapping, but not identical, receptive fields.

Retinal Ganglion Cells Exaggerate Contours

Recording of ganglion cell activity under different lighting conditions show that the retinal ganglion cells do not give information about absolute light intensity. Rather, their activity depends on the **contrast** of intensity between the light falling on the central and the peripheral parts of the receptive field. For example, for an on-center cell, a narrow beam of strong light hitting precisely the center of the receptive field while the peripheral zone is in darkness evokes maximal firing frequency.

Figure 16.8

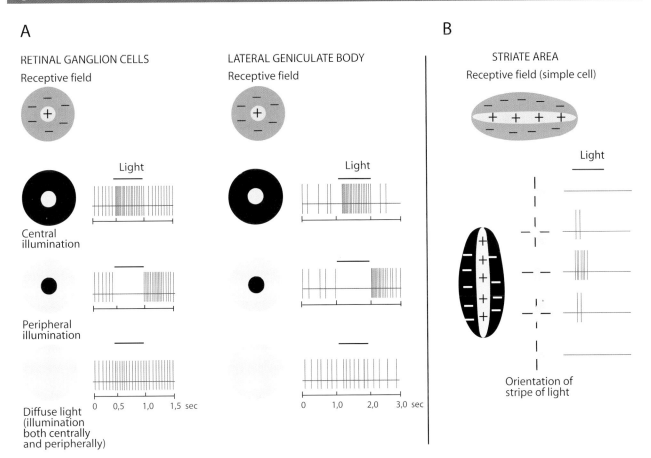

Receptive fields of cells at various levels of the visual pathways. **A:** Retinal ganglion cells and cells of the lateral geniculate body have similar receptive fields. The firing frequencies of the neurons when subjected to different kinds of light stimuli are shown in the graphs. Only cells that are excited by shining light on the central part of the receptive field are shown here (on-center field), but cells with the opposite properties—that is, inhibition from the central field and excitation from the periphery—also exist (off-center field). **B:** The receptive fields of simple cells of the striate area are typically oblong with an excitatory and an inhibitory zone. The cells are called orientation-specific because they respond preferentially to a stripe of light with a specific orientation. The figure shows only one orientation of the receptive fields, but all orientations are represented among cells of the striate area. (Based on Kuffler et al. 1984.)

This preference of the visual system for contrast in light intensity can be demonstrated, for example, by looking at a gray circular spot surrounded by black (Fig. 16.9A). Exchanging the black surrounding with a light gray makes the gray spot appear darker (even though the amount of light the eye receives from the central gray area is unchanged). This property of the visual system makes it particularly suited to detect **contours**, which are especially important for analysis of form. Our ability to judge contrasts of light intensities does not just depend on retinal mechanisms, however. For example, the brightness of an area compared with its neighbors depends on our (subconscious) judgment of how the light falls—that is, whether we assume that the area is in direct light or in shadow. Processes at the **cortical level** must cause this, since it requires assumptions of the three-dimensional form of the object and from where the light comes. If we misinterpret such conditions, we make false judgments about relative light intensities. Figure 16.9B shows that also our judgment of the color of a field depends on its context.

Visual Acuity and the Size of Receptive Fields

We know from everyday experience that in order to perceive visual details, we must direct the eyes toward an object. The visual axes have to be oriented so that light

Figure 16.9

A   B

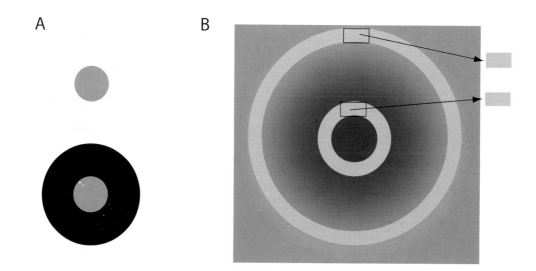

Perceived light intensity and color depend on contrast and context. **A:** The central circle reflects the same amount of light in both examples, yet we perceive the upper one as darker than the lower. **B:** Perceived color intensity differs dramatically with the context. The small colored rectangles are copied from the central and peripheral rings, respectively.

from the object falls on a small region of the retina in the back of the eye, the **macula lutea** (*macula*, spot; *lutea*, yellow). The macula is about 2 mm in diameter and has a yellowish color when viewed through an ophthalmoscope, distinguishing it from the purple color of the surrounding retina. Here the visual acuity is greatest, and it decreases steeply when moving peripherally on the retina. The **visual acuity** is expressed as the distance (in degrees) two points in the visual field must be separated by in order to be perceived as two and not one. In clinical work, visual acuity is usually determined by viewing letters of different sizes at a fixed distance (at the far point of the eye). The center of the macula has a small depression, the **fovea centralis** (Figs. 16.1, 16.2, and 16.10). The depression exists because the bipolars and the ganglion cells are "pushed" aside to enable maximal access for light to the photoreceptors. The small region is also devoid of capillaries. In the central part of the macula, only cones are present, and only in the macular part of the retina is the visual acuity sufficient to enable us to read ordinary print (e.g., a newspaper). The farther we move peripherally from the macula, the lower the visual acuity. One can demonstrate this easily by trying to determine how far out in the visual field one can recognize a face. Closely linked with these differences in visual acuity are differences in the size of the **receptive fields** of ganglion cells in the central and peripheral parts of the retina.

The Blind Spot on the Retina

Where the optic nerve leaves the eye, there is a circular area devoid of photoreceptors, appropriately called the **blind spot** (Figs. 16.1, 16.2, and 16.11.) We do not notice these blind areas of the two retinas, however, because they are not located at corresponding points (Fig. 16.3). Even when using only one eye we usually do not notice the blind spot, however. This is due to the capacity of the visual system to fill in missing parts of a visual scene (if the size of the missing part is not too large).

Figure 16.10

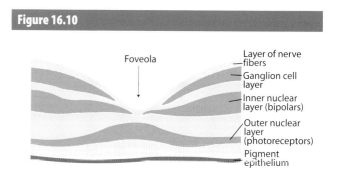

The fovea centralis. Schematized drawing of microscopic section through the posterior pole of the eye. The bipolar and the ganglion cells are "pushed" aside in the most central part of the fovea (the foveola), whereas the density of photoreceptors is at its highest in this same area.

Figure 16.11

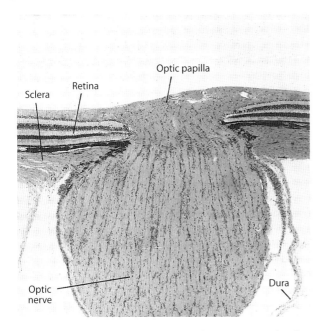

The optic nerve and the optic papillae. Photomicrograph of section through the posterior pole of the eye at the exit of the optic nerve (the blind spot). The optic nerve swells immediately outside the eye because the axons become myelinated. The ganglion cell axons are unmyelinated as long as they course through the innermost layer of the retina.

Differences between the Central and Peripheral Parts of the Retina

What is the basis for the striking differences in receptive-field size of ganglion cells in central and peripheral parts of the retina? One important factor is that the degree of **convergence** varies dramatically. There are about 100 million photoreceptors in the human retina and only 1 million ganglion cells; on the average, 100 photoreceptors connect to one ganglion cell. In the peripheral parts of the retina, however, the convergence is much greater than 100:1, whereas it is much smaller in central parts (Fig. 16.12). In the central parts of the fovea (**foveola**; Fig. 16.10), there are even 1:1 connections—that is, one photoreceptor connects to one bipolar, which is connected to only one ganglion cell. As mentioned, the rods show a much greater convergence than the cones, which is in accordance with the distribution of the rods and cones: the macula contains almost only cones, whereas the most peripheral parts contain almost only rods. The relative absence of cones in the peripheral parts of the retina (receiving light from peripheral parts of the visual field) can be demonstrated by how far out in

the visual field the color of an object can be perceived. It then appears that the visual field for color is considerably smaller than for moving objects. Another factor that contributes to the higher visual acuity in the central parts of the retina—particularly in the region of the fovea—is that the **density of photoreceptors** is higher there than more peripherally. Figure 16.13 illustrates a third contributing factor: the **dendritic arborizations** of the ganglion cells are more restricted in central than in peripheral parts of the retina, which is also important for the degree of convergence on each ganglion cell. Finally, differences between the retinal **interneurons** in central and peripheral parts of the retina play an important role.

There Are Two Main Kinds of Retinal Ganglion Cell

We described two kinds of retinal ganglion cell that differ according to whether they signal light or darkness (ON and OFF ganglion cells). There are, however, further specializations among ganglion cells that we should know about to understand the information sent from the retina to higher visual centers.

Anatomic studies showed many years ago that the retinal ganglion cells differ greatly in size. One tendency, mentioned previously, is that the **dendrites** of the ganglion cells are longer peripherally than centrally (Fig. 16.13). This relates to differences in the size of their receptive fields. However, ganglion cells with the same placement with regard to eccentricity on the retina also vary in size. It is now customary to recognize two main kinds of retinal ganglion cell, together constituting about 90% of all cells: the **M cells** and the **P cells** (ending in magnocellular and parvocellular layers, respectively, of the lateral geniculate body). As seen in Fig. 16.13, the P cells are tiny compared to the M cells, but both types are much smaller centrally than peripherally. Physiologic studies of their properties indicate that the M cells primarily signal movement and contrasts of illumination, whereas the P cells are responsible for providing information about fine features (high visual acuity) and color. Both kinds can have either ON or OFF properties and can be activated under both scotopic and photopic light conditions. This is what one would expect, because signals from rods and cones converge on the same ganglion cells (Fig. 16.7). It is nevertheless possible that the M cells play a more important role than P cells in scotopic vision.

Figure 16.12

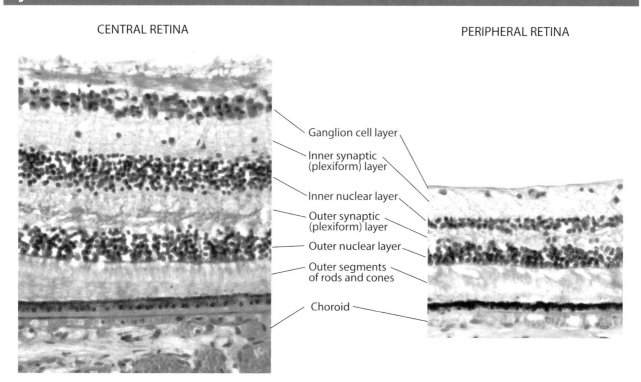

CENTRAL RETINA   PERIPHERAL RETINA

Ganglion cell layer

Inner synaptic
(plexiform) layer

Inner nuclear layer

Outer synaptic
(plexiform) layer

Outer nuclear layer

Outer segments
of rods and cones

Choroid

Central and peripheral parts of the retina. Photomicrographs illustrating how the various retinal layers differ in thickness when moving from the central to the peripheral parts of the retina. The density of ganglion cells is quite different in the two areas.

Next we discuss the organization of the pathways followed by the signals from the retina, and we will see that information from the two main types of ganglion cells is kept separate—at least to some extent—up to the cortical level.

More about Retinal Ganglion Cells

The functional properties of the two main morphological types of ganglion cells have been clarified by intracellular staining of cells that first have been characterized by their response to various kinds of light stimuli. Particularly the cat's and the monkey's retinal ganglion cells have been studied in depth. Even though cat and monkey (and presumably human) ganglion cells have several features in common—for example, with regard to the organization of their receptive fields—there are also important differences (notably that cats lack the ability to differentiate colors, and their visual acuity is much lower than in monkeys and humans). Our discussion here is based on findings in the monkey. The **M cells** (called A cells by some authors) have a large cell body and a fairly extensive dendritic tree (Fig. 16.13). The axon is relatively thick. The **P cells** (or B cells) have smaller cell bodies, a less extensive dendritic tree, and a thinner axon than the M cells. The P cells are most numerous and probably constitute about 80% of all of the ganglion cells. A major difference is that many of the P cells respond preferentially to light with a particular wavelength—that is, they are **color-specific**—whereas M cells do not have such specificity. The M cells are

more sensitive than the P cells to **contrasts** in **intensity** of illumination, however.

A further difference is that the M cells appear to respond better than the P cells to **moving stimuli**. In general, the M cells tend to respond especially when a stimulus starts and stops, whereas the P cells tend to give a signal as long as the stimulus lasts. In spite of anatomic differences between M and P cells, however, each group contains a wide variety of properties. For most properties, the two groups overlap, so that some M cells are more like typical P cells with regard to certain functional properties and vice versa.

Signals from Retinal Ganglion Cells Contribute to Optic Reflexes and Circadian Rhythms

This chapter deals primarily with parts of the visual system that enable us to perceive our surroundings—that is, we follow signals from the retina to the primary visual cortex (the striate area). The relevant pathways from M and P ganglion cells are synaptically interrupted in the thalamus (lateral geniculate body). A **third kind** of retinal ganglion cell does not fit into the M and P groups, however, because the cells send their axons to the **mesencephalon** and (to a

Figure 16.13

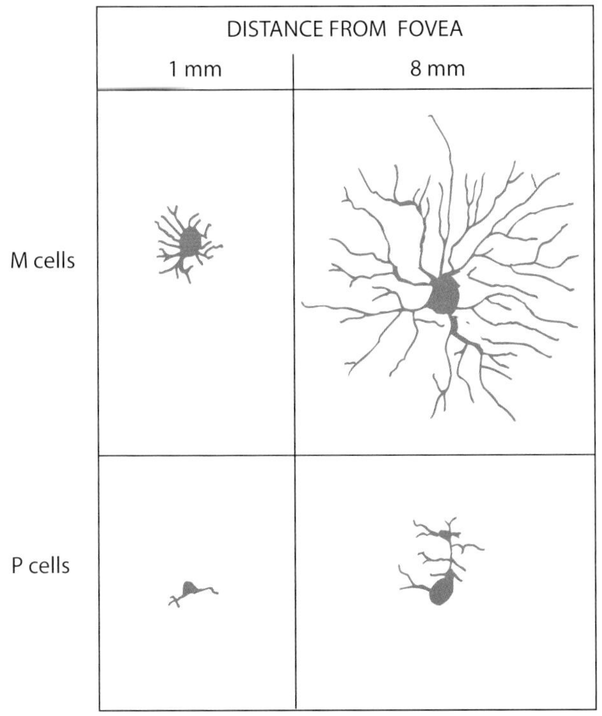

Two main kinds of retinal ganglion cells (monkey). Both types increase in size in the peripheral direction (distance from the fovea). The extension of the dendritic tree is related to the size of the receptive fields of the ganglion cells. The cells have been visualized by intracellular injection of horseradish peroxidase. (Based on Shapley and Perry 1986.)

lesser extent) to the **hypothalamus** rather than to the thalamus. These signals are used for **reflex** control of **eye** and **head movements** (Chapter 25) and for **accommodation** and control of **pupillary size** (Chapter 27). Furthermore, hypothalamic cell groups that control **circadian rhythms** are informed about ambient light (Chapter 30).

Comparing the proportion of retinal ganglion cells that sends axons to the mesencephalon in various species gives some insight into the evolution of the mammalian brain. Thus, in the cat, about 50% of the axons in the optic nerve pass to the mesencephalon, and the proportion is most likely higher in lower mammals such as the rat. In monkeys, only about 10% of all ganglion cells pass to the mesencephalon and in humans probably even less. With increasing development of the cerebral cortex, more analysis of visual information takes place at the cortical level rather than in the brain stem visual centers.

Ganglion Cells that Inform about Ambient Light

Even though "ordinary" retinal ganglion cells can inform higher centers about the level of ambient light, there are also some specialized ganglion cells that are intrinsically light sensitive (**intrinsically photoresponsive retinal ganglion cells**). The human retina contains about 3,000 such ganglion cells (0.2%), and most of them are found around the fovea. They contain a special kind of photopigment—**melanopsin**—that enable them to signal slow changes in ambient light. The fact that they send their axons to the hypothalamus makes them especially relevant for the control of **circadian rhythms**.

ORGANIZATION OF THE VISUAL PATHWAYS

The Visual Pathways

We next describe the paths followed by signals from the retina and see that information from the two main kinds of ganglion cells (M and P) are kept largely separate up to the cortical level. Figure 16.14 gives an overview of the visual pathways.

The axons of the retinal ganglion cells constitute the first link in the central visual pathways. All ganglion cell axons run toward the posterior pole of the eye, where they pass through the wall of the eyeball at the **optic papilla** (Figs. 16.1 and 16.11). They then form the **optic nerve**, which passes through the orbit and enters the cranial cavity. Here the two optic nerves unite to form the **optic chiasm** (Fig. 16.14; see also Fig. 6.13). In the optic chiasm some of the axons cross, and crossed and uncrossed fibers continue in the **optic tract**, which curves around the crus cerebri to end in the **lateral geniculate body** (*corpus geniculatum laterale*) of the thalamus (Fig. 16.15; see also Figs. 6.21 and 6.27). Here the axon terminals of the retinal ganglion cells establish synaptic contact with neurons that send their axons posteriorly into the occipital lobe. These efferent fibers of the lateral geniculate body form the **optic radiation** (*radiatio optica*) (Fig. 16.16). The optic radiation curves anteriorly and laterally to the posterior horn of the lateral ventricle and ends in the **primary visual area**, which is situated around the **calcarine sulcus** (see Fig. 6.26). The primary visual area is **area 17** of Brodmann, which is also called the **striate area**. The latter name (which we use here) refers to a white stripe in the cortex running parallel to the cortical surface. The stripe consists of myelinated fibers and is therefore whitish in a cut brain (Fig. 16.17).

Some of the fibers of the optic radiation lie in the posterior part of the **internal capsule**, where they can be damaged together with the fibers of the pyramidal tract—for example, by bleeding or infarction—thus producing a combination of weakness (paresis) of the muscles of the opposite

Figure 16.14

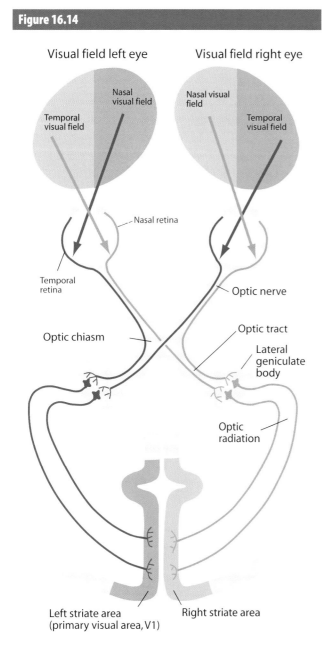

Visual field left eye   Visual field right eye

Nasal visual field

Nasal visual field

Temporal visual field

Temporal visual field

Nasal retina

Temporal retina

Optic nerve

Optic chiasm

Optic tract

Lateral geniculate body

Optic radiation

Left striate area (primary visual area, V1)   Right striate area

The visual pathways. For didactic reasons, the visual field of each eye is shown separately (cf. Fig. 16.3).

side of the body and blindness in the opposite visual hemifield (**hemianopsia**).

Not all fibers of the optic nerve terminate in the lateral geniculate body. Some fibers end in the thalamic nucleus **pulvinar** (see Figs. 6.21 and 6.22; pulvinar is discussed later in this Chapter). As mentioned, some ganglion cell axons terminate in the **mesencephalon**, especially in the **superior colliculus** and the **pretectal nuclei**, while others pass to the **hypothalamus**.

Axons from the M and P Cells Terminate in Different Layers of the Lateral Geniculate Body

The human lateral geniculate body (and that of other primates, such as monkeys) consists of six cell layers (Figs. 16.15, 16.18, and 16.19). The two ventralmost laminas (1 and 2) are composed of large cells and are therefore called the **magnocellular layers**, whereas the dorsal four are composed of small cells and are called the **parvocellular layers** (Fig. 16.18). Anatomic and physiologic studies have shown that the large retinal ganglion cells, the **M cells**, send their axons to the magnocellular layers of the lateral geniculate body, whereas the small ganglion cells, the **P cells**, send their axons (at least preferentially) to the parvocellular layers (Fig. 16.18). There is thus a division of the lateral geniculate body that largely corresponds to the functional division among retinal ganglion cells. It is now common to speak of two **parallel pathways**—M and P—from the retina to the lateral geniculate and further to the visual cortex. The significance of this is discussed later in connection with the visual cortex.

Signal Processing in the Lateral Geniculate Body: Corticothalamic Connections

Although the receptive fields of neurons in the lateral geniculate body are closely similar to those of retinal ganglion cells, the lateral geniculate is not merely a relay station. Signals from the retina are subject to modification before being forwarded to the striate area. Of special importance are strong, retinotopically organized **corticothalamic projections** from the visual cortex to the lateral geniculate. These connections most likely can control the signal traffic from the retina through the lateral geniculate and have been shown physiologically to influence the properties of the neurons. This modulation probably relates to mental states such as **motivation**, **alertness**, **expectation**, and stimulus **context**. Corticothalamic fibers may contribute to the suppression of vision of one eye in patients with **strabismus** (squint, cross-eyed); this has the obvious advantage of avoiding double vision.

In addition, the lateral geniculate receives fibers from other sources, notably from **cholinergic** cell groups of the pontine reticular formation; these connections probably regulate the signal transmission through the lateral geniculate to the striate area, in accordance with the level of consciousness and attention. Finally, a large number of GABAergic **interneurons** and numerous **dendrodendritic synapses** in the lateral geniculate presumably enable neurons with somewhat different receptive fields to influence each other.

FIGURE 16.15

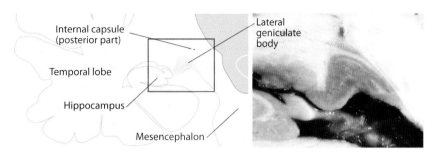

The lateral geniculate body. Drawing and photograph of frontal section through the right hemisphere. The whitish bands separating the lamellae are partly visible.

Visual Signals from One Side of the Visual Field Reach the Hemisphere of the Other Side

Figure 16.14 shows how the fibers are arranged in the **optic chiasm**. The fibers coming from the nasal halves of the two retinas cross, whereas the fibers from the temporal halves pass through without crossing. In this way, the left lateral geniculate body receives fibers from the temporal retina of the left eye and from the nasal retina of the right eye. The lateral geniculate body thus receives light from the contralateral half of the visual field. In functional terms, the crossing of signals corresponds to that taking place in the somatosensory system.

Optic nerve fibers from the two eyes are kept separate at the level of the lateral geniculate body, since three of the six layers receive fibers from the ipsilateral eye and the three others receive fibers from the contralateral eye (Fig. 16.19). After cutting one optic nerve, almost all cells in three of the layers degenerate (transneuronal degeneration), whereas the other three layers remain normal. Physiologic experiments also show that neurons within each layer of the lateral geniculate body are influenced from one eye only: these cells are **monocular**. We first encounter cells that are

Figure 16.16

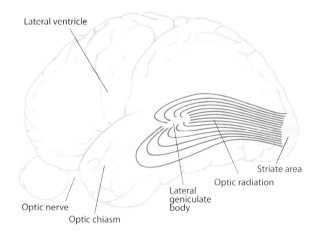

The optic radiation. The course of the fibers from the lateral geniculate body to the striate area shows how the fibers bend around the lateral ventricle and extend partly into the temporal lobe.

Figure 16.17

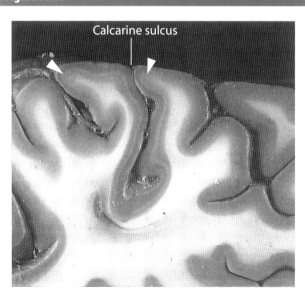

The striate area. Photograph of a section through the human occipital lobe showing the characteristic whitish stripe in layer 4 (the line of Gennari) of the striate area. Arrows mark the border between the striate area and neighboring extrastriate areas. See Fig. 33.5 for photomicrographs of thionine-stained and myelin-stained sections from the striate area.

Figure 16.18

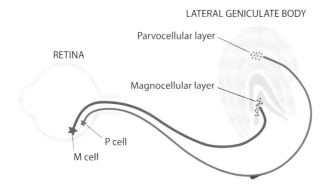

LATERAL GENICULATE BODY

Parvocellular layer

RETINA

Magnocellular layer

P cell

M cell

The lateral geniculate body. The two main kinds of retinal ganglion cells end in different layers of the lateral geniculate. (Based on Shapley and Perry 1986.)

influenced from both eyes—**binocular cells**—at the level of the striate area.

Fusion of Visual Images and Binocular Vision

Normally we perceive one image of the objects we look at, even though two (slightly different) images are formed

Figure 16.19

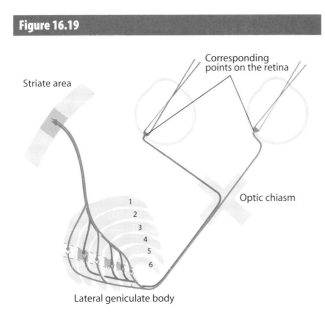

Corresponding points on the retina

Striate area

Optic chiasm

1
2
3
4
5
6

Lateral geniculate body

Fusion of the visual images. The signals from corresponding points on the two retinae end in different layers of the geniculate—that is, signals from the two eyes are kept separate at this level. The convergence of signals takes place in the striate area.

on the retina. The two images are perceived as one, and the phenomenon is called **fusion**. Fusion requires that the visual axes of the two eyes be properly aligned so that the images fall on corresponding points on the retina (Fig. 16.3). The two maculae are obviously corresponding points, and the images fall on them when we fix the gaze on a point to see it as sharply as possible. As mentioned, the signals from the two eyes are kept separate in the lateral geniculate body, but at the cortical level many cells are influenced from both eyes—that is, they are binocular (Fig. 16.19). Convergence in the cortex of signals from corresponding points in the two eyes is a prerequisite for binocular vision.

Binocular vision is not present from birth but **develops** gradually from about the age of 3 to 7 months. During this period, the movements of the eyes become coordinated, so that all movements are conjugated and the images fall on corresponding points when the gaze is fixed. There is obviously a strong (subconscious) drive in infants to obtain fusion of the retinal images.

Strabismus (Squint)

Strabismus (squint, cross-eyed) means that the visual axes of the eyes are not properly aligned, and, accordingly, the images do not fall on corresponding points. This may be due to problems with the extraocular muscles or their nervous control, or the "pressure" on the visual centers to produce fusion may be too weak. The reason for weak pressure may be reduced vision on one or both eyes (e.g., due to retinal disease or a cataract). The lack of fusion in children with a squint leads to underdevelopment or suppression of vision for the eye not used for fixation. In this manner, bothersome double vision is avoided, but even a relatively brief period of strabismus in early childhood may lead to permanently reduced visual acuity. It has been shown in monkeys that strabismus (produced experimentally) leads to a reduced number of cells in the striate area that is influenced by both eyes. In one kind of squint, the child uses the two eyes alternatively for fixation, and in such patients the visual acuity is usually conserved for both eyes.

The Visual Pathways Are Retinotopically Organized

The arrangement of the visual pathways just described concerns merely retinal halves—that is, a crude retinotopic localization ensuring that signals from different parts of the visual field are kept separate (cf. somatotopic localization within the somatosensory pathways). But the **retinotopic localization** is much more fine-grained than what appears in Fig. 16.20. Although many fiber systems of the brain are topographically

Figure 16.20

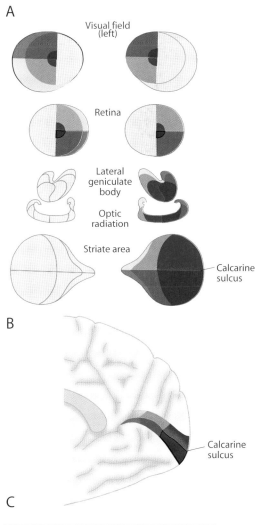

A

Visual field (left)

Retina

Lateral geniculate body

Optic radiation

Striate area

Calcarine sulcus

B

Calcarine sulcus

C

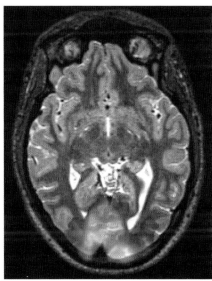

organized, no one is as sharply localized as the visual pathways, which show a true point-to-point localization.

In the **lateral geniculate body**, fibers from differently placed tiny parts of the retina end differently. Each small spot in the retina—and thus in the visual field—is "represented" in its own part of the lateral geniculate (Fig. 16.19). The retinotopic localization in the lateral geniculate is such that neurons influenced from the same part of the visual field (i.e., from corresponding points on the retina) lie stacked in a column perpendicular to the layers. This has been demonstrated with various anatomic techniques and physiologically by inserting microelectrodes perpendicular to the layers and determining the receptive fields of the cells that are encountered. The **receptive fields** of neurons in the lateral geniculate are quite similar to those of retinal ganglion cells (Fig. 16.8A).

The **thalamocortical** connections from the lateral geniculate body to the **striate area** are also organized with a precise retinotopic arrangement. This has been demonstrated, for example, by injection of a small amount of horseradish peroxidase in the striate area: retrogradely labeled cells are then confined to a narrow column that extends through all six layers of the lateral geniculate.

Mapping of the Visual Field onto the Striate Area

That all links of the visual pathways are retinotopically organized can be verified by shining light on a small spot on the retina. This evokes increased neuronal activity in a small region of the striate area, and when the light is shone on other parts of the retina, the evoked cortical activity changes position systematically. This kind of experiment has clarified how the **visual field** is mapped onto the cerebral cortex of animals. Careful examination of patients with circumscribed cortical lesions (often gunshot wounds) provides the basis for maps of the human

Retinotopic localization of the visual pathways. **A:** The striate area has been unfolded. Note that information from the upper half of the visual field reaches the part of the striate area below the calcarine sulcus, whereas the lower visual field projects above. Central parts of the visual field are represented most posteriorly and peripheral parts most anteriorly in the striate area. **B:** The extension of the striate area on the surface of the occipital lobe; most of it is buried in the calcarine sulcus. The striate area is similarly oriented in the left and the right figures. **C:** Activation of the visual cortex by flicker stimulation with light. Functional MRI, horizontal plane of sectioning. An anatomic MRI (T1 weighted) is produced and thereafter color-coded activity levels measured with blood-oxygen level dependent contrast are superimposed. Courtesy of Dr. Baard Nedregaard, Oslo University Hospital, Oslo, Norway).

visual cortex, as shown in Fig. 16.20. Electrical stimulation of the human occipital lobe confirms the retinotopic arrangement within the striate area. Stimulation with a needle electrode usually evokes the sensation of a flash of light in a certain part of the visual field. When the electrode is placed close to the occipital pole of the cerebral hemisphere, the person reports that the flash is located straight ahead, in agreement with the fact that fibers carrying signals from the macula end near the occipital pole. As the electrode is moved forward along the calcarine sulcus, the light flash is perceived as occurring progressively more peripherally in the visual field (at the opposite side of the stimulated hemisphere). If the electrode is placed above (dorsal to) the calcarine sulcus, the light occurs in the lower visual field, whereas stimulation below the calcarine sulcus elicits a sensation of light in the upper visual field. Studies in healthy humans with positron emission tomography (PET) and functional magnetic resonance imaging (fMRI) have confirmed the main features of the retinotopic organization of the striate area.

Disease processes (e.g., a tumor) involving the visual cortex may also at times elicit sensations of light because the neurons are abnormally irritated. **Epileptic** seizures originating in the visual cortex often start with a **visual aura**—that is, the muscular convulsions are preceded by bizarre patterns of light in the visual field opposite the diseased hemisphere. The characteristic, bright zigzag pattern (scintillating scotoma) preceding a **migraine** attack is caused by a wave of excitation spreading over the visual cortex.

Visual Information Can Reach the Cortex via the Superior Colliculus and the Pulvinar

Even though the "highway" from the retina to the cerebral cortex is via the lateral geniculate body, there are additional pathways. Of particular relevance is that the **pulvinar** (see Figs. 6.21 and 6.22) receives direct connections from the retina and sends efferents to parts of the visual cortex, notably to the **extrastriate visual areas** (cortical areas processing information from the striate area). Furthermore, the **superior colliculus**, which also receives fibers from the retina, sends efferents to the pulvinar and an adjacent thalamic nucleus (the **lateral posterior nucleus**; see Fig. 33.8). Thus, visual information may reach the cortex even when the optic radiation or the striate area is damaged.

Even though these visual pathways—which circumvent the lateral geniculate body—are retinotopically organized, they are apparently capable only of giving crude information about **movement** in the visual field. Thus, after bilateral damage of the striate area in monkeys, the animals react easily to moving stimuli, even though in other respects they behave as if they were blind. Studies of patients with damage at various levels of the visual pathways and of the visual cortex (localized with the use of MRI) indicate that, as long as parts of the extrastriate visual areas on the convexity are intact, the patients retain some capacity to recognize movements in the visual field. When sitting in front of a large screen with a random pattern of moving dots, patients with damage of the striate area (and surrounding areas on the medial

---

Figure 16.21

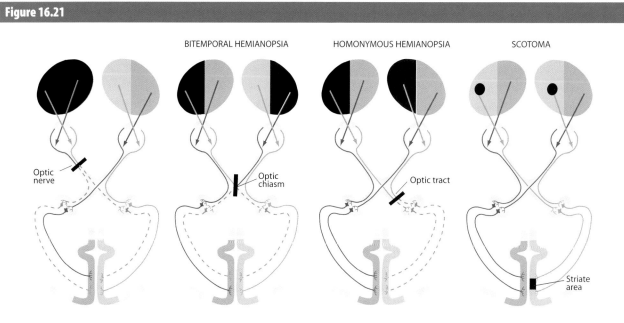

BITEMPORAL HEMIANOPSIA   HOMONYMOUS HEMIANOPSIA   SCOTOMA

Optic nerve

Optic chiasm

Optic tract

Striate area

Visual field defects after lesions of the visual pathways. The black areas indicate the blind parts of the visual field. The visual fields of the two eyes are shown separately for didactic reasons.

neurons at higher levels are devoted to the analysis of information from these parts. A disproportionately large part of the striate area treats information from the small macular region (Fig. 16.20). The **magnification factor** quantifies the relation between the cortical area devoted to different parts of the visual field. If information from all parts of the retina were to be treated with similar accuracy, the cerebral cortex would have to be several times larger. Precise control of eye movements, however, ensures that light from the most interesting part of the visual field always falls on the macula.

Interruption of the Visual Pathways

Partial damage to the visual pathways produces symptoms that confirm the arrangement of the cells and fibers at various levels of the optic system (Fig. 16.21). Interruption of the **optic nerve** prevents any visual signals from reaching the brain from that eye. If only the crossing fibers are damaged at the level of the **optic chiasm**, signals from the two nasal halves of the retinas are interrupted, and the patient is blind in the temporal parts of the visual field on both sides. This is called **bitemporal hemianopsia**. The patient may not notice this, however, because the blind part of the visual field is not experienced as darkness but rather as "nothing." The visual defect may be discovered incidentally by a tendency to bump into objects located a little to the side and perhaps by being hit by a car coming from the side when driving. This kind of visual defect may be caused by a **tumor of the pituitary** (located just below the optic chiasm). When the tumor grows, it must expand upward because it is located in a bony excavation (the sella turcica) and thus first compresses the middle part of the chiasm (Fig. 16.22). Damage to the **optic tract** produces a different clinical picture. If the damage is on the right side, visual signals from the temporal half of the right retina and the nasal half of the left retina are prevented from reaching the cortex: that is, the patient is blind in the left half of the visual field. This is called **homonymous hemianopsia**. The same visual defect occurs when the **optic radiation**, or the **striate area**, is totally destroyed. More frequently, however, there are incomplete lesions of the optic radiation (note its position in the posterior part of the internal capsule) or of the striate area, producing blind spots or **scotoma** in the opposite visual field (at corresponding points). Because of the accurate retinotopic arrangement within the visual pathways, mapping of such blind spots enables a precise determination of the site of the lesion.

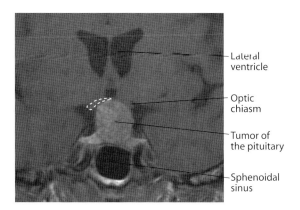

Figure 16.22

Tumor of the pituitary compressing the chiasma. Frontal MRI. The right part of the chiasma is outlined in yellow. Note how the tumor preferentially hits the middle part of the chiasma, damaging the crossing axons (cf. Fig. 16.21). (Courtesy of Dr. S.J. Bakke, Oslo University Hospital, Oslo, Norway.)

aspect of the hemisphere) reacted with movements of the eyes, apparently following the moving objects. They reported that they felt something moving in front of them, and they had some ability to identify the movement direction. They had no feeling of seeing anything, however, and when tested with perimetry, they were completely blind. This peculiar condition—termed **blindsight**—is of considerable theoretical interest in the search for the neurobiological basis of consciousness.

Central Parts of the Visual Field Are Overrepresented

In addition to the extremely precise retinotopic arrangement of the visual pathways, another important feature must be mentioned. We have explained that the density of retinal ganglion cells is considerably higher in central than in peripheral parts of the retina (particularly in the macula). This corresponds to conditions in the somatosensory system, where the density of receptors is highest at the fingertips ("the somatosensory macula"). Figure 16.20 illustrates that axons from central parts of the retina end in a disproportionally large part of the lateral geniculate body and that this overrepresentation of the central parts of the retina becomes even more marked in the striate area. Again, conditions are similar to those in the somatosensory system (see Fig. 14.8). Thus, the parts of the body and the visual field in which we have the best somatosensory and visual abilities are provided with a higher density of receptors than other parts, and, further, a much larger number of

THE VISUAL CORTEX AND THE FINAL PROCESSING OF VISUAL INFORMATION

Considerable processing of the visual information takes place in the striate area. Thus, most neurons have properties that are different from those encountered at lower levels of the visual pathways. Although it is customary to speak of "images" being formed in the brain, this is a misconception. To see an object is not to form a "picture" that other parts of the brain "look" at. Rather, there are temporally and spatially specific patterns of neuronal activity caused by the patterns of light falling on the retina. So far, however, we have only vague ideas about how the activity of the neuronal populations engaged in visual processing at the cortical level is related to our subjective visual experiences.

We next consider certain fundamental features of the functional organization of the striate area and also mention the regions surrounding it, the so-called **extrastriate visual area**s. These take part in the further processing of visual information. Thus, the visual cortex consists of much more than just the primary visual cortex (V1), the striate area, even though most of the fibers from the lateral geniculate body terminate there. Schematically, the signals from the retina first reach the striate area and, after considerable processing, are then forwarded to other cortical areas. Different aspects of visual processing such as analysis of color, form, and movement take place in at least partly different subdivisions of the extrastriate areas. Thus, damage to the striate area produces complete blindness in a part of the visual field, whereas damage restricted to extrastriate areas produces defects of restricted aspects of our visual experiences. Some of the extrastriate areas receive only indirect projections from the striate area (see Fig. 33.12).

Properties of Neurons in the Striate Area: Simple and Complex Cells

The retinal ganglion cells and cells of the lateral geniculate body have relatively simple, round receptive fields with a central zone that elicits excitation or inhibition when they are illuminated, as well as a peripheral zone with the opposite effect (Fig. 16.8B). But round spots of light are not an effective stimulus for the neurons of the visual cortex. What constitutes the adequate stimulus for the cortical cells remained a mystery for a long time. Diffuse light was not found to be effective, and neither was the kind of stimulus that so effectively affected the cells of the lateral geniculate. In 1962, however, the 1981 Nobel laureates David Hubel and Torsten Wiesel from the United States were able to show that many cells in the striate area respond briskly to elongated fields of light or

elongated contrasts between light and darkness. It was furthermore striking that many cells required that the light stimulus be oriented in a specific direction: turning a bar of light some degrees reduced the response markedly. This property was termed **orientation selectivity**. Some cells required a bar of light or a straight light/darkness transition of a specific orientation in a specific part of the visual field to respond, whereas other cells responded to a properly oriented stimulus within a larger area. Such cells thus appear to detect **contours** with a certain orientation regardless of their position within a larger part of the visual field. Hubel and Wiesel called the first type **simple cells** (Fig. 16.8B) and the latter type **complex cells**. Within each group there are several subtypes according to details of their properties. Why the properties of the complex cells are more complex than those of the simple ones may not be obvious, but presumably the terms were used because Hubel and Wiesel assumed that the properties of the complex cells could be explained by several simple cells acting on one complex cell. The properties of the simple cells, Hubel and Wiesel suggested, could be explained if several neurons in the lateral geniculate with round receptive fields in a row (together forming a stripe) converge on one cortical cell. It is, however, not yet entirely clear which neuronal interconnections underlie the properties of cells in the striate cortex.

Direction Selectivity, Disparity, and Binocular Cells

Hubel and Wiesel (1962) also discovered other fundamental properties of cells in the striate area. Among other things, cells generally respond much better to a **moving** than to a stationary stimulus. Many cells respond preferentially to a line or contour that is moving in a specific direction. Such **direction-selective** cells thus can detect not only the orientation of a contour but also the direction in which it is moving. Other kinds of specificities have also been described for cells in the striate area. For example, many **binocular cells** (cells that require input from both eyes) are sensitive to **disparity** of the images: that is, they require that the images from the two eyes are slightly different (disparate). This is always the case for images falling on corresponding points of the retina because the angle of view is different for the two eyes (except in the center of the macula) and also for images of objects that are nearer or farther from the fixation point. The ability to detect binocular disparity is important for perception of **depth** and for **stereoscopic** vision.

Modular Organization of the Visual Cortex

In addition to single cells being specific or selective with regard to their adequate stimulus, there is also a strong tendency for cells with similar properties in this respect to be located together, more or less clearly separated from cells with other properties. This is called **modular organization** (Figs. 16.23 and 16.24) and concerns properties such as orientation selectivity, wavelength (color) selectivity, and ocular dominance (i.e., which eye has the strongest influence). Such segregation of neurons in the striate area requires that fibers carrying different aspects of visual information from the lateral geniculate end at least to some extent differentially in the cortex. In agreement with this, fibers from the parvocellular layers of the lateral geniculate (Fig. 16.18) terminate deeper in lamina 4 (see Figs. 33.1 and 33.5) than fibers from the magnocellular layers.

Figure 16.23

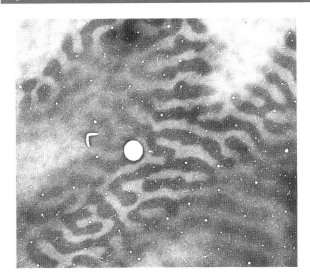

Ocular dominance columns. Photomicrograph of a section cut tangentially to the cortical surface of the striate area and stained to reveal differences in cytochrome oxidase activity. The section is from a monkey that was blind in one eye, causing reduced cytochrome oxidase activity in the regions (light stripes) of the striate area connected mainly with the blind eye. The dark stripes receive their main input from the normal eye. Magnification, ×25. (Courtesy of Dr. J.G. Bjaalie, Department of Anatomy, Institute of Basic Medical Sciences, University of Oslo.)

Figure 16.24

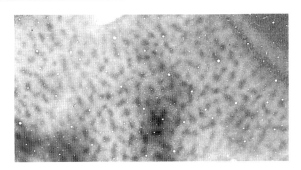

Color-specific "blobs" in the striate area. Photomicrograph of a section cut tangentially to the surface of the striate area of a normal monkey and stained to show differences in cytochrome oxidase activity. The section passes through laminas 2 to 3 and shows numerous small, darkly stained patches or blobs, which correspond to regions with color-specific neurons. Magnification, ×25. (Courtesy of Dr. J. G. Bjaalie, Department of Anatomy, Institute of Basic Medical Sciences, University of Oslo.)

More about Modular Organization

The first example of modular organization discovered by Hubel and Wiesel (1962) was the tendency for cells with similar **orientation selectivity** to be grouped together in **columns** perpendicular to the cortical surface. If we imagine that the striate area is unfolded and we are viewing it from above, the groups of cells with similar orientation selectivity are located in an irregular pattern of curving bands. This has been demonstrated with the **deoxyglucose** method, which demonstrates the neurons that are most active at a certain time. When an experimental animal is exposed for some time to parallel stripes of light, increased glucose uptake takes place in cells distributed in bands in the striate area. Another modular organization concerns **ocular dominance**. As mentioned, many cells in the striate area respond to light from corresponding points in the two retinas, but for most cells the influence is strongest from one of the eyes. The use of various tracer techniques and the deoxyglucose method has shown that neurons sharing ocular dominance are also distributed in bands within the striate area. Such ocular dominance columns can also be demonstrated in animals with monocular blindness (Fig. 16.23). A final example of modular organization concerns **color-specific** cells (strictly speaking: wavelength specific). They are not aggregated in bands but in clumps or **blobs** in laminas 2 to 3 of the striate area of monkeys. For some unknown reason, these blobs have a higher cytochrome oxidase activity than the surrounding tissue and can thus be easily identified in sections with a simple histochemical procedure (Fig. 16.24).

Extrastriate Visual Areas

As mentioned, several areas around the striate area take part in visual processing. These are collectively called the extrastriate visual areas and consist mainly of Brodmann's areas 18 and 19, which each consist of several subdivisions. In humans, fMRI studies have identified 10 extrastriate areas, each with a topographic representation of the visual field (there are probably more than 10, since 30 have been found in the monkey using methods enabling more detailed analysis than fMRI). Whereas V1 is often used for area 17 (the striate area), some of the extrastriate areas are termed V2 to V5, while others have specific names. Many of the extrastriate areas have a more or less complete representation of the visual field and are retinotopically organized, although with different degrees of precision. The interconnections between the striate area and the extrastriate areas, and among the extrastriate areas, are numerous and as a rule **reciprocal**. The complete scheme of visual association connections is therefore extremely complex and explains why it is difficult to determine the contribution of each individual area to the processing of visual information.

Why So Many Maps of the Visual Field?

It is not immediately clear why the cerebral cortex is organized so that the visual field is represented repeatedly in different parts. It may be a result of the adoption of novel functions by the visual cortex during evolution, and this probably occurs more easily by adding new areas (or duplicating old ones) than by having already existing areas take up new functions. It is presumably also a simpler solution to have several separate areas than one large area with regard to arrangement of the necessary fiber connections.

Further Processing of Visual Information: Segregation and Integration

The properties of single neurons in the striate area suggest that these neurons together are the basis for the cortical analysis of **form**, **depth**, **movement**, and **color**. Their properties, for example, fit predictions made on the basis of psychophysical experiments in humans, such as the preference for contours and for moving stimuli. Nevertheless, what is taking place in the striate area appears to be mainly a first analysis and sorting of raw data, which must be further processed elsewhere to form the basis for our conscious visual experiences. There is now much evidence of separate, or **segregated**, treatment of the various features of visual images (such as form, color, movement, and location in the

visual field) outside the striate area, and we discuss a few examples in the next section. In some way, however, different features of a scene or an object must be **integrated** to a unified visual experience. We return to this later in this chapter.

Segregation: Dorsal and Ventral Pathways (Streams) Out of the Striate Area

It has been proposed that a **ventral** stream of information concerning **object identification** ("what") passes downward from the occipital lobe to the temporal lobe, whereas another, **dorsal** stream concerned with **spatial features** and **movement** ("where") passes upward to the parietal lobe (see Fig. 16.25). This concept is partly based on results from experiments in monkeys with lesions that have been restricted to "visual" parts of either the temporal lobe or the posterior parietal cortex. Monkeys with bilateral lesions of temporal visual areas have reduced ability to identify objects; for example, they can no longer distinguish between a pyramid and a cube. In contrast, lesions of visual parts of the posterior parietal cortex reduce the ability to localize an object in space and in relation to other objects; among other symptoms, such monkeys have difficulties with performing **goal-directed movements.** It suffices with a unilateral lesion of the parietal lobe to produce deficits in

Figure 16.25

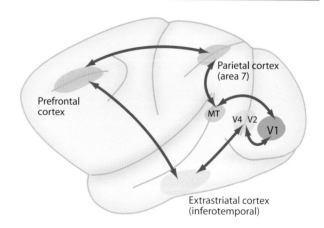

Dorsal and ventral pathways out of striate area (V1). Monkey. The ventral pathway is especially important for conscious object identification, whereas the dorsal pathway is crucial for perception of movement and space. Note convergence of information from the two pathways in the prefrontal cortex. (Based on data published by Deco and Rolls 2005.)

the contralateral half of the visual field. This resembles the symptoms occurring in humans after damage to the posterior parietal cortex, such as reduced ability to judge movements in the visual field and disturbed eye movements (see Chapter 34, under "More about Symptoms after Lesions of the Posterior Parietal Cortex"). The pathways taken by the signals from the striate area to the temporal and posterior parietal visual regions are not known in detail, but several visual areas are intercalated in the pathways (Fig. 16.25).

It is often stated without reservation that the ventral (temporal) and dorsal (parietal) streams out of the striate area segregate information from **P** and **M cells**, respectively. This is an oversimplification, however. For example, some convergence of information from M and P cells takes place already in the striate area (besides the more prominent segregation). The sum of evidence suggests that the subcortical pathways from the retina to the striate area are specialized for signaling simple stimulus features, whereas the further pathways do more advanced processing using as, a rule, information from both M and P cells.

More about Segregated Information Processing in the Extrastriate Visual Areas

Three "channels" out from the striate area (V1) have been revealed by detailed anatomic and physiologic analysis. One channel arises from cells that are predominantly influenced by the **magnocellular layers** of the lateral geniculate. The properties of these striate cells indicate that they signal **movement** and **depth** cues. Another pathway comes from cells that appear to be influenced by the **parvocellular layers** of the lateral geniculate. Accordingly, these striate cells have small receptive fields and are orientation-selective. This pathway presumably signals **forms** and **patterns** and would seem particularly important for our ability to discern visual details. A third "parvocellular" pathway originates in striate neurons that are, at least to a large extent, **wavelength-specific**, signaling information about color.

These three pathways from the striate area appear to be kept separate, at least partly, also at the next station—that is, in **area V2**, which is adjacent to the striate area. From V2, information about **movement** is channeled to **area V5** (also called the **middle temporal visual area**), whereas information about **color** is channeled primarily to **area V4**. The major outflow from V5 has been traced to the **posterior parietal cortex**. Information about forms and patterns is channeled primarily from V2 to **inferotemporal visual areas** (i.e., situated inferiorly in the temporal lobe). How far the specialization goes within each of these areas is not clear, however. The numerous interconnections among the extrastriate areas suggest that they cooperate extensively. Accordingly, single neurons in area V5, for example, are sensitive not only to movement but also to certain other visual features. Similarly, neurons in area V4 are not purely color-specific.

Color Vision and Color Opponency

We have discussed parts of the elements responsible for color vision—namely, the three kinds of **cones** with sensitivities for light of different wavelengths (Fig. 16.6). We have also emphasized that the brain must compare the degree of stimulation of three kinds of cone to "know" the wavelength composition of the light (and therefore the color of an object). Figure 16.6 shows the large overlap between the sensitivity curves of the three kinds of cone, especially between those with sensitivities in the red and green parts of the spectrum, respectively. How can we then perceive so many nuances of each color? Part of the explanation is found in how the cones are coupled to the next links in the pathway to the cortex. Thus, **retinal ganglion cells** and neurons in the **lateral geniculate body** have narrower sensitivity curves than the cones, making them better at discriminating wavelengths. Many ganglion cells and lateral geniculate cells respond to light of different wavelengths but with opposite signs—one wavelength exciting the cell, and the other inhibiting it. This phenomenon is called **color opponency** and must be due to convergence on one ganglion cell (or lateral geniculate cell) of signals from cones with different wavelength sensitivities. Some neurons are excited (ON response) by red light in the central zone of the receptive field (Fig. 16.8) and inhibited (OFF response) by green light in the peripheral zone; others are inhibited by red light centrally and excited by green peripherally; and so forth. Such combinations improve the ability to **discriminate** wavelengths in the red–green part of the spectrum. Some neurons exhibit color opponency to blue and yellow light (a combination of red and green) and others to white light (stimulation of all three kinds of cones) and darkness.

Even more complex kinds of color opponency are found among neurons in the **visual cortex**. For example, a neuron may respond with an ON response to red light and an OFF response to green light in the center of its receptive field, whereas the reverse responses are evoked from the peripheral zone (double opponency). Such neurons are found in the cytochrome-rich patches in laminas 2 to 3 of the striate area (Fig. 16.24). Together, all the color opponency neurons provide accurate information of the wavelength composition of the light hitting a spot on the retina.

Color Constancy

We take for granted that an object has a certain color, regardless of whether we see it in direct sunlight, in shadow, or in artificial light. For example, we consistently identify a banana as yellow, an apple as red, the grass as green, and so forth (although we perceive differences in nuances). This property of our visual system, called **color constancy**, is by no means self-evident. Thus, the wavelength composition of the light reflected from an object depends not only on the physical properties of the surface but also on the light shining on the object. Different light sources produce light with quite different wavelength composition. The light received by the eye from an object thus differs markedly under different lighting conditions.

Color constancy is obviously of great **biologic importance**. The color of an object gives us essential information as to its nature, but only if the color is an invariant, typical property. For example, we know that a yellow banana is edible, whereas green or brown ones are not. Even under quite different illuminations, we easily make this kind of choice based on color.

We do not fully understand how the brain accomplishes this remarkable task, although it must depend on processing at the cortical level. Color constancy occurs only if the object we look at is part of a **complex, multicolored scene**. Experiments with patterned, multicolored surfaces show that the composition of the light reflected from one part of the visual scene may be changed considerably without changing the color perceived by an observer. If the same square is seen against an evenly dark background, however, the perceived color changes according to the composition of the reflected light—for example, from green to white. This must mean that under natural conditions the brain determines the color of an object by comparing the wavelength composition of the light from its surface with the composition of light from all other surfaces in the visual field.

Afterimages

If we look at a red surface for a few seconds and then move to a white, we see a green surface where we just saw the red. This is called an **afterimage**. The afterimage of yellow is blue, and for white it is black. This phenomenon can be partly explained by selective bleaching of a particular kind of cone. For example, a red light bleaches mainly the cones with wavelength sensitivity in the red part of the spectrum. When the eye then receives white light, the "red" cones are, for a short while, less sensitive than the others. This creates a relative dominance of signals from "green" cones, and the surface is perceived as green. What we have said so far might suggest that the color of the afterimage depends only on the light first hitting the retina. It is not that simple, however. The afterimage depends on the color perceived by the subject, not the absolute wavelength composition—that is, **color constancy** occurs also for afterimages. The afterimage effect can also occur when looking for a while at a moving object and then

at a stationary one. We then perceive an **illusory movement** of the stationary object in the opposite direction.

Perceptual Mistakes

There is obviously no absolute correlation between a visual stimulus and the perception it evokes. Of course this is not specific to seeing but pertains to the other senses as well. Fortunately, relationships between certain patterns of stimuli and external events are reasonably constant. Therefore, we usually make the right decisions by relying on our interpretation (our percept) of the stimuli (the color of a traffic light, the movements of a snake, the contours of a horse, and so forth). Perceptual mistakes are usually due to certain evolutionary-based priorities in how our brains treat sensory information: we attend to what is judged as **salient** at the expense of all other information. Magicians exploit such perceptual "weaknesses" to create expectations that, for example, divert our attention away from what they do not want us to see.

Lesions of the Extrastriate Areas: Visual Agnosia

Humans with lesions of the **temporal extrastriate areas** show various forms of reduced ability to **recognize objects** (agnosia). A patient may be unable to recognize faces, another may have no problem with faces but cannot recognize fingers (finger agnosia), and so on (see Chapter 34, under "Lesions of the Association Areas: Agnosia and Apraxia"). High-resolution fMRI in humans and recording from single neurons in monkeys indicate that a region in the **fusiform gyrus** contains a particularly high proportion of **face-specific** neurons (Fig. 16.26). Nevertheless, recordings with multiple-surface electrodes in patients (to localize epileptic foci) suggest that several separate, small areas in the inferior temporal cortex participate in **face recognition**. These areas appear to be parts of a mosaic of areas with different specializations. This agrees with observations after lesions of extensive parts of the inferotemporal extrastriate areas: such patients are deficient in several specific kinds of object recognition and suffer from not only **prosopagnosia** (inability to recognize faces; Greek: *prosopon*, face). Selective loss of **color vision** (**achromatopsia**) after lesions restricted to a region below the calcarine sulcus (in the **lingual gyrus**) has been convincingly documented (Fig. 16.26). This corresponds most likely to **area V4** in monkeys. Patients with unilateral lesions in this region are reported to see everything in the opposite half of the visual field in black and white, whereas the other half has normal colors.

Damage at the junction between the occipital and the parietal lobes can produce selective impairment of the ability to recognize **movements** (**akinetopsia**). One patient with a bilateral lesion of this region could not see moving objects; when the same objects were stationary, however, he could easily describe their form and color, and he could judge depth in the visual scene.

Patients with selective loss of **depth perception** after cortical damage have been described. To such patients other people look completely flat, as if made from cardboard; patients can recognize

Figure 16.26

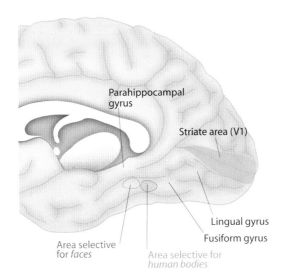

Subdivisions of the extrastriate visual areas that are selective for recognition of human faces and human bodies, respectively. Surface marking is based on high-resolution fMRI from normal persons. These two areas could not be discerned with standard fMRI with lower resolution. The representation is simplified. Thus, there may be more than one area specialized for faces, and neurons related to specific categories may not be as clearly separated as shown here. (Based on data published by Schwarzlose et al. 2005.)

their color, contours, and shading, however. The exact site of the lesion in such patients has not been determined, but PET studies indicate that tasks requiring depth perception activate several areas in the cerebral cortex (and in the cerebellar hemispheres) and that these areas overlap with areas involved in other visual tasks.

Integration of Visual Information: One Final Area?

Despite the fact that there is much evidence of separate processing in the visual cortex of different aspects of visual information, we must remember that at some level a synthesis has to occur. Information about form, position, movement, and color must in some way be linked together. After all, the color "belongs" to a certain object, with a certain form and position and with a certain speed and direction of movement. Our percept is unitary, although the brain first has already "dissected" out and analyzed the bits and pieces of information in the light falling on the retina. What does integration of information mean in the context of sensory processing? One might think that there must exist one final, site (area) in which all aspects of visual information are brought together, but **anatomic** data do not favor the

existence of such cortical areas. Even in the **prefrontal cortex**, visual information about "what" and "where" is treated separately (in conjunction with coupling of visual features of objects to voluntary movements).

There are also theoretical problems with the notion of a **final integrative area**. Thus, although our conscious experience is unitary, it consists of components to which we have separate, conscious access. For example, a car may be characterized by its color, by its shape, or by its movements. The components are kept separate yet are linked in such a way that we perceive them as belonging together. Another theoretical problem with a final integrative area is where to "place" awareness of the visual image. As expressed by the British neurobiologist Semir Zeki (1993): "If all the visual areas report to a single master cortical area, who or what does that single area report to? Put more visually, who is 'looking' at the visual image provided by that master area?"

Role of the Striate Area in Visual Awareness and Visual Imagery

We mentioned patients with **blindsight** previously (under "Visual Information Can Reach the Cortex via the Superior Colliculus and the Pulvinar"). Such patients have no awareness of having seen anything, yet they can respond to movement in the visual field. In such cases, visual information reaches the extrastriate areas that are specialized for analysis of movements without going through the striate area. We may then ask whether conscious visual experience requires that visual information first go through the **striate area**—in other words, is activation of the striate area necessary for visual awareness? One approach to this question has been to study brain activity with the PET technique while subjects imagine visual scenes, such as a red car or their home street. In such situations, the subject has retrieved the information from memory and "sees" the scene with closed eyes. Which parts of the brain are then specifically activated? It appears that largely the same extrastriate areas are activated during **visual imagery** as when seeing. The PET data are conflicting as to whether the striate area is activated with visual imagery, but the fact that patients with cortical blindness (damage to the striate area) are able to imagine visual scenes strongly suggests that the striate area is not necessary for visual imagery. Also, clinical observations suggest that visual imagery and seeing may not use identical cortical structures. Thus, a few patients have been reported who could recognize objects when seeing them but could not imagine the same objects. The reverse situation has also been described.

Visual Awareness and Synchronized Network Activity

We have treated integration at early stages of the visual processing, such as cells in the striate area responding to contours with a certain orientation regardless of where it occurs within a larger part of the visual field. Further integration produces more complex properties, so that cells respond only when several characteristics coincide (such as a contour with a specific orientation moving in a certain direction). Such and more complex integration of data need not occur on single cells, however; it may also occur by coordinated activity in separate neurons that are synaptically linked (neuronal networks). As mentioned, it is noteworthy that the many visual areas are so extensively interconnected. For example, the striate area receives connections from most of the areas to which it projects, and the same holds for many extrastriate areas and their relations to other cortical areas. Presumably, our **conscious visual experience** depends upon the total pattern of neuronal activity in many, interconnected cortical areas at any moment. **Synchronized, oscillatory** activity of neuronal groups receiving the same kind of information (e.g., about the direction of movement) may play an important part and has been shown to occur in cortical areas.

Functional MRI studies suggest that an extended **network** connecting ventral (temporal) visual areas and parts of parietal and prefrontal areas (Fig. 16.25; see also Fig. 33.12) is especially active in conjunction with visual **awareness**. A possible common denominator for awareness of sensory information in general was formulated as follows by Zeman (2004, p. 324): "awareness occurs as the result of physiologically appropriate interactions between neural systems which serve sensation, memory, and action; activity which remains within a single system . . . can influence behavior but will not enter awareness."

In conclusion, both clinical and brain imaging studies clearly show that extensive parts of the cerebral cortex are involved in conscious visual experience. It should be noted, however, that visual information that is not consciously perceived can nevertheless be used for preparation of voluntary (conscious) movements.

Subconscious (Implicit) Use of Visual Information

A striking example was published by Goodale and Milner in 1992. A woman suffered damage to parts of her occipital lobes (with sparing of the striate cortex) because of carbon monoxide poisoning. Afterward she was unable to recognize objects (**visual agnosia**). For example, she could not decide whether an object was oriented vertically or horizontally, nor could she show the size of the object with her fingers. When asked to grasp it, however, she accomplished this easily and with normal preparatory adjustment of the fingers. Thus, she could adapt her grip to specific visual features, yet she had no awareness of these features. Obviously, the parts of the brain preparing voluntary, **goal-directed movements** have access to information about shape, size, and orientation, no matter whether or not these features are consciously perceived.

Development of Normal Vision Requires Proper Use

There may be causes other than a squint for lack of normal visual development. For example, if the eye does not receive proper stimulation because errors of refraction produce a retinal image that is out of focus or because light for some reason does not reach the retina, vision does not develop normally. In humans, the first 2 to 3 years (in particular the first year) are especially important in this respect; lack of **meaningful use** of the eye even for a short period may then cause permanently reduced visual acuity (as discussed in Chapter 9). Animal experiments furthermore show that, contrary to what might be expected, vision is better preserved if both eyes are covered for a period than if only one is covered. This is so because the two eyes "compete" during the early development of the visual system. If only one eye is used, it acquires an advantage and takes over neurons in the visual cortex that normally would have been used by the other eye.

The Auditory System

The sense of hearing is of great importance in higher animals—not least in humans, for whom speech is the most important means of communication. The adequate stimulus for the auditory receptors is **sound waves** with frequencies between 20 and about 20,000 Hz. The sensitivity is greatest, however, between 1,000 and 4,000 Hz and declines steeply toward the highest and the lowest frequencies; that is, a tone of 15,000 Hz must be much stronger than a sound of 1,000 Hz to be perceived. The range of frequencies to which the ear is most sensitive corresponds fairly well to the range of frequencies for human speech. The **frequency** of sound waves determines the pitch, whereas the **amplitude** of the waves determines the intensity.

Many animals can perceive sound over a much wider range of frequencies than humans can. For example, dogs can hear a whistle hardly noticed by humans, and bats use extremely high-pitched sounds for echolocation. Sound waves pass through the air to the tympanic membrane, which transmits them via a chain of three tiny bones to the **cochlea.** The sensory cells—the **hair cells**—of the cochlea are low-threshold mechanoreceptors sensitive to the bending of stereocilia on their surface. From the cochlea, the signals are conducted to the **cochlear nuclei** in the brain stem through the eighth cranial nerve, the **vestibulocochlear nerve**. This nerve also carries signals from the sense organ for equilibrium—the vestibular apparatus— that anatomically and evolutionarily is closely related to the cochlea. Functionally, however, these two parts have little in common, and we describe the sense of equilibrium together with other aspects of vestibular function in Chapter 18.

From the cochlear nuclei, the **auditory pathways** carry signals to **the inferior colliculus** (and some other brain stem nuclei). Neurons in the inferior colliculus send their axons to the **medial geniculate body** of the **thalamus**. Thalamocortical axons reach the **primary auditory area** (A1) situated on the upper face of the temporal lobe (buried in the lateral sulcus). The auditory pathways from one ear reach both hemispheres, in contrast to the almost complete crossing of somatosensory pathways. Further processing of auditory information takes place in cortical areas surrounding A1 in the temporal lobe. Outward connections from these areas ensure integration of auditory information with other sensory modalities. Nuclei in the brain stem receiving signals from both ears with a time difference are crucial for our ability to **localize sounds**.

THE COCHLEA

The Cochlea Is Part of the Labyrinth

The **labyrinth** consists of an outer bony part surrounding an irregular canal in the temporal bone and an inner **membranous part** following and partly filling the canal (Figs. 17.1, 17.2, and 17.3). The membranous canal is filled with a fluid called the **endolymph** (Figs. 17.4). Between the membranous and the bony parts is a space filled with a fluid called the **perilymph** (Figs. 17.1 and 17.4).

The labyrinth has two main parts. One is the cochlea, and the other is the vestibular apparatus, consisting of three semicircular ducts and two round dilatations (Figs. 17.1 and 17.2). Here we consider only the organ of hearing, the cochlea. The **membranous part** of the cochlea—the **cochlear duct**—forms a thin-walled tube with a triangular shape (in cross section), surrounded by the bony part of the cochlea (Figs. 17.4 and 17.5). The duct forms a spiral with two and a half to three turns (Figs. 17.2, 17.3, and 17.4). The lowermost wall of the cochlear duct is formed by the **basilar membrane** (*membrana basilaris*), which is suspended between the two facing sides of the bony canal (Figs. 17.4 and 17.5). At the inner side of the turns, the basilar membrane is attached to a bony prominence the **bony spiral lamina** (*lamina spiralis ossea*)—that follows the cochlea in its spiraling course (Figs. 17.4 and 17.5). The sensory epithelium, forming the **organ of Corti**, rests on the basilar membrane (Figs. 17.4, 17.5, and 17.6). The length of the cochlear duct, and thus of the basilar membrane, is about 3.5 cm (Fig. 17.7). The thin **vestibular membrane** forms the

Figure 17.1

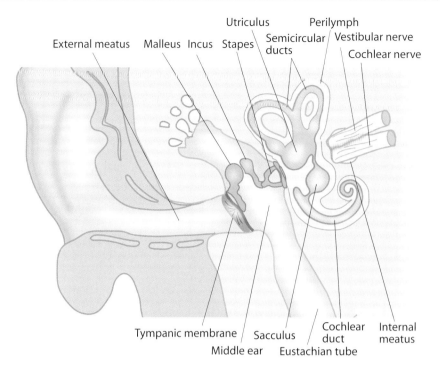

The ear. The middle ear has three ear ossicles, and the inner ear has the membranous labyrinth (located in the temporal bone). The Eustachian tube connects the middle ear with the pharynx.

upper wall of the cochlear duct (Figs. 17.4 and 17.5). The third, lateral, or outer wall of the cochlear duct lies on the bony wall of the canal and is formed by a specialized, stratified epithelium, the **vascular stria** (Fig. 17.5). As the name implies, there are **capillaries** among the epithelial cells. The vascular stria controls the composition of the endolymph.

The room outside the cochlear duct consists of two parallel canals. The one situated below the basilar membrane is

Figure 17.2

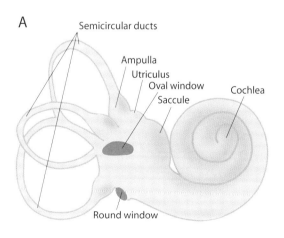

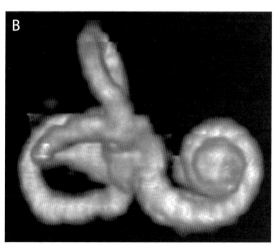

A: *The membranous labyrinth with its vestibular part (the semicircular ducts, the saccule, and the utricle) and the auditory part (the cochlea).* The stapes is attached in the oval window. **B:** The fluid in the labyrinth visualized via three-dimensional reconstruction of MRIs. (Courtesy of Dr. Einar Hopp, Oslo University Hospital, Oslo, Norway.)

Figure 17.3

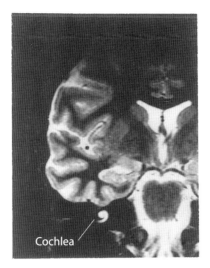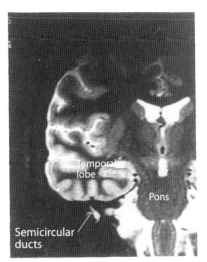

The labyrinth. Two closely spaced, frontal MRIs. The fluid-filled cochlea **(left)** and semicircular canals **(right)** are clearly seen just below the temporal lobe (the image is weighted so that water appears white). (Courtesy of Dr. S.J. Bakke, Oslo University Hospital, Oslo, Norway.)

the **scala tympani,** and the one above the vestibular membrane is the **scala vestibuli** (Figs. 17.4 and 17.5). Both have openings, or windows, in the bone facing the middle ear (Figs. 17.2 and 17.7). The **oval window** (*fenestra vestibuli*) is situated at the end of the scala vestibuli, whereas the **round window** (*fenestra cochleae*) is at the end of the scala tympani. The stapes and a thin membrane of connective tissue close the windows, respectively (Fig. 17.7).

Figure 17.4

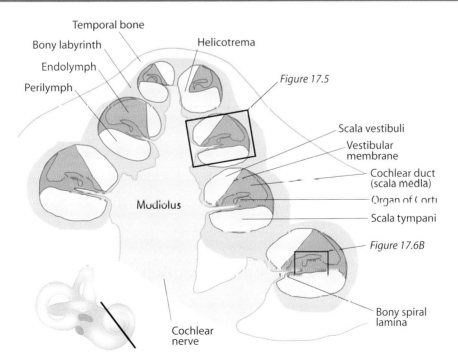

Section through the cochlea.

Figure 17.5

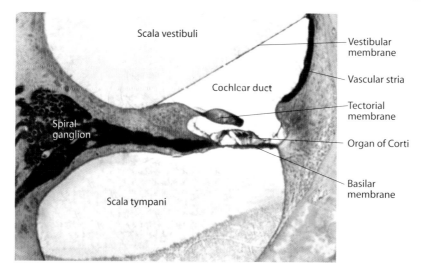

Section through the cochlea. Photomicrograph. Cf. Fig. 17.4.

The Perilymph, the Endolymph, and the Endocochlear Potential

The composition of the endolymph and of the perilymph differs: the concentrations of sodium and potassium ions in the perilymph are similar to those in the cerebrospinal fluid (i.e., similar to those in the extracellular fluid), whereas the concentrations of these ions in the endolymph are like those found intracellularly. Thus, the cilia of the sensory cells—surrounded by the endolymph (Fig. 17.5)—are embedded in an unusual extracellular fluid with K^+ as the dominating cation. (The protein concentration, however, is much higher in the perilymph than in the endolymph and the cerebrospinal

Figure 17.6

A

B

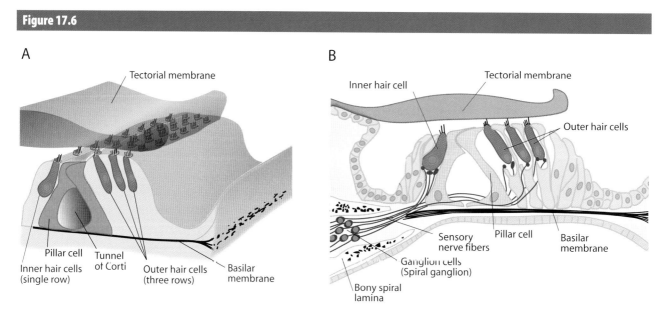

The organ of Corti. **A:** Three-dimensional representation of a short segment of the organ of Corti (the whole organ extends the full length of the cochlear duct). The inner hair cells are in a single row, and the outer hair cells are in three parallel rows. The pillar cells appear to change their form in relation to loud sounds, possibly to prevent damage of hair cells. **B:** Cf. Fig. 17.4. Note that only the tallest stereocilia of the outer hair cells are in contact with the tectorial membrane.

Figure 17.7

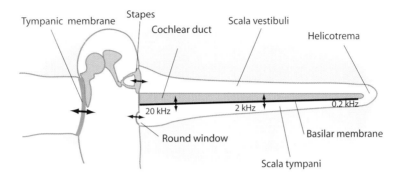

The middle ear and the cochlea. The cochlear duct is pictured as if straightened (length about 3.5 cm). The oscillations of the stapes are transmitted to the fluid in the scala vestibuli and from there to the cochlear duct. Different tone frequencies set different parts of the basilar membrane in motion. Note that the highest frequencies stimulate the hair cells near the base of the cochlea, whereas the lowest frequencies stimulate hair cells near the apex (near helicotrema). (Based on Fettiplace and Hackney 2006.)

fluid.) The **vascular stria** is responsible for the high K⁺ concentration of the endolymph. The high K⁺ concentration creates a potential of about 90 mV between the endolymph and the perilymph, called the **endocochlear potential** (the endolymph is positive in relation to the perilymph). The special composition of the endolymph and the endocochlear potential are of crucial importance for the transduction mechanism of the hair cells, as discussed later in this chapter.

In experimental animals, atrophy of the vascular stria causes **hearing loss**, and the severity seems to be proportional to reduction of the endocochlear potential. There is further evidence that—in addition to loss of hair cells— atrophy of the vascular stria can contribute to **age-related hearing loss** in humans.

How Sound Waves Are Transmitted to the Sensory Cells in the Cochlea

Conduction of sound waves from the air to the receptor cells in the cochlea occurs through the **external ear** (the auricle and the external auditory meatus) and the middle ear or **tympanic cavity** (Fig. 17.1). Sound waves hitting the skull can also be transmitted through the bone directly to the receptors. This kind of transmission, however, is very inefficient with regard to airborne sound waves and therefore plays no role in normal hearing (bone conduction of sound waves is used for testing the function of the cochlea and also for certain hearing aid devices).

Sound waves hit the eardrum or **tympanic membrane** located at the bottom of the external meatus (Fig. 17.1). The

eardrum consists of a thin, tense connective tissue membrane covered by a thin layer of epithelium on both sides; it is richly supplied with **nociceptors**, like the tight skin of the inner part of the external meatus. The three **ossicles** form a chain through the middle ear and connect the eardrum with the oval window (Fig. 17.1). The **malleus** (the hammer) has a shaft that is attached to the inner side of the eardrum. The head of the malleus connects to the **incus** (the anvil) by a joint, and the incus is further connected to the **stapes** (the stirrup) by a joint. The basal plate of the stapes inserts in the oval window, thus closing the scala vestibuli (Fig. 17.7). The sound waves make the eardrum and the ossicles vibrate with the frequency of the waves, and thus the movement transmits to the fluid in the cochlea. Because the area of the eardrum is so much larger than that of the basal plate of the stapes, the **pressure** per square unit increases 20 times. This amplification mechanism increases the sensitivity for sound dramatically, compared to a situation without the ossicles. Normally, even the slightest movement of the eardrum is sufficient to cause stimulation of the receptors in the cochlea; sound waves with **amplitude** of only 0.01 nm suffice to produce the weakest perceptible sound with the frequency to which the ear is most sensitive. If the sound waves were to be transmitted directly from the air to the fluid in the cochlea, a large proportion would be reflected without reaching the sensory cells of the cochlea. The sound would have to be much stronger to be perceived in such a situation. This is the case when diseases of the middle ear destroy the ossicles or stiffen their joints and thus eliminate the amplification mechanism. The ensuing hearing loss is called **conduction deafness**. A prerequisite for the free movement of the eardrum is that the pressure be equal on the two sides. This is ensured by the **Eustachian tube** (*tuba auditoria*), which connects the middle ear cavity with the pharynx (Fig. 17.1).

When the **stapes** is pressed (slightly) into the **oval window**, the pressure of the sound waves is transmitted directly to the fluid (the perilymph) in the scala vestibuli. Because water is incompressible, the sound waves can cause movement of the fluid only because the room can expand at some other point. The thin, compliant membrane that covers the **round window** allows such expansion. The membrane is pressed outward (into the middle ear) each time the stapes is pressed into the oval window. Movement of the perilymph in the scala vestibuli transmits immediately to the endolymph in the cochlear duct through the thin **vestibular membrane**. The movement thus propagates to the basilar membrane, which is pressed downward, and transmits the movement to the perilymph in the scala tympani. In short, movements of the stapes in and out of the oval window—in pace with the sound waves—produce corresponding movements of the basilar membrane. Movements of the basilar membrane stimulate the receptor (hair) cells.

Next we describe how the receptor cells are arranged in the organ of Corti and the mechanism by which movements of the basilar membrane lead to excitation of the receptor cells.

Sound Pressure Is Measured in Decibels

The **amplitude** of sound waves determines the **sound pressure**—that is, the pressure of air molecules on the tympanic membrane. The most intense sound that the human ear can perceive is about 10^{12} times stronger than the weakest. A logarithmic scale is used for sound pressure. One decibel (dB) represents the pressure necessary to produce the weakest perceptible sound, whereas just below 130 dB represents the strongest (the pain threshold is at 130–140 dB). A 10 dB increase means that the sound pressure has increased 10 times, and a 30 dB increase equals a 1,000 times sound pressure increase. Ordinary speech produces a sound pressure between 30 and 70 dB. The dB scale gives relative measures of intensity because the sensitivity of the ear differs for different frequencies.

The Organ of Corti

The receptor cells in the cochlea are called **hair cells** because they are equipped with sensory hairs, or **stereocilia**, on their apical surface (Figs. 17.6 and 17.8; see also Chapter 18, under "More about Vestibular Hair Cells"). Along the basilar membrane, there are two populations of receptor cells: one formed by the **outer hair cells** and the other by the **inner hair cells** (Fig. 17.6). The inner hair cells, closest to the bony spiral lamina, form a single row, while the outer hair cells form three parallel rows. There

---

Figure 17.8

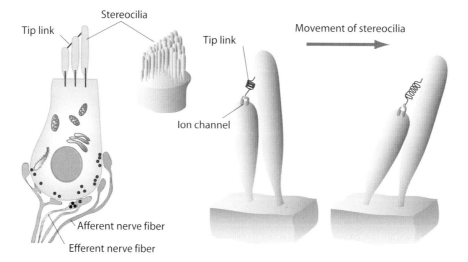

Inner hair cell. **Left:** Compare with Fig. 17.6. Note the arrangement of the stereocilia. The basal part of the hair cell is contacted by afferent (sensory) fibers and a few efferent fibers. Depolarization of the hair cell releases neurotransmitter from vesicles near the nerve terminals. **Right:** The most likely mechanism of sensory transduction in hair cells. The tip link pulls open the ion channel when the stereocilia are deflected. The tip link is thought to act like a spring that gates the opening of the channel. (Based on Pickles and Corey 1992.)

are approximately 3,500 inner and 15,000 outer hair cells in the human cochlea. The two kinds of cells differ in both morphology and innervation. Many more sensory nerve fibers contact the inner than the outer hair cells, whereas the reverse situation exists for the efferent innervation. There is good evidence that the inner hair cells are responsible for signaling sound, whereas the outer hair cells regulate the sensitivity of the sense organ.

Supporting cells surround the hair cells. Two rows of especially large supporting cells, the **pillar cells**,[1] separate the inner and outer hair cells and form the **tunnel of Corti**. Above the hair cells lies a thick plate, the **tectorial membrane**, which is indirectly attached to the bony wall of the cochlea (Figs. 17.5 and 17.6). Sensory (afferent) nerve fibers of the **eighth cranial nerve** contact the basal parts of the hair cells (Figs. 17.6 and 17.8). The cell bodies of the sensory neurons are located in the **bony spiral lamina** close to the midportion of the cochlea (the **modiolus** (Figs. 17.4, 17.5, and 17.6B). **Efferent nerve fibers** also contact the hair cells (Fig. 17.8), enabling the central nervous system (CNS) to control the sensitivity of the auditory receptors.

Deflection of the stereocilia, caused by movement of the basilar membrane, produces **receptor potentials** in both inner and outer hair cells. The further events differ, however: in the inner hair cells, depolarization facilitates transmitter release, whereas depolarization stimulates contractile activity in the outer hair cells.

The Inner Hair Cells and Mechanoelectric Transduction

Unlike the stereocilia of the outer hair cells, those of the inner hair cells are not in direct contact with the tectorial membrane (Fig. 17.6B). How then can the sound waves lead to deflection of the stereocilia of the inner hair cells? Most likely, movement of the fluid surrounding the stereocilia is sufficient, causing the stereocilia to move back and forth, in pace with the vibrations of the basilar membrane. The stereocilia are stiff, due to their content of actin filaments. Thus, each cilium moves like a rod around its point of insertion in the top plate of the hair cell (Fig. 17.8). Further, the stereocilia are coupled so that they all move together. Thereby, the sensitivity of

each hair cell becomes much higher than if the stereocilia moved independently.

The stereocilia are of unequal length and are orderly arranged from the shortest to the longest (Fig. 17.8).[2] This structural polarization corresponds to a functional one: bending of the stereocilia toward the longest cilium **depolarizes** the hair cell, whereas the opposite movement **hyperpolarizes** it. The depolarization produces a graded **receptor potential**. Thus, bending the stereocilia one way increases the frequency of firing in the afferent nerve fibers. Depolarization of the hair cell is most likely caused by opening of **mechanosensitive cation channels** near the tip of the stereocilia.

The mechanism for **channel opening** appears to be as follows. The stereocilia are interconnected near their tips by a thin protein thread called a **tip link** (Fig. 17.8). The tip links attach to the channel proteins and open the channels by a direct pull when the stereocilia are deflected. The depolarization is presumably mediated by K^+ ions entering the hair cell, since the endolymph that surrounds the stereocilia contains a very high concentration of K^+ and low Na^+. In addition, the **endocochlear potential** speeds the flow of cations because it adds to the membrane potential of the stereocilia. The required movement of the stereocilia is minimal: a barely perceptible sound moves the tip of each stereocilium about 1 nm (1/100,000,000 mm), whereas the strongest perceptible sound moves the stereocilia about 1 μm—that is, corresponding to the thickness of the stereocilium.

Depolarization leads to release of **glutamate** from the basal part of the inner hair cells. This transmits the signal to the sensory nerve endings (acting on AMPA receptors). Release of sufficient amounts of the transmitter elicits action potentials in the sensory nerve fibers, and the signals are transmitted to the brain stem (see Fig. 12.2). When the stereocilia move back and forth, the ensuing receptor potential of the hair cell follows a sinus curve; that is, the membrane potential oscillates in pace with the vibrations of the basilar membrane. Because the receptor potential modulates the transmitter release, the action potentials conducted in the sensory fibers follow the frequency of the sound waves.

The Outer Hair Cells Amplify Sound Waves

The motion of the basilar membrane differs from that expected of a passive mechanical structure. There must be

---

1. The pillar cells and other supporting cells in the organ of Corti appear to contribute to control of cochlear sound sensitivity. In animals exposed to loud sounds, the form and mutual positions of the supporting cells change in pace with changes in cochlear sensitivity. This may be a mechanism to protect the hair cells.

---

2. Vestibular hair cells have an extra tall kinocilium (non-motile) marking the highest point in the row of stereocilia (see Fig. 18.6). This disappears from the cochlear hair cells shortly after birth.

mechanisms intrinsic to the cochlea that can **amplify the vibrations** of the basilar membrane almost 100 times. Much evidence points to the outer hair cells as the **motors** of the amplification; that is, they can rapidly transmit mechanical energy to a very narrow strip of the basilar membrane.

Because the stereocilia of the outer hair cells are attached to the tectorial membrane, their deflection by basilar membrane vibration seems easy to explain. (Although only the tallest stereocilia attach to the tectorial membrane, the linking of the stereocilia to each other makes them move together as a unit.) When the basilar membrane vibrates, the hair cells are displaced relative to the tectorial membrane, which is relatively immobile because it is anchored to the bony wall. Thus, the stereocilia are moved back and forth in pace with the frequency of the sound waves. The receptor potential initiates **contractile** activity, changing the form of the cell.[3] The ensuing fast contractions of the outer hair cells move the basilar membrane, producing both an **amplification** of the vibrations and a narrowing of the vibrating part, which sharpens the **tuning** of the **frequency curve**. Together these changes ensure more precise signal transmission. Whether the amplification is due solely to deformation of the outer hair cell body (elongation and shortening) or movements of the cilia also contribute is not settled.

Efferent Innervation Protects the Hair Cells

The **efferent fibers** arise in the **superior olivary complex**, located in the rostral part of the medulla (Fig. 17.10), and form the **olivocochlear bundle**. The fibers end predominantly on the outer hair cells and release **acetylcholine** (and most likely ATP) that hyperpolarizes the cells by binding to muscarinic receptors. The activity of the efferent fibers increases with increasing sound levels, thus reducing the active movements of the outer hair cell stereocilia, which in turn produces less amplification and broader tuning of the frequency curve. Accordingly, animal experiments show that stimulation of the efferent fibers reduces the signal frequency of the afferent fibers from the inner hair cells. This **feedback** mechanism protects against hair cell loss in animal experiments with overexposure to loud noise. The efferent innervation also seems to protect against loss of synapses on the inner hair cells caused by prolonged,

moderate noise exposure (in this instance, the damage is probably due to excess glutamate release causing neurotoxicity). The strength of the cochlear feedback control varies among individuals, and it has been suggested that a weak feedback control may be a risk factor for **age-related hearing loss**.

The Ear Produces Sound: Otoacoustic Emissions

The ear actually emits faint sounds—**otoacoustic emissions**—that appear to be produced by the contractions of the outer hair cells. A microphone in the external meatus can record such sounds, which can occur spontaneously or be evoked by a click. The hearing system works in reverse, as it were: the outer hair cells move the basilar membrane, which in turn moves the fluid in the cochlea; this moves the ossicles, which then move the tympanic membrane that produces the sound. The phenomenon is used diagnostically—for example, in infants—to decide whether the cochlea functions normally.

Different Frequencies Are Registered at Different Sites along the Basilar Membrane: Tonotopic Localization

The ordered arrangement of neurons and nerve fibers signaling different pitches of sound (frequencies) is called **tonotopic localization** (cf. somatotopic localization in the somatosensory system and retinotopic localization in the visual system). As discussed later, the auditory pathways are tonotopically organized all the way from the cochlea to the cerebral cortex. The tonotopic localization in the cochlea has been demonstrated in several ways. After receiving lesions restricted to a small part of the organ of Corti (which extends along the full length of the basilar membrane), experimental animals no longer react to sound in a certain, narrow range of frequencies (pitches), whereas they react normally to sounds of other frequencies. In humans, similar selective deafness may occur after prolonged exposure to noise, for example, in factories. Anatomic examination of the cochlea after death in such persons has shown that the hair cells have disappeared in a restricted region on the basilar membrane, the position of the region differing with the frequency to which the person was deaf. The tonotopic localization has been determined in detail by recording the response of single hair cells to sounds of different frequencies. Each hair cell is best activated by tones within a very narrow range of frequencies. Together, the hair cells and the sensory fibers leading from them cover the total range of frequencies we can perceive.

---

3. The voltage-sensitive contractile protein **prestin** expands or compresses the cell body in response to changes of the membrane potential. The effects of manipulating the *prestin* gene (e.g., studying the effects on hearing of making the gene nonfunctional in knockout mice) suggest that this protein is of critical importance for the amplification mechanism.

The **tonotopic** localization is such that the tones with the **highest pitch** (highest frequencies) are registered by the hair cells closest to the oval window (i.e., on the basal part of the basilar membrane), whereas the lowest frequencies are registered at the top of the cochlea (i.e., at the apical part of the basilar membrane) (Fig. 17.7). This can be explained, at least partly, by the physical properties of the basilar membrane, as proposed by the German physicist Hermann Helmholtz in the nineteenth century. The basilar membrane is most narrow basally and becomes progressively wider in the apical direction. The fibers of the basilar membrane are oriented transversely to the long axis of the basilar membrane (Fig. 17.6) and are therefore longer apically than basally. In analogy with the strings of an instrument (e.g., a piano), basal parts would be expected to vibrate with a higher frequency than apical parts. This is the main basis of the **resonance theory** of Helmholtz, which postulates that each position along the basilar membrane corresponds to a certain frequency. Although later research has shown that even a pure tone makes large parts of the basilar membrane vibrate, the region in which the maximal amplitude occurs is very narrow. This appears to be caused by the amplification produced by contractions of the outer hair cells, as discussed earlier. Thus, the hair cells differ in accordance with their position on the basilar membrane, so that their thresholds are lower for certain frequencies than for others.

Cochlear and Brain Stem Implants to Restore Hearing

When deafness is due to loss of hair cells without affection of the afferent nerve fibers, hearing can be restored by a so-called **cochlear implant.** During surgery, a thin, insulated electrode is inserted along the basilar membrane. The insulation is removed at about 20 points, enabling electric stimulation of the cochlear nerve fibers at these sites. Hence a range of frequencies can be transmitted to the brain; in accordance with the tonotopic localization along the basilar membrane (the frequency resolution is of course inferior to what is possible with a normal number of hair cells). A microphone and microprocessor transform the sound waves to electric signals that are sent to the electrode.

In **children** who are **born deaf,** a cochlear implant can enable development of speech and speech comprehension. Most of the children are able to attend normal school classes, provided that they receive intensive training afterward. The implant must be inserted as early as possible and not later than 3 to 4 years of age. If the cortical networks necessary for analysis and use of sounds are not developed before this age, they cannot develop later, probably because the auditory cortex has been taken over by other systems. Indeed, there is evidence from functional magnetic resonance imaging (fMRI) studies that visual stimuli may activate the auditory cortex in congenitally blind persons. This corresponds to the situation in children who are born blind and later regain sight (e.g., by removing a cataract), as discussed in Chapter 9. In **deaf adults,** who had normal hearing earlier, a

cochlear implant can restore hearing so they can comprehend speech. In this situation, the networks responsible for sound processing were presumably established in early childhood and remained essentially intact even after a period without hearing. However, intense training is required after surgery in order to make sense of the foreign sounds provided by the implant. Further, the longer the time from loss of hearing to implantation, the poorer the prospect of a satisfactory result.

When deafness is due to destruction of the **cochlear nerve**, a cochlear implant will of course have no effect. In some such patients, restoration of hearing has been attempted by implanting an array of electrodes over the ventral **cochlear nucleus**. Otherwise, the strategy is similar to that used in cochlear implants. The success so far has been much more limited than with cochlear implants, however.

Current experiments in animals explore the possibility of restoring hearing by genetic, **stem cell,** and molecular strategies—either to rescue ailing hair cells (and spiral ganglion cells) or to replace dead ones.

THE AUDITORY PATHWAYS

Distinctive Features of the Central Auditory System

The anatomic organization of the central auditory pathways has some unusual features that are different from other sensory systems we have discussed so far. More nuclei are intercalated in the auditory pathways, and these nuclei have extensive and complicated interconnections. In addition, some fibers cross the midline at several levels of the auditory pathways. These features make the auditory pathways more difficult to study than other sensory pathways. The crossing at several levels also renders hearing examinations of limited practical value for determining the site of lesions in the CNS.

Conduction Deafness and Sensorineural Hearing Loss

The most common causes of hearing loss are diseases of the middle ear, either because they compromise the conduction of sounds to the cochlea or because they destroy the neural elements of the cochlea or the eighth nerve. The first kind is called **conductive deafness** and the second **sensorineural (or nerve) deafness**. Transmission of sound to the cochlea can be reduced or abolished by middle ear infections that damage the eardrum or the ossicles. In **otosclerosis**, the basal plate of the stapes becomes fixed in the oval window and therefore cannot transmit sounds. Less frequently, lesions of the central auditory pathways cause hearing loss; this kind, called **central deafness**, is considered later in this chapter.

To **distinguish** between conductive and sensorineural deafness, one can compare the threshold for sounds conducted through the air with sound conducted through the bones of the skull. In the **Rinne test**, a vibrating tuning fork is first applied to the mastoid process and then a little away from the external ear. Normally, the sound is heard much better when it is conducted through the air than through the bone; however, in conductive deafness caused by destruction of the eardrum or the ossicles, the bone-conducted sound is heard best. In the **Weber test**, the vibrating tuning fork is applied to the forehead in the midline. Normally, the sound is heard equally in both ears; in conductive deafness, it is heard best in the deaf ear, whereas in sensorineural deafness it is heard best in the normal ear. The reason for the lateralization to the deaf ear in conduction deafness is not clear. It is possible that the airborne sound masks the bone-conducted sound on the normal side.

Destruction of the cochlear nerve or the cochlear hair cells, that is, **peripheral lesions**, produces hearing loss of the ear on the same side (the same happens, of course, with a lesion of the cochlear nuclei). The **hair cells** may be damaged by noise and by certain drugs. There is also a steady loss of hair cells with **aging**, particularly near the base of the cochlear duct (high frequencies). Destruction of the **cochlear nerve** may be caused by a tumor in the internal auditory meatus (Fig. 17.1), called **acoustic neuroma** or Schwannoma (arising from the Schwann cells of the eighth cranial nerve). As the tumor grows, it compresses the cochlear, the vestibular, and the facial nerves (all passing through the internal meatus). Symptoms may therefore be caused by irritation (in the early phase) or destruction of all of these nerves. Thus, the first symptoms may be due to irritation of the cochlear nerve, causing ringing in the ear (tinnitus) and sometimes vertigo due to irritation of the vestibular nerve, but gradually deafness develops. As the tumor grows, it compresses the brain stem with additional symptoms from the trigeminal nerve and ascending and descending long tracts. The cochlear nerve may also be compressed or torn by **skull fractures** passing through the temporal bone. Peripheral lesions of the auditory system, in addition to causing unilateral deafness, also reduce or eliminate the ability to **localize** the source of a sound.

The Cochlear Nerve and the Cochlear Nuclei

The part of the eighth cranial nerve conducting signals from the cochlea is called the **cochlear nerve**. Most of the fibers are afferent and have their cell bodies in the **spiral ganglion**, which is located in the bony spiral lamina (Figs. 17.4, 17.5, and 17.6). From the spiral ganglion the fibers pass through the midportion of the cochlea (the modiolus, Fig. 17.4) and through the **internal acoustic meatus** (Fig. 17.1) to the **cerebellopontine angle** (Fig. 17.9; see also Fig. 27.1). There the nerve enters the two **cochlear nuclei**— the **dorsal** and the **ventral**—located laterally on the medulla (Figs. 17.9 and 17.10; see also Fig. 27.2), external to the inferior cerebellar peduncle (see Fig. 24.2). After entering the nuclei, the cochlear nerve fibers divide and end in precise **tonotopic** order in several parts of the nuclei. The tonotopic localization has been demonstrated, for example, with

microelectrode recordings that make it possible to determine the response of single fibers and neurons to tones of different frequencies.

For more information about the **efferent fibers** of the cochlear nerve, see "Efferent Innervation Protects the Hair Cells" earlier in this chapter.

Ascending Pathways from the Cochlear Nuclei

From the cochlear nuclei, the auditory signals are transmitted to the **inferior colliculus** (mainly of the opposite side). The pathway formed by the ascending fibers from the cochlear nuclei is called the **lateral lemniscus** (Figs. 17.9 and 17.10). Many of the fibers end in other nuclei—such as the **superior olivary complex**—that send fibers to the inferior colliculus. Neurons in the inferior colliculus send their axons to the **medial geniculate body** of the thalamus (Figs. 17.9 and 17.10; see also Figs. 6.21 and 6.22). The fibers form an oblong elevation at the dorsal side of the mesencephalon, the **inferior collicular brachium** (*brachium quadrigeminum inferius*). The efferent fibers from the medial geniculate body end in the **auditory cortex** located in the temporal lobe (in the superior temporal gyrus; Figs. 17.10 and 17.11).

Figure 17.9

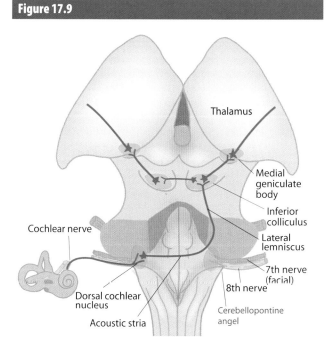

Nuclei of the auditory pathways. Signals from the cochlea of one side reach the medial geniculate bodies of both sides (although not shown in the figure).

Figure 17.10

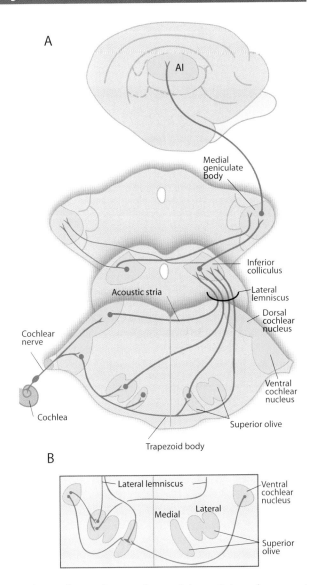

A

AI

Medial
geniculate
body

Inferior
colliculus

Acoustic stria

Lateral
lemniscus

Dorsal
cochlear
nucleus

Cochlear
nerve

Ventral
cochlear
nucleus

Cochlea

Superior olive

Trapezoid body

B

Lateral lemniscus

Ventral
cochlear
nucleus

Medial   Lateral

Superior
olive

Parallel ascending auditory pathways, Schematic based on experimental studies of the cat. **A:** The connections are bilateral, so that the AI on one side receives signals from the cochleae of both sides. **B:** Some main connections of the superior olive. Note that signals from both ears reach the medial part of the superior olive. This arrangement is of importance for localization of sound.

The ascending fibers from the medial geniculate body are located in the posterior part of the **internal capsule**. At all levels, the auditory pathway is precisely, **tonotopically** organized, with cells responding to sounds of different frequencies arranged in parallel lamellae.

Even though the central auditory pathways are predominantly crossed, there is a significant uncrossed component. Therefore, unilateral damage to the pathways does not produce a clear-cut hearing deficit. The ability to **localize** from where a sound comes may be reduced, however.

The Auditory Pathways Consist of Functionally Different Components

Efferent fibers from the cochlear nuclei take different routes (Fig. 17.10A). Fibers from the **dorsal cochlear nucleus** pass in the **acoustic stria** dorsal to the inferior cerebellar peduncle and then cross through the reticular formation and join the **lateral lemniscus** (Figs. 17.9 and 17.10). Most fibers from the **ventral cochlear nucleus** pass ventrally and cross to the other side in the **trapezoid body** in the lowermost part of the pons (Fig. 17 10A). Some of these fibers end in the **superior olivary complex** of both sides, whereas others continue rostrally in the lateral lemniscus to the **inferior colliculus**. The functional significance of these parallel paths out of the cochlear nuclei is not fully understood, but animal experiments show that single cells in the dorsal and ventral nuclei have different properties. Schematically, many cells in the **ventral nucleus** respond to sound stimuli much like the primary afferent fibers of the cochlear nerve, whereas cells in the **dorsal nucleus** have more complex response properties. For example, cells in the dorsal nucleus are often excited by sound with one particular frequency and inhibited by those of another frequency. It has been suggested that the dorsal nucleus forwards signals that are important for **directing attention** toward a sound, whereas information from the ventral nucleus is important for, among other tasks, **localizing** a sound.

Experimentally, two components of the ascending auditory pathways have been identified. One is called the **core projection** and is a pathway for auditory signals only. It is precisely tonotopically localized at all levels and terminates in the **primary auditory cortex (AI)**. The core projection is synaptically interrupted in the central parts of the inferior colliculus and specific parts of the medial geniculate body. The other component is called the **belt projection**. It is synaptically interrupted in the peripheral parts of the inferior colliculus and terminates in the **cortex surrounding the AI**. The cells of this pathway are influenced by visual and somatosensory stimuli in addition to auditory ones. The belt projection is thought to be important for **integrating** of auditory information with other kinds of sensory information.

Generalizations to conditions in humans on the basis of studies done in other species must be made with particular caution, however, as species differences appear to be greater for the auditory system than for other sensory systems. This may presumably be related to the great differences that exist among species with regard to how sound is used as a source of information. For example, certain nuclei that are large in the cat are very small in humans and vice versa.

Sound Localization

It is not enough that the CNS analyzes the sound frequencies and on this basis interprets the meaning of the sound (e.g., who or what produced the sound). Locating the source of a sound is another important but difficult task of the auditory

Figure 17.11

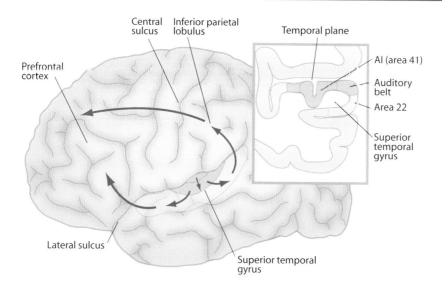

The human auditory cortex. The figure shows in a simplified form the concentric arrangement of the auditory areas and how the connections spread out from the AI, finally reaching the prefrontal cortex (there are reciprocal connections at all levels, although not shown here). Dorsal and ventral pathways from auditory areas to the frontal lobe are indicated. The ventral pathway is thought to deal with identification of sounds and their meaning, whereas the dorsal pathway primarily deals with aspects of sound localization and movements. The **inset** shows a frontal section through the temporal lobe and the distribution of the auditory areas.

system. To be able to judge the distance and direction to a sound source (e.g., a potential prey or a danger) is obviously of vital importance to most animal species. The precision of our ability to localize sound is formidable: humans can distinguish sounds separated by no more than 2 degrees. To do this, central parts of the auditory system must be able to detect temporal differences of 11 microseconds between sounds reaching the two ears.

Unilateral damage to the **auditory cortex** reduces the ability of experimental animals to locate sounds coming from the opposite side. Thus, a cat with such a lesion does not move toward its prey sending out a brief sound (e.g., a mouse). The head and eyes, however, move toward the prey—even after bilateral damage of the auditory cortex—showing that nuclei at lower levels of the auditory pathways can locate the sound and elicit appropriate reflex movements.

Concerning location of sounds in the **horizontal plane**—that is, to the right or left of the midsagittal plane—basic computations occur in the first synaptic relay after the cochlear nuclei, the **superior olive** (Fig. 17.10). We are less certain regarding mechanisms for location of sounds in the vertical plane, although the **dorsal cochlear nucleus** is probably involved. Neurons in the **inferior colliculus** respond specifically to sound from a certain direction, and the inferior colliculus probably contains a **map** of our **auditory space**.

The Superior Olive and Sound Localization

The **superior olivary complex** (superior olive) is located in the lower part of the pons in the trapezoid body (Fig. 17.10). A striking feature is that most neurons are influenced from both ears, which led to the assumption that the superior olive is particularly important in localizing the origin of a sound. When a sound hits the head from the right side, it will reach the right ear slightly before it reaches the left, because the head is in the way. The sound will also be slightly weakened before reaching the left ear. Psychophysical experiments in humans indicate that side differences in both time and intensity are used by the auditory system to localize sounds. The **time difference** is most important for localizing sounds of **low frequencies**, whereas **intensity differences** are most important for sounds of **higher frequencies** (above 4,000 Hz).

The superior olivary complex consists of several, tonotopically organized subdivisions. The lateral part receives afferents from the cochlear nuclei of both sides and projects bilaterally to the inferior colliculi. Most cells in the lateral part are excited by signals from the ear of the same side and inhibited by signals from the contralateral ear (via interneurons). The cells respond best when the sounds hitting the two ears are of different intensities. Consequently, the **lateral part** of the superior olive is assumed to use intensity differences for the analysis of sound localization.

The **medial part** of the superior olive appears to be particularly important in localizing **low-frequency sounds**. It receives afferents from a particular subdivision of the ventral cochlear nucleus of both sides (Fig. 17.10B). Each cell has two long dendrites oriented transversely. One dendrite receives signals from the right ear and the other from the left. These cells are very sensitive to small time differences in synaptic inputs to the two dendrites and are most sensitive to sounds with low frequencies. The efferent fibers of the medial part pass to the central nucleus of the inferior colliculus on the same side.

Descending Control of the Auditory Pathways

Descending fibers exist at all levels of the auditory pathways. At the lowest level, the efferent fibers in the cochlear nerve, forming the **olivocochlear bundle,** exert a negative feedback to the hair cells, as discussed previously. At the highest level, numerous fibers pass from the **auditory cortex** to the medial geniculate body (like other thalamic nuclei) and to the inferior colliculus. Other fibers descend from the **inferior colliculus** to the nuclei at lower levels. The descending connections are, at least in part, precisely organized and can therefore be expected to selectively control subgroups of neurons in the auditory pathways (e.g., neurons transmitting information about a certain frequency).

There are many inhibitory **interneurons** in the nuclei of the auditory pathways, and both γ-aminobutyric acid (**GABA**) and **glycine** are used as transmitters for such interneurons. Physiologic experiments show that the central transmission of auditory signals can be inhibited, probably at all levels from the cochlea to the cerebral cortex. The censoring of the sensory information that is allowed to reach consciousness is perhaps even more pronounced in the auditory system than in other sensory systems. Selective suppression of auditory information is necessary if we are to **select** the relevant sounds among numerous irrelevant ones. Such mechanisms are most likely at work when, for example, at a cocktail party with numerous voices we are nevertheless able to select and pay attention to only one of them.

The brain must be able to distinguish between sounds that are generated externally and sounds we produce ourselves. Indeed, auditory neurons are inhibited during **vocalization**. Although the exact mechanisms are unknown, this most likely involves interpretation of **corollary discharge**—that is, copies of the motor commands producing the sounds are sent to the auditory cortex (cf. .the inhibition of sensory signals produced by our own movements, discussed in Chapter 14 under "The Brain Controls the Transmission of Sensory Signals").

Auditory Reflexes: Orienting and Protecting

The ascending auditory pathways convey signals that enable the conscious perception of sounds. In addition, auditory information is used at a subconscious level to elicit reflex responses. The **reticular formation** receives collaterals from the ascending auditory pathways, and such connections mediate the sudden muscle activity provoked by a strong, unexpected sound—that is, a **startle response**. Other auditory signals pass to the nuclei of the facial and trigeminal nerves, which innervate two small muscles in the middle ear: the **stapedius** and **tensor tympani muscles**. Contraction of these muscles dampens the movements of the middle ear ossicles and thereby protects the cochlea against sounds of high intensity. Paresis of the **facial nerve** often is accompanied by hypersensitivity to sounds, or **hyperacusis**.

Other, more complex reflex arcs mediate automatic, orienting **movements of the head and eyes**, and even the body, in the direction of an unexpected sound. The centers for such reflexes are probably located in the inferior and superior **colliculi**. The inferior colliculus sends fibers to the superior colliculus, which has connections to the relevant motor nuclei in the brain stem and spinal cord. Further, **integration** of auditory, visual, and somatosensory information takes place in the **superior colliculus**, so that the final motor response is appropriate for the organism as a whole.

THE AUDITORY CORTEX

The cortical auditory areas are less studied than the visual areas, and important aspects of human hearing are still poorly understood. While the auditory cortical areas are organized according to the same general principles as the other sensory areas, notable differences exist. Thus, the auditory system shows a more pronounced parallel organization than, for example, the visual system. This is particularly evident in the auditory pathways and intercalated nuclei but also concerns the cortical areas. Further, more information processing takes place at lower levels in the auditory than in other sensory systems. While the auditory cortex is not crucial for the ability to identify single sounds, it is required when different sounds must be put together into a meaningful whole.

Core and Belt Areas

The **primary auditory area** consists of several tonotopically organized subdivisions (in contrast to the striate area that consists of one retinotopically organized representation of visual field). We use the term **AI** for this auditory **core region,** which is situated on the upper face of the temporal lobe in a region called the **temporal plane** (Fig. 17.11). In humans, Brodmann's **area 41** is thought to correspond to area AI of monkeys and other animals. Several other auditory areas are arranged concentrically around AI (in the monkey about 15 such areas have been identified; cf. organization of extrastriatal visual areas). The areas closest to AI form a belt-like region and have therefore been termed the **auditory belt.** The belt region receives thalamocortical afferents from parts of the medial geniculate body other than the AI, while its main afferents come from the AI. Outside the auditory belt we find additional auditory areas that receive processed auditory information from the auditory belt but no afferents from the medial geniculate body. Here starts integration of auditory and other sensory modalities. These areas are probably located within area 22 of Brodmann (Fig. 17.11; see also Fig. 33.4). There appears to be several **parallel channels** from the core region to the belt region and further on to area 22 (similar to the organization of parallel pathways out of the striate area)—each conveying different aspects of auditory information. There are, however, numerous interconnections among areas, thus suggesting that the functional segregation cannot be absolute.

Subdivisions of the Primary Auditory Area

In monkeys, three areas in the superior temporal gyrus receive tonotopically organized projections from the ventral part of the medial geniculate body. One is the "classical" AI area; the two others adjoin AI rostrally (termed R and RT). We include them in the term AI because all three show structural features typical of primary sensory areas, such as a well-developed lamina 4 consisting of densely packed, small neurons (see Fig. 33.5) and dense afferent projections from a specific thalamic nucleus. The tonotopic arrangement in AI is such that the highest frequencies are represented caudally and the lowest rostrally, whereas the opposite arrangement appears to exist in area R.

Properties of Neurons in Primary Auditory Cortex

Fibers from the **medial geniculate body** end with precise tonotopic localization in the AI (Figs. 17.10 and 17.11).

Accordingly, single neurons in the AI respond to sounds with a narrower frequency range than neurons in other auditory areas (sharper tuning). Although many neurons in the AI depict **simple**, physical features of sounds (such as pitch and amplitude), others have surprisingly **complex** properties. While neurons at lower levels are as a rule specific to a certain frequency, cortical neurons are often sensitive to multiple, harmonically related frequencies. Furthermore, some neurons respond best to a sound when the frequency is increasing or decreasing. Other neurons are influenced from both ears but often such that they are excited by signals from one ear and inhibited from the other. Further, the response of many neurons (as in other primary visual areas) depends on the **context** of a stimulus. It even seems that the **object** with which a sound is associated modulates the activity of many AI neurons.

Asymmetrical Organization of the Auditory Cortex in the Temporal Plane

The auditory cortical areas appear to be asymmetrical in most humans. Thus, according to several MRI and postmortem studies the so-called **Heschl's gyrus**—containing the AI—is larger on the left than on the right side, and the same holds for **area 22** adjacent to the AI in the temporal plane (some studies did not find such asymmetries, however). Intrinsic (horizontal) connections in area 22 show a higher number of separate clusters of terminal fibers on the left than on the right side, which presumably enables a more fine-grained analysis. It has furthermore been reported that fibers in the white matter are more heavily myelinated in the left than in the right temporal plane, enabling faster processing. Such anatomic differences are compatible with evidence that the left auditory cortex has a higher degree of temporal sensitivity needed for optimal **speech** discrimination. The right auditory cortex appears to be better than the left in the discrimination of pitch, **melody**, and sound intensity.

Further Treatment Outside the Primary Auditory Cortex

As mentioned, the **auditory belt** receives its main afferents from the AI. The tonotopic localization is less sharp than in the AI. Many neurons appear to respond best to **species-specific sounds** (e.g., sounds of speech in humans). Other neurons seem to code the **localization** of a sound source, while others combine information about speech sounds and their source (wherefrom and from what). With regard to perception of voices and music, the analysis of **temporal patterns** is of particular importance.

The areas outside the AI show **functional specializations**. Thus, at least partly different subregions of the auditory belt deal with "**what**" (the frequency composition of the sounds) and "**where**" (the localization in space of the sound source). Functional MRI studies show, for example, that especially caudal parts of the auditory cortex are activated by moving sounds, while speech-relevant sounds primarily activate rostral parts.[4] Further, there is evidence from both experimental animals and humans that the further projections to the **frontal lobe** are divided into a **ventral** pathway for "what" and a **dorsal** pathway for "where" (Fig. 17.11). This seems to correspond to the organization of visual corticocortical connections into dorsal and ventral pathways or streams (see Fig. 16.24). Projections to the prefrontal cortex enable transformation of auditory information into actions. How far the subdivision of tasks between a ventral and a dorsal pathway goes is nevertheless not clear. Thus, many neurons in posterior parts of the auditory cortex, supposed to be specialized for spatial tasks, respond to various aspects of speech.

Damage to Central Parts of the Auditory System and Acoustic Agnosia

Restricted lesions of the auditory pathways or the auditory cortex—**central lesions**—usually produce no clear-cut symptoms. As mentioned, this is because the connections from the cochlear nuclei to the cerebral cortex are bilateral (although with a contralateral preponderance). Patients with bilateral damage of the auditory cortex are reported to be able to perceive sounds and even discriminate tones with different pitches and intensities (even though not necessarily with normal speed and precision). This corresponds to findings made in monkeys. The ability to recognize and interpret tones in particular patterns, however, is reduced or abolished. Such patients are unable to recognize familiar sounds such as laughter, a bell that tolls, sounds of various animals, and so forth. They are furthermore unable to understand the speech of other people, even though they can speak and read themselves. This is called **acoustic agnosia**.

Tinnitus—A Phantom in the Ear?

Tinnitus refers to a ringing or buzzing sensation in one or both ears in the absence of acoustic stimuli. It was formerly thought to result from signals coming from the cochlea, but this has not been confirmed. On the contrary, persistent tinnitus is usually associated with hearing loss, and interrupting the auditory nerve has not proved to be a cure. It seems likely that tinnitus can arise due to an unsuccessful adaptation in central auditory networks to loss of afferent input (loss of afferent input from hair cells have been shown to occur even if the hearing threshold remains normal). There is evidence from animal experiments that hearing loss is associated with central hyperexcitability—perhaps as an expression of **homeostatic plasticity**. If this plasticity for some reason goes awry, excitability changes might lead to spontaneous firing in auditory networks leading to perception of sounds. Indeed, tinnitus has been likened to phantom phenomena occurring after limb amputations.

---

4. Clinical observations in humans also support specializations among the auditory areas outside the AI. For example, in some patients after bilateral, partial lesions of the superior temporal gyrus, speech comprehension may be preserved while the perception of **prosody** (speech melody) and **music** may be impaired.

18 The Sense of Equilibrium

OVERVIEW

The sense of equilibrium, narrowly defined, depends on signals from sense organs that record the position and movements of the head. Such receptors are found in the **vestibular apparatus** in the inner ear. Together with the cochlea they form the **labyrinth**. As the cochlear duct, the vestibular labyrinth is filled with **endolymph.** The vestibular labyrinth consists of three **semicircular ducts** (canals) and two small expansions, the **saccule** and the **utricle. Cristae** equipped with hair cells are found in expansions of the ducts and respond to movements of the endolymph. Movements of the endolymph arise when the head rotates, and the hair cells thus signal **angular acceleration.** The semicircular ducts are oriented in three, mutually perpendicular planes. Hair cells in the saccule and utricle are found on flat surfaces called saccular and utricular **maculae.** The stereocilia of the hair cells are embedded in a gelatinous substance containing **otoliths.** These tiny stones ensure that the hair cells respond to gravitational forces and thus record the position of the head in space.

Afferents from the vestibular apparatus end in the **vestibular nuclei** in the upper medulla and lower pons. From there, signals flow in three main directions: to the **spinal cord,** to neuronal groups controlling **eye movements,** and to the **cerebellum.** These connections mainly control automatic responses aimed at maintaining the upright position (**postural reflexes**) and fixation of visual targets (**vestibulo-ocular reflexes**). In addition, vestibular signals reach several small areas in the **cerebral cortex.** Thereby, signals from vestibular receptors contribute to our conscious **awareness** of the position of the body in space.

The vestibular apparatus is not the only source of sensory information for maintaining equilibrium, however, and neither does it provide all necessary information. **Visual information** and signals from somatosensory receptors (**proprioceptors** and **cutaneous receptors**) also contribute. To control the upright, bipedal position of the human body, the brain needs information not only of the position of the head in space (provided by the vestibular receptors) but also of the head's position in relation to the body and the mutual positions of the major body parts. Distributed networks process all information needed for the motor system to issue proper commands to maintain balance and ensure the postural adjustments during goal-directed movements. Indeed, the experience of **dizziness** and disequilibrium can have many causes other than dysfunction of the vestibular apparatus. To analyze such problems one must take into account all factors that contribute to maintenance of our upright position.

Postural control and the role of vestibular signals in the control of eye movements are also discussed in Chapter 22 and Chapter 25, respectively.

STRUCTURE AND FUNCTION OF THE VESTIBULAR APPARATUS

The Vestibular Part of the Labyrinth

Unlike the cochlea, the vestibular apparatus does not depend on the external ear and the tympanic cavity to function. Like the cochlear duct with the organ of Corti, the **membranous labyrinth** containing the vestibular receptors is embedded in the temporal bone and surrounded by a space containing **perilymph** (Fig. 18.1; see also Fig. 17.1). The membranous labyrinth is filled with **endolymph.**

The vestibular part of the labyrinth consists of two small vesicles, the **utricle** and the **saccule**, and three circular tubes connected to the utricle, the **semicircular ducts** (see Fig. 17.1). Each of the semicircular ducts has a swelling, the **ampulla**, in the end close to the utriculus (Fig. 18.1). The ducts are oriented in three planes perpendicular to each other. In the erect position and with the head in a neutral position, the lateral semicircular duct lies approximately in the horizontal plane, whereas the posterior and the anterior ducts are oriented vertically (Fig. 18.1).

Figure 18.1

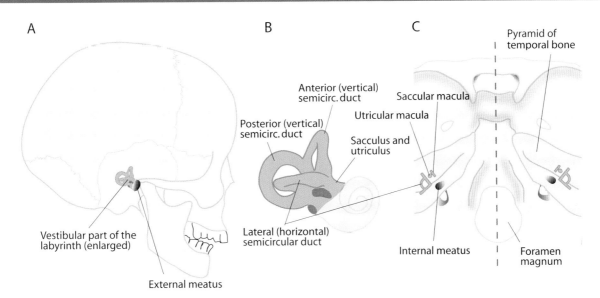

A

B

C

Pyramid of temporal bone

Anterior (vertical) semicirc. duct

Saccular macula

Posterior (vertical) semicirc. duct

Utricular macula

Sacculus and utriculus

Vestibular part of the labyrinth (enlarged)

Lateral (horizontal) semicircular duct

Internal meatus

Foramen magnum

External meatus

The vestibular apparatus. **A:** The position of the labyrinth in the temporal bone. **B:** The vestibular part of the labyrinth is colored more darkly than the auditory part. Note the orientation of the semicircular ducts in relation to the conventional planes of the body. **C:** The base of the skull, as viewed from above, with the vestibular apparatus projected to the surface of the pyramid of the temporal bone. Note the orientation of the saccular and utricular maculae.

Sensory epithelium with **hair cells** (Figs. 18.2 and 18.3) is found at five locations in the vestibular labyrinth. The hair cells are similar to those in the cochlea, except that they are equipped with a long **kinocilium** not present on cochlear hair cells (compare Figs. 18.6 and 17.8). In each of the ampullae of the semicircular ducts, there is a transversely oriented elevation, the ampullar **crista** (Fig. 18.2). Hair cells with long cilia (Fig. 18.4) are present between the

Figure 18.2

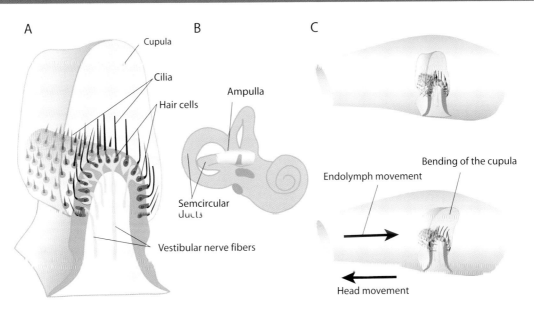

A

B

C

Cupula

Cilia

Hair cells

Ampulla

Semcircular ducts

Vestibular nerve fibers

Bending of the cupula

Endolymph movement

Head movement

The ampullar crista. **A:** Three-dimensional drawing showing the relationship between the crista, the hair cells, and the cupula. (Based on Wersäll 1956.) **B:** The labyrinth with the position of the crista in the horizontal semicircular duct. **C:** Movement of the endolymph deflects the cupula and the stereocilia of the hair cells. See text for further details.

Figure 18.3

A

UTRICULAR MACULA

Otolith membrane

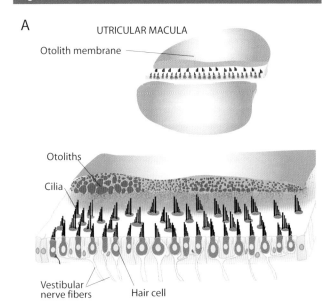

Otoliths

Cilia

Vestibular
nerve fibers   Hair cell

B

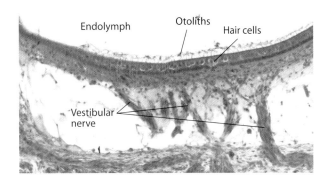

Endolymph   Otoliths   Hair cells

Vestibular
nerve

The utricular and saccular maculae. **A:** The utricular macula. Note the polarization of the hair cells. The otoliths are embedded in a gelatinous substance that covers the hair cells (otolith membrane). (Based on Lindeman 1973.) **B:** Photomicrograph of a section through the sacculus with the macula.

Figure 18.4

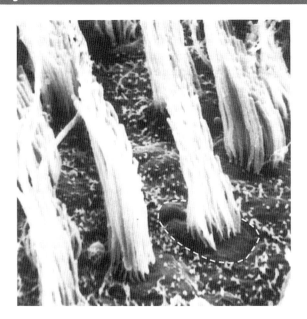

Sensory (hair) cells of the utricular macula. Scanning electron micrograph. The apical surface of one sensory cell is indicated. Magnification, ×10,000. Compare with Fig. 9.2B. (Courtesy of Dr. H. Lindeman, Oslo University Hospital, Oslo, Norway.)

Figure 18.5

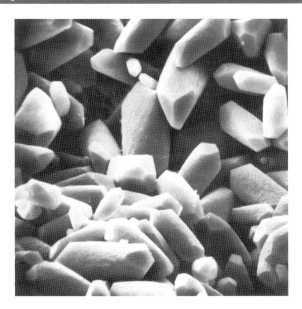

Otoliths from the utricular macula. Scanning electron micrograph. Magnification, ×2,100. (Courtesy of Dr. H. Lindeman, Oslo University Hospital, Oslo, Norway.)

epithelial cells that form the crista. The cilia project into a jellylike mass, the **cupula**. In the utricle and the saccule there are small patches of hair cells like those in the ampullae, the utricular and saccular **maculae** (Figs. 18.3 and 9.5). The macular hair cells are also covered by a jellylike mass, which is special because of its content of small "stones," the **otoliths** (Figs. 18.3 and 18.5). The otoliths are crystals of calcium salts. The utricular macula lies in approximately the same plane as the lateral semicircular duct (i.e., horizontally in the neutral position), whereas the saccular macula is oriented almost vertically (Fig. 18.1C).

More about Vestibular Hair Cells

The vestibular and cochlear hair cells have the same basic properties (see Chapter 17, under "The Inner Hair Cells and Mechanoelectric Transduction"), although there are some structural differences. On the apical end of the cells there are 50 to 110 **stereocilia** and one longer and thicker **kinocilium** (Fig. 18.6). The stereocilia are unusually long microvilli and contain actin filaments like other microvilli. The kinocilium contains microtubuli (like cilia of the respiratory epithelial cells). The stereocilia are arranged regularly in accordance with their height (Figs. 18.3, 18.4, and 18.6). This structural **polarization** of the receptor cells corresponds with a functional polarization. Thus, bending of the stereocilia toward the kinocilium increases the firing frequency of the sensory fibers in contact with the cell, whereas bending in the opposite direction reduces the firing frequency. This is because the receptor cell is depolarized or hyperpolarized by bending of the cilia. The receptor potentials of the hair cells induce release of **glutamate**, which depolarizes the afferent nerve fibers. Deflection of the cilia perpendicular to the direction of the polarization produces no response, whereas oblique displacements give a reduced response compared with a stimulus that is properly aligned with the polarization. This means that a given **firing frequency** of an afferent fiber is **ambiguous**; it can be caused by a weak stimulus in the direction of the polarization or a stronger obliquely oriented one. Further, a given firing frequency may be caused by moving the head forward (e.g., walking) or tilting the head backward. This may be why the hair cells in the maculae are arranged differently with regard to the orientation of the polarization axes, so that all the cells together cover 360 degrees (Fig. 18.6B). This ensures that the information received by the brain about head position in space is unambiguous. This requires, of course, that the brain is able to compare the magnitude of the signals from various parts of the maculae to reach a conclusion.

The Adequate Stimulus for the Semicircular Ducts Is Rotation of the Head

Flow of the fluid (the endolymph) inside the semicircular ducts displaces the cupula, thereby bending the cilia (Fig. 18.2). This activates or inhibits the sensory cells, depending on the direction of bending. Rotational movements of the head produce flow of the endolymph in the semicircular ducts. This is explained by the inertia of the fluid: when the head starts to rotate, the fluid "lags behind," and when the rotation stops, the fluid continues to flow for a moment (like the water in a bowl that is rotated rapidly for a couple of turns). If the head rotation continues at even velocity, the fluid and the head will after a short time move with the same speed and in the same direction, which means that the cilia are not bent. Thus, it is clear that not every rotational movement is recorded by the receptors of the semicircular ducts: alteration of the velocity of the rotational movement—that is, positive or negative **angular acceleration**—is the adequate stimulus for the semicircular duct receptors. Thus, these receptors have **dynamic sensitivity**. Linear acceleration does not affect (or affects only slightly) the semicircular ducts. By linear displacement of the head—a **translatory** movement—without concomitant rotation, there is no stimulation of the semicircular duct receptors. An example of linear acceleration is a car that starts or brakes on a flat, straight road. If the road goes up and down and is curved, rotational accelerations of the car (and the heads of its passengers) are superimposed on the linear ones.

The orientation of the semicircular ducts ensures that rotation of the head in any conceivable direction produces change of activity of the receptors in one or more of the ducts. The brain monitors the rotational movements of the head by reading the pattern of activity produced by all the receptors. The semicircular ducts of both sides must

Figure 18.6

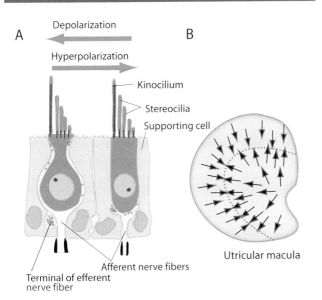

Sensory cells of the vestibular apparatus. **A:** Two types of hair cells with different shapes and relations to the afferent nerves. Note the polarization of the cilia. **B:** The utricular macula, as viewed from above. Arrows indicate the direction of polarization of the sensory cells in the various parts, which altogether cover all directions of deflection of the sensory hairs.

function normally to supply the brain with the necessary information. A pair of ducts (e.g., the right and left lateral ones) gives **complementary signals** to a given rotation—that is, increased signal frequency from the one and reduced from the other.

Sacculus and Utriculus Signal the Position of the Head and Linear Acceleration

The small **otoliths** have higher specific weight than the endolymph and the substance in which they are embedded and are therefore more influenced by gravitational forces. Taking as an example the utricular macula, which in the neutral head position is oriented horizontally (Fig. 18.1), a change of head position tilts the macula, and the otoliths pull the cilia in that direction. Different angles of tilt produce different patterns of activity of the macular hair cells. Due to their different orientations in space, the utricular and saccular hair cells together provide information about all possible head positions. The **utricle** records especially **lateral tilt** (i.e., head positions that vary around a sagittal axis), whereas the **saccule** probably records mainly flexion—extension of the head (i.e., movement in the cervical joints around a transverse axis). Its ability to provide information about the position of the head at any one time (in the absence of movement) shows that the vestibular apparatus has **static sensitivity**. This property depends on the presence of receptors that adapt slowly or not at all, so that they give a constant signal as long as a certain position is maintained. The static sensitivity of the vestibular apparatus depends, as we have seen, on the force of gravity and disappears in a state of weightlessness (such as in space travel). Because the static sensitivity is a property of the utricle and the saccule, these parts of the vestibular apparatus are called the **static labyrinth**. We will see, however, that this part of the labyrinth also has dynamic properties.

The **dynamic sensitivity** of the utricle and the saccule is seen when their activity is recorded during **linear acceleration**. The response increases (i.e., the firing frequency of the afferent fibers) with increasing acceleration. This is again explained by the inertia of the otoliths. On linear displacement of the head with changing velocity, as in a car that is accelerating, the otoliths lag behind and thereby bend the cilia backward (in relation to the direction of the movement). The opposite happens when the car slows down; the otoliths continue to move for a moment and bend the cilia forward (cf. the forces acting on a loose object in a car when the car speeds up or slows down).

Two Channels from the Vestibular Apparatus to the Brain

Recordings from vestibular ganglion cells have identified two kinds of responses. One kind of ganglion cell, conducting from hair cells in the central parts of the cristae and maculae, fire with an irregular pattern. Furthermore, such ganglion cells have **phasic** properties (responding preferentially to fast and brief head movements) and high conduction velocity. The other kind, leading from hair cells in the periphery of the sensory epithelium, fire action potentials regularly, conduct slowly, and are especially sensitive **to slow movements** (static properties). There are also two kinds of vestibular receptor cells, which are found both in the cristae of the semicircular ducts and in the maculae of the saccule and utricle (Fig. 18.6A). One kind, the **type 1** cell, is bottle-shaped, whereas the **type 2** cell is slender. The sensory fibers (the peripheral process of the vestibular ganglion cells) end differently on the two cell types (Fig. 18.6A). The sensory fibers from the ganglion cells end differently on the two kinds: the type 1 cells are almost encapsulated by a large terminal, forming a calix, whereas the type 2 hair cells are contacted by several, small nerve endings. It is therefore reasonable to assume that the phasic ganglion cells lead from the type 1 hair cells, and the type 2 hair cells lead from the other (static) kind of ganglion cell. Such a relationship is at least not absolute, however, since type 1 and 2 hair cells are present both centrally and peripherally in the sensory epithelium.

The **functional** significance of two different channels from the vestibular apparatus to the brain may be that one channel serves to provide a quick and forceful response to fast body movements (great danger of imbalance), while the other channel provides precise information during slow movements.

THE VESTIBULAR NUCLEI AND THEIR CONNECTIONS

The vestibular system differs from other systems in its high degree of **multisensory integration**. Thus, signals from the semicircular ducts and from the saccular and utricular maculae—that is, information about movements and head positions—converge in the vestibular nuclei and in the cerebellum. Further, integration of visual, proprioceptive, and vestibular signals occurs at all levels—from the first synapses of the primary afferent fibers in the brain stem to the cerebral cortex. This is obviously necessary because the vestibular signals are of little behavioral value on their own. The position and movements of the head must continuously be related to the positions and movements of the eyes and of the body. Accordingly, vestibular stimulation does not evoke a conscious "vestibular"

Figure 18.7

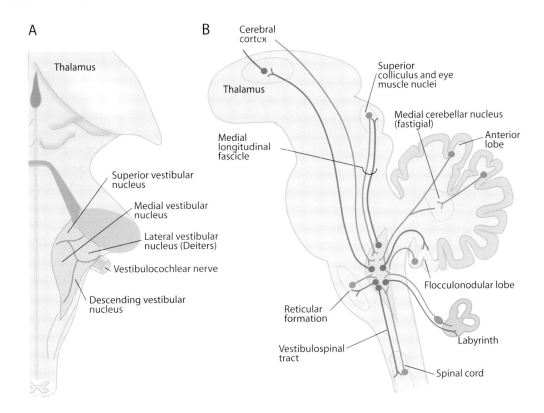

The vestibular nuclei. **A:** Location of the nuclei in a dorsal view of the brain stem. **B:** The main afferent and efferent connections. Note reciprocal connections with the spinal cord, the cerebellum, the reticular formation, and the nuclei of the extraocular muscles and other visually related nuclei of the mesencephalon. Note also ascending connections to the thalamus (and from there to the cerebral cortex) and descending connections from the cerebral cortex to the vestibular nuclei.

sensation that can be easily distinguished from other sensory modalities.

The Vestibular Nuclei and Primary Afferent Fibers

The primary afferent fibers of the eight cranial nerve end in various parts of the **vestibular nuclei**.[1] The collection of large and small vestibular nuclei is collectively called the **vestibular complex**. It covers a large area in the floor of the fourth ventricle and consists of four large nuclei and several small cell groups. (Not all cell groups within the vestibular complex receive primary vestibular fibers, however, and are therefore not vestibular, strictly speaking.) Figure 18.7A shows the location of the four major nuclei: the **superior**, the **lateral** (or nucleus of Deiters), the **medial**, and the **descending** (or inferior).

Primary afferent vestibular fibers divide into an ascending and a descending branch when entering the brain stem. Together, they end in large parts of the vestibular complex and in parts of the cerebellum (see Fig. 24.4). Although terminations of fibers from the ampullar cristae and the maculae overlap in the vestibular nuclei, they also show notable differences in distribution. Thus, afferents from the **cristae** (i.e., from the semicircular ducts) end in the **superior nucleus** and the rostral part of the **medial nucleus** but not in the lateral nucleus, whereas the fibers from the **utricular and saccular maculae** end in the **lateral nucleus** but not (or only sparsely) in the superior nucleus. In agreement with the distribution of primary afferents, neurons in the superior

---

1. There are also **efferent cholinergic fibers** in the vestibular nerve, ending in contact with the vestibular receptors (Fig. 18.6A). The efferent fibers come from a small cell group in the lower pons just lateral to the abducens nucleus. The projection is bilateral and ends diffusely. Rotational head movements evoke efferent activity, with mainly excitatory effects on the vestibular primary afferents. Although its functional role is still unknown, one possibility is that the efferent innervation increases regularity of afferent firing.

nucleus respond best to rotational head movements (angular acceleration), whereas the cells in the lateral nucleus are particularly sensitive to static head position. Nevertheless, physiologic studies show that a substantial proportion of neurons in the vestibular nuclei integrate information about angular acceleration and static position/linear acceleration.[2]

The Vestibular Nuclei Receive Afferents from Regions Other than the Labyrinth

The physiologic properties of neurons in the vestibular nuclei are not copies of those of the primary afferent fibers. This is due to convergence on the cells of various kinds of afferents (such as fibers from the semicircular ducts and the utricle) and by interconnections between the nuclei (e.g., commissural fibers linking the two sides). Further, the vestibular complex receives afferents from other parts of the central nervous system (CNS), especially the **spinal cord,** the **reticular formation,** certain mesencephalic nuclei, and the **cerebellum.** Afferents from the mesencephalon arise, for example, in the **superior colliculus,** and the cerebellar fibers come from both the flocculonodular lobe and the anterior lobe (Fig. 18.7B; see also Fig. 24.4) and contribute to adaptation of vestibular reflexes to changed conditions, for example during growth of the head, wearing of glasses, and learning of new movements.

The vestibular nuclei receive signals from the **cerebral cortex** (mainly indirectly via the reticular formation but also through some direct fibers). The **corticovestibular** fibers arise in parts of the cortex, such as the primary somatosensory cortex (**SI**; areas 2 and 3a) and the **insula,** which receive converging information from the labyrinth and proprioceptors. The vestibular nuclei are also influenced from the **posterior parietal cortex,** which is concerned with spatial orientation and goal-directed movements. Presumably, these cortical regions are important for building internal representations of the position and movements of the body, necessary for the control of movements. Accordingly, physiologic experiments show that **vestibular reflexes—** the **vestibulospinal** ones in particular—are modulated in conjunction with voluntary movements. In this way, the reflex responses are subordinated to the overall plan for the

movements, presumably by way of corticovestibular connections (among others).

Efferent Connections of the Vestibular Nuclei

Schematically, the vestibular nuclei (and therefore also the vestibular receptors) act on three main regions (Figs. 18.7B and 18.8), namely **motoneurons** in the **spinal cord,** motoneurons in the **nuclei of the extraocular muscles,** and the **cerebellum.** Accordingly, information from the vestibular apparatus is used primarily to influence muscles that maintain our **upright position** (equilibrium) and muscles that produce **eye movements.** The latter movements ensure that the retinal image is kept stationary when the head moves.

Most of the fibers to the **spinal cord** come from the **lateral vestibular nucleus** and form the **lateral vestibulospinal tract.** The fibers descend in the ventral funiculus on the same side as the nuclei from which they come. In the ventral horn they end—in part monosynaptically—on alpha (α) and gamma (γ) **motoneurons** (Fig. 18.8A). The tract is somatotopically organized, so that various body parts can be selectively controlled. The vestibulospinal tract has strong effects on the muscles that contribute to equilibrium and posture (see also Chapter 22, under "Vestibulospinal Tracts"). As mentioned, the lateral nucleus receives afferents from the utricular macula; these provide information about the static position of the head in space and thereby indirectly about the position of the body. Change of body position also changes its center of gravity, with a resulting need to adjust muscle tone to maintain equilibrium.

A smaller, **medial vestibulospinal tract** arises in the medial vestibular nucleus. It also descends in the ventral funiculus and acts on motoneurons. The fibers do not reach below the upper thoracic segments, however, and are thought to be of importance primarily for **head movements** elicited by the vestibular receptors.

Fibers to the **nuclei of the extraocular muscles** arise mainly in the **superior** and **medial nuclei,** which receive many primary afferent fibers from the semicircular ducts (Fig. 18.8B). The fibers leave the nuclei medially and join to form a distinct fiber bundle, the **medial longitudinal fasciculus,** which is located close to the midline below the floor of the fourth ventricle (Figs. 18.7 and 18.8; see also Fig. 6.18). Some of the fibers cross to the other side as they ascend. They end in the abducent, the trochlear, and the oculomotor nuclei and are precisely organized. In addition to the direct connections in the medial longitudinal

---

2. For example, a study in the cat with electric stimulation of separate divisions of the vestibular nerve found that about one-third of all neurons received convergent inputs from the vertical semicircular canal and sacculus/utriculus. Another one-third received convergent input from sacculus and utriculus and one-fifth from the horizontal canal and sacculus/utriculus.

Figure 18.8

A

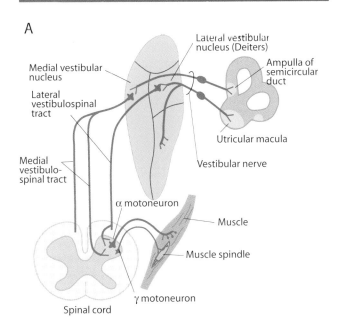

B

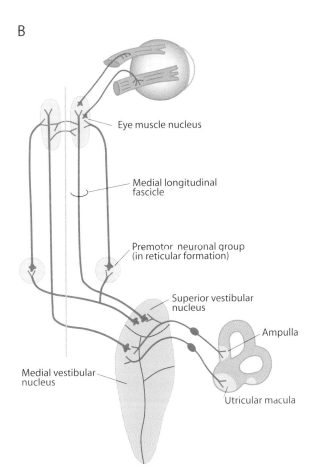

Main features of vestibular connections. **A:** Descending connections acting on α and γ motoneurons in the spinal cord. The medial vestibulospinal tract reach only cervical levels. **B:** Ascending connections controlling eye movements.

fasciculus, there are **indirect pathways** from the vestibular nuclei to the eye muscle nuclei via the **reticular formation** (Fig. 18.8B). We return to this later when discussing vestibular reflexes.

Vestibulocerebellar fibers (arising in the medial and descending vestibular nuclei) end primarily in the **vestibulocerebellum** (Fig. 18.7; see also Fig. 24.4). Fibers from the vestibulocerebellum to the vestibular nuclei can adjust the gain (sensitivity) of the **vestibulo-ocular reflex**, as discussed next (see also Fig. 25.4).

Connections to the **thalamus** from the vestibular nuclei have been demonstrated anatomically and end in the ventral posterolateral nucleus and nearby nuclei. Physiologically, scattered neurons in a fairly large region respond to signals from the vestibular apparatus. This probably explains why vestibular signals reach several discrete regions of the cerebral cortex.

VESTIBULAR REFLEXES: CONTROL OF EYE MOVEMENTS AND BODILY POSTURE

The special problems encountered in space journeys aroused great interest in the mechanisms that underlie vestibular reflexes. As with other parts of the brain that are comprehensively investigated, conditions turn out to be more complex than initially thought. Here we discuss only a few salient points. There are two kinds of reflexes that are elicited from the vestibular apparatus: **vestibulo-ocular reflexes** that control eye movements and so-called **labyrinthine reflexes** mediated by the vestibulospinal tracts controlling bodily postures (especially the upright position). Among these reflexes is the **vestibulocollic reflex,** mediated by the medial vestibulospinal tract. The reflex serves to stabilize the position of the head in space, but its functional role is less well understood than that of the vestibulo-ocular reflex, which stabilizes the eyes during head movements.

In general, signals from the utricle and the saccule elicit **tonic** reflex effects, whereas **phasic** reflex responses are caused by signals from the semicircular ducts when the stimulus is rotation of the head (angular acceleration) and from the utricle or saccule when the stimulus is linear acceleration. Because the vestibular receptors inform only about the head, other receptors must inform about the movements and positions of other bodily parts. To control our upright position, the brain must integrate these various sources of information and issue commands that are appropriate for the whole body. Therefore, the labyrinthine reflexes must operate in concert with other postural reflexes; we discuss these together next.

Vestibulo-Ocular Reflexes

There are several vestibulo-ocular reflexes, mediated by reflex arcs of various complexities. This topic is also discussed in Chapter 25 dealing with the control of eye movements. In general, the vestibule-ocular reflexes ensure that the **image is kept stationary** on the retina when the head moves (rotates).

The simplest vestibulo-ocular reflex is mediated by a chain of three neurons (Fig. 18.8; see also Fig. 25.5):

1. Primary afferent fibers from the cristae of the semicircular ducts

2. Neurons in the vestibular nuclei that send their axons to the nuclei of the extraocular muscles (passing in the medial longitudinal fasciculus)

3. Motoneurons in these nuclei, which send their axons to the extraocular muscles

In addition, there are other pathways from the vestibular nuclei to the nuclei of the extraocular muscles that are synaptically interrupted in the reticular formation and some other brain stem nuclei (Fig. 18.8B).

A movement of the head in any direction is accompanied by a **compensatory movement** of the eyes in the opposite direction and with the same velocity as the head movement. Rotation of the head produces movement of the endolymph inside the semicircular ducts. Taking a rotation in the horizontal plane (turning the head from one side to the other) as an example, mainly the lateral semicircular duct records the movement and elicits a compensatory eye movement in the horizontal plane.

When the head movement is relatively small, the eyes move with exactly the same velocity as and in the opposite direction of the head, and the image is kept in the same position on the retina all the time. When the head movement becomes pronounced enough that it becomes impossible to keep the image stationary even with maximal excursion of the eyes, a fast, or **saccadic**, movement occurs in the same direction as the head movement. Then the gaze is fixed again on the object, and another slow movement follows (as long as the head continues to move in the same direction). Such an alternation between slow and fast saccadic eye movements is called **nystagmus**. In this case, the nystagmus is produced by stimulation of the

semicircular ducts (rotation of the head) and is therefore called **vestibular nystagmus**. Movement of the surroundings can also elicit nystagmus when the head is stationary. This **optokinetic nystagmus** occurs, for example, when a train-passenger watches the landscape pass by (nystagmus is discussed also in Chapter 24, under "Cerebellar Lesions and Eye Movements," and in Chapter 25, under "Kinds of Eye Movement").

Vestibular Signals Must Be Integrated with Other Sensory Modalities for Control of Eye Movements

As mentioned, the vestibular nuclei receive afferents from sources other than the labyrinth, such as nuclei in the mesencephalon, the reticular formation, and the cerebellum. Some of these sources mediate visual information that can modify the vestibular reflex responses. This convergence of various inputs seems logical. Thus, to achieve optimal control of the eye movements, the responsible neural cell groups must receive and integrate vestibular information about movements of the head, visual signals about movements of the image on the retina, and proprioceptive signals about movements of the eyes relative to the head.

Vestibular Stimulation Produces Nystagmus and Falling Tendency

When an upright person rotates fairly rapidly a few times around his or her axis and then stops, the eyes can be seen to move rapidly one way (saccade) and slowly the other for some seconds afterward. Obviously, the rotation has induced **nystagmus**. By using special instruments, we can see that nystagmus is also present at the start of the rotation but in the opposite direction of that after the rotation has stopped. When the person rotates to the right, the saccade movement is to the right and the slow movement is to the left, as if the person fixes his or her gaze on a stationary point and then moves the eyes rapidly when this point is slipping out of the visual field. The eyes then move to a new fixation point, and the same sequence of events is repeated. This **postrotatory nystagmus** is caused by stimulation of the receptors in the semicircular ducts. As mentioned, at the start of the movement the inertia of the endolymph makes it lag behind, thereby bending the cilia of the receptor cells, whereas the endolymph continues to flow for a moment after the rotation has stopped. The person who had just stopped rotating feels as if he or she were still rotating but now in the opposite direction. The direction of the nystagmus corresponds to the **illusion** of such a rotation—that is, with the saccade phase to the left after a rotation to the right. If the rotation of the body continues for some time, the nystagmus disappears and the person gets dizzy (cf. ballet dancers who deliberately ensure that the head does not move with even velocity during pirouettes; this way they have sufficient time for fixation so that the brain gets information to determine the orientation of the body in space).

After stopping the rotation, the person is also unsteady and tends to fall to one side, especially if asked to keep his or her eyes closed. Further, the arm deviates to the right if the person is asked to point straight ahead (with eyes closed). This is called **postrotational past pointing**. After the rotation stops, the illusion of the opposite movement (i.e., the person feels he or she is turning to the left) causes the past pointing to the right: the person feels that the room is moving to the right.

The postrotational effects on postural muscles are mediated via the **vestibulospinal tracts** (Fig. 18.8A) and show that the receptors of the semicircular ducts also influence the spinal cord and the postural muscles, not just the cranial nerve nuclei and the extraocular muscles.

Nystagmus, falling tendency, and past pointing can also be produced by irrigation of the external auditory meatus with hot or cold water. The change of temperature makes the endolymph flow in the semicircular ducts and thus produces stimulation of the receptors. Such a **caloric test** is used clinically to examine the function of the vestibular labyrinth and the conduction of signals to the brain stem.

Various **diseases** affecting the vestibular receptors or the signal pathways to the motoneurons of the extraocular muscles (the vestibular nerve, the vestibular nuclei, the medial longitudinal fasciculus, and the cerebellum) can produce nystagmus in the absence of vestibular or visual stimulation. This is called **spontaneous nystagmus**. In certain cases, the nystagmus may be present only in certain positions of the head (**positional nystagmus**).

Neck and Labyrinthine Reflexes

The vestibular receptors inform about the position and movements of the head in space, whereas neck proprioceptors can inform about the position and movements of the body in relation to the head. Based on information from both kinds of receptors, the brain can decide whether the head is moving in isolation or whether it moves together with the rest of the body. Obviously, different kinds of postural responses are needed in these two situations. The **labyrinthine reflexes** are elicited by stimulation of the sensory receptors of the **semicircular ducts** and the **utricle** of the labyrinth. In the **neck reflexes**, the response is a change of muscle tension, especially in the extremities supporting upright stance, induced by a change in the position of the head relative to the body (such movements take place primarily in the upper cervical joints). The labyrinthine reflexes, when operating alone, produce muscle contractions in the trunk and extremities that serve to keep the position of the head constant. The neck reflexes, as mentioned, serve to keep the position of the body constant in relation to the head. The latter is a prerequisite for the labyrinthine reflexes

to function properly; the vestibular apparatus can provide information only about the position of the head in space and not about its position in relation to the body. Thus, the labyrinthine reflexes work on the assumption that the head has a constant position relative to the body, and the neck reflexes ensure that this position is constant.

The reflexes may be either **tonic** or **phasic**. A phasic neck or labyrinthine reflex consists of a rapid, transient change of muscle tension in postural muscles as a response to a change of posture (usually a disturbance of the equilibrium). We experience phasic labyrinthine reflexes when we trip over something, and a coordinated set of compensatory movements occurs before we consciously perceive what is going on. In a tonic reflex, the change of muscle tension lasts as long as the new position is maintained.

Vestibulospinal tracts are the most likely candidates for mediation of the labyrinthine reflexes. The **reflex center** of the neck reflexes is located in the medulla, and the effects on the motoneurons are most likely mediated by both the **reticulospinal** and vestibulospinal tracts.

More about the Neck and Labyrinthine Reflexes

Studies of **decerebrate**, four-legged animals have elucidated the neck and labyrinthine reflexes (the brain stem is transected just below the red nucleus in the mesencephalon). To demonstrate clearly the **neck reflexes** in decerebrate animals (mostly cats have been studied), the vestibular receptors must have been eliminated. Then, when the head is bent backward (extension of the neck), the muscle tension is increased in the extensor muscles of the forelimbs and decreased in the extensors of the hind limbs. Forward bending of the head (flexion) induces the opposite pattern of changes (extension of the hind limbs and flexion of the forelimbs). Tilting the head sideways increases the extensor tone on the same side and reduces it on the other side, as does turning the head sideways. These changes of the muscle tone aim at reestablishing the position of the body relative to the head. The receptors for these reflexes are located near the upper cervical joints, because they disappear after transection of the upper three cervical dorsal roots. **Muscle spindles** are the most likely candidates, but joint receptors may also contribute. As mentioned, the functional role of the neck reflexes cannot be understood when observed in isolation, however. Only in conjunction with the labyrinthine reflexes are their effects appropriate for the whole body.

To demonstrate clearly the **labyrinthine reflexes**, the neck reflexes must have been eliminated by cutting the upper dorsal roots (in a decerebrate animal). It then appears that the effects produced by the labyrinthine reflexes are the opposite of those of the neck reflexes when the latter act alone. Thus, bending the head backward elicits flexion of the forelimbs and extension of the hind limbs and vice versa when the head is bent forward. The purpose of these changes of muscle tone is to bring the head back to the position held before the movement—that is, to keep the position of the head in space constant. Provided the neck reflexes ensure that the body stays in a constant position relative to the head, the labyrinthine reflexes will serve to maintain both the position of the head in space and the upright position of the whole body. The labyrinthine reflexes are shown clearly when the experimental animal stands on a platform that can be tilted in various directions. Tilting the platform forward increases the extensor tone in the forelimbs and decreases the tone in the hind limbs. Tilting the platform sideways increases the muscle tone in the extensors on the side to which the tilt is directed. Both responses are obviously appropriate for the maintenance of body balance. When the platform is moved quickly in one direction and then back, the reflex response is transient (**phasic reflex**). When the platform is maintained in the new position, the altered muscle tone is upheld (**tonic reflex**).

When **both reflexes work together** in an intact organism, backward bending of the head, for example (with movement taking place only in the upper cervical joints and no change of body position), produces no change in muscle tension of the extremities. The tendency of the labyrinthine reflexes to produce forelimb flexion and hind limb extension is canceled by the opposite tendency of the neck reflexes. In contrast, when the same movement of the head is produced by a backward movement of the whole body (with no movement of the head relative to the body, such as a horse that is rearing), the labyrinthine reflexes act alone to produce extension of the hind limbs and flexion of the forelimbs. Another example is an animal standing on a platform tilting forward with no movement of the head relative to the body. In that case, the labyrinthine reflexes produce forelimb extension and hind limb flexion. This is an appropriate response to maintain balance when standing on a downhill slope. However, if the position of the head in space is kept constant and the body is moved in relation to the head, the neck reflexes act alone. An example is a cat jumping down from a table: the neck is extended (keeping the head position constant), producing extension of the forelimbs, which is appropriate for landing.

Postural Reflexes: Various Receptors Contribute

In order to control posture and balance, the CNS must receive sufficient information about positions and movements in various body parts as well as the nature of the support surface. This information enables the brain to compute the position of the center of gravity and the movements needed to keep it in the right position relative to the supporting base. All sense organs providing information about the position and movements of the body may contribute. This concerns proprioceptors, cutaneous receptors, the vestibular apparatus, and vision, all representing independent information channels. The signals are analyzed in the CNS, which in response initiates **postural reflexes**, that is, automatic, coordinated contractions of muscles that maintain our upright position. Postural reflexes can thus be elicited from the vestibular apparatus (labyrinthine reflexes), from proprioceptors (neck reflexes, stretch reflexes), from

cutaneous receptors (notably in the sole of the foot), and by moving visual stimuli.

The contribution of various receptors to control of the upright position is not static, however, but varies with the kind and magnitude of a postural perturbation and not the least its context.[3] Even if the total information delivered through all the sensory channels is often more than needed, some of it may be unreliable in a particular situation. In general, it seems that if one source is unreliable, its contribution tends to be ignored, and information from other sources becomes more important. Therefore, the relevant brain networks must be able to select which ones to "listen to" among the various information channels. For example, somatosensory information from the sole of the foot is less reliable when the support surface is slippery than when it is firm and even. Further, proprioceptive information eliciting a reflex contraction of a muscle may in one situation help maintain balance while in another situation cause imbalance. Visual information may be unreliable if we are in an environment with moving objects, because it may be difficult to distinguish own movements from those of the surroundings. Persons with loss of vestibular function manage well as long as they can see, but they have serious problems in maintaining the body's equilibrium in the dark. We also treat postural reflexes in Chapter 22 in conjunction with the control of automatic movements.

More about Receptor Types and Their Contribution to Postural Control

Persons standing on a platform that can be tilted or moved forward or backward have often been used in studies of postural control. In this situation, the experimenter can control the direction, speed, and amplitude of perturbations, and specific kinds of sensory information can be removed temporarily. In addition, patients with loss of one or the other kind of receptor have been studied extensively.

Signals from **muscle spindles**—providing rapid information about joint position and movements—are important for postural control. This is, for example, evident from persons who lose the proprioceptive sense (cf. Chapter 13, under "Clinical Examples of Loss of Somatosensory Information"). Further evidence that muscle spindles play a role for posture comes from experiments with **vibration** (activating Ia afferents) of leg muscles and neck muscles. Such vibration elicits postural adjustments, which are appropriate, considering that the brain

---

3. There furthermore seems to be **individual variation** among normal subjects with regard to which kind of information they rely on for the reflex adjustments in quiet standing. In a study of healthy volunteers, only half of the subjects increased their body sway when their eyes were closed. This suggests that persons differ with regard to how much they rely on visual information to stabilize the quiet standing position.

"believes" that the muscles are being stretched. The signals are obviously interpreted as if the center of gravity were moving. In this case, the muscle spindle information is not primarily used at the segmental level for quick postural responses but is integrated with other inputs at higher levels. Platform experiments further support that the contribution of muscle spindles to postural control does not depend mainly on simple, **spinal reflexes** (i.e., reflex contractions in response to muscle stretch that do not depend on higher levels). When the platform is suddenly displaced backward (without tilting), the body first sways forward with movement primarily at the ankle joints. The balance is regained mainly because the calf muscles at the back of the leg contract (muscles of the hip, the back, and the neck also contribute, especially if the displacement is large). The first part of the contraction of the leg muscles occurs so early after the perturbation that a reflex must mediate it. (Somewhat later there is also a voluntary contraction, which contributes to the final outcome of the postural adjustment.) In this case, a reflex elicited by stretch of muscle spindles in the calf muscles would seem appropriate. In another situation, however, such a reflex would worsen the balance: if the platform is suddenly tilted backward, the calf muscles are stretched (as in the former example), but the center of gravity is now displaced backward instead of forward. Consequently, a contraction of the calf muscles would worsen the imbalance. To regain balance, the muscles at the front of the leg must contract as rapidly as possible, in spite of being shortened by the tilting of the platform. Thus, whether a segmental, spinal reflex is elicited depends on the situation, and inappropriate reflex responses to stretch are generally suppressed. Indeed, for the functionally important reflex response in the leg muscles (starting about 90 msec after the balance perturbation), signals from proprioceptors around the **vertebral column** may be more important than signals from leg muscle spindles. Thus, the contraction of the leg muscles correlates less with their own length change than with the displacement of the trunk.

Signals from **cutaneous** low-threshold mechanoreceptors in the **sole of the foot** seem to contribute to the reflex contractions of the leg muscles in platform experiments. The dorsal column–medial lemniscus pathway transmits such signals very rapidly. Presumably, the brain determines the center of pressure by calculating the difference between the pressure applied to the heel and the forefoot. The center of pressure informs about the position of the body center of mass. Patients with **neuropathies** who have reduced sensibility in the sole of the foot witness the importance of this input for postural control and for normal gait.

Vision also contributes to adjustment of muscle tone with the purpose of maintaining body equilibrium. Platform experiments indicate that the muscle contractions in response to a movement of the platform depend on whether the subject can see that the body moves in relation to the surroundings. If the experimental setup is such that it appears as though the surroundings do not move (i.e., they are made to move in the same direction as the head), the earliest reflex contractions of the legs are weaker than when the sense of vision also informs about the movement. We do not fully know the pathways involved, but the final commands are probably sent from the vestibular nuclei in the vestibulospinal tract.

In platform experiments with moderate postural perturbations, signals from **vestibular receptors** seem not to be essential for the corrective contractions of leg muscles (ankle strategy).

With larger perturbations, however, vestibular information contributes to contractions of hip muscles (hip strategy). When visual information is eliminated, signals from the utricle and the saccule are indeed necessary for the proper orientation of the body in space, as can be shown in animals whose otoliths have been removed. An **unexpected fall** from some height elicits a postural reflex that depends on information from the vestibular apparatus. The fall initiates a contraction of the muscles of the leg as an appropriate preparation to the landing. The contraction begins about 75 msec after the start of the fall and can therefore occur before landing (and thus before a stretch reflex can be elicited). The latency is also too short for the contraction to be voluntary. Animal experiments indicate that the receptors of this reflex are located in the labyrinth (probably in the saccular macula).

Goal-Directed Movements Require Central Control of Postural Reflexes

Reflex responses occur too early after a balance perturbation to be caused by conscious decisions. Indeed, the main advantage of a reflex response is that it occurs so rapidly. Nevertheless, even automatic movements are subject to central control. The response to a perturbation challenging our upright position is strongly modulated by expectation and the context in which the perturbation occurs. In general, the individual reflex responses are subordinate to an overall, coordinated motor plan designed to attain a certain goal. For example, if the shoulder is not kept stable, precise movements of the hand are impossible, and if the trunk is not stabilized, control of the shoulder is impossible. The sensitivity of the reflex centers is continuously up- or down- regulated, so that the reflex responses are appropriate for the goals of the whole organism.

In **infants**, comprehensive, high-level motor programs have not yet developed and, accordingly, some postural reflexes operate "on their own." This concerns some vestibular reflexes, the grasp reflex, and others. In comatose patients with lesions of the upper brain stem, exaggerated postural reflexes may appear spontaneously—usually with a strong dominance of extensor tone. This condition is called **decerebrate rigidity**.[4]

---

4. In four-legged animals, a corresponding condition can be evoked by transection of the brain stem in the mesencephalon. In these animals the muscular rigidity is caused by enhanced firing of vestibulospinal and reticulospinal neurons that activate α motoneurons in the cord. This conclusion is based on, among other data, the idea that electrical stimulation of the lateral vestibular nucleus (Deiters) enhances the rigidity whereas destruction reduces it. Obviously, vestibulospinal and reticulospinal neurons are normally subject to tonic inhibition from higher levels of the CNS.

Disequilibrium, Dizziness, and Vertigo

Berthoz and Viaud-Delmond (1999, p. 709) give a concise yet comprehensive description of dizziness: "Dizziness is characterised by a marked distortion of self-world relations and reflects a discrepancy between internal sensation and external reality. Spatial disorientation, as well as dizziness, can be due to a peripheral problem in any of the sensory modalities; or, it may be due to a central problem, involving not one particular sensory modality but rather the integration and weighting of the different modalities and their relation with memory." Certainly, **disequilibrium** and **dizziness** can arise because one of the usual channels of sensory information is lost or malfunctioning—that is, dizziness of peripheral origin. **Vertigo**—with the very distinctive illusion of movements (usually rotation), either of the body in relation to the surroundings or vice versa—should be distinguished from other kinds of dizziness. True vertigo is usually caused by labyrinthine disease, whereas dizziness without vertigo may have various causes. For example, considerable loss of proprioceptors and vestibular receptors is common in elderly people and may contribute to dizziness. Abnormal stimulation of certain receptors may also provoke dizziness and imbalance. Perhaps the problems arise not so much because of lack of information as from a **conflict** between the various sensory inputs: the internal model expects a certain relationship between them so that if the composition of inputs is altered, it takes some time to update the internal model. The updating presumably depends on use, as do plastic changes in general—that is, improvement depends on specific training of the impaired functions. Elderly people suffering from dizziness may easily enter a vicious cycle: they need increased amounts of balance training because of reduced sensory inputs or central processing capacity, yet they move less than before because they are afraid of falling. Dizziness is also

a common symptom in many **psychiatric** disorders, and it is a transient reaction in certain situations, as with strong **emotions**. In such cases, malfunctioning receptors are hardly responsible. Rather, the cortical networks for spatial orientation may have a reduced ability to integrate the various sensory inputs—perhaps because inputs from networks related to emotions and memories disturb them.

Unilateral **destruction** of the **vestibular apparatus** in humans usually gives very disturbing symptoms, dominated by dizziness, spontaneous nystagmus, nausea, and disequilibrium. The symptoms generally vanish with time, mainly due to central excitability changes that level out the unequal inputs from the two sides. The normalization of eye movements seems to be due, at least partly, to the patient learning to use **proprioceptive** signals instead of vestibular ones. Thus, in monkeys with unilateral damage of the labyrinth, signals from neck muscle spindles initiate an almost normal vestibulo-ocular reflex when the head rotates.

CORTICAL NETWORKS FOR POSTURAL CONTROL AND BODY REPRESENTATION

Several Areas Receive Vestibular Signals

Vestibular signals reach several small areas in the cortex, as shown electrophysiologically in monkeys and with imaging methods in humans (Fig. 18.9). The **parietal insular vestibular cortex** (**PIVC**) is of particular interest (as the

Figure 18.9

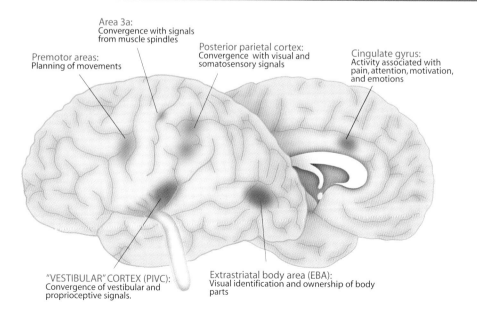

Area 3a:
Convergence with signals from muscle spindles

Premotor areas:
Planning of movements

Posterior parietal cortex:
Convergence with visual and somatosensory signals

Cingulate gyrus:
Activity associated with pain, attention, motivation, and emotions

"VESTIBULAR" CORTEX (PIVC):
Convergence of vestibular and proprioceptive signals.

Extrastriatal body area (EBA):
Visual identification and ownership of body parts

Cortical areas receiving signals from the vestibular apparatus (red) and one area related to body image (blue). The locations of regions are only approximations, based on extrapolation from fMRI data published by Bottini et al. 2001 and Astafiev et al. 2004.

name implies, it lies at the junction between the parietal lobe and the insula).[5] The PIVC contains neurons that are activated by signals from both the semicircular canals (head rotation) and from proprioceptors around the upper cervical joints. Because, in addition, the neurons are influenced by visual signals, it seems likely that they integrate all kinds of **movement-related information**. Signals from the labyrinth would thus contribute to the awareness of bodily posture and movements in space. Indeed, clinical studies indicate that stroke patients with balance problems most often have a lesion affecting the parieto-temporal junction. Furthermore, lesions in this region have been reported to result in denial of ownership of the contralateral hand. Neurons in other parts of the cortex that are activated from the labyrinth have properties similar to those in PIVC. This concerns neurons in **area 3a** (muscle spindle input), **area 2** (joint receptor inputs), and the **cingulate gyrus**. An area close to the PIVC in the **posterior parietal cortex** integrates vestibular and optokinetic information. Vestibular activation furthermore occurs in the **premotor cortex** (and in some other areas). The various "vestibular" cortical areas are interconnected and send efferent fibers to the vestibular nuclei, as mentioned earlier.

The PIVC has been suggested to form the "nave" of a **central vestibular network**, which also includes nodes in SI, the premotor cortex, and the cingulate gyrus.

Body-Related Networks in the Cerebral Cortex

As mentioned, vestibular information seems to be processed in a distributed cortical network, not in a single center. This network integrates several kinds of sensory information related to extrapersonal space and the body. It is connected with and overlaps other networks—notably those that control movements but also networks related to attention, emotions, and pain. By feeding into this network, vestibular receptors contribute to, but are not solely responsible for, our awareness of body orientation and movements in space. Other specialized regions of the cortex process

other aspects of body-related information. For example, two extrastriatal visual areas appear to be specialized for recognition and analysis of human bodies and body parts. We mentioned the **fusiform body area** in Chapter 16 (see Fig. 16.26), which is particularly activated by recognition of whole human bodies (rather than body parts). Another similar area in the occipital lobe—the **extrastriatal body area** (EBA; Fig. 18.9)—responds especially to body parts (e.g., when the person looks at an arm or a hand). Active movement of the body part modulates the EBA activity even when the body part is not seen, and this may enable this region to help decide whether the hand belongs to the person or someone else (body ownership).

This discussion suggests that a distributed cortical **network** is responsible for superior postural control—that is, the coordination of muscular activity to maintain upright position and ensure postures needed for successful goal-directed movements. The network interconnects widely separated nodes that integrate various kinds of bodily information (Fig. 18.9).

Ownership, Body Image, and Body Scheme

Together, multiple, interconnected regions enable us to be aware of our bodies; they provide us with a feeling of **ownership** and a sense of **agency** (i.e., the experience that *I* am moving my hand, not someone else). They also, presumably, form the basis of **internal models** representing stored information of the neuronal processes needed for specific actions (grasping a glass of water, descending a staircase, and so forth). **Body image** and **body scheme** are terms often used for two different aspects of internal bodily representations. Body image concerns our conscious perception of the appearance of our body, with regard to its form, size, and other characteristics. Body scheme concerns spatial representations of our body parts that do not enter awareness. Body scheme provides a basis for actions and is continuously **updated** during movements.

Human experiments indicate that self-initiated movement is the dominant source of our feeling of **ownership**. Thus, we recognize body parts as our own by the actions they perform, not only through sensory feedback. This fits with peculiar sensations often arising from immobilized limbs—for example, the leg may be perceived as changing size and position. Stroke patients sometimes deny the ownership of a paralyzed limb. Presumably, such phenomena are caused by the lack of updating and a mismatch between motor commands and sensory feedback.

---

5. Imaging studies in humans do not agree on where to place the PIVC and other presumptive vestibular-activated areas. For example, some find that PIVC includes posterior parts of the insula, while others limit it to a region just posterior to the insula. Such discrepancies are most likely due to differences in experimental conditions. It is very difficult to rule out that cortical activation evoked by caloric, galvanic, or optokinetic stimuli—applied to stimulate vestibular receptors—are due to concomitant stimulation of somatosensory or visual systems.

Putting it simply, **body image** concerns the "what" whereas **body scheme** concerns the "how." At least superficially, the distinction between body image and body scheme resembles the distinction between the ventral and dorsal pathways of the visual system: the ventral pathway processes explicit, conscious knowledge about objects, whereas the dorsal pathway deals with implicit knowledge about an object's spatial characteristics and its relation to action.

Unity and Coherence

Normally, ownership and agency are self-evident: I do not doubt the hand is mine and that I am moving it. The transformation of intention into action is effortless and requires no knowledge of the internal operations underlying it. Further, I always experience my body as a unity: I have a "natural" sense of coherence. Nevertheless, these self-evident "facts of life" depend on a complex interplay among numerous specialized regions of the brain. There is no single area responsible for our sense of unity, ownership, or agency. Indeed, there are numerous clinical examples that body image and body scheme are more fragile than we usually assume. Thus, after a stroke, the patient may deny ownership of an arm, not recognize that the arm is paralyzed, or even experience that someone else is moving the arm. In addition, strong emotions and mental illnesses (e.g., schizophrenia) may disturb body image or body scheme. Immobilization of joints—presumably producing a mismatch between motor

commands and sensory feedback—may cause bizarre experiences of positions and movements of the extremity.

Motion Sickness

Many people suffer from this condition characterized by nausea, vomiting, dizziness, and autonomic disturbances like cold sweat and low blood pressure. Presumably, the symptoms arise because of **conflict** between motor commands and sensory information (from the semicircular ducts, the maculae, the proprioceptors, and vision); that is, there is a **mismatch** between the sensory information and what was expected based on prior experience. Usually, our own movements produce sensory signals, whereas, when sitting in a car, signals from vestibular receptors are passively produced and are not accompanied by the expected pattern of proprioceptive signals. Such theories do not explain all aspects of motion sickness, however.

Animal experiments confirm that stimulation of vestibular receptors can produce several **autonomic effects**, by connections from the vestibular nuclei to the reticular formation and then to preganglionic autonomic neurons. Signals from the sacculus and utriculus are probably particularly important for the occurrence of motion sickness, judging from studies of persons exposed to weightlessness during space travels. The **cerebellum** (especially the nodulus and uvula in the posterior vermis) also seems to play a role. Thus, after removal of the posterior vermis in animals, provocations must be much stronger to produce motion sickness.

The **symptoms** of motion sickness resemble those evoked by ingestion of certain poisons (see Chapter 27, under "The Vomiting Reflex") and involve some of the same central structures (indeed, labyrinthectomized dogs show decreased susceptibility to many emetic drugs). This concerns the **solitary nucleus** in the medulla, as well as the pathways that control the preganglionic autonomic neurons and motoneurons responsible for emptying the stomach.

OVERVIEW

The chemical senses of smell and taste enable us to recognize a vast number of different molecules in our surroundings. Obviously this gives us very important information that triggers a range of responses—from avoiding poisonous food to enjoying the fragrance of a rose. Both senses depend on binding of molecules to specific **chemoreceptors**. These receptors are very sensitive, thus permitting recognition and discrimination of molecules in extremely low concentrations (in air or in fluids). **Stereospecificity**—that is, the shape of the ligand determines which receptor it binds to—is another common property of the chemoreceptors for taste and smell. The transduction mechanisms—that is, how the stimuli translate to graded receptor potentials—are similar for receptors for taste and smell because they (with some exceptions) are coupled to **G proteins** (as are photoreceptors and many neurotransmitter receptors).

The **olfactory system** differs from other sensory systems in certain respects: the **sensory cells**—located in the upper nasal cavity—are neurons with an axon that goes directly to the **olfactory bulb** (part of the central nervous system). Further, the signals in the **olfactory tract** destined for the cerebral cortex are not synaptically interrupted in the thalamus but go directly to the **primary olfactory cortex** (piriform cortex) in the medial temporal lobe near the uncus.

The taste (gustatory) receptor cells are found in taste **buds** scattered over most of the tongue. The sensory cells are equipped with receptors identifying four basic **taste qualities** (sweet, salty, sour, and bitter). In addition, a fifth quality called *umami* (Japanese: savory, meaty) is evoked by glutamate binding to specific receptors. Signals from the taste buds are transmitted in the **facial** (intermediate) and **glossopharyngeal** nerves to the **solitary nucleus** in the upper medulla. From there signals are distributed to other brain stem nuclei important for food intake and digestion and to higher levels such as the **hypothalamus**, the **amygdala,** and the primary taste area in the anterior part of the **insula**. Integration of olfactory and gustatory information takes place in the **orbitofrontal cortex** (and some other places). Here information from the chemical senses is processed in a broader context with the aim to facilitate appropriate behavior.

THE OLFACTORY SYSTEM

The sense of smell does not play the same important role for adult humans as the senses of hearing and vision. This does not mean that the sense of smell is insignificant in daily life, and the loss of smell reduces quality of daily life. The capacity of the olfactory system is indeed impressive: it has been estimated that humans can detect and discriminate more than 400,000 **odorants** (compounds in gaseous form). The smell we associate with, for example, an apple, consists of perhaps 100 different odorants, but we nevertheless experience it as one sensory experience. Obviously the olfactory system recognizes a vast number of unique odorant patterns that we learn to associate with specific objects. Our ability to identify a certain smell is also highly trainable.

The perception of odors is special due to its close association with memories and with emotions and moods. Presumably this explains why we usually remember odors so well. An enormous industry devoted to producing perfumes and other fragrances shows that, for humans, the sense of smell has an important role in interpersonal communication.

The Sense of Smell and Evolution

Going back in the evolution of the species, we find that smell is the earliest of the senses. To understand the evolution of the brain, knowledge of the "olfactory brain" or **rhinencephalon** has been important because in the early, primitive vertebrates almost the whole cerebrum was devoted to the processing of olfactory signals. In higher vertebrates, new parts of the cerebrum emerged that gradually and completely overshadowed the phylogenetically old parts. The organization of the central pathways and nuclei that process olfactory information reflects the fact that this system developed earlier than the parts of the cortex (the neocortex) that treat other sensory modalities. The term "olfactory brain" for these older parts is unfortunate, however. In higher vertebrates, large parts of the regions corresponding to the rhinencephalon in lower animals have nothing to do with the sense of smell but have taken on other important functions, with the hippocampus (see Chapter 32) the most striking example. This was a common occurrence during evolution: structures that were no longer used for one function formed the basis for the development of new capacities. Thus, the parts treating olfactory signals have not developed in pace with the rest of the brain during evolution and are therefore relatively much smaller in humans than in, for example, cats and dogs. In absolute terms, however, the differences are not so marked.

Receptor Cells for Smell

The special receptor cells for smell are located in the mucous membrane of the upper part of the nasal cavity, the **olfactory epithelium**. The total number of receptor cells has been estimated to be about 10 million in humans, and the cells are constantly renewed. Because they are in fact primitive neurons, they are exceptions to the rule that neurons that die are not replaced. The olfactory epithelium is pseudostratified and consists of supporting cells and so-called basal cells besides the receptor cells (Fig. 19.1). The **supporting cells** probably insulate the receptor cells electrically, so that signals are not propagated from one cell to another. The **basal cells** divide mitotically and probably give rise to the receptor cells. The **receptor cells** are bipolar and send a dendrite-like branch toward the epithelial surface and an axon through the base of the skull to the olfactory bulb. The dendrite ends with an expansion densely covered with **cilia** (Fig. 19.1). Because the cilia are embedded in the **mucus** that covers the epithelium, only substances dissolved in the mucus can act on the receptor cells. Many **odorants** (odorous substances) are hydrophobic, however; that is, they do not dissolve easily in water. Therefore, we assume that mechanisms—such as transport proteins—exist to bring hydrophobic odorants through the mucus. Several families of **odorant**-binding proteins have in fact been identified in the mucus. It is probable that each protein binds specifically to certain odorants and may serve to concentrate the odorant in the proper part of the olfactory epithelium (i.e.,

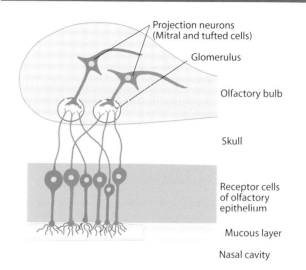

Figure 19.1

The olfactory epithelium and connections to the olfactory bulb. Neurons (receptor cells) in the olfactory epithelium have cilia embedded in mucus. The central process (axon) of the receptor cells end on mitral cells in the glomeruli of the olfactory bulb. The axons from neurons sharing odorant specificity tend to converge on one or a few glomeruli in the olfactory bulb. Thus, the glomeruli show some odorant specificity. (Based on Mombaerts 1996.)

the part containing the receptors specific for the particular odorant). The odorant-binding proteins may also help remove the odorant so that the receptors quickly regain their sensitivity. Specialized glands produce the mucus, which consists of several layers.

How Large is the Olfactory Epithelium?

The **area of the olfactory epithelium** is obviously not easy to determine in humans. Thus, figures in the literature vary from 1 to 5 cm² (the total area of the nasal cavity is about 60 cm² on each side). This variation may be at least partly due to a patchy distribution of the epithelium and age-related loss. Thus, while in the fetus the epithelium is continuous and covers a large proportion of the nasal cavity, it is gradually replaced by respiratory epithelium in a patchy fashion. Further, the epithelium may be more anteriorly located than first thought. A combined histological (biopsies) and electrophysiologic study located the anterior border of the olfactory epithelium at the level of the anterior end of the middle turbinate—1 to 2 cm anterior to what was formerly believed (Leopold et al 2000).

Transduction Mechanism

Experiments with a large number of odorants suggest that the shape of the molecule, rather than its chemical composition, determines how it smells (stereospecificity). This **stereochemical theory** of smell proposes that the receptor sites on the receptor cells have different shapes and that only molecules with a complementary shape fit into the receptor site. Binding of the molecules (odorants) to specific **odorant receptor proteins** (**ORs**) in the membrane of the cilia evokes a **receptor potential**. This involves activation of G proteins and cyclic AMP. Increased intracellular cyclic AMP opens Na⁺-selective cation channels and thus depolarizes the cell. The ORs share structural features with photoreceptors and β adrenergic receptors. In contrast to photoreceptors, however, the olfactory receptors produce action potentials. The action potential arises in the initial segment of the axon and is transmitted to the olfactory bulb.

The Olfactory Receptor Cells Express an Enormous Repertoire of Receptor Molecules

What is the basis of our ability to discriminate several thousand different odors? The olfactory system is special by the expression of a large number of specific **ORs**, coded by the largest vertebrate gene family comprising around 1,000 genes (only the immune system can recognize more different molecules). Human ORs express "only" about 350 different ORs on the surface of the cilia, while rodents and lower primates express many more, probably because a large fraction (60%–70%) of the human odorant-receptor genes appears to be **pseudogenes** (genes that are not expressed). In rodents, the proportion of pseudogenes is only about 5%. Presumably this evolutionary increase in the number of pseudogenes may reflect diminished importance of olfaction in higher primates.

Although each olfactory receptor cell expresses only one kind of OR, electrophysiologic recordings show that the individual olfactory cell responds to several odorants. This is because each OR can bind to several odorants (with closely similar 3D-structure), and each odorant can bind to multiple ORs. Thus, each odorant evokes a complex pattern of activity among the odorant receptor cells.

Central Pathways for Olfactory Signals

Like other sensory cells—for example, those in the inner ear and in the taste buds—the olfactory receptor cells are surrounded by supporting cells. In other respects, however,

the olfactory receptor cells are different from other sensory receptors, showing a more primitive arrangement. Thus, the olfactory cells themselves send a process (an axon) centrally, whereas in the inner ear, for example, a peripheral process of a ganglion cell contacts the receptor cell. The unmyelinated axons of the olfactory cells form many small bundles, together constituting the **olfactory nerve** (the first cranial nerve; Fig. 19.2). The bundles pass through the base of the skull close to the midline in the anterior cranial fossa— through the **lamina cribrosa** of the ethmoid bone. The olfactory nerve enters the **olfactory bulb** (Figs. 19.1 and 19.2; see also Fig. 6.13), located just above the nasal cavity under the frontal lobe. In the olfactory bulb, the unmyelinated olfactory nerve fibers establish synaptic contacts with the dendrites of **projection neurons**, notably the so-called **mitral** and **tufted cells** (Fig. 19.1). These send their axons

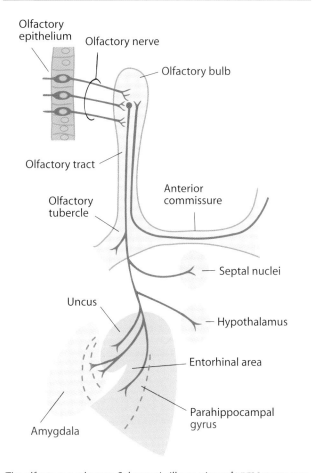

Figure 19.2

The olfactory pathways. Schematic illustration of some main connections. In the upper left are the olfactory receptors in the nasal mucosa, sending their central processes to the olfactory bulb. The neurons of the olfactory bulb send their axons to the cortex and various nuclei in the vicinity of the tip of the temporal lobe.

to the brain through the **olfactory tract** (Fig. 19.2). The synaptic contacts between the olfactory nerve fibers, and the bushy dendrites of the projection neurons are collected in small, round aggregates, called **glomeruli** (Latin: *glomerulus*, small ball of thread). Each projection neuron as a rule has one primary dendrite that ramifies within one glomerulus.

The Olfactory Bulb

The structure of the olfactory bulb is complex. It is not a simple relay station but rather a small "brain" in itself, carrying out substantial processing of the sensory information reaching it. In this sense, there are similarities with the retina, and both are parts of the central nervous system that have been "moved" outside the brain. There is some evidence that the olfactory bulb is of decisive importance for the **discriminative** aspect of olfaction, or the ability to distinguish different odors. Thus, lesions of nuclei in which the fibers from the olfactory bulb terminate do not appear to impair simple olfactory discrimination.

As mentioned, the axons from the receptor cells synapse with the dendrites of the **mitral** and **tufted cells**. The **glomeruli** form complex arrangements involving several dendrites and processes of interneurons. In humans there are about 5,000 glomeruli in each olfactory bulb, but the number declines with **age**, and only a few are said to remain in very old persons. Besides projection neurons, the olfactory bulb contains numerous small **granule cells**, forming a separate layer. They are interneurons that interconnect the projection neurons by way of **dendrodendritic synapses** (the granule cells lack axons). The granule cells are believed to mediate **lateral inhibition** in the olfactory bulb, and this is analogous to the horizontal cells of the retina. Like the horizontal cells, the granule cells are **electrically coupled**.

Many **neurotransmitters** are found in the olfactory bulb. The mitral cells most likely use glutamate, whereas the granule cells release γ-aminobutyric acid (GABA). Other interneurons are believed to be dopaminergic. In addition, norepinephrine and glycine are present in some neuronal processes.

There are also **efferent fibers** in the olfactory tract, as shown anatomically. Accordingly, electrical stimulation of the olfactory cortex can influence (primarily inhibit) the signal transmission through the olfactory bulb. Some of the efferent fibers release norepinephrine and are involved in synaptic changes in the olfactory bulb related to a certain kind of **learning** (see later discussion).

The Terminal Areas of the Olfactory Tract

In contrast to pathways for other sensory modalities, which are synaptically interrupted in the thalamus, fibers from the olfactory bulb pass directly to the cortex. Another difference concerns the cortical lamina in which the fibers terminate: olfactory fibers terminate in the outermost layers, whereas thalamocortical fibers terminate mainly in deeper layers. Most of the efferent fibers from the olfactory bulb

Figure 19.3

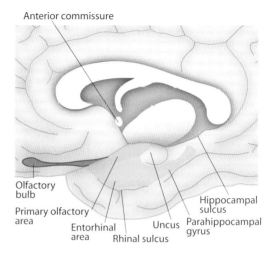

The olfactory cortex. The medical aspect of the cerebral hemisphere. The primary olfactory cortex is located in the uncus. The olfactory cortex in humans most likely also encompasses parts of the entorhinal area.

end at the medial aspect of the **temporal lobe**—partly in the **cortex** and partly in the **amygdala** (Figs. 19.2 and 19.3). The amygdala is located just below the cortex in the tip of the temporal lobe (Fig. 19.2; see also Figs. 31.1 and 31.3). In the cortex, fibers terminate both in the so-called **piriform cortex** in the **uncus** and in the adjoining parts of the **entorhinal area** (Figs. 19.2 and 19.3). The fibers to the amygdala end only in the corticomedial nuclear group, which sends efferent fibers to the **hypothalamus**. (The amygdala is discussed further in Chapter 32.) The cortical regions in the temporal lobe that receive direct fibers from the olfactory bulb are called the **primary olfactory cortex** (Fig. 19.3). Single neurons in this region respond preferentially to specific combinations of odorants; that is, afferents from many glomeruli with different specificities must converge on each cortical neuron.

Two Channels from the Olfactory Bulb to the Olfactory Cortex

The **mitral cells** and **tufted cells** have different properties and project to largely separate targets. For example, tufted cells respond to much lower concentrations of odorants than mitral cells. They also show different patterns of activity in relation to the **sniff cycle** (inhalation–exhalation): the tufted cells are activated earlier than the mitral cells. Finally, the tufted cells project in a patchy pattern to restricted (anterior) parts of the olfactory cortex, whereas single mitral cells project in an apparently diffuse manner to most parts of the olfactory cortex. The functional meaning of two parallel information channels may perhaps be that the tufted-cell pathway provides rapid information about odors associated with danger (e.g., the smell of a fox, which means danger to a rodent), whereas the mitral cells provide a means to bind together and put the early specific input into a proper context.

The Olfactory Pathways and Odor Discrimination

The sensory systems treated in the previous chapters all have an orderly anatomic arrangement of pathways and neuronal groups. We speak of somatotopic, retinotopic, and tonotopic patterns and take for granted that these phenomena represent prerequisites for sensory discrimination. Again, the olfactory system turns out to differ from the other sensory systems: sharp topographic arrangement is not a feature of the olfactory system, in spite of our ability to discriminate an enormous number of different smells.

At the lowest level, there is admittedly *some* topography within the sheet of olfactory epithelium. Thus, different receptor genes are expressed in somewhat different parts of the **olfactory epithelium**, as shown with the *in situ* hybridization technique. Four zones differing with regard to receptor–gene expressions exist in rodents, and axons from these zones end differentially in the olfactory bulb. Still, this is a very crude topography compared with the enormous repertoire of specific odorant receptors (and also the point-to-point precision in the visual pathways). A more pronounced segregation occurs in the **glomeruli**, however, as each glomerulus receives afferents from receptor cells with the same or closely similar specificity. This implies that axons from receptor cells with quite different positions in the olfactory epithelium converge in one glomerulus. The glomerular specificity appears not to be inborn, however, but results from **use-dependent plasticity**. Thus, in neonatal mice each glomerulus receives axons with different specificities. This condition persists if use of the olfactory system is prevented by closure of the nostrils shortly after birth.

In spite of the specificity of the glomeruli, however, no clear topographic pattern has been found in the connections from the olfactory bulb to the **olfactory cortex**. Accordingly, cortical neurons responding to a given odor are dispersed widely in the olfactory cortex—there is no "odorotopic" organization. Obviously, a spatial code is not crucial for our discriminative abilities. Much research effort is devoted to elucidating the codes used by the olfactory system to read out the pattern of neuronal activity sent to the olfactory cortex from the olfactory bulb. One important feature may be the exact **timing** of spikes emanating from the glomeruli (temporal code). Another possible salient feature may be the **rate** of spikes transmitted.

Uncinate Fits and Déjà Vu

Lesions affecting the uncus and the immediately surrounding cortex can be accompanied by subjective olfactory experiences (often unpleasant). Such sensations often occur as so-called **uncinate fits**, which frequently also include a peculiar feeling of experiencing the events in a dream—**dreamy state**. Often the patients feel that they have experienced the event before (**déjà vu**). Such uncinate fits may develop into an epileptic seizure, and the condition is regarded as a form of **epilepsy**.

Further Processing Outside the Primary Olfactory Cortex

The olfactory cortex and the amygdala forward olfactory signals to other parts of the brain. Connections to other parts of the cortex serve to **integrate** olfactory with other kinds of sensory information, leading to the analysis of its meaning. From the primary olfactory cortex, direct fibers reach nearby areas on the underside of the frontal lobe, the **orbitofrontal cortex**. In addition, this part of the cortex might receive olfactory information indirectly by way of connections from the **mediodorsal thalamic nucleus**, which receives fibers from the amygdala. The orbitofrontal cortex receives converging projections from many cortical areas, such as visual and **somatosensory** association areas; parts of the insula in receipt of **taste** information; and areas related to **emotions, motivation,** and **memory**. Such connections are generally reciprocal; that is, the sending areas receive information from the orbitofrontal cortex, which presumably concerns the broader meaning of the olfactory information.

One important pathway for olfactory signals reaches parts of the **hypothalamus**. These hypothalamic parts are involved in control of appetite, digestion, and feeding behavior (among other functions). Since also the orbitofrontal cortex sends fibers to the hypothalamus (among other areas), this part of the brain receives both relatively "pure" olfactory information from the amygdala and highly processed information that has been analyzed regarding its meaning for the organism.

The olfactory nuclei (not the olfactory bulb) on the two sides are interconnected by fibers running through the anterior commissure (Fig. 19.2). Thus, olfactory information from both sides of the nasal cavity is treated in each hemisphere.

Significance of Olfactory Signals for Social Communication and Behavior

Olfactory signals are perhaps more important for human communication than we realize. Humans are highly social animals, and especially body odors provide salient information, although not necessarily consciously perceived. For example, experiments clearly show that humans can "smell" fear in others, and other emotions may be communicated by chemical signaling. It seems that odor molecules in **sweat** are particularly important in this respect. However, also other body secretions may be relevant. Thus, the odor of female **tears** has been shown to reduce the sexual appeal of female faces to men and also to reduce testosterone levels (emotional tears and reflexive tears caused by local irritation differ in composition). It should be emphasized, however, that while these phenomena are convincingly documented, their importance for human behavior is less clear. Thus, the effects are demonstrated in controlled, experimental situations designed to study effects in isolation. In real life, the chemosignals act in complex and varying contexts and mental states. For example, olfactory communication always occurs together with other forms of communication (somatosensory, visual, verbal) that usually would be expected to be much more decisive with regard to human behavior.

With regard to the more direct impact of olfaction on behavior, connections to the hypothalamus—both direct and indirect via the amygdala—are of special importance for eating and for behavior directed at acquiring **food**. **Sexual** reflexes and sexually related behavior are also influenced by olfactory signals, although more so in lower mammals than in humans.

The structural basis for these phenomena is complex and not known in detail. Olfactory connections to the amygdala are most likely of importance, not only because the amygdala acts on the hypothalamus but also because it acts on parts of the prefrontal cortex involved in control of emotions and emotional behavior.

Olfactory Imprinting

Olfactory sensations in certain **sensitive** (critical) periods of development can induce lasting changes of behavior—specifically,

learning. This phenomenon is called **olfactory imprinting**. One example concerns **sheep** that establish a strong bond to the lamb shortly after the birth. This depends on odors of the lamb that are present in the amniotic fluid. The mother must be exposed to the odor(s) during the first 4 to 12 hours for the bond to develop. The migration of **salmons** for thousands of miles is an almost incredible example of how memory of odors can control behavior. At 2 years of age, the salmon is imprinted by odors at its birthplace, and these odors guide it when returning "home" several years later. Imprinting by smell or taste can occur also before birth. If **pregnant rabbits** are fed a diet with certain aromatic substances, their offspring prefer foods containing these substances. This happens even if they grow up with a substitute mother on a different diet.

Olfactory imprinting is related to synaptic changes in the **olfactory bulb** (and most likely other places as well). Simultaneous arrival of olfactory signals and signals in **norepinephrine**-containing afferents seems to be necessary for lasting synaptic changes to occur. In the previous example with sheep, more mitral cells responded to odors from the lamb after imprinting.

Pheromones

The term "pheromone" was introduced by Karlson and Lüscher in 1959 (p. 55) and defined as "substances which are secreted to the outside by an individual and received by a second individual of the same species, in which they release a specific reaction, for example, a definite behaviour or a developmental process." Some use the term **signature odor** of mixtures of odor molecules that we learn to use to recognize other individuals, with the term "pheromone" restricted to substances that elicit stereotyped endocrine and behavioral responses.

In animals—rodents have been most studied—several substances in body fluids (such as urine and saliva) have pheromone activity and influence a wide range of social interactions, such as sexual behavior, aggression, recognition of other individuals, and so forth. After destruction of the sense organ for pheromone recognition, rodents show, for example, reduced sexual activity and territorial defense. Pheromones may be volatile substances (small molecules) that move easily with the air, or they may be heavier molecules (peptides) that are exchanged among individuals only by close contact. In general, it seems that the volatile pheromones act as signals for sexual attraction or warning of impending danger, whereas the peptide pheromones are of special importance for recognition among individuals.

The Vomeronasal Organ and Human Pheromones

The **vomeronasal organ** is a tubular structure in the nasal septum with an anterior opening. It is well developed in rodents, whereas it seems to disappear before birth in humans. It contains sensory cells like those in the olfactory epithelium, expressing a distinct class of receptor molecules (in higher primates, the genes coding for these receptors have become nonfunctional). In rodents, the sensory cells send their axons to the **accessory olfactory bulb**, and from there connections continue to cortical structures that partly overlap those treating signals from the olfactory epithelium.

Even though the vomeronasal organ is lacking, there is evidence of pheromone-like actions in humans, where pheromones presumably act via receptors in the olfactory epithelium (in rodents pheromones act via both the vomeronasal organ and the olfactory epithelium). For example, synchronization of the **menstrual cycle** in women living close together is believed to be mediated by pheromones. Especially volatile substances present in armpit **sweat** seem to act as pheromones in humans. For example, some studies suggest that male armpit sweat may influence female menstrual cycle and mood. Mothers (but not fathers) seem to be able to recognize their babies by smell.

The significance of pheromones for human social behavior and development is controversial. It is safe to say, however, that they would play a minor role compared with their effects in rodents and other animals. In a broader context, pheromones are just one means of social communication. As concluded by Swaney and Keverne (2009, p. 239), "the evolution of trichromacy [color vision] as well as huge increases in social complexity have minimised the role of pheromones in the lives of primates, leading to the total inactivation of the vomeronasal organ … while the brain increased in size and the behavior became emancipated from hormonal regulation."

Disorders of Olfaction

Loss or reduction of the sense of smell (**anosmia** or hyposmia) is quite common and may cause a marked reduction in quality of life. Some people are born without a sense of smell (**congenital anosmia**). In these, the condition is associated with a small or missing olfactory bulb. Most cases of anosmia are acquired, however, and caused by upper respiratory tract infections, nasal diseases, head trauma, or toxic substances. Some people suffer from abnormal, unpleasant olfactory sensations (**phantosmia**), usually associated with diseases that cause loss of smell.

GUSTATORY SYSTEM (THE SENSE OF TASTE)

The sense of taste enables us to judge the nutritional composition of foods and helps us avoid ingesting poisonous substances. In addition to such prosaic survival functions, taste is of course a rich source of pleasure. However, much of what we experience as taste is in reality brought about by stimulation of **olfactory receptors**. This happens primarily by expiratory airflow through the nose while eating (compare the reduced sense of taste during a common cold). We nevertheless interpret this olfactory stimulation as taste (a further example of the importance of central interpretations of sensory signals for our conscious perception). In addition, signals from oral **thermoreceptors** and **mechanoreceptors** contribute to what we experience as a unitary sensory phenomenon. Finally, **nociceptors** activated by spicy food (such as chili peppers) contribute to taste perception.

Taste Receptors

The true taste signals come from **chemoreceptors** in the taste buds that are located primarily in the epithelium of the tongue (Fig. 19.4). The taste buds are concentrated along the lateral margins of the tongue and the root of the tongue and are found in small elevations of the mucous membrane called **papillae**. The largest (vallate) papilla lies along a transverse line posteriorly on the tongue (Fig. 19.5).[1] The **taste buds** are composed of approximately 100 elongated sensory cells and supporting cells (Fig. 19.4). The **sensory cells** of the taste buds are constantly renewed; each cell lives probably only about 10 days. They have long **microvilli** at their apical surface, protruding into a small opening in the epithelium, the **taste pore**. Here substances that are dissolved in the saliva contact the membrane of the sensory cell. Terminal endings of sensory (afferent) axons contact the basal ends of the sensory cells. Binding of the tasty substances to receptors in the membrane of the sensory cells depolarizes the cell and thus produces a **receptor potential** (as in other sensory cells). **ATP** released from the basal aspect of the sensory cell binds to ionotropic **purinoceptors** (P_{2x}) in the sensory nerve endings and produces action potentials.

Two Kinds of Taste Receptor Cell

There are two kinds of receptor cell in the taste buds. Unexpectedly, it seems that the kind that expresses taste receptors in high concentrations do not contact sensory fibers, whereas the other kind, expressing fewer taste receptors, makes direct contact. Therefore, several taste cells probably work together as

---

1. There are also some taste buds on the soft palate, which are innervated by the intermediate nerve. The few taste buds present on the most posterior part of the tongue and on the upper side of the epiglottis are innervated by the vagus nerve. Extralingual taste receptors are believed to protect the airways from aspiration of fluids.

Figure 19.4

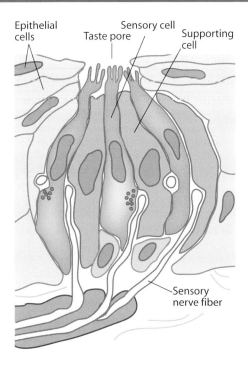

Taste bud. Semischematic drawing based on electron micrographs. The receptor molecules for taste substances sit in the membrane of the receptor cell cilia. In the taste pore, the receptors are exposed to substances dissolved in fluids.

a unit with some cells responsible for transduction while others transmit signals to the sensory fibers. Indeed, the taste cells seem capable of mutual communication by way of gap junctions and release of neurotransmitters (ATP, serotonin, and others).

Taste Qualities

We usually distinguish four elementary **taste qualities**: **salty**, **sour**, **sweet**, and **bitter**. In addition, **umami** taste has more recently been included as a fifth quality. The receptors evoking the umami quality detect **L-glutamate**. Indeed, the sodium salt of glutamate is widely used as a flavor enhancer. There are probably many more specific receptors than basic taste qualities. Especially bitter-tasting substances appear to be detected by several specific receptors. This seems reasonable, as bitter taste often is associated with poisonous foods, and their recognition would provide special survival value. **Fat** is very important for the tastiness of foods. It therefore seems a paradox that no specific receptors are known, even though the texture of fat—detected by low-threshold mechanoreceptors in the oral cavity—appears to play a role

Figure 19.5

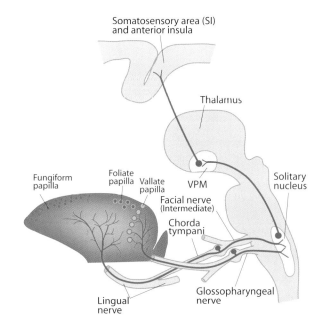

Pathways for taste signals. The various kinds of papilla contain taste buds. In the solitary nucleus, taste information is integrated with somatosensory signals from the oral cavity. The solitary nucleus receives additional input from the viscera via the vagus nerve (not shown in the figure).

for taste perception. However, now binding of long-chain **fatty acids** to the apical membrane of taste cells have been demonstrated, and, furthermore, we know that fatty acids act on taste-cell ion channels.

Each of the basic taste qualities is most easily perceived (have the lowest threshold for identification) in a particular **region of the tongue**: sweet at the tip of the tongue, then salty, sour, and bitter more posteriorly, in that order. Such differences are only relative, however, and humans are able to perceive all qualities from either the anterior and posterior part of the tongue. Accordingly, receptors for all taste qualities have been identified in all parts of the tongue equipped with taste buds.

Taste Experiences

Our varied **taste experiences** must depend on central integration of signals from different taste receptor, olfactory signals, and somatosensory information from the oral cavity. As a rule, we accept easily food that tastes sweet, umami, or moderately salty, whereas food that tastes bitter, sour, or very salty is rejected. This favors the choice of nutritious food, while potentially toxic substances are avoided. In general, sweet receptors signal calorie-rich food while umami signals protein-rich food. In an evolutionary perspective, such preferences give meaning. Thus, until quite recently the struggle for life meant primarily finding enough energy-rich food. With easy access to as much tasty food as we like in affluent Western societies, however, such preferences are less adaptive.

Individual Differences in Taste Perception

The intensity of taste experiences varies among people. This was first thought to concern bitter taste in particular, but later findings indicate that some people experience *all* taste qualities more intensely than others. Several factors seem to contribute to such individual differences. One difference concerns the **density of taste receptors** on the tongue (shown for the fungiform papillae), which appears to be higher in so-called **supertasters**. Twin studies suggest that genetics is most important to explain differences in sour taste, whereas environmental factors play a decisive role for differences in salty taste. Furthermore, **central processing** may enhance or reduce signals from taste receptors, leading to different intensity of sensation. Possibly supertasters may experience all sensory modalities more intensely. Thus, a study reported co-variation of taste sensitivity on the tongue and discriminative cutaneous sensation.

Flavors Act on Ion Channels and on G Protein–Coupled Receptors in the Apical Membrane

Sweet and bitter substances and glutamate act mainly or only on **G protein–coupled receptors**. A number of genes code for sweet, bitter, and umami receptors. The identity of the taste cell receptors for detection of salty and sour substances is still a matter of controversy.

It was originally thought that no specific receptors were required for **sour** and **salty** substances, because they can act on ubiquitous H^+ and Na^+ ion channels. The specificity of the salt and sour sensing sensory cells could perhaps be explained by the fact that the cell is exposed to fluid in the mouth only at the apical membrane, since the cells of the taste bud are interconnected with **tight junctions** (*zonula occludens*) that seal the lateral membranes off from the taste pore. Nevertheless, conditions have proven not to be that simple, and numerous candidate ion channels and receptor proteins have been implicated without final proof of their role. Furthermore, sour taste is evoked not only by protons (H^+ ions) but also by weak **organic acids**. These penetrate

the cell membrane and act presumably by acidifying the interior of the cell. In fact, the organic acids (like acetic acid in vinegar) evoke a stronger response than inorganic acids (like hydrochloric acid) at the same proton concentration.

Sweet substances and **umami** act on members of the same family of G protein–coupled receptors (**T1R**), which also includes metabotropic glutamate receptors and $GABA_B$ receptors. One kind of the T1R receptor binds several different sweet substances, while another binds amino acids. In humans, this receptor is selective for **glutamate** (in rodents it binds several kinds of amino acids).

Bitter substances act on another G protein–coupled receptor family than sweet and umami (**T2R**). Whereas only three genes code for T1R, about 30 code for T2R. Each variety of T2R recognizes only a few bitter substances, but each sensory cell expresses several kinds of the T2R. Thus, each cell can recognize a wide variety of bitter substances.

Why Cats Do Not Like Sweets

Cats do not express the gene coding for one of the sweet receptors (T1R2). This may explain why cats show little interest in sweet foods: they probably receive no taste perception from them. In an evolutionary perspective, sweet receptors are much more important for primates that feed on fruits and berries than for carnivores that feed primarily on meat. **Aspartame**, used as an artificial sweetener, binds in humans to the T1R2 receptor and therefore gives a sweet sensation. In mice, this receptor is slightly different and unable to bind aspartame. Consequently, mice are unable to detect aspartame in their food. Similar genetic **polymorphisms** may perhaps explain why humans differ concerning their propensity for sweets. Panda bears seem to lack the receptor for umami, which may reflect that their diet is entirely vegetarian.

Modulation of Taste-Cell Sensitivity

Various factors, such as hormones and neurotransmitters, and neuropeptides modulate the sensitivity of the sensory cells. These substances can be released from basal cells in the taste buds or enter from the blood. The basal cells of the taste buds contain **serotonin** (among other substances). Although its function is not clear, serotonin increases the sensitivity of the sensory cells to taste stimuli. Depression and anxiety are commonly associated with reduced taste sensation. One study found reduced sensitivity for all taste qualities (but especially sweet) in deeply depressed patients. The sense of taste returns when the depression resolves. Low levels of monoamines in the taste buds may explain these findings, as suggested also by the finding that selective serotonin-reuptake inhibitors (SSRIs) reduce the threshold for detecting flavors by 20% to 30% in normal persons.

Vasopressin (the antidiuretic hormone) and **aldosterone**—both protect the blood volume by acting on ionic transport across the renal tubular epithelium—increase the response of the taste cells to sodium chloride (by acting on Na^+ channels).

Specificity of Taste Cells and Primary Afferent Units

Each sensory cell in the taste buds appears to respond rather specifically to one kind of taste substance (sweet, sour, bitter, or umami). The further transmission of signals in the primary afferent fibers is less specific but retains some segregation. Thus, primary taste afferents (sensory units) fall into two broad categories, **specialists** or **generalists**, depending on degree of specificity. The specialist sensory units respond best to stimulation with one category of substances, whereas the generalists respond to several with about the same threshold. This conclusion is based on recordings from single afferent fibers in several animal species. In agreement with the existence of specific primary afferents, stimulation of one kind of sensory unit (e.g., sweet specific) evokes behavior in agreement with the nature of the stimulus. The specific response to electric stimulation of the sensory units remains even though their properties are changed (by genetic manipulation) so that they no longer express the appropriate receptor. Thus, the central connections of the sensory unit determine the behavioral response evoked upon stimulation of a sensory unit, even if its receptor expression has been changed from, for example, sweet to bitter. This implies the existence of mechanisms ensuring that, when the sensory cells are renewed, they retain their "line" to the brain. On the other hand, each sensory fiber must be able to recognize "its" kind of sensory cell among many others of different kinds. Thus, each sensory fiber branches and supplies several taste buds and several sensory cells in each taste bud.

Pathways for Taste Signals and the Primary Taste Area

The **intermediate nerve** (accompanying the **facial nerve**) contains the taste fibers from the anterior two-thirds of the tongue, whereas the fibers from the posterior third follow the **glossopharyngeal nerve** (Fig. 19.5). All taste fibers end in the rostral part of the **solitary nucleus**. The neurons in the solitary nucleus send their axons to several areas, thus mediating reflex effects, coordination of the activity of visceral organs, and perception of taste. Fibers pass to the visceral efferent nuclei of the **salivary glands** and to the dorsal motor (parasympathetic) nucleus of the **vagus**. Such connections mediate reflex secretion of saliva and gastric juice (and other digestive fluids). Some of the cells in the solitary

nucleus send their axons to the **hypothalamus**. This enables taste signals to influence the higher autonomic centers. Furthermore, the solitary nucleus projects to the **parabrachial area** in the pons, which send signals on to the **amygdala.** This may contribute to the linking of taste signals with emotions and the quick decision to avoid or approach a certain food. Finally, direct fibers from the solitary nucleus end in the **thalamus**, enabling taste signals to reach the cerebral cortex. The synaptic interruption in the thalamus is in the ventral posteromedial nucleus (**VPM**) (Fig. 19.5; see also Fig. 14.6), which serves as a relay for signals from the face in general. Taste signals are transmitted from the thalamus to the **face region** of the primary somatosensory cortex (**SI**), close to the representation of the tongue (see Fig. 14.8) and the anterior part of the **insula**. Together, these areas comprise the **primary taste area** (Fig. 19.6).

Organization of the Primary Taste Area

Our ability to discriminate the five basic taste qualities and innumerable complex tastes raises the question regarding which kind of code is used for taste discrimination. Is it a **labeled line** organization creating a **chemotopic (gustotopic) map** at the cortical level (like the retinotopic map in the striate area), or is the organization more like that found in the olfactory system, with no apparent orderly representation of receptor specificities at the cortical level? Sensory units responding to the elementary taste qualities are, as mentioned, to some degree segregated in the first link of the taste pathways. However, considerable convergence occurs at the next station in the taste pathway, namely in the **solitary nucleus.** While most solitary nucleus neurons respond to several taste qualities, a few respond specifically to sweet or bitter substances. In the **primary taste area** in the insula, even fewer neurons appear to be specific to one taste quality. Further, many neurons receive convergent inputs of taste and other sensory modalities, so that integration of taste and, for example, olfaction starts at the first cortical station. Indeed, it seems neurons in the primary taste area integrate taste information with other sensory modalities as well as with contextual and emotional information.

While a **chemotopic** or "gustotopic" organization in the primary taste area has not been documented in neurophysiologic studies of primates, recent studies in rodents showed clear separation of the different taste qualities in the cortex. Furthermore, a functional magnetic resonance imaging study reported slightly different locations of cortical

Figure 19.6

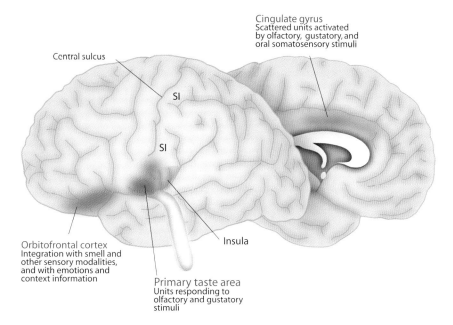

Cortical regions processing information from taste receptors. These regions may constitute a "flavor network" responsible for our experience and discrimination of flavors. The density of taste-responsive units is low in all regions. In contrast to primary visual and auditory cortices that contain only modality-specific units, the primary taste area contains neurons integrating several sensory modalities, notably olfactory and oral somatosensory stimuli.

responses to different flavors in humans. (The interpretation of such data is uncertain, however, because the distribution of response may have been influenced by other factors than taste that varied during the experimental sessions.)

In conclusion, it is possible that the human gustatory cortex has some degree of chemotopic localization, although the most salient feature seems to be convergence of many inputs onto single neurons. In any case, it is highly unlikely that a crude gustotopic localization alone can explain our discriminative capacities. It seems more likely that discrimination mainly depends on simultaneous analysis of the activity pattern in many sensory units—so-called **population coding**.

Signal Transmission from Taste Buds Is Modulated in the Brain Stem

The response of neurons in the solitary nucleus to signals from taste buds depends on several other inputs to the solitary nucleus. For example, the response is inhibited by distension of the **stomach**. This is mediated by signals transmitted from the stomach by the **vagus nerve**. Further, solitary neurons respond to alterations in blood levels of **insulin** and **glucose** (presumably by way of descending fibers from the hypothalamus). The solitary nucleus receives descending fibers from the **amygdala**, probably mediating conditioned **aversion** to certain flavors. Finally, the cortical taste area sends fibers to the rostral part of the solitary nucleus,

enabling the signal traffic to be modulated by **context** and **expectation** already at the brain stem level.

Further Cortical Processing

Our **conscious experience** of taste is due not just to stimulation of taste receptors, as mentioned. Furthermore, numerous taste cells with different specificities are presumably always stimulated while eating or drinking. The synthesis in the cerebral cortex of all these varied signals forms the basis of our subjective experience of taste. As mentioned, convergence of olfactory and taste signals takes place in the anterior part of the insula. A higher level of integration occurs in the **orbitofrontal cortex** where taste, smell, and other sensory modalities meet (Fig. 19.6). Thus, responses of neurons in the orbitofrontal cortex to flavors depend on whether or not the animal is hungry. This may be caused by connections from cortical areas related to **motivation**—that is, areas that may inform about the significance of a sensory stimulus. That our subjective sensory experience is determined not only by the stimulus holds for all sensory systems. Nevertheless, the emotional influence on the sensory experience is probably more marked for taste and smell than for other modalities. We know from everyday experience, for example, how the same smell or taste may be experienced as pleasant in one situation and nauseating in another.

Conditioned Taste Aversion

Taste is an important learning signal; it may be of vital importance to learn rapidly the association between a taste and its significance—that is, whether it signals something edible or poisonous. Survival of wild animals depends upon their ability to learn such association at the first trial, establishing a stable **conditioned taste aversion** to dangerous foods. Nausea is a very efficient learning signal when evoked by food intake. By just trying a small portion of the food, the animal usually can survive and learn to never again try the same potential food. The close coupling in the solitary nucleus of gustatory information with signals from the stomach most likely is involved in establishing the associations between flavors and their significance. Other neuronal groups believed to participate in conditioned taste aversion are found in the **parabrachial area** (pons), the **amygdala**, and the **orbitofrontal cortex**.

PART FOUR

Motor Systems

The cell groups and tracts in the central nervous system that control the activity of the skeletal muscles compose the **motor systems**. We may also use the term **somatic** motor systems to distinguish them from the systems that control smooth muscles and glands.

Although the motor systems consist of several interconnected parts, we first discuss some general aspects (Chapter 20). Then we explain the peripheral **(lower) motor neurons** (Chapter 21) and the **central (upper) motor neurons** (Chapter 22). These parts are directly involved in mediating the commands from the motor centers to the muscles and are necessary for the initiation of voluntary movements; paralysis ensues when they are damaged. Next we discuss the **basal ganglia** (Chapter 23) and the **cerebellum** (Chapter 24), which have their main connections with the central motor nuclei and are necessary for the proper execution of movements rather than for their initiation. The **control of eye movements** is covered separately in Chapter 25 due to the distinctive features of this system.

This chapter discusses the close interdependence of what we, somewhat arbitrarily, term the "motor systems" and other "systems" of the brain. For example, normal motor control and especially motor learning depend heavily on **sensory information**. Large parts of the cerebral cortex in the parietal and frontal lobes are engaged in transformation of sensory information into action. Further, the purpose of movements is often not movement per se but movements performed to collect sensory information. Without precise control of our fingers, lips, tongue, and eyes, sensory information would be severely degraded. This also concerns the chemical senses (olfaction and taste). For example, sniffing is a prerequisite for optimal detection of smells. We furthermore need to be able to scan our environments with our eyes, and our fingers move swiftly and accurately back and forth over objects we need to identify. Movements are also crucial for the brain's body "representations" that form the basis of our **body image** and the feeling of **ownership** and **agency**. The close interaction between movements and **cognition** is witnessed by the high degree of sharing of nodes between networks serving motor control and cognitive tasks.

We further discuss **classification of movements** with regard to velocity and whether they aim at stabilizing or moving parts of the body. Finally, we discuss how we can classify movements according to degree of voluntary control, from fully automatic reflex movements to the most consciously controlled skilled movements of the fingers.

The Term *Motor System* Lacks Precision

We usually include only restricted parts of the nervous system in the term "motor system(s)," namely the parts that are most closely linked with the execution of movements and that produce pareses or abnormal movements when injured. This definition obviously concerns the lower motor neurons in the cord and brain stem as well as the upper motor neurons in the motor cortex. In addition, the basal ganglia and the cerebellum are traditionally included among the motor systems because their destruction produces clear-cut motor symptoms, even if they are not necessary for the initiation of movements. Nevertheless, signals from parts of the brain not usually considered motor are necessary for the execution of meaningful, goal-directed movements. Thus, many parts of the central nervous system (CNS) may be considered motor in the sense that they are necessary for the proper functioning of the narrowly defined motor systems. Some of these regions are usually considered part of the sensory systems, as they are crucial for the processing of sensory information (e.g., the posterior parietal association areas, discussed in Chapters 14 and 34, which process visual and somatosensory information but also issue commands to motor areas). Other parts of the brain, which are usually classified as "cognitive," are nevertheless indispensable for performance of purposeful movements (e.g., parts of the prefrontal cortex involved in the early stages of movement planning and in the mediation of motivated behavior). On the other hand, parts that we include in the motor systems, notably the basal ganglia and the cerebellum, participate in nonmotor tasks. The basal ganglia, for example, play prominent roles in emotional and cognitive functions. Likewise, recent research, for example, functional magnetic resonance imaging studies in humans strongly suggest that the cerebellum participates in sensory and cognitive functions.

In conclusion, at the higher levels of the CNS, it becomes somewhat arbitrary whether we classify regions as sensory, motor, cognitive, or emotional: these concepts are too narrow to encompass the complex tasks undertaken by large parts of the cerebral cortex and many related subcortical nuclei.

Sensory Feedback Is Crucial for Movement Control

For the motor systems to function, they must cooperate closely with the sensory systems. For example, during most movements, the motor centers need constant information from receptors in muscles, around joints, and in the skin about whether the movement is progressing in accordance with the plan. Further, visual information is often crucial for the proper execution of movements. Such **sensory feedback** information enables the CNS to adjust and correct the command signals issued to the muscles either during the movement or during the next time the movement is performed. In Chapter 13 (under "Clinical Examples of Loss of Somatosensory Information") we discussed the importance of sensory feedback for movement execution; for example how a hand devoid of sensory innervation becomes virtually useless (see also Chapter 14, under "Functions of the Dorsal Column–Medial Lemniscus System").

Learning new skills depends critically on reliable sensory information. Indeed, we perform unfamiliar movements slowly to allow sufficient time for sensory feedback.

Movements in the Service of Sensation

Many movements—notably of the hands, mouth, and tongue—are executed to collect sensory information. Indeed, the hand is a sensory organ in its own right. For example, we use delicate, exploratory finger movements to judge the form, surface, consistency, and so forth of objects. Losses of muscle coordination or of hand sensation have equally devastating consequences for hand function. In addition, eye movements are entirely devoted to assist the brain in the acquisition of visual information, and head movements aid the auditory system. As aptly formulated by the Israeli neuroscientist Ehud Ahissar (2008, p. 1370), "Without eye movement, the world becomes uniformly gray; without sniffing, only the initial changes in the odor environment are sensed; and without finger or whisker motion, objects cannot be identified."

Motor Systems and Self-Recognition

Movements play an important role in the experience and ownership of our bodies. For example, experiments in human volunteers show that self-recognition (e.g., "this hand belongs to me") is significantly better during a self-generated movement than when depending on proprioceptive and visual information alone. Our **body scheme** and **body image** (cf. Chapter 18) depend on regular **updating** by sensory information provided by our own, purposeful movements. If there is a mismatch between movement commands and sensory feedback, misconceptions of the body regularly occur (e.g., after amputation, deafferentation, immobilization of joints, and so forth).

CLASSIFICATION OF MOVEMENTS

Stabilizing and Moving

Before we describe the motor systems, some comments on movements in general are pertinent. First, muscle contraction may not necessarily elicit movement (i.e., alter the position of one or more joints); just as often, muscle activity is used to prevent movement—for example, muscles maintain our **posture** by counteracting the force of gravity. In preventing movement, the muscles may be said to **stabilize** a joint (against external forces) and to have a postural function. Further, movement in one part of the body—for example, in an arm—requires that muscles in other parts contract to prevent the body balance from being upset. Therefore, a muscle in one situation may be used as a mover and in another situation as a stabilizer.

Contractions: Concentric, Isometric, and Eccentric

Whether or not a movement is to occur depends on the magnitude of the force produced by the muscle contraction and the external forces acting on the joint. When the external force is smaller than the muscle force, the muscle shortens and a movement occurs; this is called **concentric** or **isotonic contraction**. When the external forces equal the force of the muscle contraction, no movement occurs; this is called **isometric contraction**. When the external force is greater than the opposing force produced by the muscle contraction, the muscle lengthens; this is called **eccentric contraction**.[1] Eccentric contraction occurs, for example, with the thigh muscles when we walk down a staircase, as the muscles brake the movement produced by the weight of the body.

Ramp and Ballistic Movements

Movements may be classified by the **speed** with which they are performed. **Ramp movements** are performed relatively slowly. The crucial point is that the movement is slow enough to enable sensory feedback information to influence the movement during its execution. **Ballistic movements** are very rapid, and their characteristic feature is that they are too fast to enable feedback control: the name derives from analogy with a bullet shot out of a gun.

Automatic and Voluntary Movements

Movements may also be classified according to whether they are **voluntary** or **automatic**; automatic movements take place without our conscious participation. In reality, this is much too crude a distinction: there is a gradual transition from what Hughlings Jackson (1884) termed the most automatic to the least automatic movements. The **most automatic** movements are basic, simple reflexes, such as the retraction of the arm from a noxious stimulus. Locomotion is an example of a semiautomatic movement—that is, the basic pattern is automatic, but starting and stopping and necessary adjustments may require conscious (voluntary) control. The **least automatic** movements are precision grips with the fingers and delicate manipulatory or exploratory movements such as writing, drawing, playing a musical instrument, and so forth. Equally precise voluntary control exists for the muscles of the larynx, the tongue, and some of the facial muscles. We know that the degree to which a movement is automatic changes with **learning**: in the beginning a new movement requires full voluntary control, and in the process of learning the movement becomes more automatic. When playing a well-rehearsed musical piece on the piano, for example, we do not need to pay attention to the fingers and their movements.

As a rule, the most automatic movements require only the use of relatively simple **reflex arcs** at the spinal level; participation of higher motor centers is not necessary. Somewhat less automatic and more complex movements such as ventilation, locomotion, and postural control depend, in addition, on the participation of neuronal groups in the brain stem. Such movements do not require our attention directed toward them but can be subjected to voluntary control. The least automatic movements depend on the participation of the highest level—the **cerebral cortex**—to coordinate and control the activity of motor centers in the brain stem and spinal cord. The vast number of neurons and the plasticity of the human brain enable learning of an almost infinite repertoire of voluntary movements. Also, these features ensure great **flexibility** in how motor tasks are solved. The same task may be solved in different ways, and we can continuously adapt to novel challenges. The great adaptability and flexibility of movements distinguish humans from most animals. Most animals are highly specialized for a limited number of motor tasks, controlled by stereotyped motor programs that develop according to a fixed pattern.

---

1. This term may seem confusing, since *contraction* literally means "shortening" (Latin: *contractio*, the act of drawing together). Strictly speaking, it is therefore self-contradictory to call lengthening of a muscle a *contraction*. In common usage, however, contraction implies merely that the muscle is actively working with dynamic interactions between the contractile muscle proteins (actin and myosin).

21 The Peripheral Motor Neurons and Reflexes

OVERVIEW

The peripheral or lower motor neurons (motoneurons) constitute the final and only connection between the central nervous system (CNS) and the muscles. If they are destroyed, paralyses of the muscles ensue. There are two types of lower motor neurons—α **motoneurons** innervating the extrafusal muscle fibers and γ **motoneurons** supplying the muscle spindles. The motoneurons are arranged in **columns** in the spinal cord; each column supplies one or a few muscles with synergetic actions. Each column extends through two or more segments, so that each muscle receives fibers from at least two spinal segments. An α motoneuron and all the muscle fibers it innervates is called a **motor unit**. Large muscles consist of a few hundred to more than a thousand motor units. Muscle fibers are classified according to ATPase activity into **type 1** and **type 2** fibers. In general, type 1 fibers have the highest endurance whereas the type 2 fibers contract with the highest velocity and force. The muscle fibers of one motor unit are all of the same fiber type.

A **reflex** is an involuntary response to a stimulus, which is mediated by the nervous system. The motoneurons are parts of **reflex arcs,** consisting of receptors that capture the stimulus, sensory neurons conducting signals to the CNS, a reflex centrum (e.g., in the spinal cord), and an effector (muscle or glandular cells). In this chapter, we discuss the **flexion reflex** and **stretch reflexes** in particular. Stretch reflexes are of two main kinds: the **monosynaptic** stretch reflex (routinely tested by a tendon tap) and the polysynaptic, **long-latency** stretch reflex. Both consist of a muscle contraction in response to muscle stretch (the muscle spindle is the receptor). We also discuss the **resting tone of muscles** (muscle tone), and how it may vary in health and disease. Finally, we treat the ability of peripheral nerves to **regenerate** after severance.

MOTONEURONS AND MUSCLES

The **peripheral motor neurons** are nerve cells that send their axons to skeletal muscles. Another term is **lower motor neurons**. These are the motoneurons in the ventral horn of the spinal cord and in the somatic motor cranial nerve nuclei. There are two kinds: α **motoneurons** innervate the extrafusal muscle fibers, whereas the γ **motoneurons** innervate the intrafusal muscle fibers of the muscle spindle (see Figs. 13.6 and 13.7).

The motoneurons of the ventral horn (Fig. 21.1) and in the cranial nerve nuclei are easily recognized in microscopic sections because of their large size and the big clumps of rough endoplasmic reticulum (rER) in the cytoplasm of their cell bodies (see Fig. 1.2). The rich content of rER indicates that the neurons have a high protein synthesis. These proteins are, for example, enzymes for transmitter synthesis and metabolism and various kinds of membrane proteins. The vast surface of the motoneurons with their large dendritic tree and long axons presumably explains why motoneurons contain more rER than most other neuronal types.

Ventral Roots and Plexuses

The axons of the motoneurons leave the spinal cord through the **ventral roots** and continue into the **ventral** and **dorsal branches** (rami) of the spinal nerves to innervate skeletal muscles of the trunk and the extremities (see Figs. 6.5 and 6.7). Correspondingly, the axons from the **cranial nerve motor nuclei** supply the muscles of the tongue, pharynx, palate, larynx, and face, as well as the extraocular muscles. The axons of all the motoneurons located in one spinal segment leave the cord through one ventral root and continue into one spinal nerve. The ventral branches of the spinal

Figure 21.1

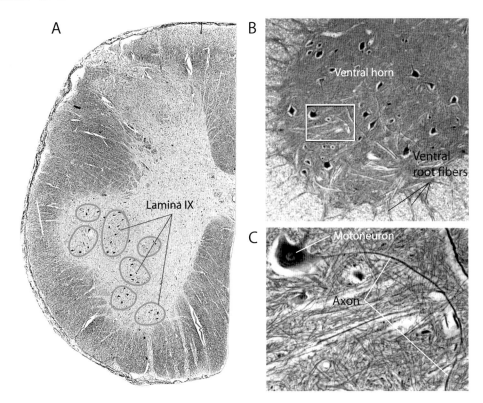

Motoneurons. **A:** Photomicrograph and drawing of a transverse section of the (lumbar) spinal cord. The motoneurons are collected in groups (columns) that together form the lamina IX of Rexed (outlined in orange). **B:** Photomicrograph of a transverse section through the human lumbar enlargement, Bodian's silver impregnation method. Cell bodies and axons are black. Due to shrinkage, the cell bodies are surrounded by a light zone. Bundles of motor axons can be seen penetrating the white matter. **C:** Higher magnification of a motoneuron and the first part of its axon; from the framed area in B.

nerves form **plexuses** so that the motor axons from one spinal segment are distributed to several peripheral nerves (Fig. 21.2).

The Final Common Path and Synaptic Contacts on Motoneurons

Contraction of skeletal muscles can be elicited only by signals conducted in the axons of motoneurons. If these axons are interrupted, the muscles become **paralyzed.** The peripheral motor neurons thus constitute the **final common path** for all signals from the CNS to skeletal muscles (the term "final common path" was introduced by the British neurophysiologist and Nobel laureate Sir Charles Sherrington). The motoneurons may be compared with the keys of a piano on which higher levels of the CNS can play. As we describe later in this chapter, many parts of the CNS cooperate in determining the activity of the motoneurons and thus the contraction of our muscles.

Each motoneuron probably receives about 30,000 nerve terminals—some forming excitatory synapses, others inhibitory; some with fast synaptic actions, others with slow modulatory ones. The sum of these influences determines whether and with what frequency the motoneurons send action potentials to the muscles. That we can perform such a wide variety of movements is due to the ability of the CNS to select precisely, by way of the motoneurons, the combinations of muscles to be used and to determine the speed and force with which they are to contract.

How Do the Complicated Plexuses Arise?

About 20 *Hox* genes control the specification of motoneurons with regard to their peripheral target (muscle). In addition, expression of recognition molecules and guidance receptors in the peripheral tissues is required for axons to find their target. When looking at the intricate trajectory of branches from motoneurons in one segment (Fig. 21.2), the task of creating a precise topographic relationship between spinal cord motoneurons and muscles seems daunting. It should be recalled, however, that at the time of outgrowth in early embryonic life, the distances are

Figure 21.2

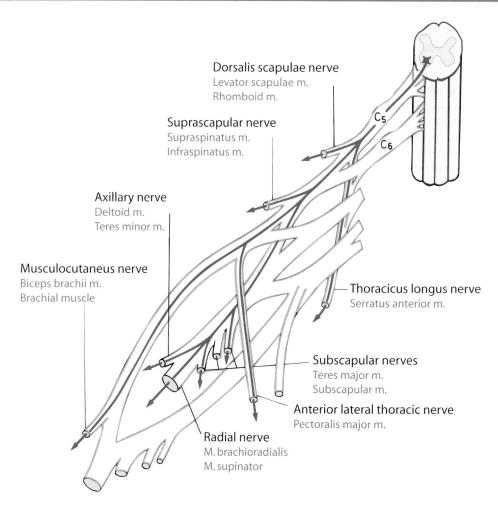

The brachial plexus. Axons of motoneurons in one spinal segment (C_5 is used as an example) are distributed to several peripheral nerves to supply various muscles of the arm. Each muscle also receives motor fibers from other segments, although they are not shown here.

small and trajectories of axonal growth are usually fairly straight. The complicated pattern of the plexuses (Fig. 21.2) arises later in development.

Neurotransmitters

The motoneurons use **acetylcholine** as a transmitter, and the synthesizing enzyme **choline acetyltransferase** can be demonstrated immunohistochemically in the motoneurons and in their terminals. Motoneurons also contain the neuropeptide **calcitonin gene-related peptide (CGRP)**. There is experimental evidence that CGRP influences the synthesis of acetylcholine receptors (AchRs) of the muscle cells. The level of CGRP in the motoneurons is under the influence of descending connections from higher levels of the CNS; when such connections are transected, the level

of CGRP drops. Thus, activity of central motor pathways may contribute to the regulation of AchR density at the neuromuscular junction. If so, this may be one of several means by which the CNS can influence the properties of muscle cells.

Motoneurons Are Collected in Columns

The motoneurons are collected in groups, which form **Rexed's lamina IX** in the spinal cord (Fig. 21.1A; see also Fig. 6.10). The dendrites of the motoneurons do not respect the boundaries of lamina IX, however, and extend far in the transverse and in the rostrocaudal directions—for example, into lamina VII, where many interneurons are located (see Fig. 6.12). The rostrocaudal (longitudinal) extension of the dendrites enables dorsal root fibers from several segments

Figure 21.3

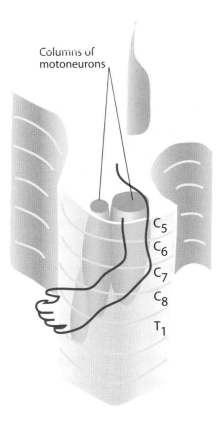

Columns of motoneurons

C5
C6
C7
C8
T1

Columnar arrangement of motoneurons. Schematic of the somatotopic localization of the motoneuronal columns innervating the arm, located in the spinal segments C_5–T_1. Motoneurons supplying the intrinsic muscles of the hand are located most caudally (C_8–T_1) and most dorsally in the ventral horn.

How Was the Localization of Motoneurons in the Cord Determined?

The anatomic organization of motoneurons has been studied via transection of muscle nerves in experimental animals. A **retrograde reaction**, which is easily seen through a microscope, occurs in the cell bodies of the motoneurons. Studies using retrograde transport of **tracer substances** have detailed the picture considerably. Study of patients with **poliomyelitis** has provided information about conditions in the human cord (the poliovirus infects and kills motoneurons). Because the distribution of paralyzed muscles usually has been determined before death, it can be compared with the distribution of cell loss among the motoneuron groups in the cord and brain stem.

Motoneuron Columns Are Somatotopically Distributed in the Ventral Horn

Groups of motoneurons that supply **axial muscles**—that is, muscles of the back, neck, abdomen, and pelvis—are located most medially within the ventral horn, whereas motoneurons supplying muscles of the **extremities** lie more laterally. This explains why the ventral horn is broader (extends more laterally) in the segments of the cord that send fibers to the extremities (i.e., C_5–T_1 and L_1–S_2; compare Figs. 6.8, 6.10, and 6.11). There is also a further somatotopic organization: motoneurons supplying **proximal muscles** of the extremities (the shoulder and hip) are located more ventrally than those supplying the **distal muscles** (the hand and foot). This is shown in Figure 21.3, which also shows that the proximal muscles are supplied from motoneurons located more rostrally than those supplying the distal muscles. For example, the shoulder muscles are mainly innervated by the upper parts of the brachial plexus (C_5–C_6), whereas the lowermost segments (C_8–T_1) innervate the intrinsic muscles of the hand.

Motoneurons Are of Functionally Different Kinds

As mentioned, the α and γ motoneurons supplying one muscle lie together within one column in the ventral horn. In a microscopic section of the cord it can be seen that the motoneuron cell bodies vary in size (Fig. 21.1; see also Fig. 1.2). As in other parts of the nervous system, the neurons with the largest cell bodies have the thickest (and thus the fastest conducting) axons. The **γ motoneurons** are the smallest within a group, while the **α motoneurons**—although larger

to act on each motoneuron. The dendritic tree increases the surface of the motoneurons enormously, and, not surprisingly, the vast majority of the nerve terminals contacting motoneurons are axodendritic.

Three-dimensionally, the motoneurons are collected in longitudinally oriented **columns** (Fig. 21.3). Each column contains the α and γ motoneurons to one muscle or a few functionally very similar (synergistic) muscles. Within a column supplying more than one muscle, the motoneurons to each muscle are at least partly segregated. As a rule, each column extends through more than one segment of the cord. Consequently, each muscle receives motor fibers through more than one ventral root and spinal nerve. **Destruction of one root** or spinal nerve only for example, by disk protrusion in sciatica or by a tumor growing in the spinal canal—will not produce paralysis of a muscle but only a more or less pronounced paresis (weakness).

than the γ motoneurons—vary considerably in size. Such **size** differences are related to differences among the muscle cells supplied by the α motoneurons. Briefly stated, the smallest α motoneurons control delicate movements with little **force**, whereas the largest motoneurons come into play only when a movement requires great force. The large α motoneurons also have a much higher maximal **firing frequency** than the small ones, and the large ones tend to fire in brief bursts with a high frequency, whereas the small α motoneurons tend to go on firing for a long time with a low frequency. These differences in **firing pattern** reflect that the large motoneurons are used for forceful, rapid movements of short duration, whereas the small motoneurons can uphold a moderate muscular tension for a long time. For these reasons, we apply the term **phasic α motoneurons** to the large ones, and **tonic α motoneurons** to the small ones. The properties of the α motoneurons are discussed further when we deal with the motor units.

The Motor End Plate and Neuromuscular Transmission

After entering the muscle, the α-motoneuron axon divides into many thin branches or collaterals. Each of these terminal branches contacts one muscle cell only. Each muscle cell is thus contacted by only one branch from one α motoneuron. Such a branch ends on the muscle cell approximately midway between its ends, forming the **motor end plate**, where the signal transfer from nerve to muscle takes place (Figs. 21.4 and 21.5). Within the end-plate region, the axonal branch divides further and forms up to about 50 nerve terminals (boutons), each establishing synaptic contact with the muscle cell. The postsynaptic side at this **neuromuscular junction** is somewhat special compared to synapses in the CNS, as **junctional folds** and a thin **basal lamina** are intercalated between the presynaptic and postsynaptic membranes (Fig. 21.5B). The boutons contain **acetylcholine**, and the postsynaptic membrane contains **acetylcholine receptors** of the **nicotinic** type. The density of acetylcholine receptors is much higher in the end-plate region than elsewhere on the muscle cell surface, which is appropriate because only at the end plate is the muscle cell normally exposed to acetylcholine.

During **embryonic development**, however—before the nerve fibers growing out from the cord have reached the muscle cells—the acetylcholine receptors are evenly distributed all over the muscle membrane. Only after establishment

Figure 21.4

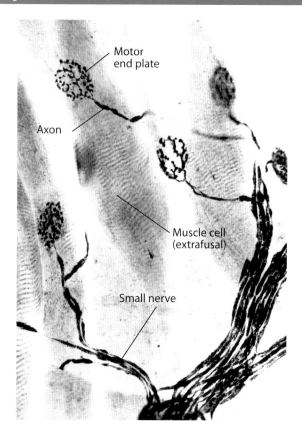

Motor end plates. Photomicrograph of skeletal muscle cells and a small bundle of nerve fibers innervating the cells. The tissue is stained with gold chloride to darken the nerve fibers and their terminal boutons. Each motor end plate consists of numerous small boutons. Four end plates are seen here. Magnification, ×500.

Figure 21.5

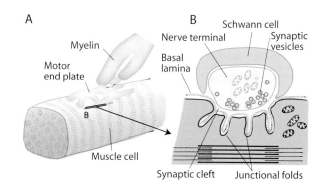

The motor end plate. **A:** Schematic showing how the myelinated nerve fiber loses the myelin sheath before it ramifies in the end-plate area, each terminal branch ending in a nerve terminal. Each muscle cell has only one end plate. **B:** Section through one of the nerve terminals in **A**, based on electron microscopic observations. The synaptic cleft contains a thin basal lamina, and the postsynaptic membrane is thrown into deep folds (junctional folds).

of properly functioning synaptic contacts are the receptors redistributed to attain the mature pattern. During development, spinal motoneurons transiently express the neuropeptide **galanin**, which presumably influences the synapse formation at the motor end plate.

An action potential propagated along the axon of the motoneuron depolarizes all the boutons and elicits release of acetylcholine. The transmitter binds to the acetylcholine receptors, and, as at other excitatory synapses, this depolarizes the postsynaptic membrane. This change in the membrane potential is called the **end-plate potential**. Because of the large number of nerve terminals formed by one terminal fiber, enough transmitter is released by a single nerve impulse to depolarize the muscle cell membrane to the threshold for an action potential. The action potential is propagated over the whole surface of the muscle cell and elicits a brief contraction. The enzyme **acetylcholinesterase** rapidly terminates the action of acetylcholine by degrading it. The enzyme is present in the synaptic cleft and the junctional folds.

Neuromuscular Transmission Can Be Disturbed by Poison and Disease

Various drugs and naturally occurring poisonous substances can influence the signal transmission at the neuromuscular junction and produce involuntary muscle contractions or muscle paralysis. The South American Indian poison **curare** and similar synthetic substances paralyze the muscle cells by blocking the acetylcholine receptors. Such drugs are often used during abdominal surgery to obtain sufficient muscle relaxation. Several kinds of **snake poisons** act by blocking acetylcholine receptors and thereby paralyze the victim. The **botulinum toxin** (produced by a microorganism growing in certain kinds of spoiled food) paralyzes the muscles by preventing the release of acetylcholine from the nerve terminals at the motor end plate. A similar mechanism sometimes produces muscle weakness in patients with **cancer**; apparently substances preventing release of acetylcholine are produced in the body.

The disease **myasthenia gravis** is characterized by excessive fatigability of striated muscles, which is caused by **autoantibodies** binding to the acetylcholine receptors. Thus, there are fewer than normal acetylcholine receptors available at the neuromuscular junction and release of acetylcholine opens fewer ion channels, leading to less than normal depolarization. The probability of evoking an action potential in the muscle cell membrane is consequently reduced. Drugs that inhibit the acetylcholine esterase, such as **pyridostigmine**, may lessen the symptoms. With this inhibition, the transmitter has a longer time to act, and the probability of evoking an action potential is increased. Typically, the muscles of the head are most severely affected, producing symptoms such as double vision (due to paresis of extraocular muscles) and involuntary lowering of the upper eyelids (ptosis). The voice becomes weaker while speaking, and swallowing may become difficult. In addition, the respiratory muscles are usually affected.

The Force of Muscle Contraction Is Controlled by the Motoneurons

A single presynaptic action potential at the motor end plate elicits only a brief contraction, a **twitch**, of the muscle cell (Fig. 21.6). The twitch lasts only for about one-tenth of a second. However, if another action potential follows shortly after the first one—that is, before the tension produced by the first twitch is over—the tension produced by the muscle is upheld and, furthermore, may increase considerably. This is called **summation**. Up to a limit, the tension produced by the muscle cell increases with increasing frequency of action potentials; that is, the **force** produced by the muscle cell is determined by the **firing frequency** of the motoneuron. Whereas the twitch is the response of the muscle cell to a single nerve signal, **tetanic contraction** is the term used of the muscle response to a train of signals with the highest frequency to which the muscle cell can respond (Fig. 21.6). The tetanic tension is thus the maximal force the muscle cell can produce. (One may, as shown in Fig. 21.6, differentiate between unfused or incomplete tetanus at submaximal firing frequencies and fused or complete tetanus at the maximal firing frequency. The term "tetanus," as used here, refers to the complete tetanus.)

There Are Functionally Different Kinds of Striated Muscle Fiber Types

In both animals and humans, the skeletal muscles are composed of different kinds of muscle cells or muscle fibers (these terms are used interchangeably). The most clear-cut evidence is provided by the fact that in some species certain muscles have a dark color (**"red" muscles**), whereas other muscles are light (**"white" muscles**)—for example, the almost white breast muscles and the dark leg muscles of the chicken. Such muscles are composed of muscle fibers of only one (or predominantly one) kind, and we classify the muscle cells as either white or red. The color difference is due to differences in the content of **myoglobin**, which is red (closely related to hemoglobin) and transports oxygen within the muscle cell. Further study showed that white and red muscle cells differ with regard to **endurance**—that is, how long they can maintain tension. This is mainly due to differences in the capacity to take up oxygen and to **aerobic ATP production** (oxidative phosphorylation). As one would expect, the red muscles have the highest endurance.

let the sensory axons degenerate) and counting the muscle cells. An average seems to be around 150 muscle cells per motoneuron, with a range of from less than 10 to more than 1,000. As might be expected, the **smallest motor units** are found in muscles that are used for delicate movements, which we must be able to control very precisely. Examples are the intrinsic muscles of the hand, the muscles of the larynx, the facial muscles, and the extraocular muscles. The **largest motor units** occur in large muscles used for movements of considerable force and with less precise control, such as the muscles of the back, the abdomen, and the thigh. Within one muscle, however, the motor units also vary in size.

There is also a relationship between the **size of a motor unit** (in terms of number of muscle fibers) and the size of its **motoneuron**. Thus, the motoneurons with the largest cell bodies and the thickest axons as a rule belong to the largest motor units. This fits with the use of large motor units for fast and forceful movements: the large motoneurons have the highest maximal firing frequencies, and their axons conduct the signals to the muscles with a minimal delay.[1]

Muscle cells belonging to different motor units lie **intermingled** in the muscle, as is obvious in sections stained to identify fiber types (Fig. 21.7). Correspondingly, muscle cells belonging to one motor unit spread over a considerable part of the total cross-sectional area of the muscle.

Motor Units and Fiber Types

Muscle cells belonging to the same motor unit are all of the same **fiber type**. Thus, they not only contract simultaneously but also share properties with regard to **contraction velocity**, maximal **force**, and **endurance**. In general, the smallest motor units consist of **type 1** fibers, whereas the largest ones consist of **type 2B** fibers. This further increases the difference between large and small motor units with regard to their maximal force; not only are there more muscle cells in the large units, but each cell also develops more force. Recruitment of one extra motor unit with type 1 fibers adds just a little extra to the total tension of the muscle, which thus can be graded finely (like an electrical

switch with many small steps to vary the heat of a stove). As one might expect, such motor units are used for precisely controlled movements of small force. Recruitment of a large motor unit consisting of type 2 fibers, in contrast, gives a comparatively large increase in the total tension of the muscle (the switch has large steps). Such motor units are recruited only when large force production is needed. Often this concerns fast movements because high acceleration requires a large force.

Fiber Types and Kinds of Movement

The fiber type used for a particular kind of movement has been studied by the so-called **glycogen-depletion technique**. By prolonged use, all of the muscle fibers of a motor unit deplete their stores of glycogen, as evident in histochemically treated frozen sections of a small piece of muscle tissue (obtained by biopsy). The type 1 muscle fibers are depleted first when the force exerted is low—that is, no type 2 fibers are recruited. When the force is very high, however, the type 2 fibers are depleted first; although type 1 fibers are also recruited, because of their high endurance, they are not depleted during the short period in which a maximal force can be maintained.

Electromyography

As mentioned, muscle contraction is elicited by an action potential that is propagated along the muscle cell membrane. Like action potentials of nerve cells, the muscle cell action potential can be recorded with an electrode. This is called **electromyography** (EMG) and is performed either with an electrode placed on the skin overlying the muscle—a surface EMG—or with a thin needle electrode inserted into the muscle. The surface method gives an impression of the total electrical activity of the muscle, whereas needle electrodes sample the activity of a small part of the muscle. Because the EMG is a measure of the electrical activity and not of the mechanical activity of the muscle, it is not well suited to measure muscle-force production. In some instances of prolonged activity, the muscle force may decline (**fatigue**) in spite of constant or even increasing EMG activity—with the declining force caused by changed conditions in the muscle itself—whereas muscle action potentials are evoked normally by the nerve to the muscle. In other instances, however, muscle fatigue during prolonged activity is due to declining firing frequency of the motoneurons (central fatigue).

When recording from a normal muscle at the start of a very weak, voluntary contraction, the EMG shows regular, single potentials due, presumably, to the activity of only one motor unit. As the force increases, more potentials occur in the EMG, reflecting the recruitment of more motor units. At a certain level of force, the potentials are so frequent that the picture becomes unclear—that is, it is impossible to recognize a further increase of the EMG activity. This occurs not only because of recruitment but also because of the increase in the frequency of action potentials for each motor unit.

---

1. The relationship between motoneuron size and motor unit properties is not absolute, however. Motoneurons of the same size may have different maximal firing frequencies. Further, motoneurons of the same size may innervate muscle cells with different contractile properties. The latter is probably because the motoneuron firing frequency (and firing pattern) influences the contractile properties of the muscle cells.

EMG is a valuable tool for studying the participation of various muscles in normal movements: for example, to determine the timing of contraction in muscles of the leg during walking. EMG also aids in the diagnosis of diseases of the peripheral motor neurons and of the muscles themselves, as in determining whether a disease affects the motoneurons or the muscle. If the motoneurons are put out of action, the EMG activity will be reduced or absent, whereas in a disease that affects the contractile apparatus of the muscle, the EMG may be normal. In addition, in cases of injury to peripheral nerves, it can be ascertained whether the lesion is complete (no EMG activity) or incomplete (even though there may be no visible movements).

Gradation of Muscle Force: Recruitment and Frequency

As we know, the force of muscular contraction can be finely graded within very wide limits, from a barely perceptible contraction to a tension that is high enough to tear the muscle loose from its insertion. This depends on the ability of the CNS to control the activity (the level of excitation) of the motoneurons. There are two means by which the force of muscle contraction can be gradually increased. One means is to bring more and more α motoneurons to send action potentials to the muscle. This is called **recruitment**, because more and more motor units—and thus muscle fibers—are called into action. The other means is by increasing the **firing frequency** of the motoneurons already recruited and thereby increasing the force developed by each motor unit. Thus, the force exerted by each motor unit (as by each muscle cell) can be graded from the small and brief tension produced by a single twitch to full **tetanic tension** (Fig. 21.6).

When a muscle contraction is initiated, the small motoneurons are always recruited first, and with increasing force the larger ones are recruited successively. This is called the **size principle of recruitment** and was demonstrated by the American neurophysiologist E. Henneman (1965). The excitability of the motoneurons is inversely related to their size; thus, the small motoneurons are more easily excited to the threshold for initiation of action potentials than are the large ones. This is presumably related to differences both in membrane properties of the motoneurons and in the density of excitatory synapses. The size principle ensures selection of the motor units that are best suited for a particular kind of movement.[2]

Recruitment during Movements with Different Force Requirements

The number of motor units that are recruited at the beginning of a voluntary contraction depends on the force requirement. If **maximal force** is needed (as with a movement of maximal speed), most or all motor units are recruited almost simultaneously. Nevertheless, the small ones are activated slightly before the large ones because the small motoneurons reach the threshold for eliciting action potentials first. Thus, the order of recruitment is maintained (according to the size principle) when maximal force is required. To produce the maximal force, besides recruiting as many motor units as possible, the central motor centers must increase the firing frequencies of the motoneurons to the maximal: a muscle develops maximal force when all motor units are recruited and contract tetanically (complete tetanus). Such a contraction, however, can be maintained for only a short period before the muscle fatigues. The situation is different when a movement requires **low force**. Consider, for example, an isometric contraction that should last as long as possible (i.e., the force must be kept constant). Here, more than half the motor units are recruited at the beginning of the contraction (judging from animal experiments).[3] Because a relatively large fraction of the motor units is recruited, the required force is achieved with a low firing frequency, so that the motor units can work for a long time without fatigue. If the contraction continues, however, some motor units fatigue and "fresh" ones are recruited to maintain constant force. Finally, in some cases so many small or medium large motor units are fatigued that the largest motor units must be recruited to prevent a drop of force. This recruitment pattern is only valid, however, when the contraction force is so low that the blood flow is not impeded (even at 25% of maximal voluntary contraction force the blood flow is significantly reduced).

REFLEXES: GENERAL ASPECTS

When a response to a stimulus is automatic (involuntary), and the response is mediated by the nervous system, we call it a "reflex." Many of the tasks of the nervous system are

2. In spite of the general validity of the size principle for recruitment of motoneurons, experiments with the use of biofeedback (EMG) during voluntary movements indicate that humans can to some degree select among the low-threshold motor units, probably depending on the ability of higher motor centers to focus excitation among motoneurons with presumably the same size.

3. There are, however, large differences among human muscles with regard to the proportion of motor units that are recruited early. In intrinsic hand muscles, for example, most of the units are recruited even at low forces, whereas in the biceps brachii new units are recruited until maximal force.

carried out automatically or reflexly—that is, independent of conscious interaction. This, of course, frees the higher levels of the brain from handling numerous trivial everyday tasks. The distinction between reflex movements and those initiated voluntarily are not always as clear-cut as it might seem from this definition, however. We discussed in Chapter 20 that movements are best classified on a continuous scale from the most automatic to the least automatic. Here we discuss mainly some spinal reflexes that are examples of the **most automatic movements**. Chapters 18 and 22 discuss somewhat less automatic movements, such as postural reflexes and locomotion. Reflexes involving cranial nerve nuclei are discussed in Chapter 27, and some visceral reflexes are covered in Chapter 29.

Even though reflexes differ in many respects, they nevertheless share some **fundamental properties**. Reflexes are stereotyped and constant because the same stimulus always gives the same kind of response. With increasing strength of the stimulus, however, the response usually increases in strength or magnitude. The reflexes are **inborn**: we do not need to learn them from experience. (One example that illustrates the need for inborn motor behavior is the sucking reflex in the newborn child.) Many reflexes occur in large groups of animal species; all mammals, for example, have several reflexes in common. In general, the reflexes are appropriate and useful and ensure that the individual adapts to the environment. Reflexes are also fundamental for reproduction.

Some reflexes are simple with regard to both the stimulus and the response, like the blink reflex (closing of the eye when something touches the cornea). Others are much more complex and require cooperation of many structures, like the swallowing reflex. Some reflexes involve lower parts of the CNS only (spinal cord and brain stem), whereas others involve the higher parts (even the cerebral cortex). Some reflexes are mediated by a chain of only two or three neurons and others by complicated and extensive neuronal networks.

Even though reflexes are independent of our will, some of them can be **suppressed voluntarily** (e.g., the reflexes for emptying the bladder and the rectum). Other reflexes take place without our being aware of them and with no possibility of influencing them voluntarily (like most of the reflexes related to the control of visceral functions).

Conditioned Responses (Reflexes)

True reflexes should not be confused with another kind of automatic behavior, **conditioned** reflexes or, better termed, conditioned responses. In conditioned responses the stimulus evoking a true reflex response (the unconditioned stimulus) is replaced—by learning—by another stimulus. This learning occurs when the unconditioned stimulus (e.g., a puff of air on the cornea, which elicits a blink reflex) is regularly preceded by another kind of stimulus (e.g., a tone; the conditioning stimulus). After some time, the conditioning stimulus will elicit the reflex response even when it is not followed by the unconditioned stimulus. The classical examples are the experiments of the Russian physiologist Pavlov, in which gastric secretion was produced in a dog by ringing a bell (conditioned stimulus). During the learning phase, the bell was always followed by food being presented (unconditioned stimulus). There are many examples from daily life of such conditioned behavioral responses, and conditioning is an important kind of learning. The **cerebellum** appears to be important for conditioning of movements, such as the blink reflex but also movements that involve skeletal muscles.

Some Reflexes "Disappear" during Development

Some reflexes are present only during certain phases of development, such as the **sucking reflex** and the **grasping reflex** in infants. When the reflexes disappear, they are no longer needed and would only disturb voluntary, goal-directed movements. The reflex arcs do not disappear, but higher levels of the CNS suppress the reflex response. That the nervous apparatus persists is witnessed by the persistence or reappearance of primitive reflexes in brain-damaged children and adults.

The Reflex Arc and Basic Features of Reflexes

The structural basis of a reflex is a **reflex arc** (Fig. 21.9), which consists of the following links:

1. A **receptor**, which records the stimulus and "translates" it to action potentials

2. An **afferent link** (a primary sensory neuron), which conducts the action potentials to the CNS

3. A **reflex center**, in which the signals from the receptor may be modified (increased or decreased) by signals from other receptors and other parts of the CNS, where after signals are issued to effectors

4. An **efferent link** (neurons with axons passing out of the CNS), which conducts action potentials to the organ producing the response

Figure 21.9

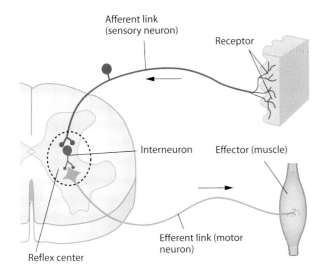

Reflex arc. Schematic. All reflex arcs contain the same elements. The figure shows a spinal reflex arc, with cutaneous nerve endings as receptors and a skeletal muscle as effector. The reflex center has in this example two synapses (a disynaptic reflex).

5. An **effector**, which may be skeletal (striated) muscle, cardiac muscle, smooth muscle (in the wall of vessels and visceral organs), or glands

Reflexes with their reflex center in the spinal cord are called **spinal reflexes**. **Brain stem reflexes**, as the name implies, have their center in the medulla, pons, or mesencephalon; **cortical reflexes** have a reflex center that involves parts of the cerebral cortex. Some reflex arcs are simple, while others that involve coactivation of several muscle groups may be highly complex—with reflex centers that include neurons in the brain stem and in the cord. Most reflex centers include links of several synaptically coupled neurons; such reflexes are called **polysynaptic**. If only one synapse is intercalated between the afferent and the efferent link, the reflex is called **monosynaptic**.

Modulation of Reflex-Center Excitability

Although a reflex response is mediated each time by the same set of neurons, the **excitability** of these neurons can be modified from higher levels of the CNS. This is necessary to adapt individual reflexes to the overall plan for bodily movements. Reflex movements that operate on their own would disturb normal voluntary movements. **Modulation** of the excitability of the reflex center can be exerted by presynaptic inhibition of primary

afferent fibers, by postsynaptic excitatory of inhibitory actions on interneurons and motoneurons, and by efferent control of the sensitivity of some kinds of receptor (cf. γ motoneurons).

SPINAL REFLEXES: THE FLEXION REFLEX AND STRETCH REFLEXES

Here we discuss two different spinal reflexes and their reflex centers in the cord. The first—the **flexion** or **withdrawal reflex**—serves to protect the body; the second, the so-called **stretch reflex** (or rather "stretch reflexes," since there are several varieties), automatically adjusts muscle tension during postural tasks and voluntary movements.

The Flexion Reflex

The flexion reflex is evoked by activation of **nociceptors** in the skin and underlying tissues. For example, when a foot hits a sharp object while walking, the whole leg is immediately withdrawn away from the object (Fig. 21.10). In this case, one or more interneurons are intercalated between the terminals of the afferent sensory fiber and the motoneurons producing the response—that is, the reflex is **polysynaptic**. That this is a reflex is clear from, among other things, the fact that it may be elicited even when the spinal cord is transected above the reflex center. The flexion reflex disappears in deep unconsciousness. For surgery, anesthesia must be sufficiently deep to abolish flexion reflexes.

As mentioned, the **receptors** for the flexion reflex are nociceptors. The **stimulus** usually hits a small spot on the skin, whereas the **response** involves a complex array of muscles (such as extensors of the ankle, flexors of the knee and the hip; Fig. 21.10). Contraction of the muscles in the leg that is withdrawn, however, is not sufficient. Muscles of the other leg must also contract (primarily extensor muscles) to prevent loss of balance. Thus, the stimulus must be distributed to motoneurons in many segments and on both sides of the cord. This happens by way of ascending and descending collaterals of the primary sensory fibers and by way of spinal interneurons (Fig. 21.10). In response to a simple stimulus, a purposeful, harmonious movement occurs, requiring that all the muscles contract at the right time and with the right force. The synaptic couplings in the cord underlying this response must be both complex and precise.

Figure 21.10

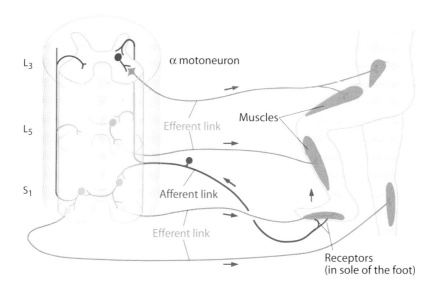

The flexion (withdrawal) reflex. Highly simplified. In this case, several synapses are intercalated between the afferent and the efferent links of the reflex arc. Here nociceptors in the sole of the foot are activated (by walking on a sharp object). The signals are conducted centrally in a sensory fiber (red), which sends out several collaterals and, via interneurons and propriospinal fibers, activates α motoneurons at several segmental levels of the cord. In turn, the motoneurons make many muscles contract to lift the foot off the ground (away from the painful stimulus). At the same time, extensor muscles are activated in the other leg to maintain balance.

A Flexion Reflex Can Be Evoked from Low-Threshold Receptors

Under certain circumstances, several kinds of receptor in the skin, around the joints, or in muscles can elicit a flexion reflex. Common to these receptors is that their signals converge on **interneurons** that excite **flexor motoneurons**. The sensory fibers from such receptors are therefore termed **flexor reflex afferents** (FRAs). Their effects have been most studied in so-called spinal animals (the cord is transected and isolated from the rest of the CNS). Many FRAs lead from low-threshold mechanoreceptors (e.g., group II muscle afferents), while others lead from nociceptors. Normally, the convergence of FRAs on interneurons is believed to ensure necessary **feedback** during ongoing movements—perhaps **rhythmic movements** (e.g., walking) in particular. The term "flexor reflex afferents" is therefore not quite appropriate because many of the FRAs do not normally evoke the protective flexion reflex. In patients with **transverse lesions of the cord** the situation is different, however. Then changes in reflex movements occur in body parts that have been innervated from the cord below the lesion, including forceful and long-lasting contractions of flexor muscles. Such contractions can be elicited by innocuous stimuli, including stimulation of low-threshold mechanoreceptors and thermoreceptors (e.g., a cold washcloth). This is most likely due to abnormal excitability of **interneurons** in receipt of FRA inputs produced by the lack of supraspinal control (see also Chapter 22, under "Spasticity: Possible Mechanisms").

Stretch Reflexes

Under certain circumstances, a muscle responds with a contraction when it is being stretched. (It is easy to see by oneself that stretching a muscle does not always produce a contraction.) When the latency of the contraction is too short to be voluntary, we call this a **stretch reflex**. The most obvious purpose of such a reflex might be to keep the muscle length constant. **Receptors** for stretch reflexes are the **muscle spindles**. Stretch reflexes have been much studied due to their relation to movement control.

We speak of different stretch reflexes because muscle contraction occurring as a result of muscle stretching usually consists of several phases of contractions, each with a different latency as recorded by EMG. The reflex **latency** is the time between the stimulus and the response (between stretch and contraction). It results from the conduction time from the muscle spindles to the spinal cord, the delay at the synapse(s) intercalated between the muscle spindle afferent fibers and the α motoneurons, the conduction time from the motoneurons to the muscle, and the synaptic delay at the motor end plate. Measurement of the latency between the stimulus and the response makes it possible to decide whether a muscle contraction is the result of a **monosynaptic** stretch reflex or whether other—**polysynaptic**—pathways are involved. The monosynaptic stretch reflex, with only one synapse intercalated between the afferent and the efferent link, is the simplest reflex with the shortest latency (Fig. 21.11). Each intercalated synapse increases the latency by a few milliseconds. Thus, muscle contractions occurring with longer latencies after stretching the muscle indicate that there are more neurons intercalated between the afferent link (the sensory fibers) and the motoneurons. That some stretch reflex responses have longer latency than others may not be due only to more synapses intercalated in the reflex center, however. Thus, while the fast monosynaptic reflex depends on signals in the thick group Ia fibers (see Figs. 13.6 and 13.7), slower-conducting group II muscle spindle afferents may contribute to reflex responses with longer latencies.

We discuss the monosynaptic and the polysynaptic stretch reflexes separately next. Much remains to be clarified, however, concerning the role of the stretch reflexes in movement control.

The Monosynaptic Stretch Reflex

The **patellar reflex** (Fig. 21.11)—tested routinely as part of a clinical examination—is probably the best-known example of a stretch reflex. The **stimulus** is a tap on the patellar ligament (the tendon of the quadriceps muscle). The **response** is a contraction of the quadriceps muscle, thus producing a brief extension movement at the knee joint. The reflex arc is shown schematically in Fig. 21.11, and it can be seen that only one synapse is intercalated in the reflex center—that is, the reflex is **monosynaptic**. The **receptors** are the muscle spindles in the quadriceps muscle that is stretched; the **afferent link** is constituted by the Ia fibers, which end in the spinal cord with some collaterals ending directly (monosynaptically) on the α motoneurons supplying the quadriceps muscle. The axons of the α motoneurons constitute the **efferent link**, which at the motor end plate activates the extrafusal fibers of the quadriceps muscle (the effector). For the patellar reflex, the **latency** between the stimulus and the start of the contraction (as recorded with EMG) is about 30 msec, and a slightly shorter latency pertains to reflexes in the upper arm muscles because of a shorter peripheral pathway—for example, the **biceps reflex** has a latency of about 25 msec.

To evoke a muscle contraction through this simple reflex arc, the muscle must be stretched rapidly—that is, by phasic stretching. The actual lengthening produced by the stimulus may be very little; the salient point is the **velocity** of stretching. As discussed in Chapter 13, the group Ia afferents of the muscle spindles are especially sensitive to the velocity of stretching, so that even a brief stimulus, such as stretching the muscle only a fraction of a millimeter, produces a brisk response. A tap on a tendon with a reflex hammer produces this kind of stimulus, although it is far from being a natural stimulus. Because both the stimulus and the response last only for a very short time, we use the term **phasic stretch reflex**.

The monosynaptic stretch reflex can be elicited in most skeletal muscles but much more easily in some muscles than in others. There are also **individual differences**: in some healthy persons, phasic stretch reflexes cannot be elicited.

The Jendrássik Maneuver and Strengthening of the Monosynaptic Stretch Reflex

As mentioned, in some healthy persons the monosynaptic reflex cannot be elicited by ordinary tendon taps with a reflex hammer. Absent stretch reflexes may also be due to lesions of the

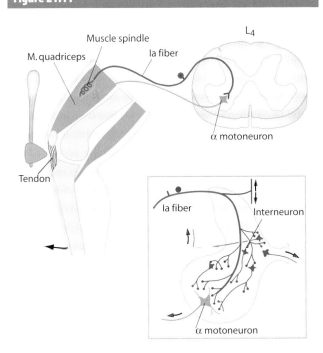

Figure 21.11

Stretch reflex. The patellar reflex is used here as an example of a monosynaptic reflex—that is, with only one synapse intercalated between the afferent and the efferent link. The stimulus is a tap on the patellar ligament below the patella, which stretches the muscle. The response is a brief muscle contraction. **Bottom right:** The Ia fiber from the muscle spindle contacts the motoneurons monosynaptically, but it also contacts many interneurons. Some of these are excitatory, mediating a polysynaptic activation of some motoneurons; other interneurons are inhibitory, mediating inhibition of other motoneurons.

A striking property of the long-latency stretch reflex is that the strength of the response depends to a very high degree on whether the muscle is relaxed or **active** at the time of stretching. If the muscle is relaxed or only slightly active when stretched, there is usually no long-latency reflex response at all. Further, the strength of the response depends on **prior instruction** to the subject with regard to whether to resist the imposed stretch or to let go. When the person is asked to let go when an imposed movement (at an unpredictable time) stretches the muscle (e.g., an imposed extension at the elbow that stretches the biceps muscle), the reflex response is much smaller than when the person is asked to resist the imposed movement. Thus, the magnitude of the reflex response seems to be adapted to what is functionally appropriate in a particular situation.

A further characteristic of the long-latency stretch reflex is that the strength of the response may change during **learning** of a motor task. Thus, by repeated trials, the reflex response becomes weaker in muscles in which a contraction in response to stretching is functionally inappropriate and stronger in muscles in which a contraction is appropriate. This learning effect, or adaptation of the stretch reflex, occurs only in connection with the particular learned movement; in connection with other movements, the reflex response of the muscle is unaltered.

As mentioned, the **monosynaptic stretch reflex** is also subject to similar learned, task-related modulation, but the changes appear to be smaller than those obtained with the long-latency reflex. Although synaptic changes are widespread in the cord, altered **presynaptic inhibition** of the Ia terminals on the α motoneurons seems to be of particular importance for modulation of the monosynaptic stretch reflex.

Is the Long-Latency Stretch Reflex Mediated by the Cerebral Cortex?

The exact central pathway followed by the impulses mediating the long-latency stretch reflex has been much debated. Indirect data indicate that the reflex pathway may involve the motor cortex of the cerebral cortex (therefore, the term "long-loop stretch reflex" is often used). In support of a **transcortical** route are observations that the reflex is weakened or abolished by lesions of the descending motor pathways or by lesions of the dorsal columns (presumably carrying the signals from the muscle spindles to the cerebral cortex). Further, the reflex is often weakened after lesions of the **cerebellum**. But such findings may also be explained by a purely spinal reflex that is under strong supraspinal control.

More decisive evidence of a transcortical route for the long-latency stretch reflex—at least regarding certain muscle groups—comes from observations in a few patients with a peculiar inborn abnormality of the pyramidal tract. These persons always perform **mirror movements** of the hands; asked to flex the index finger of the left hand, they always flex the right index finger as well (more proximal movements, e.g., of the shoulders, are performed normally). This behavior appears from electrophysiologic studies to be caused by branching of individual pyramidal tract axons to supply motoneurons of both sides of the spinal cord. Thus, stimulation of the hand region of the motor cortex of one hemisphere causes symmetrical movements of both hands (unlike the normal situation, in which such stimulation always causes movements of the opposite hand only). When eliciting stretch reflexes in such subjects, the monosynaptic reflex occurs only on the same side as the stretch is applied (as normal), whereas the long-latency stretch reflex occurs in both hands after a unilateral stimulus. The latter observation is hard to explain unless the reflex arc of the long-latency reflex involves the pyramidal tract.

These findings may not pertain to long-latency stretch reflexes in all muscle groups. For example, the reflexes appear to be transcortical for distal arm muscles but not (or to a lesser degree) for proximal arm muscles and muscles in the foot. For these latter muscles, the long-latency reflex may be elicited by **group II muscle afferents**, which conduct with about half the velocity of group Ia fibers.

The Function of Stretch Reflexes

One might think that the stretch reflexes—which, after all, are relatively simple—are well understood with regard to their functional roles. For example, the muscle spindles and the motoneurons are among the best-characterized receptors and central neurons, respectively. Nevertheless, we still do not fully understand the role of the stretch reflexes in the control of voluntary movements and in the control of posture and muscle tone. We discuss here only some possible functions.

As mentioned, one likely task of the stretch reflex is to ensure that the **length** of a muscle is kept constant. In many situations, this is of obvious importance—for example, in the upright position when some external perturbation threatens the **body balance**. The sudden displacement of the center of gravity forward stretches the extensor muscles of the back and thus might elicit a stretch reflex tending to resume the former position. It is furthermore an obvious advantage that such a corrective contraction occurs as quickly as possible. Making such an adjustment depend only on voluntary contraction would lengthen the latency fourfold, with the danger of the corrections occurring too late. Also while **walking**—when external perturbations may disturb the programmed pattern of muscular activity—stretch reflexes may contribute to rapid adjustments. Nevertheless, it is not clear to what extent stretch reflexes really participate in such adjustments. (See Chapter 18, under "More about Receptor Types and Their Contribution to Postural Control.")

Another situation in which stretch reflexes may be of importance is during slow, **precise voluntary movements** when the external opposing forces change unpredictably. Again, the advantage would be that the adjustment of muscle tension occurs much earlier than can be achieved by voluntary action alone. (See Chapter 13, under "Proprioceptors, Balance, and Voluntary Movements.")

Stretch Reflexes May Correct for Change in External Resistance during Precision Movements

Studies of slow movements of the thumb by the British neurologist David Marsden have shed light on the contribution of stretch reflexes during precision movements. The subject is asked to flex the thumb with a constant speed against an external opposing force of constant magnitude. The EMG of the flexor pollicis longus muscle is recorded continuously. The external force is then changed suddenly at unpredictable times during the movement—either increased or reduced. When the external force is increased, the movement is immediately slowed down. Because of the **α–γ coactivation** (see Chapter 13, under "Muscle Spindles in Humans and α–γ Coactivation"), the frequency of signals from the muscle spindle increases. The α–γ coactivation ensures that, as the muscle shortens due to the activation of the α motoneurons, the spindle midportion is stretched. This upholds the firing of muscle spindle afferents in spite of the shortening, which otherwise would have led to reduced firing. To keep up with the steadily shortening muscle, the firing of the γ motoneurons must also increase steadily. When the movement is suddenly halted or slowed down, the firing frequency of the γ motoneurons continues increasing, in anticipation of further shortening of the muscle. Thus, for a moment, the firing of the muscle spindle afferents increases more than what is appropriate with regard to the actual length of the muscle. This increases the excitation of the γ motoneurons, and their firing increases, thus increasing the force of the muscle contraction. The result is that the increased external force is rapidly compensated for, and the original speed of the movement is resumed.

When the opposing external force is suddenly reduced, the opposite events take place. The speed of the flexion movement of the thumb increases, and the firing frequency of the spindle afferents decreases for a moment, thus reducing the firing of the α motoneurons and the force of contraction. The speed of movement is adjusted.

It is probable that the stretch reflex functions in this manner especially during **slow precision movements** when we cannot accurately predict the external force at all times. The sensitivity of the muscle spindles is kept at a high level, so that they may record even the slightest perturbations and ensure that the activity of the α motoneurons is adjusted appropriately.

Cutaneous Receptors and the Precision Grip

In some situations, stimulation of low-threshold skin **mechanoreceptors** causes reflex muscular contraction. For example, when (during a precision grip with the fingers) the object slips, a reflex increase of the grip force occurs. The latency from the start of the slip to the muscular response is only 60 to 80 msec—that is, too short to be mediated by a voluntary command. Examination of patients with reduced cutaneous sensation but normal motor apparatus suggests that loss of such rapid, reflex adjustment of the grip force is partly responsible for their difficulties with precision movements (see Chapter 13, under "Clinical Examples of Loss of Somatosensory Information").

Central Modulation of Reflexes

It should be clear from the preceding discussion that stretching of a muscle does not necessarily elicit a reflex contraction. Many factors influence whether there will be a response, such as the velocity of stretching and whether the muscle is active when being stretched. Further, the response depends heavily on whether a reflex contraction is functionally appropriate. Such **gain modulation** of the stretch reflex is mediated by descending connections from higher levels of the CNS (e.g., from the motor cortex). It appears to be exerted mostly by a precise control of the excitability of specific sets of **spinal interneurons**, which are intercalated in particular reflex arcs. In addition, **presynaptic inhibition** may very selectively "switch off" the input from specific sets of receptors. Thus, reflex arcs may be "opened" or "closed" in accordance with the need of the overall plan for movements (Fig. 21.15). Obviously, the motor programs in the cerebral cortex and the brain stem specify not only the muscular activity but also the gain of spinal reflex arcs at any moment.

Also, the gain of the **flexion reflex** is under some degree of supraspinal control. This is evident during walking, when a flexion reflex may cause a fall. Thus, noxious stimulation of the sole of the foot elicits a brisk flexion reflex if the leg is in the swing phase, whereas the response is weak or absent when the foot is used for support. Interestingly, this kind of modulation appears not to be present in four-legged animals, presumably because their balance is less vulnerable to changing the support of one leg only.

Examples of Stretch Reflex Modulation during Voluntary Movements

Reflex modulation has been studied most during **locomotion** in humans and is found in several muscle groups. Thus, the strength of reflex contractions in many leg muscles depends on whether the leg is in the swing or in the stance phase. In the ankle flexors (*musculus triceps surae*), for example, stretch reflexes are weak or of the muscle. It should be noted that in **diseases** affecting motor neurons, the muscles exhibit more or less pronounced changes of their viscoelastic properties.

In conclusion, individual differences in resting muscle tone among healthy persons may in some cases be caused by differences in the degree of relaxation. In addition, there are most likely individual differences with regard to the passive viscoelastic properties of the muscles.

Changes of Muscle Tone in Disease

Pathologically changed muscle tone is called **hypotonia** when it is lower than normal and **hypertonia** when higher than normal. Of course to recognize abnormal muscle tone one must first be able to decide what is normal, but from the preceding discussion, it should be clear that "normal muscle tone" is not a precise, well-defined concept. The decision as to whether a muscle has a normal tone is based largely on the subjective judgment of the examiner. This judgment, of course, depends on experience. Whereas hypertonia may be identified with reasonable certainty and even measured in semiquantitative terms by stretching the muscles, the decision as to whether a muscle has abnormally low tone is more difficult. As mentioned, a normal, fully relaxed muscle will have a very low tension when tested by stretching. Some authors believe that when paretic or paralytic muscles feel softer and more flaccid than normal muscle, it is because of lack of voluntary contraction, which probably occurs to some extent during passive movements and palpation. Indeed, experiments measuring the resistance to passive stretching of normal and alleged hypotonic muscles did not show consistent differences. The experiments were performed by measuring the falling time of the leg (passive flexion of the knee) in healthy persons with the ability to relax fully (determined with EMG) and in patients with pareses of the quadriceps muscle (clinically judged as hypotonic). On the other hand, the individual differences in falling time—that is, muscle tone—among the normal subjects were fairly large, presumably because of differences in the passive viscoelastic properties, as discussed previously.

Nevertheless, with **peripheral pareses**, rapid changes of the passive viscoelastic properties of the muscles may occur, which may help explain why the paretic muscles feel softer on palpation. After damage to peripheral motoneurons, the muscles waste rapidly, reducing the muscle volume to sometimes only 20% to 30% of normal in about 3 months. The metabolism of muscle cells is obviously dramatically altered by loss of contact between nerve and muscle.

Muscle Cramps and Plateau Potentials

Cramps are sudden, involuntary, and painful muscle contractions. The person notices that a part of the muscle becomes tight. Cramps may occur in **healthy people** during sleep, in pregnancy, and after fatiguing muscular exercise. Cramps may also occur in diseases such as **neuropathies, amyotrophic lateral sclerosis** (ALS), and **vascular diseases**. Stretching the muscle is often the most efficient way to stop the contraction. **Exercise-associated muscle cramps** in particular have been subject to much research and speculation. Three possible explanations are most commonly considered: dehydration, electrolyte depletion, and altered neuromuscular control. The latter seems to have the best scientific support. The fact that cramps cannot be induced in a curarized muscle (curare blocking the neuromuscular transmission) strongly suggest that, whatever the cause, it is not to be found in the muscle cells. With regard to neuromuscular control, some data indicate that local factors induce spontaneous depolarization of the nerve endings, while the best evidence favors abnormal behavior of the α motoneurons. For example, it was shown many years ago that the kinds of cramps mentioned here can be caused by high-frequency **firing of α motoneurons**. An interesting possibility is that cramps arise because of the motoneurons' ability to form **plateau potentials**, as characterized by a stable depolarized state (see Chapter 3, under "Plateau Potentials," and Chapter 22, under "Monoaminergic Pathways from the Brain Stem to the Spinal Cord" and "Spasticity: Possible Mechanisms"). In this state, a brief excitatory input can trigger a train of action potential lasting for many seconds or even minutes. Experimentally, a brief train of signals in Ia fibers from the muscle spindles can cause sustained motoneuron firing and cramps, possibly because of induction of plateau potentials, but any excitatory input would presumably have the same effect. The plateau potential can be terminated by a brief hyperpolarizing synaptic input.

Whether plateau potentials occur in muscle cramps in humans is unknown, but if they do, why they are induced at rest in some healthy persons needs to be explained. Conceivably, increased extracellular K^+ due to intense motoneuronal firing during endurance exercise may elicit plateau potentials. Another possibility is that plateau potentials are triggered by altered inputs to motoneurons during muscular fatigue—for example, by increased muscle spindle afferent activity and reduced presynaptic inhibition. That stretching and sometimes massage terminates cramps might be due to stimulation of afferent inputs that inhibit motoneurons (via interneurons). Ia afferents are unlikely to be activated in this situation, as they respond poorly to slow stretching of the muscle. Electrical stimulation of the tendon inhibits experimentally evoked muscle cramps, suggesting that stretching of the cramped muscle works by activation of 1b afferents from the tendon organ.

So-called **writer's cramp** is a task-specific **focal dystonia** of the hand. The cramp usually occurs when trying to do a task that requires fine-motor movements. In this case, it is believed that basal-ganglia dysfunction lies behind the abnormal motoneuronal firing.

Abnormally increased muscle tone, or **hypertonia**, would imply that the muscles continuously have an increased tone, in spite of attempts to relax. As mentioned, many healthy persons are not able to relax completely, at least not in an examination situation, and the line between normal and pathologically increased muscle tone may not be easy to draw. Fairly characteristic disturbances of muscle tone do occur in certain diseases of the CNS, however.

Spasticity and Rigidity

The term **spasticity** is used in clinical neurology of a condition in which there is increased resistance against the rapid stretching of muscles. Spasticity occurs after damage to the descending motor pathways from the cerebral cortex to the motoneurons (Fig. 21.16) and is probably due primarily to changed excitability among spinal interneurons (spasticity is discussed in more depth in Chapter 22). By palpation, the muscles may feel normal or hypotonic, and there may not be increased resistance against slow, passive movements. The increased resistance to rapid stretch is most likely caused by abnormally brisk monosynaptic stretch reflexes, whereas the long-latency stretch reflexes are weaker than normal.

Rigidity is the term used to characterize the increased muscle tone occurring in **Parkinson's disease** (Chapter 23). Even with very slow, passive movements, an increased, "cogwheel"-like resistance is felt by the examiner. This may be caused by increased **long-latency stretch reflexes** that are elicited by abnormally slow movements.

Along with rigidity and spasticity, there is evidence of changed passive **viscoelastic properties** (in addition to the changed stretch reflexes). Thus, in patients with moderately severe Parkinson's disease, increased resistance to slow elbow extension was found, even though there was no EMG activity of the biceps muscle (which was being stretched). In some spastic patients, increased resistance even to slow stretching of relaxed leg muscles was present, but only when the spasticity had lasted for more than a year. Thus, it seems as though an altered pattern of signals from the motoneurons—like those occurring in diseases with rigidity or spasticity—may change the passive, viscoelastic properties of the muscles.

INJURY OF PERIPHERAL MOTOR NEURONS AND REGENERATION

When all motoneurons (or their axons) supplying a muscle are destroyed, the muscle cannot be made to contract: it is **paralyzed** (Fig. 21.16). Both voluntary and reflex movements are abolished. If not all of the motoneurons (or their axons) supplying a muscle are destroyed, the muscle can still contract, although with less speed and force than normal. This is called a partial paralysis, or **paresis**. The muscle cells that no longer receive signals from the motoneurons undergo **atrophy**—that is, they become thinner and eventually disappear if no reinnervation takes place (see later discussion).

Peripheral and Central Pareses

The muscle weakness caused by the loss of the α motoneurons or their axons (**lower motor neurons**) is called a **peripheral paralysis** (paresis) to distinguish it from a **central paralysis** caused by interruption of the central motor pathways (the upper motor neurons). Central pareses are discussed in Chapter 22. Suffice it here to mention that in central pareses the spinal reflex arcs are intact (Fig. 21.16). This means that flexion reflexes and stretch reflexes can be elicited. Characteristic of peripheral pareses—apart from the weakened or abolished voluntary contractions—is that the muscles are flaccid, reflex movements are weakened or abolished, and muscle wasting progresses rapidly and becomes marked.

In cases of peripheral pareses, the **distribution** of affected muscles may tell us where the disease process is located. For example, the distribution will differ depending on whether the lesion is located in the spinal cord, in the plexuses formed by the spinal nerves, or in the peripheral nerves more peripherally (Fig. 21.2). As a rule, one muscle

Figure 21.16

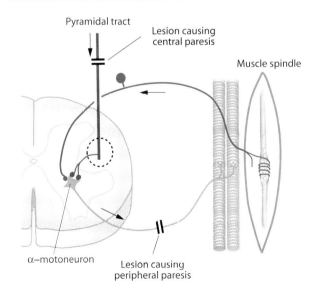

Peripheral and central pareses. Lesions of the motoneurons produce peripheral pareses, characterized by loss of both voluntary and reflex contractions. Central pareses—characterized by loss of voluntary movements but retained reflex contractions—ensue when descending corticospinal pathways are interrupted.

22 The Motor Cortical Areas and Descending Pathways

OVERVIEW

This chapter deals with the control of complex, purposeful movements—from those that are largely automatic to those that require our full attention. The most direct control is exerted by **upper motor neurons** in the cerebral cortex and the brain stem that send fibers to end in direct synaptic contact with the **lower motor neurons** (motoneurons) or with interneurons that, in turn, contact the motoneurons. (The basal ganglia and the cerebellum—both necessary for proper motor control without being responsible for movement initiation—are discussed in the next two chapters.) The **pyramidal tract** is the only **direct** pathway from the cerebral cortex to the lower motor neurons in the brain stem and the spinal cord. The pyramidal tract is indispensable for the ability to perform precise, voluntary movements of the hands (requiring fractionate finger movements), whereas more proximal movements can be performed although with less speed and precision in the absence of the pyramidal tract. For the latter kind of movement, several **indirect** pathways—synaptically interrupted in the brain stem—are especially important. The **corticoreticulospinal** pathways are important for maintaining the upright position (posture), for orienting movements of the body toward external events, and for fairly crude, stereotyped voluntary movements of the extremities. Nevertheless, both the direct and the indirect pathways participate, to a varying degree, in virtually all voluntary movements. The sharing of tasks among them is such that cell groups in the brain stem can largely on their own control many automatic movements, whereas the participation of the cortex increases with increasing degrees of voluntary control.

Reticulospinal and vestibulospinal pathways are of special importance for the more **automatic movements**, such as postural adjustments and locomotion. Rhythmic movements, such as locomotion and respiration, depend on the activity of **rhythm generators** in the spinal cord and the brain stem. With regard to locomotion, there is most likely one spinal rhythm generator for each extremity. Supraspinal control of locomotion depends on a **mesencephalic locomotor region** (MLR). A contribution from the motor cortex is necessary if the ground is uneven and unpredictable.

We also discuss **motor cortical areas**—that is, areas that participate in planning and organizing movements. Many parts of the cortex are motor in this respect, but we usually restrict the term to the **primary motor cortex** (MI) in the precentral gyrus, the **premotor area** (PMA) just in front of MI, and the **supplementary motor area** (SMA) on the medial aspect of the hemisphere. The MI gives origin to a large part of the pyramidal tract fibers and has monosynaptic connections with the motoneurons in the brain stem and spinal cord. The PMA and SMA act largely by "instructing" the MI what to do. Whereas lesions of the MI produce pareses, lesions of the PMA and SMA cause difficulties with initiation of movements and with purposeful movements that require coordinated sequences of muscle contractions. **Posterior parietal cortex** and regions in the **prefrontal cortex** are necessary for transforming sensory information into action and for selection of actions that are behaviorally appropriate.

The final part of the chapter deals with symptoms resulting from **damage** to the central motor pathways. The main characteristics of central pareses—such as **hyperreflexia** (spasticity) and **loss of dexterity**—are described and some tentative explanations offered.

THE PYRAMIDAL TRACT (THE CORTICOSPINAL TRACT)

The pyramidal tract is of crucial importance for our ability to perform precise, voluntary movements. The tract consists of axons of neurons with their cell bodies in the cerebral cortex, as indicated by its other name, the **corticospinal tract**. The axons descend through the internal capsule, the crus cerebri (*cerebral peduncle*), the pons, and the medulla

what we regard as the most important components in control of voluntary movements.

Figure 22.1

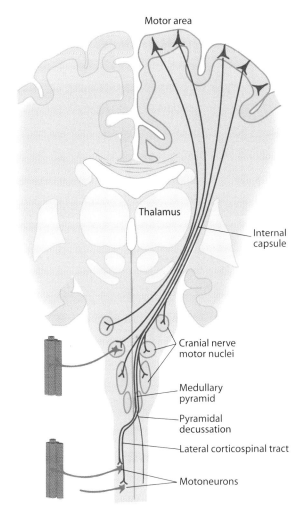

Motor area

Thalamus

Internal capsule

Cranial nerve motor nuclei

Medullary pyramid

Pyramidal decussation

Lateral corticospinal tract

Motoneurons

Direct corticobulbar and corticospinal pathways (the pyramidal tract). The corticospinal tract is mainly crossed, whereas many of the cranial nerve nuclei receive crossed and uncrossed corticobulbar fibers. Note the crossing of the corticospinal tract in the lower medulla.

(Figs. 22.1, 22.2, and 22.3A). Most of the fibers cross to the other side in the lowermost part of the medulla and continue downward in the lateral funiculus of the cord, to finally establish synaptic contacts in the spinal gray matter.

"The Extrapyramidal System"

Customarily, a division has been made between the pyramidal (corticospinal) tract and other nuclei and tracts involved in motor control. The latter have often been collectively called the "**extrapyramidal system**." So many parts of the brain contribute in different ways to motor control, however, that lumping them together in a "system" confuses more than it clarifies. Therefore, we do not use the term "extrapyramidal" here but rather describe

Fibers also leave the pyramidal tract on their way through the brain stem, to reach cranial nerve motor nuclei (Figs. 22.1 and 22.3A). Such fibers form part of the **corticobulbar tract** (other corticobulbar fibers reach the red nucleus, the pontine nuclei, the reticular formation, the colliculi, the dorsal column nuclei, and other nuclei).

The pyramidal tract derives its name from the **pyramid** of the medulla, which is formed by the fibers of the corticospinal tract (see Figs. 6.15 and 6.16). Strictly speaking, therefore, the term "pyramidal tract" encompasses only the fibers destined for the spinal cord and not those bound for the cranial nerve motor nuclei. Nevertheless, for practical reasons both groups are usually included in the term.

Origin of the Pyramidal Tract

The cell bodies of all neurons of the pyramidal tract lie in the cortical **fifth layer** (lamina V; compare Figs. 22.4 and 33.1) and are called **pyramidal cells**. The name refers to the shape of the cell body (see Figs. 1.1, 33.1, and 33.6).

A large proportion of the fibers of the pyramidal tract comes from neurons with their cell bodies in the **precentral gyrus**—that is, **area 4** of Brodmann (Figs. 22.4 and 22.5; see also Fig. 33.4). This region is called the **primary motor area** (MI) because muscle contractions can most easily (with the weakest current) be elicited from this part of the cerebral cortex. The **somatotopic organization** of the MI (Fig. 22.5) has been verified in humans with various kinds of stimulation and imaging techniques (electric and magnetic stimulation, positron emission tomography [PET], functional magnetic resonance imaging [fMRI]). It corresponds roughly to the somatotopic pattern in the primary somatosensory cortex (SI; see Fig. 14.8). We return to the MI later in this chapter.

It was originally thought that all fibers of the pyramidal tract came from area 4 and from only the cells with the largest cell bodies, the **giant cells of Betz**. The number of Betz cells, however, is much too low to account for the number of axons in the pyramidal tract (about 1 million in humans). More recent studies with retrograde transport of tracer substances (Fig. 22.4) have largely clarified the origin of the pyramidal tract in various animals. In the monkey, numerous cells in area 4, in addition to the Betz cells, contribute to

Figure 22.2

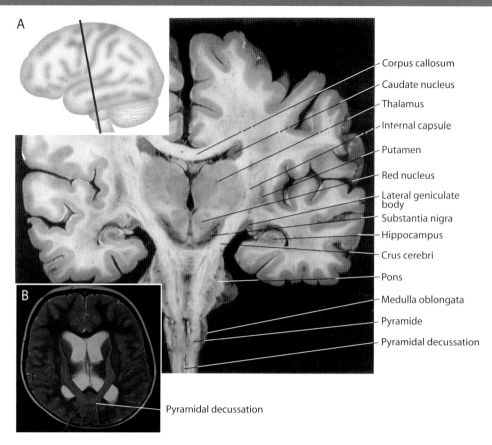

A

Corpus callosum
Caudate nucleus
Thalamus
Internal capsule
Putamen
Red nucleus
Lateral geniculate body
Substantia nigra
Hippocampus
Crus cerebri
Pons
Medulla oblongata
Pyramide
Pyramidal decussation

B

Pyramidal decussation

Course of the pyramidal tract through the internal capsule and the brain stem. **A:** Frontal, unstained section through the brain and brainstem. Longitudinal bundles of myelinated fibers are evident in the crus, the pons, and the medullary pyramid. Compare with Fig. 22.13. **B:** MRI tractography showing the course of the pyramidal tract (blue) and its decussation in the medulla. Oblique-horizontal plane of sectioning. (Courtesy of Dr. Baard Nedregaard, Oslo University Hospital, Oslo, Norway.)

Figure 22.3

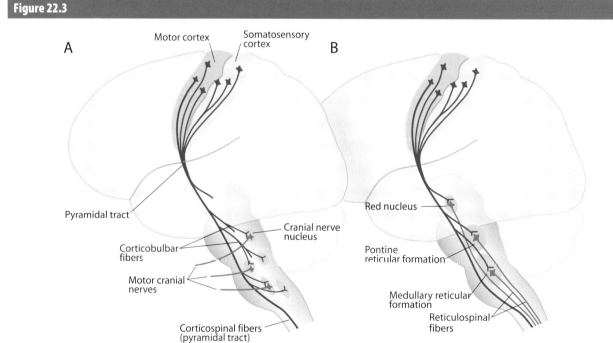

A

Motor cortex
Somatosensory cortex

B

Pyramidal tract
Cranial nerve nucleus
Corticobulbar fibers
Motor cranial nerves
Corticospinal fibers (pyramidal tract)

Red nucleus
Pontine reticular formation
Medullary reticular formation
Reticulospinal fibers

Direct and indirect motor pathways to the spinal cord. **A:** The pyramidal tract passes directly from the cerebral cortex to the motoneurons in the brain stem (corticobulbar fibers) and in the spinal cord (corticospinal fibers). **B:** Nuclei in the brain stem with efferent connections acting on motoneurons. Indirect corticospinal pathways are established by corticofugal connections to the brain stem nuclei.

Figure 22.4

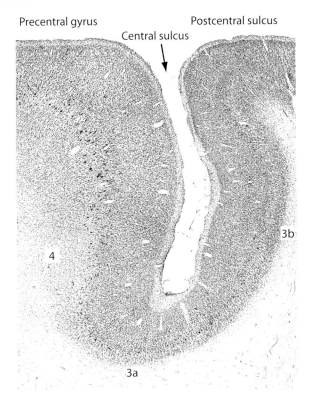

The central region with MI (primary motor area) and SI (somatosensory area). Photomicrograph of a section perpendicular to the central sulcus (monkey). There is a notable difference in thickness between the MI and the SI. The dark dots in the deep parts of the cortex (in layer 5) are the cell bodies of pyramidal tract cells that have been retrogradely labeled by an injection of a tracer substance (horseradish peroxidase) in the spinal cord. There are more labeled cells in the MI than in the SI.

Figure 22.5

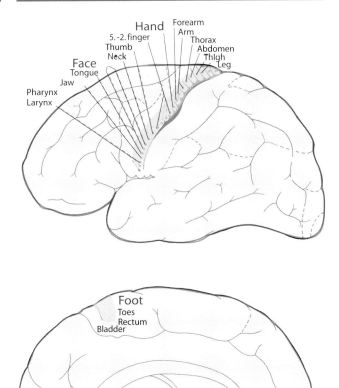

Somatotopic organization of the motor cortex. The points indicate the sites from which muscle contraction in a particular body part was produced by weak electrical stimulation. (Based on Foerster 1936.)

Figure 22.6

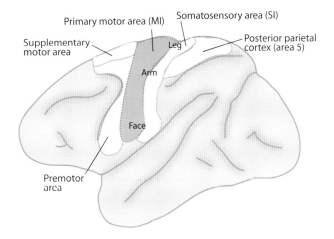

Cortical regions giving origin to the pyramidal tract. Based on experimental studies in monkeys with retrograde transport of tracer substances (cf. Fig. 22.4). The MI has the highest density of pyramidal tract neurons, that is, neurons that are retrogradely labeled from the spinal cord. Lower densities of labeled neurons occur in the SI, SMA, PMA, and posterior parietal cortex.

the pyramidal tract, as do many cells in areas outside area 4. Although the relative contribution from various areas differ among researchers, it seems that about two-thirds of all fibers arise in front of the central sulcus—that is, in area 4 and **area 6** (PMA and SMA in Fig. 22.6), whereas the rest comes from the **SI** (areas 3, 1, 2), **SII**, and parts of the **posterior parietal cortex** (area 5). A considerable fraction of the fibers from the SI arise in **area 3a**—that is, the part of the SI adjacent to area 4 (Fig. 22.4) that receives an input from muscle spindles.

Muscle contractions can also be elicited from the areas outside the MI, such as the SI, by electrical stimulation, but the stimulation must be more intense than in area MI. This reflects that the pyramidal tract fibers from the SI and the other regions outside area 4 have less direct access to the motoneurons than the neurons in area 4. The pyramidal tract fibers coming from the SI and area 5 are probably more concerned with the control of sensory signal transmission than with the initiation of movements.

Course and Crossing of the Pyramidal Tract

As mentioned, the pyramidal tract passes downward through the **internal capsule**. It occupies a posterior position (Fig. 22.7A), as judged from observations after small lesions (Fig. 22.13) and stimulation during brain surgery of the internal capsule in humans. (It was formerly assumed that the pyramidal tract fibers were spread over a large part of the "posterior leg" of the internal capsule.) Fibers governing the muscles of the face are believed to lie most anteriorly and the leg most posteriorly. Experimental studies in monkeys indicate that descending fibers from the **PMA** and **SMA** lie in the "knee" region (genu) and the "anterior leg" of the internal capsule, respectively. The internal capsule contains many other fibers than those of the pyramidal tract; the latter constitute only a minority. For example, **sensory fibers** ascend from the thalamus to the cortex, and descending fibers from the cortex reach the thalamus, the reticular formation, and other cell groups of the brain stem. Further, in the anterior part of the internal capsule lie the **pallidothalamic** fibers (related to motor functions of the basal ganglia), and posteriorly (in the lower part) the **optic radiation** passes through on its way to the occipital lobe. Therefore, **damage** of the internal capsule—such as an infarction caused by occlusion of an artery—may produce sensory and other deficits

Figure 22.7

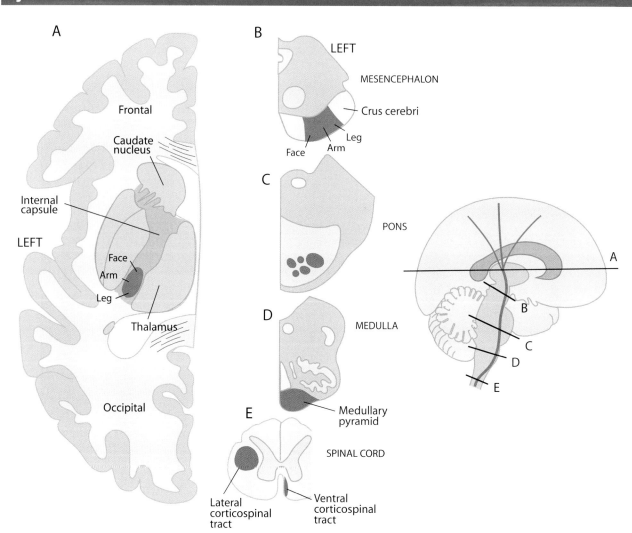

Position and somatotopic pattern of the pyramidal tract at various levels. **A:** Horizontal section (cf. Fig. 6.30). **B–E:** Transverse sections. Compare with Figs. 14.2, 14.3, and 14.4 showing the positions of the somatosensory tracts at the same levels.

in addition to pareses of the muscles of the opposite body half (capsular **hemiplegia**).

In the **mesencephalon**, the pyramidal tract fibers distribute over the middle two-thirds of the crus and mix with other descending fibers (Fig. 22.7B). As mentioned, all of the corticospinal fibers are collected within the **medullary pyramid** (Fig. 22.6D; see also Fig. 6.17). At the caudalmost level of the medulla, most of the corticospinal fibers **cross** the midline and continue in the **lateral funicle** of the cord as the **lateral corticospinal tract** (Figs. 22.7E and 22.8). A small contingent continues, without crossing, downward in the ventral funicle as the **ventral corticospinal tract**. Some uncrossed fibers may also pass in the lateral funicle (Fig. 22.8).

Pyramidal-tract actions on the muscles of the **distal extremities** are mediated almost exclusively by fibers that

cross in the lower medulla. This is supported by studies in humans with transcranial magnetic stimulation of the motor cortex. The small contingent of uncrossed (and doubly crossed) fibers mentioned earlier can influence mainly **axial muscles**—that is, muscles of the back, the thorax, and the abdomen. This is in accordance with their termination medially in the ventral horn (Fig. 22.8; also see Fig. 21.3).

The pyramidal tract fibers that control the **muscles of the head** (the face, tongue, pharynx, and larynx) leave the corticospinal fibers in the brain stem to end in or close to the motor and sensory cranial nerve nuclei (Figs. 22.1 and 22.3). Apart from the facial muscles of the lower part of the face, muscles of the head generally receive both crossed and uncrossed pyramidal tract fibers. Thus, when the pyramidal tract fibers are interrupted in the internal capsule, there are seldom clear-cut pareses of the muscles of the tongue, the pharynx, and the larynx, whereas the corner of the mouth hangs down on the opposite side of the lesion.

Individual Variations in the Position and Crossing of the Pyramidal Tract

There are considerable individual variations in both the distribution of the pyramidal tract fibers in the spinal white matter and the percentage of uncrossed fibers. Nathan et al. (1990) reexamined these clinically important matters and found, for example, that the corticospinal fibers are more widely distributed in the lateral funicle than is depicted in textbooks. Thus, such fibers are usually found also ventral to the level of the central canal (Fig. 22.7E is probably reasonably accurate in this respect). Equally important for the interpretation of symptoms in patients with spinal cord injuries is that the anteroposterior location of the lateral tract shows considerable individual variations.

The majority of the corticospinal fibers cross in most individuals, and it is customary to say that there are about **15% uncrossed** fibers. The great individual variations emphasize that this is only an average number, however. Indeed, in a few individuals the pyramidal tract is completely crossed with all fibers located dorsally in the lateral funicle, or it is completely uncrossed with all fibers in the ventral funicle. As a rule, most of the uncrossed fibers continue in the ventral funicle as the ventral corticospinal tract (Fig. 22.5), whereas some join the crossed fibers from the other side in the lateral funicle (Fig. 22.8). Some fibers cross twice, and many individuals have a small crossed, ventral component. The division of uncrossed fibers between the lateral and the ventral funicles varies among individuals.

Finally, although usually not acknowledged, in about 75% of the population the pyramidal tract is **asymmetric**: the lateral and the ventral components are both larger on one side than on the other (most often on the right side). This asymmetry presumably arises because a larger proportion of the fibers from (usually) the left hemisphere cross than from the right hemisphere. Thus, the lateral (crossed) tract becomes larger on the right side than on the left, whereas the ventral (uncrossed) tract becomes smaller on the left side.

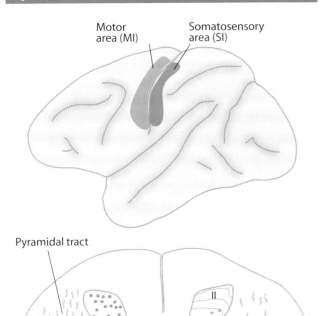

Terminal regions of the pyramidal tract. Based on experiments in monkeys with anterograde transport of radioactively labeled amino acids after injections in various parts of the MI and the SI. Corticospinal fibers from the MI end more anteriorly in the gray matter of the cord than those from the SI. The uncrossed fibers end predominantly medially in the ventral horn—that is, in contact with the motoneurons that supply axial and proximal muscles. (Based on Ralston and Ralston 1985.)

with an **internal model** of the motor task facing us. The sensory information serves to update the internal representations so they fit the present situation. Internal models are thought to serve as frames of reference for the continuous monitoring and adjustment of our posture. Selection of an overall motor response is done on the basis of the central processing of the sensory information. However, the final motor command depends not only on the sensory signals but also on the **context** in which they arise. Therefore, a certain sensory input can elicit very different postural responses in different situations. Mainly **reticulospinal** and **vestibulospinal** fiber tracts mediate the final postural commands.

The postural reflexes operate on a **feedback** basis: they are responses to movements that have already started. In conjunction with voluntary movements, however, commands about postural adjustments are issued in **advance**. From prior experience, the brain has determined which adjustments will be needed to keep balance during, for example, an arm movement. This is called **feedforward** or **anticipatory** control and is presumably based on the presence of internal models for well-rehearsed movements.

Development of Postural Control

Postural control is developed during childhood, starting as soon as the balance is challenged by the upright position. Although anticipatory control probably starts to develop very early, the first attempts at postural corrections depend heavily on feedback information. The corrections are large and inaccurate (ballistic). By constantly challenging the limits of its balance, the child improves both his or her use of feedback information and anticipatory control—improving skills by **experimentation**. This presumably goes together with establishing and refining the **internal models** of various skills. The development is not monotonous; there appear to be alternating periods with overreliance on one or the other strategy until the adult pattern is established around age 10 to 12. The adult pattern is characterized by flexible postural responses based on a full integration of feedback and anticipatory control strategies.

The Grasp Reflex

The grasp reflex is usually regarded as one of the postural reflexes. It is normally expressed only in infants during the first 6 months and disappears by 12 months. It consists of the fingers firmly grasping an object that touches the palm. After damage of the frontal lobes (presumably, in particular, the **supplementary motor area** [SMA]), the reflex may reappear in adults. The

strength of the grasp reflex depends on the position of the body, reflecting that its purpose is to cling to the mother when she moves about (thus, the reflex is of less functional importance in humans than in monkeys).

Control of Locomotion and Rhythm Generators

The upright locomotion of humans requires somewhat different movements than in animals walking on four legs; the demands on postural control are quite different. Certainly, the large size of the human brain has enabled many processes—which in lower animals are controlled from the spinal cord and the brain stem—to be controlled from the cerebral cortex. Nevertheless, with regard to basic mechanisms, the neural control of locomotion is probably very similar in humans and in other mammals. The following account is largely based on data obtained from animal experiments.

Fairly normal locomotion can be produced in animals (such as cats) even when the spinal cord is isolated from the brain stem and the brain. This can be observed on a treadmill when the paws touch the moving ground (the animal has to be supported since there are no postural reflexes). **Central rhythm (pattern) generators** must, therefore, exist in the cord and be able to produce rhythmic, alternating leg movements in the absence of any command signals from higher levels. The rhythm generators consist of complicated spinal **networks** of interneurons with excitatory and inhibitory interconnections, eventually controlling the activity of the motoneurons. Some of the neurons within the network appear to have **pacemaker properties**; that is, they fire brief trains of action potentials with silent periods between, without receiving a rhythmically alternating input.

The rhythm generator does not depend on sensory input from the moving parts to produce the motoneuron activity typical of locomotion. Thus, the rhythmic motoneuronal activity continues even after complete paralysis of the muscles (e.g., after cutting the ventral roots). This is called **fictive locomotion**, and the pattern of motoneuronal activity is strikingly similar to that observed during normal walking in intact animals. This does not mean that sensory inputs are without significance for locomotor control, however. The activity of the rhythm generators can indeed be modified by **sensory signals** from the peripheral receptors providing information about how the movements are proceeding. **Inhibitory interneurons** can contribute to the rhythmic pattern of activity by inhibiting the antagonists when the agonists have reached their maximal activity. **Renshaw cells** (see Fig. 21.14) probably contribute by shortening impulse trains from the motoneurons and at the same time increasing the excitability of antagonist motoneurons. There is most likely one rhythm generator for each extremity. Long **propriospinal fibers** that interconnect the forelimb and hind limb generators ensure that their activities are coordinated.

Rhythm Generators in the Human Cord

The presence of rhythm generators in the **human** spinal cord is indicated by the occurrence of locomotion-like movements in **anencephalic infants** (born without most of the brain). In normal infants, walking movements of the legs can be elicited in the first few months (if the infant is held under the arms and the feet are made to touch the floor). This ability usually disappears, to reappear when the infant starts to crawl at about 8 months. Locomotor movements can be elicited in patients with complete **transverse lesions** of the cord if the body is supported and the feet hit a treadmill. The locomotor pattern is more normal with high than with low spinal lesions, suggesting that the network controlling human walking is not restricted to the lumbosacral cord. Presumably, the lumbosacral rhythm generators depend on cooperation with similar networks in the cervical cord (as in four-legged animals).

Central Control of Locomotor Movements

Several parts of the brain contribute to a **network** that can modify the activity of the spinal rhythm generators. The most direct influence comes from parts of the reticular formation, but the basal ganglia, the cerebellum, and the cerebral cortex also contribute. Electric stimulation of a region in the mesencephalic reticular formation produces rhythmic locomotor movements in animals.[3] This **mesencephalic locomotor region** (MLR) is situated just ventral to the inferior colliculus on the pontomesencephalic junction. The **pedunculopontine nucleus** (PPN) is another name applied to this part of the mesencephalon (although the MLR and PPN are probably overlapping but not identical). Most likely, the effects on spinal motoneurons from the MLR are mediated by reticulospinal fibers, since they are abolished by cutting the ventral and ventrolateral

funicles. Further, many reticulospinal neurons are rhythmically active in pace with walking movements.

The **basal ganglia** have reciprocal connections with the PPN and appear to modulate locomotor movements without initiating them. The characteristic **gait** disturbances in **Parkinson's disease** may possibly be explained by dysfunction of these connections (see Chapter 23, under "The Basal Ganglia Act on the Brain Stem: Pedunculopontine Nucleus and Superior Colliculus"). In addition, the **cerebellum** (particularly the vermis) influences locomotor movements, and cerebellar lesions may produce an **ataxic** gait. The cerebellar effects are probably mediated by connections from the medial (fastigial) cerebellar nucleus to the medullary reticular formation (see Fig. 24.6).

Connections from the **motor cortex** (especially the pyramidal tract) are of increasing importance for the control of locomotion as the ground becomes more uneven and unpredictable—that is, as each step has to be controlled individually. Thus, after destruction of the motor cortex, cats can still walk fairly normally on an even surface but are helpless when required to walk along a ladder or a narrow bar. Other parts of the cerebral cortex than the motor cortex are also involved when the locomotor pattern needs to be modified. For example, the **posterior parietal cortex** receives visual information about the location of obstacles and integrates this with information of the state of the body. Accordingly, a PET study showed activation of the posterior parietal cortex when a person imagined walking in a field with obstacles.

MOTOR CORTICAL AREAS AND CONTROL OF VOLUNTARY MOVEMENTS

Motor Networks

We do not fully know how the appropriate corticospinal neurons are selected to produce a purposeful movement. The decision to initiate a particular movement is certainly not made in the MI, and it is not likely to be caused by activity in one particular neuronal group. Cognitive processes are expressions of activity in **distributed networks** of cortical neurons. Likewise, many parts of the cerebral cortex and interconnected subcortical nuclei are responsible for motor control. While the final movement command issues from the MI, the **decision to move** is mediated to MI from other parts of the cortex. Accordingly, brain-imaging methods such as PET and fMRI have shown that large parts of the cortex are activated in relation to voluntary movements. Further, when sensitive methods are used to record the

---

3. Rhythmic locomotor movements can be elicited by stimulation of the so-called **subthalamic region**, which is close to the posterior hypothalamus. It is not clear, however, whether the effect is due to stimulation of passing fibers rather than neurons in the subthalamic region itself.

and with learning new ones. Efference copies also reach cortical regions that are responsible for the **sense of effort** (see Chapter 13, under "Perception of Muscle Force"), and regions that enable us to distinguish sensory information that arises as a result of our own movements from such that is due to external events. Efference copies are also important for updating the **body scheme** and for our perception of bodily **ownership** (see Chapter 18, under "Body-Related Networks in the Cerebral Cortex"). Consequently, damage to the motor cortex is not identical to damage of the pyramidal tract—many neuronal groups besides the motoneurons lose crucial information.

Properties of Single Neurons in MI

Many cells in the MI become active (or increase their firing frequency) immediately before a voluntary movement starts, as shown with microelectrode recordings. In contrast, most cells in the SI become active after movement onset, indicating that they are activated by sensory signals from the moving parts but do not contribute to the initiation of the movement. Some pyramidal tract neurons (corticospinal neurons) increase their activity only in relation to the **start** of a movement, whereas others are active during the entire movement. The firing frequency of some neurons correlates with the **force** of muscular contraction. In the MI of a monkey sitting quietly waiting for a signal to move, some corticospinal neurons fire continuously. This probably means that the motor cortex not only initiates and controls movements but also determines the **readiness** of selected motoneuronal groups by keeping them slightly depolarized (below the threshold for initiation of action potentials). This enables the motoneurons to respond more quickly to a "go" signal from the motor cortex or from subcortical levels, such as the reticular formation, the vestibular nuclei, and sensory signals through the dorsal roots (e.g., from muscle spindles). At the same time that a corticospinal neuron excites motoneurons of synergistic muscles, motoneurons of antagonistic muscles are inhibited (via inhibitory interneurons mediating reciprocal inhibition).

The MI Controls Movements via Monosynaptic and Polysynaptic Pathways

Most if not all **pyramidal tract** fibers ending monosynaptically on the motoneurons come from the MI, which explains why the threshold for eliciting movements by electrical stimulation is lower there than in any other part of the cortex.[5] Accordingly, the movements evoked by very weak

electrical stimulation of the motor cortex are mediated by the pyramidal tract. Such movements occur in the opposite body half and can be limited to a few muscles in distal parts of the extremities and the face. Increasing stimulus strength recruits more muscles and more proximal ones. These effects are most likely mediated by **polysynaptic** pyramidal tract connections (via spinal interneurons) and by **corticoreticulospinal** pathways. Muscles that are often used simultaneously on both sides of the body, such as the muscles of the back and the abdomen, can be relatively easily activated **bilaterally** (on both sides) by stimulation of the MI of one side. Movements of the fingers, however, can be evoked only from the opposite (contralateral) MI, which reflects that the fingers are used independently and usually differently on the two sides. The anatomic basis of this is the complete crossing of the pyramidal tract fibers that control distal muscles, as mentioned earlier. Similar conditions pertain to the **commissural fibers** that interconnect the MI of the two hemispheres: only parts of the MI representing the trunk and the proximal parts of the extremities are interconnected. The large areas representing the distal muscles are devoid of commissural connections, presumably as an expression of the independent use of the two hands (see Fig. 33.13).

Epileptic Seizures Starting in the MI

The so-called **Jackson epileptic seizures** (described in Chapter 14) illustrate the somatotopic pattern within the MI (Figs. 22.5 and 22.12). The abnormal discharges of the neurons start at one site in the MI and spread out in a regular manner. Thus, the muscular cramps start in one part of the body—for example, the foot—and spread to the lower leg, then to the thigh, the abdomen, the shoulder, and so forth. Nearly always, the fits start around the mouth, in the tongue, the thumb, or the big toe. This is best explained by the fact that the cortical neurons controlling these parts occupy the largest volume of the MI and have the largest proportion of monosynaptic corticomotoneuronal connections.

Functional Organization of the Primary Motor Area: Task-Oriented Rather than Muscle-Oriented

As with the SI, a disproportionally large part of the MI is devoted to control of the **hand** (especially the thumb and the index finger), the **lips**, and the **tongue** (Fig. 22.12). In comparison, very small parts of the MI contain neurons that control muscles of the back and the abdomen. The number of cortical neurons that are involved with the motor control of a particular body part depends on the

---

5. Near the end of the nineteenth century, electrical stimulation of area 4 in dogs produced the first firm evidence of specializations within the cerebral cortex. Before that, the existence of functional localization in the cerebral cortex was hotly debated.

Figure 22.12

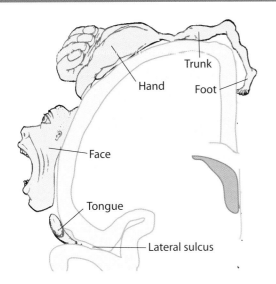

Relative size of the regions of the MI representing various body parts, as revealed by electrical stimulation of the exposed human MI. (Based on Penfield and Rasmussen 1950.)

This conclusion has received support from experiments with **micro-stimulation** of the monkey motor cortex. In contrast to most previous studies, long trains of stimuli lasting for about 500 msec were used, similar to the timescale of normal reaching movements. Such stimulation evoked coordinated movements and postures that involved many joints. Notably, the movements resembled purposeful movements—such as opening the mouth and, at the same time, shaping the hand and moving it to the mouth. In other words, the motor cortex is organized to optimize **task performance**, not to control individual muscles or joints. As an example, destruction of the cat's motor cortex does not affect single-joint movements but rather complex, multijoint movements, such as stretching the paw toward a goal.

Precise and Flexible Recruitment of Pyramidal Tract Neurons

Several observations show that the **selection of corticospinal neurons** can be extremely precise and varied. First, one corticospinal neuron can be active when a certain hand muscle is used for a precision grip, whereas it is much less active or inactive when the muscle is used for a more crude grasping movement. Other corticospinal neurons must therefore be responsible for producing the required force from the muscle in the latter situation. Second, human subjects can quickly learn to recruit one **specific motor unit** among many others when given **biofeedback** (seeing the EMG pattern of the muscle). This suggests an almost incredible ability to focus excitation from the motor cortex on certain spinal motoneurons. Considering the precision of movements required of a violinist, a watchmaker, or a neurosurgeon, these observations become perhaps less surprising.

The Supplementary Motor Area (SMA)

The SMA is located in front of the MI on the medial side of the hemisphere (Fig. 22.10). It sends fibers to both the spinal cord and the reticular formation. Thus, the SMA contributes to both direct and indirect corticospinal pathways. Spinal projections from the SMA (and PMA) end primarily on interneurons in the intermediate part of the spinal gray matter—that is, relatively far from the motoneurons. These spinal projections may therefore serve to prepare the spinal networks for the motor commands from the MI,

variety and precision of the movements rather than on the size of the part.

Focusing on the properties of single cells led to the view that pyramidal tract neurons were collected in groups controlling muscles around single joints (somewhat like the arrangement in the spinal cord where motoneurons are collected in groups related to single muscles; see Fig. 21.3). However, further studies have not supported this interpretation. Thus, pyramidal tract neurons controlling **motoneurons of one muscle** usually spread over a relatively large cortical area (although respecting the rough somatotopic pattern shown in Fig. 22.5). For example, within the motor hand region, pyramidal tract neurons that control different joints of the hand are intermingled. Thus, every small patch of the motor cortex contains neurons that control several different muscles. We also know that each pyramidal tract axon acts on more than one muscle (although with a stronger action on some than on others). Therefore, the explanation regarding why we can do isolated movements of single joints cannot be that each pyramidal tract neuron is specified for one movement only. A particular movement is specified by the collective activity of a large neuronal **population** rather than by a narrow tuning of a few neurons. Further, such populations appear to be related to **initiation of purposeful movements** involving several joints rather than to isolated, single-joint movements (consider how seldom our movements involve one joint only).

rather than initiating movements on their own. The SMA also sends many fibers to the MI, and this pathway is probably most important for its influence on motor control. This assumption is primarily based on results obtained by microelectrode recordings in monkeys and on brain imaging in humans. **Afferents** to the SMA come from—among other sources—the **prefrontal cortex** and the **posterior parietal cortex** (see Figs. 34.3 and 34.4).

The neuronal activity in the SMA of humans appears to increase especially in relation to somewhat complex movements. As mentioned, a series of simple flexion–extension movements of a finger increases the activity mainly in the MI hand area, not in the SMA (Fig. 22.11). When the task is to perform a series of movements in a specified **sequence**, however, there is also increased activity in the SMA. It appears that the activity increases first in the SMA and then in the MI. Increased activity in the SMA is not related to the movement itself, as it is sufficient that the person **imagines** the performance of a complex movement. Observations of the kinds discussed here have led to the suggestion that the SMA is important for organizing and planning **complex movements** and for mediating an appropriate **motor response to sensory stimuli**.

Damage of the SMA in humans usually produces severe motor impairments. Typically, the spontaneous use of the contralateral hand is abolished for weeks to some months; this condition is sometimes termed **motor neglect**. Another and more enduring problem is difficulty with the **simultaneous use of both hands** to solve a task. Monkeys with a lesion of the SMA show similar symptoms. For example, when a piece of food is stuck in a hole in a Plexiglas plate, a normal monkey easily retrieves it by pushing with one finger from above and collecting the piece with the other hand from below. After damage to the SMA, the monkey pushes from above with both hands. This is not due to the kind of incoordination seen after cerebellar damage but to loss of the ability to make different body parts cooperate in the execution of a specific task. That the **grasp reflex** is disturbed for some time after damage to the SMA may presumably be due to a disruption of normal integration of somatosensory stimuli and motor responses.

Additional Motor Areas on the Medial Wall of the Hemisphere

Several smaller motor areas have been identified adjacent to the SMA on the medial wall. This concerns the so-called **presupplementary motor area** (pre-SMA) and the **cingulate motor area** (consisting of three small areas buried in the cingulate sulcus).

These areas differ from the SMA with regard to connectivity and by their association with somewhat different aspects of motor control. The pre-SMA seems to be particularly active in relation to the performance of **novel** movement sequences but less so in relation to well-rehearsed movements. The cingulate motor area may be involved in **reward-based** movement control.

The Premotor Area

The PMA occupies the largest part of area 6 on the convexity of the hemisphere (Fig. 22.10). Like the SMA, the PMA receives **afferents** from the **prefrontal cortex** and the **posterior parietal cortex**, although not from identical parts. Parts of the PMA also receive afferents from **extrastriate visual areas**. The PMA probably sends fewer **efferent** fibers to the spinal cord than the SMA but has strong connections with the **reticular formation**, the **red nucleus**, the **basal ganglia**, and the **cerebellum**. As with the SMA, however, the connections from the PMA to the **MI** are probably those most directly related to the motor functions of the PMA. As indicated in Fig. 22.10, the PMA consists of a dorsal (PMd) and a ventral (PMv) subdivision that differ with regard to connectivity and functional properties.

Evolutionary Increase of Area 6

Assuming that area 6 of humans corresponds functionally to area 6 in monkeys, the SMA and PMA increased in size during **evolution**. Thus, areas 4 and 6 are of approximately the same size in monkeys (Fig. 22.8), whereas area 6 is much larger than area 4 in humans (see Fig. 22.10, see also Fig. 33.4).

Experiments in monkeys indicate that the PMA is important for the control of **visually guided** movements, such as the proper orientation of the hand and fingers when they approach an object to be grasped. The PMA thus performs **visuomotor transformations** of signals coming especially from the posterior parietal cortex. In monkeys, many cells in the PMA change their activity about 60 msec after a light signal that the monkey is trained to respond to with a certain movement. The activity of the PMA neurons continues until just before the movement starts, even when the monkey is trained to wait for many seconds after the signal before actually performing the movement. Thus, the PMA appears to hold the **intention** to move and the motor plan in standby until it is appropriate to start. Furthermore, the PMA is important for the ability to adapt a goal-directed movement to **altered external conditions**. For example, monkeys with lesions of the PMA have difficulties moving the hand around a transparent obstacle to reach an object and persistently use the direct approach, bumping into the obstacle. (After damage to the MI, the handling of an object is clumsy and insecure, but the ability to avoid an obstacle is not lost.) Interestingly, humans with lesions of the prefrontal cortex exhibit a similar tendency to continue a certain movement when first started, even though the movement is unsuccessful in achieving its goal. This phenomenon is called **perseveration.**

Mirror Neurons

In the ventral part of the **PMA** (PMv) and in the **posterior parietal cortex,** certain neurons are active not only when a monkey performs a certain movement but also when it is watching another monkey performing the same movement. Such **mirror neurons** respond particularly well to the use of tools, and they may even respond to the sound produced by an action. Although identified with certainty only in monkeys, mirror neurons probably exist in the human brain as well, as judged from fMRI studies. It is believed that the perceived action of the other person is automatically simulated by the mirror system without being actually carried out. The system of mirror neurons is probably involved in **learning by imitation** and in the "reading" of other persons' **motor intentions.** Some argue that the mirror system is also responsible for mind reading in a wider sense, that is, perception of others' intentions and the communicative content of movements (called **social cognition**). Others question this so-called "motor theory of social cognition." As said by Jacob and Jeannerod (2005, p. 22), "we grant that simulating an agent's movements might be sufficient for understanding his motor intention, but we ... argue that it is not sufficient for understanding the agent's prior intention, his social intention, and communicative intention." Certainly, identical movements may result from very different intentions and for different purposes. Another system that collects much more varied information than the mirror system seems necessary for social cognition (notably association areas in the superior temporal sulcus, the amygdala, and the orbitofrontal cortex).

Ownership and Agency—Depending on Motor Areas?

Intuitive feelings of ownership of our bodies and of being responsible for our actions depend on distributed brain networks involving the posterior parietal cortex, the prefrontal cortex, and several other regions (see Chapter 18, under "Body-Related Networks in the Cerebral Cortex"). Integration of different sensory modalities is one important task of these networks, but we also know that voluntary movements play an important role in bodily awareness. It is therefore not unexpected that motor areas participate in networks related to ownership and agency. For example, the sense of **agency** (experiencing oneself as responsible

for an action) seems to depend on activity in the SMA, as judged from observations of patients with brain damage. Thus, some patients with lesions affecting the SMA show the so-called **alien (anarchic) hand syndrome.** The hand makes purposeful movements, for example grasping an object, without the patient's intention. The person recognizes the limb as his own but has apparently no control over its actions and no feeling of having initiated the movements (loss of agency).

The feeling of **ownership** ("this arm is mine; it is a part of me") seems to be related to activity in the PMA. This has been shown experimentally with the so-called **rubber hand illusion.** A rubber hand is aligned with the hand of the test person, but only the rubber hand is visible. When the experimenter strokes the rubber hand synchronously with the unseen hand, the test person after some time feels that the rubber hand is part of his or her body. Simultaneous with this experience of ownership, the activity in the PMA increases (as shown in fMRI).

Motor Imagery

Do we use the same parts of the brain when we imagine a movement as when we perform it? Many studies with brain-imaging methods, such as PET and fMRI, have addressed this question. Most agree that overall the same **cortical networks** are activated in both situations. This holds true for the PMA, parts of the prefrontal cortex, the basal ganglia, lateral parts of the cerebellum, and the posterior parietal cortex. Some studies also show increased activity in the MI, although considerably less than in relation to movement execution. In agreement with such data, magnetic stimulation of the MI most easily evokes contraction of the muscles involved in the imagined movement (data are conflicting, however, whether spinal motoneurons also show similar facilitation during motor imagery). There are dissimilarities in the SMA, however, where somewhat different subregions are active in motor imagery than in real movements. Further, inferior parts of the prefrontal cortex are active only during imagery, so perhaps this region is responsible for the **suppression** of movements. The same neuronal processes seem to underlie imagined and real movements, as indicated by the fact that they take the same time from start to end. Patients with **lesions** of the **motor cortex** can still imagine movements in the paretic side, but, just like the real movements, the imagined ones are slower than normal. Patients with **Parkinson's disease** likewise exhibit similar slowing and reduced amplitude of real and imagined movements. After lesions of the **posterior parietal cortex**, however, the imagination of movements seems to be more affected than their execution.

Learning and the Motor Cortex

Brain-imaging studies show that higher association areas in the prefrontal and posterior parietal cortices are active during learning of new motor skills. As movements become more automatic, the activity decreases in these areas, presumably because of use-dependent plastic changes. We mentioned that the **pre-SMA** might be particularly engaged in learning new sequential movements. Further, animal experiments and human brain-imaging data show that plastic changes occur in the MI during motor learning (see Chapter 4, under "Spines Are Crucial for Synaptic Plasticity"). Both long-term potentiation (**LTP**) and long-term depression (**LTD**) can be induced in the cerebral cortex, and motor learning appears to be associated with strengthening of **horizontal connections** within the MI thereby coupling functionally related neurons. Thus, pyramidal cells in laminas II and III strengthen their synaptic couplings with neurons in other parts of the motor cortex during skill-learning in rats. Further, the connections are specific for the body parts that are used in the motor performance.

In humans, the finger representation in MI increases during 1 week of intense **piano training** of a specific sequence, as judged from threshold changes to magnetic stimulation of various parts of the motor cortex. Changes were obtained both with real movements and with mental training (motor imagery), although the effect was largest with real movements. In a group of right-handed elite **badminton** players, the stimulation threshold was lower and the hand area was larger in the left than in the right motor cortex (such differences were not found in a group of recreational players). Many more similar examples of plastic changes associated with learning of skills have now been published.

The Posterior Parietal Cortex and Voluntary Movements

The posterior parietal cortex consists of a mosaic of smaller areas with different specializations (see Fig. 34.4). Here we limit ourselves to two main subdivisions. **Area 5** is of particular importance for processing somatosensory information (received from the SI), whereas **area 7** also receives information from visual cortical areas (see Figs. 33.12 and 34.3). Many neurons in these areas are active in relation to movements, as shown by Vernon Mountcastle (1975) and others. One kind of neuron is active before goal-directed, reaching movements, such as when a monkey stretches its hand toward a banana. Such neurons do not become active, however, in relation to a movement in the same direction but without a specific aim or in relation to a passive movement. Other kinds of neurons increase their activity in relation to exploratory hand movements, such as when a monkey studies a foreign object. In area 7, some neurons increase their activity only when the monkey stretches its hand toward an object that it also looks at. Broadly speaking, it appears that area 5 (and parts of area 7) represent movements in a proprioception-based coordinate system, whereas most of area 7 relies more on

visual information. Ample connections from the posterior parietal cortex to the SMA and PMA (see Fig. 34.3) are crucial for the planning and preparation of goal-directed movements occurring in these areas.

Indeed, **damage** to the posterior parietal cortex also produces motor disturbances. There are no pareses, however, but rather difficulties with the execution of more complex movements. Patients with such lesions may be unable to open a door or handle previously familiar tools such as a screwdriver or a can opener. They also have difficulties with proper orientation of the hand in relation to an object, and they easily miss an object even though they see it clearly. This kind of symptom is called **apraxia** (see also Chapter 34, under "Lesions of the Association Areas: Agnosia and Apraxia"). Interestingly, similar symptoms may occur after lesions of the frontal lobes anterior to the MI, presumably reflecting the intimate connections between the posterior parietal cortex and the frontal lobes.

SYMPTOMS CAUSED BY INTERRUPTION OF CENTRAL MOTOR PATHWAYS (UPPER MOTOR NEURONS)

The term **central paresis** is used for a muscle weakness that is caused by interruption of the central motor pathways that conduct signals from the **upper motor neurons** in the cerebral cortex (especially the MI) to the **lower motor neurons** (motoneurons) in the brain stem and spinal cord. Only the pyramidal tract travels directly; the other pathways are indirect, with synaptic interruption in the brain stem. We have discussed that the various pathways take care of somewhat different aspects of motor control. The term **upper motor neuron syndrome** is often used for the clinical picture resulting from interruption of the central motor pathways, to differentiate it from the **lower motor neuron syndrome** (peripheral pareses) resulting from destruction of the motoneurons (including their axons; see Fig. 21.16).

Mechanisms underlying recovery after damage to the upper motor neurons are discussed in Chapter 11, under "Studies of Recovery after a Stroke in Humans."

"Negative" and "Positive" Symptoms

Although pareses are present in both, peripheral and central pareses differ in other respects. In peripheral pareses, the symptoms are all **negative**, in the sense that they represent **loss of function**, such as reduced or abolished muscle power, resting tone, and reflex contractions. There is also marked and rapid wasting of the muscles. In central pareses **positive symptoms** also occur—that is, there are symptoms caused by hyperactivity of neurons, such as increased reflex responses and resting muscle tone. Such differences are understandable when considering that the peripheral motor neurons are still functioning in central paresis (see Fig. 21.16). The motoneurons can be activated by signals from various receptors through the dorsal roots, from spinal interneurons, and from any remaining descending pathways, even though they cannot be brought into action voluntarily. Because the motoneurons still send signals to the muscles in a patient with central pareses, muscle wasting is modest, in contrast to that in peripheral pareses. Generally speaking, the positive symptoms occurring after damage to upper motoneurons are due to **hyperexcitability** of neuronal groups in the spinal cord, thus producing abnormal muscle contractions (e.g., on innocuous stimuli such as moving or touching a limb). Because the reflex arc is intact, reflexes such as the stretch reflex and the flexion reflex can still be elicited, and, typically, the reflex responses are stronger than normal in patients with central pareses (**hyperreflexia**). Although typically the reflex responses are weak or absent shortly after a stroke, and especially after a transverse lesion of the cord (spinal shock), patients recover in some days or weeks. Especially the **monosynaptic stretch reflex** (as tested with a tendon tap) becomes hyperactive on the affected side.[6] In addition, most patients develop an increased reflex response to passive movements of the affected limbs—that is, to stretching of the paretic muscles. This reflex response depends on the **velocity of stretch**, so that slow movements typically do not elicit any contraction. In some patients, however, especially in those with spinal trans-section or multiple sclerosis, even slow movements or innocuous cutaneous stimuli may provoke prolonged and painful **muscle spasms**.

The Plantar Reflex and Other Reflexes that Are Changed in Upper Motor Neuron Lesions

Interruption of descending central motor pathways, as in capsular hemiplegia, also produces changes of reflexes other than the stretch reflexes. The so-called **plantar reflex**,

elicited by stroking with a pointed object in a forward direction along the sole of the foot (especially the lateral margin), is inverted (Fig. 22.13). Instead of the normal response, which is a flexion movement of the great toe (and the other toes), the great toe extends (moves upward). This phenomenon, with extension instead of flexion of the great toe, is called the **sign of Babinski** and is a sensitive indicator of damage of corticospinal pathways.

More about the Sign of Babinski

Studies of patients subject to **cordotomy** (cutting parts of the lateral funicle to achieve analgesia) indicate that the sign of Babinski occurs only if the lesion affects the pyramidal tract. Further, electrophysiologic studies indicate that Babinski's sign is due to hyperexcitability of the reflex center in the cord, so that the extensor hallucis longus muscle is recruited together with the ankle extensors. EMG recordings and experiments with nerve blocks show that the flexors of the great toe are still active but that they are overcome by the greater force exerted by the extensors.

For example, increased intracranial pressure and unilateral herniation with compression of the descending motor fibers in the mesencephalon may invert the plantar reflex at an early stage (this will occur with the foot contralateral to the herniation, due to the crossing of the pyramidal tract in the lower medulla). An inverted plantar reflex may also occur during general anesthesia and in other conditions with reduced cerebral activity. In patients with central pareses, the **threshold** for eliciting the plantar reflex is lowered, and it can be elicited from a wider area than normally. Further, the response may include a complete flexion reflex

Figure 22.13

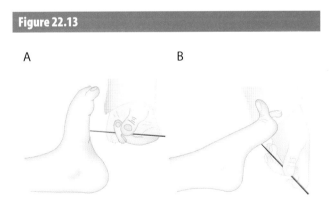

A   B

Inverted plantar reflex in central pareses (sign of Babinski). **A:** The normal plantar reflex is plantar flexion of all the toes when a pointed instrument is moved along the sole of the foot (from the heel to the toes). **B:** In a patient with central pareses (damage of the pyramidal tract) the big toe moves upward (dorsiflexion).

---

6. The **long-latency stretch reflex** appears to be weaker than normal in patients with an upper motor neuron syndrome, as judged from the EMG response to carefully graded muscle stretch and vibratory stimuli. This fits with other data suggesting a transcortical route for the long-latency stretch reflex, as discussed in Chapter 21.

of the lower extremity with flexion in the hip and knee and dorsiflexion in the ankle.

In **newborn children,** the plantar reflex is inverted and can remain so until the age of 2 (although most infants respond with plantar flexion of the big toe by 12 months). This is most likely due to the dependence of the "normal" reflex on the integrity of the pyramidal tract, which is not fully myelinated until between 12 and 24 months of age.

Reduction or absence of the so-called **abdominal reflex** is also typical of upper motor neuron lesions. The normal reflex response is a unilateral contraction of abdominal muscles upon stroking the skin with a pointed object.

The so-called **clasp-knife reflex** or phenomenon occurs in some patients with lesions of upper motor neurons: the examiner imposes a brisk stretch of a muscle (e.g., the biceps muscle by extension of the elbow), eliciting the typical reflex contraction, which stops the movement. If the examiner then keeps a steady force against the contracting muscle, the contraction suddenly yields. This involuntary stop of contraction is due to stimulation of high-threshold muscle afferents that inhibit the motoneurons (formerly, signals from tendon organs were believed to be responsible, but this has not been confirmed in animal experiments).

Other Features of the Upper Motor Neuron Syndrome

Even though central pareses can be produced by lesions located anywhere between the motor cortex and the motoneurons, the most common cause is interruption of the descending fibers by a thrombosis or bleeding in the internal capsule (Fig. 22.14). The pareses then affect the muscles of the opposite half of the body (hemiparesis, hemiplegia). The term **capsular hemiplegia** is commonly used for this condition. In such patients—in contrast to those who suffer a transverse lesion of the cord—fibers descending from cell groups in the brain stem (the reticular formation and the vestibular nuclei) can still activate the motoneurons. This may explain why resting muscle tone is typically increased in some muscle groups in patients with capsular hemiplegia (Fig. 22.15). Thus, in the arm, the increased tone affects the flexors so that the arm is kept flexed at the elbow, whereas the extensors of the leg are affected (interruption of motor pathways in the cord result in increased resting tone of flexors also in the leg).

An important feature of pareses in hemiplegia is that the **velocity** with which voluntary movements can be performed is reduced more than the isometric force (i.e., speed of movements is reduced more than strength). This is called **retardation** and concerns particularly fine finger movements and movements of the lips and tongue, whereas larger movements are less severely affected. Writing, tying, buttoning, and similar delicate movements may be impossible for a patient with capsular hemiplegia, or the movements are performed only very slowly and clumsily. This **loss of dexterity** is due to the loss of direct corticospinal fibers (the pyramidal tract), which are necessary for independent finger movements. Movements lose their rhythm and fluency. The **fatigability** is also abnormally great—that is, the muscular force drops quickly when a voluntary movement is repeated several times. The patient experiences a dramatic increase in the **mental effort** needed for voluntary movements: movements that before the stroke required no mental effort can afterward be performed only with the utmost concentration and strain.

Changes in Contractile and Passive Muscle Properties

Changes in the **contractile properties** of the paretic muscles also occur in hemiplegic patients. Thus, in the intrinsic muscles of the hand, the fatigability of type 1 muscle cells is increased and the contraction velocity of the type 2 fibers is reduced. Such changes will presumably contribute to the slowness and increased fatigability in patients with central pareses. Further, the passive, **viscoelastic properties** of muscles can change gradually after damage to the upper motor neurons. That is, resistance to stretch may be increased without concomitant muscle contraction, and the range of joint motion may be restricted. The latter phenomenon is called **contracture** and is due to change of connective tissue elements in muscle, tendons, and joint capsules that are kept in a shortened position. Several studies show that it is difficult clinically, when evaluating muscle tone, to distinguish the contribution of reflex hyperexcitability from changes in passive muscle properties. This is of some practical importance; for example, drugs used to treat spasticity such as **baclofen** (which reduces the excitability of motoneurons) or **botulinum toxin** (which paralyzes muscles) cannot reduce increased muscle tone due to altered passive muscle properties.

The "Pyramidal Tract Syndrome"

Formerly, all of the motor symptoms occurring in capsular hemiplegia were thought to be caused by damage to the

Figure 22.14

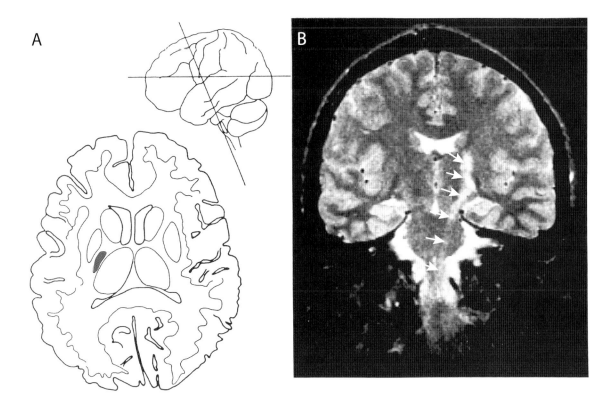

Infarction in the internal capsule with degeneration of the pyramidal tract. The patient, a 19-year-old man, suddenly became hemiplegic, probably due to occlusion of a brain artery by an embolus from the heart. **A:** Drawing of a horizontal CT showing the localization of the infarction (red) in the posterior limb of the internal capsule (cf. Fig. 6.30). Seven months after the stroke, the lesion measured 5 × 16 mm. **B:** Frontal MRI 4 months after the stroke, with the degenerated pyramidal tract (arrowheads) shown as whitish (cf. Fig. 22.2). It can be followed from the internal capsule through the pons and into the medulla. Immediately after the stroke, the patient had pareses on the right side, most marked for finger movements. He recovered completely. PET studies in this patient after recovery showed that finger movements of the right hand were associated with increased activity in the left motor cortex and PMA and bilaterally in the SMA, cingulate gyrus, and insula (in normal controls only the motor cortex show increased activity with isolated finger movements; cf. Fig. 22.11). The patient made involuntary mirror movements of the left fingers when using the right ones. (From Danek et al. 1990. Reproduced with permission from Oxford University Press.)

pyramidal tract, and the term "pyramidal tract syndrome" is still widely used. Closer study suggests, however, that not all symptoms can be explained by damage to the pyramidal tract. As discussed under "Function of the Pyramidal Tract as Judged from Functional Deficits after Lesions" earlier in this chapter, lesions limited to the corticospinal tract in the pyramid seem to produce difficulties with fractionated finger movements as the dominant or only permanent symptom In monkeys, spasticity ensues after lesions of the motor and premotor cortex but not after complete lesions of the medullary pyramid. To complicate matters, however, hyperreflexia and spasticity have been reported in a few patients with (most likely) pure lesions of the pyramid. Nevertheless, the weight of evidence favors the view that in capsular hemiplegia motor symptoms other than loss of dexterity arise from destruction of other corticofugal pathways than the pyramidal tract. It seems likely that interruption of the **corticoreticulospinal pathways** is important for

the more severe symptoms after a capsular lesion than after one limited to the medullary pyramid, including the development of spasticity.

We should also keep in mind that a lesion of the internal capsule might interrupt tracts of importance for motor control other than the corticospinal and corticoreticular ones. Thus, many fibers acting (directly or indirectly) on the **cerebellum** and on the **basal ganglia** are usually destroyed, and this probably contributes to the clumsiness of voluntary movements. Further, many patients with capsular hemiplegia have **sensory symptoms** in addition to the motor ones, either because the thalamus itself is affected or because the ascending fiber tracts conveying sensory signals from the thalamus to the cortex are interrupted (e.g., visual field defects). Reduced or altered cutaneous sensation and kinesthesia therefore also contribute to the motor symptoms.

Figure 22.15

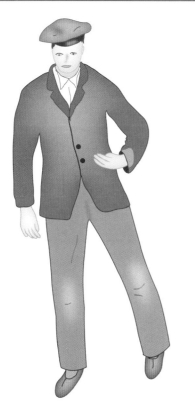

Hemiplegia of the left side. Note the characteristic position of the arm with flexion in the elbow and wrist. The paretic leg is moved laterally in a semicircle during the swing phase to keep the foot off the ground (circumduction).

Spasticity

The term **spasticity** refers to the positive symptoms in patients with upper motor neuron lesions. Some use the term to include all positive symptoms—that is, hyperreflexia, increased muscle tone, and muscle spasms. Others define spasticity more narrowly, restricting it to the velocity-dependent increase of resistance to muscle stretch.[7] Sometimes the term is used without specification to encompass all symptoms included in the upper motor neuron syndrome. This unfortunate situation was described as follows by Landau (1987, p. 721): "The word spasticity has been so carelessly used that it has become necessary to redefine it for particular contexts."

---

7. As defined by J. . Lance (cited in Landau, 1987, p. 722), "Spasticity is a motor disorder characterized by a velocity-dependent increase in tonic stretch reflexes (muscle tone) with exaggerated tendon jerks, resulting from hyperexcitability of the stretch reflex, as one component of the upper motor neuron syndrome."

The term **spastic paresis** is often used interchangeably with "central paresis." However, the most constant and characteristic positive symptom in central pareses (as part of the upper motor neuron syndrome) is the exaggerated velocity-dependent stretch reflex. Increased resting tone and contractions or spasms elicited by slow movements or cutaneous or other stimuli are more variable but functionally much more important symptoms. Spasticity, narrowly defined, is therefore of limited help when trying to determine a stroke patient's **functional impairment**. Since each of the positive symptoms can vary among patients with similar lesions, it seems inappropriate to use "spasticity" as a collective term without further specification. This point is further supported by the fact that muscle tone and reflex responses in the individual patient are highly **context dependent**. Thus, the symptoms vary with the patient's general condition, mental state, body position, and, not the least, whether he or she is at rest or moving.

Spasticity: Possible Mechanisms

The development of spasticity—widely defined as the positive symptoms that occur after a lesion of the upper motor neurons—is due mainly or solely to **excitability changes in the cord** leading to exaggerated motor responses to signals from receptors, other parts of the cord, and remaining supraspinal pathways. It is highly likely that **plastic processes**, for example, in the form of accidental **collateral sprouting**, contribute to excitability changes. The more precise mechanisms underlying spasticity are not known, however. To complicate matters, there is evidence that the mechanisms differ among spastic patients with similar lesions.

A priori, it seems likely that the loss of descending corticospinal fibers results in decreased activity of **inhibitory interneurons,** and many studies have been performed in humans to determine the excitability of specific kinds of interneurons. As discussed earlier in this chapter, the pyramidal tract modulates reflex responses by specific actions on several kinds of spinal interneurons. Several studies have shown reduced activity of the interneurons mediating **reciprocal inhibition** (see Fig. 21.13) in spastic patients, both after spinal cord lesions and in capsular hemiplegia. This would help explain the occurrence of hyperreflexia. For example, when testing the Achilles reflex with a tap on the tendon, a monosynaptic stretch reflex is elicited in the calf muscles (ankle plantar flexors). Normally the reciprocal inhibition prevents a stretch reflex from being elicited also in the antagonists—that is, the ankle dorsiflexors. If the reciprocal inhibition is reduced, however, a reflex contraction of the ankle dorsiflexors can occur; in turn, this may produce a new reflex contraction in the plantar flexors and so forth. When a single tap on the tendon elicits repeated contractions, it is termed **clonus**.

Another possible factor in spastic patients may be reduced **recurrent inhibition** of α motoneurons by **Renshaw cells** (see Fig. 21.14). When ankle dorsiflexors contract, for example, Renshaw cells inhibit the motoneurons to the ankle plantar flexors, so there is less chance of eliciting an unwanted stretch reflex. Reduced activity of the Renshaw cells in such situations would contribute to the occurrence of clonus in spastic patients. Reduced recurrent inhibition has indeed been found in some spastic patients with spinal lesions, although not in hemiplegic patients. Conversely, reduced activity in inhibitory interneurons activated from **tendon organs** (Ib afferents) has been found in hemiplegic patients but not in patients with spinal lesions.

There is also evidence of reduced activity of interneurons mediating **presynaptic inhibition** of Ia afferent terminals. This would lead to a stronger than normal excitatory effect of muscle stretch (particularly rapid stretch) on the α motoneurons. This appears not always to be present in spastic patients, however. For example, one study found reduced presynaptic inhibition in the arm but not the leg of hemiplegic patients. Reduced **postactivation depression** has been observed in patients with spasticity due to various causes. Postactivation depression means that the postsynaptic effect diminishes when action potentials in muscle spindle primary afferents follow each other with brief intervals. It is probably due to less transmitter being released. There is evidence that this phenomenon contributes to spasticity.

A permanently increased **excitability of the motoneurons** themselves has not been found in patients with spasticity due to stroke; it may occur, however, when spasticity is caused by a spinal injury. The intrinsic properties of the motoneurons might nevertheless be changed after a stroke, because **plateau potentials** may be more easily induced, as judged from animal experiments. As mentioned under "Monoaminergic Pathways from the Brain Stem to the Spinal Cord," when a plateau potential is induced in a motoneuron, it goes on firing for seconds to minutes without further stimulation. After a spinal transection in rats, plateau potentials disappear but return in the course of some months. Interestingly, when plateau potentials reappear, they can be induced by a variety of innocuous stimuli and appear to be closely related to the degree of spasticity. Whether lowered threshold for inducing plateau potentials plays a part in humans with spasticity remains to be determined, however.

It was formerly assumed that increased signal traffic from the muscle spindles—due to increased γ **motoneuron** firing— explained the increased stretch reflex responses in spasticity. Microneurographic recordings have not verified this, however, since the firing frequency of Ia afferent fibers was not found to be increased in spastic patients compared with normal controls.

In conclusion, the reflex hyperexcitability and increased muscle tone in patients with the upper motor neuron syndrome may arise from changes of several inhibitory mechanisms in the spinal cord, although few if any of the changes seem to be present in all patients. Possibly, varying combinations of disturbed inhibitory mechanisms, reduced postactivation depression, and perhaps an abnormally low threshold for eliciting plateau potential produce symptoms that are indistinguishable clinically. Yet, to select the right treatment, it would be crucial to know which mechanisms are disturbed in each patient.

Figure 23.3

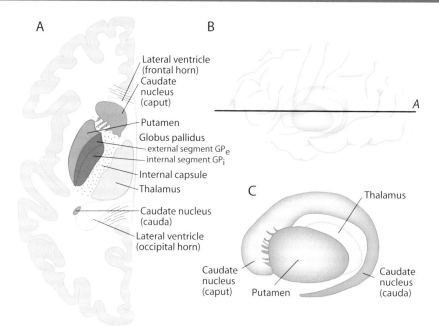

Shape and position of the basal ganglia. **A:** Part of a horizontal section through the hemisphere, as shown (**B**) with a line in drawing of the hemisphere (cf. Fig. 6.30 showing the whole section). **C:** Left putamen and caudate nucleus; lateral aspect.

Figure 23.4

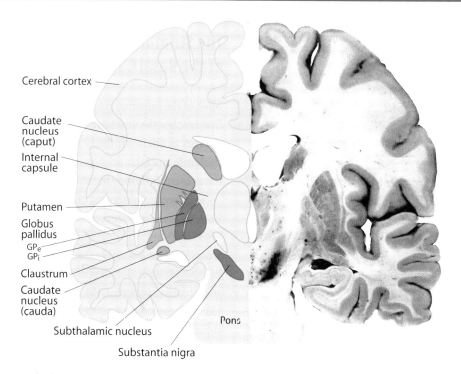

The basal ganglia seen in the frontal plane.

Figure 23.5

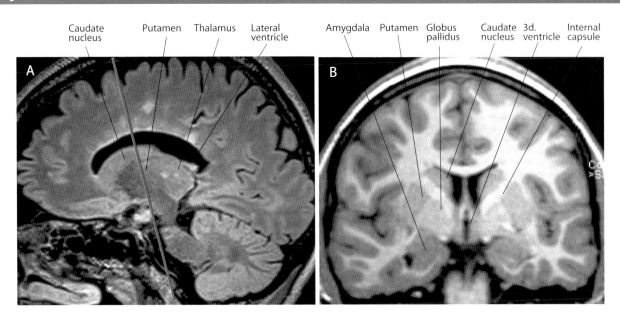

MRI of the basal ganglia. **A:** Parasagittal section; red line shows approximate position of the section in B. **B:** Frontal section. (Courtesy of Dr. S. J. Bakke, Oslo University Hospital, Oslo, Norway.)

information reaching the caudate nucleus may concern, for example, earlier stages in the chains of neural events leading to a decision about which movements are appropriate in the situation.

Figure 23.6

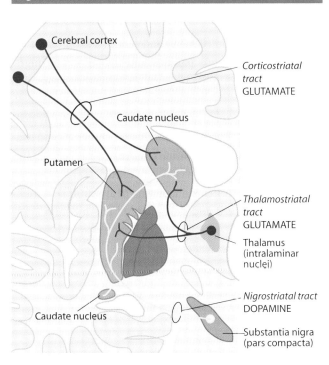

The main afferent connections of the striatum.

The striatal afferents from the **intralaminar thalamic nuclei** (Fig. 23.6) are numerous and are believed to transmit information to the striatum about stimuli that need special attention, while ongoing movements are halted to enable shift of activity.

Dopaminergic striatal afferents to the dorsal striatum arise in the **pars compacta** of the **substantia nigra**, whereas the ventral striatum receive such fibers from more scattered dopaminergic cells in the **ventral tegmental area** (VTA) dorsal to the substantia nigra (Fig. 23.8). The VTA also sends dopaminergic fibers to the prefrontal cortex.

Additional, quantitatively minor afferent contingents to the striatum come from the serotonergic **raphe nuclei** in the brain stem, among several other sources.

Thalamostriatal Connections: Goal-Directed Learning?

The thalamostriatal projections have marked effects on striatal-neuron excitability. The main sources of thalamostriatal fibers are the **centromedian** (CM) and **parafascicular** (Pf) nuclei. In addition, projections arise in the specific thalamic nuclei. Thus, while the **ventral anterior nucleus** (**VA**) and the **ventrolateral nucleus** (**VL**) send their main efferents to the cerebral cortex, they also send many fibers back to the striatum. The projection from the intralaminar nuclei has been most studied. Broadly, the CM projects to the sensorimotor part of the striatum, whereas the Pf supplies the associative parts. A major input to the CM and Pf comes from the globus pallidus (internal segment) and the substantia nigra (*pars reticulata*) in the form of collaterals of fibers ending in the specific thalamic nuclei. Thus,

Figure 23.8

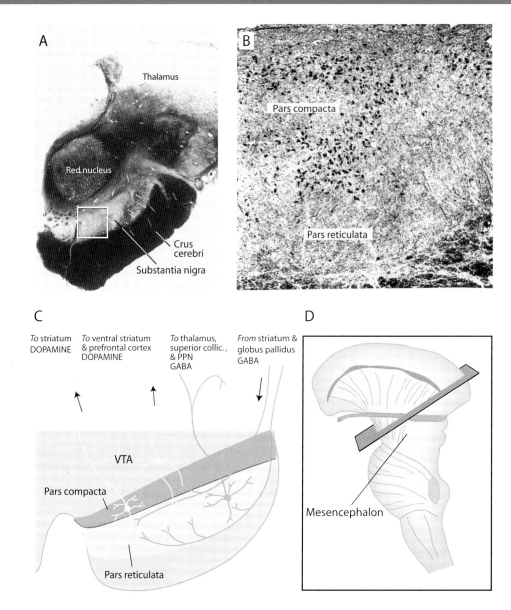

The substantia nigra. **A:** Photomicrograph of transverse section through the mesencephalon (myelin stain). Inset (**D**) shows plane and position of the section. The photomicrograph is from the section shown in Fig. 6.21. **B:** Higher magnification of framed area. The cells of the pars compacta are clearly seen as dark dots. The dark color is due to their content of pigment. **C:** The two parts of the substantia nigra differ structurally and with regard to connections. Afferent fibers to the pars reticulata contact the dendrites of the dopaminergic neurons in the pars compacta.

Compartments in the Striatum: Striosomes and Matrix

The various cell types, neurotransmitters, and afferent connections are not evenly distributed throughout the striatum. One example is the **mosaic** pattern that appears after staining to demonstrate **acetylcholine esterase**. Poorly stained patches called **striosomes** are embedded in a heavily stained **matrix**. The matrix can be further subdivided by visualization of various transmitters and their receptors. Cholinergic interneurons and medium spiny neurons are found within both the matrix and the striosomes, and the two main kinds do not appear to be clearly segregated, either. However, corticostriatal fibers terminating in the striosomes and in the matrix come from deep and superficial parts of layer 5, respectively. Thus, cortical information to neurons in the two compartments would be expected to differ slightly, even when coming from the same cortical area. Also, the further projections appear to differ with regard to exact termination and patterns of arborizations.

The Basal Ganglia Act on Premotor Networks in Thalamus and Brain Stem

The efferent connections of the basal ganglia may be summarized as follows. The internal segment of the globus pallidus and the substantia nigra send the information processed in the basal ganglia to premotor networks in the thalamus, the mesencephalon, and the superior colliculus. Here we use the terms premotor and **premotor networks** in a rather loose sense about neuronal groups acting either directly on motoneurons or on the motor cortex. Such premotor networks are found in the spinal cord, the reticular formation, and the thalamus. Neurons of the thalamic VL nucleus, for example, are considered premotor due to their direct projection to the motor cortex. Premotor networks organize the activity of motoneurons to produce purposeful actions, not merely isolated movements. Thus, the effects exerted by the basal ganglia on other parts of the nervous system are mediated primarily by efferent fibers from the **pallidum** and the **substantia nigra**. These nuclei receive their main afferents from the striatum (Figs. 23.7 and 23.10). In this manner, the pallidum and nigra process information from the striatum before it is sent to premotor networks. The efferents from the striatum are **topographically organized**, so that subdivisions of the striatum are connected with specific parts of the pallidum and the nigra.

The Substantia Nigra

The substantia nigra and some of its connections have been mentioned several times, and we return to this subject when dealing with Parkinson's disease, in which the nigra plays a crucial role. A collective treatment of the main features of the substantia nigra is therefore pertinent at this stage.

The substantia nigra can be divided anatomically into two parts, the **pars compacta** and the **pars reticulata** (Figs. 23.8A and 13.11A). The **dopaminergic nigrostriatal** neurons are located in the pars compacta, whereas the **GABAergic nigrothalamic** neurons are located primarily in the pars reticulata (Fig. 23.8C). The compacta is richer in cells than the reticulata, whereas the latter (as the name implies) is dominated by dendritic arborizations. The compacta neurons contain pigment (**neuromelanin**), which makes the nigra visible as a dark band in the cut human mesencephalon (see Fig. 23.4). The pars reticulata, located ventral to the compacta, is lighter.

The **efferent** connections of the **pars compacta** (Fig. 23.11A) pass primarily to the striatum (with a smaller contingents to the subthalamic nucleus and some other nuclei). This is the largest dopaminergic pathway in the brain, and the nigra is the largest collection of dopamine-containing neurons. **Pars reticulata** send GABAergic fibers to the **thalamus** (VA, mediodorsal nucleus [MD]). In addition, it projects to the **superior colliculus** (Fig. 23.11A), which control coordinated eye and head movements, and to the **PPN**, involved in control of gait and posture. The nigral

neurons sending their axons to the thalamus, and the superior colliculus are found in largely separate parts of the pars reticulata.

The **afferent** fiber connections of the nigra (Fig. 23.11B) arise in numerous cell groups, but quantitatively the most important input comes from the **striatum**. This projection shows some topographic organization; for example, afferents from the putamen and caudate nucleus end differently. Even though most striatonigral fibers terminate in the pars reticulata, cells in the compacta can also be influenced because their long dendrites extend into the reticulata (Fig. 23.8C). As mentioned, GABA is the transmitter for the striatonigral fibers, exerting **inhibitory** effects on the cells in the nigra. **Excitatory** afferents to the nigra arise in the **subthalamic nucleus** and the **pedunculopontine nucleus** (PPN) in the mesencephalon (glutamate). Afferents with **modulatory** effects come from the locus coeruleus (norepinephrine) and the raphe nuclei (serotonin). Additional afferents arise in the **ventral striatum** and the **bed nucleus of the stria terminalis**, presumably mediating signals related to motivation, attention, and mood. An important link in the latter pathways is the **habenula** (especially the lateral nucleus). Electric stimulation of the lateral habenula effectively suppresses activity of dopaminergic neurons, presumably by activating inhibitory interneurons.

Pathways from the Globus Pallidus and the Substantia Nigra to the Cerebral Cortex

As mentioned, the **globus pallidus** consists of two parts, an **external** (GP$_e$) and an **internal** (GP$_i$) segment (Figs. 23.3 and 23.4). Both segments receive their main **afferents** from the striatum, with additional inputs from the subthalamic nucleus. Whereas the fibers from the striatum exert inhibitory actions in the GP$_i$, the subthalamic afferents are excitatory. The balance between these two inputs therefore to a large extent determines the activity of the GP$_i$ neurons. The main part of the **efferents** from GP$_i$ goes to the thalamus and the substantia nigra (*pars reticulata*), whereas the GP$_e$ projects mainly to the subthalamic nucleus. Many of the **pallidothalamic fibers** pass through the internal capsule (Fig. 23.10) and can therefore be damaged by lesions in this region (this should be kept in mind when analyzing the symptoms occurring after capsular infarctions, as discussed in Chapter 22).[4] In the thalamus the pallidal fibers end in the **VA** and in parts of the **VL** (Fig. 23.7). The VL and VA send their main efferents to the cerebral cortex but also fibers back to the striatum. In more detail, the VA sends efferent fibers to the premotor area (PMA) and the prefrontal

---

4. The efferent fibers from the pallidum to the thalamus form two bundles, the **ansa lenticularis** and the **fasciculus lenticularis**. They arise from somewhat different parts of the internal pallidal segment and fuse to form the **fasciculus thalamicus** after having traversed the internal capsule. In addition, a **pallidotegmental** fiber bundle ends in the PPN.

Figure 23.11

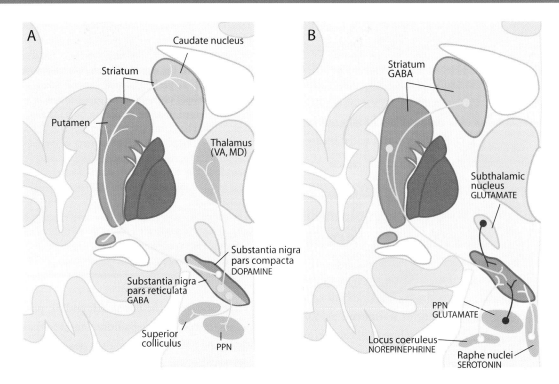

Main connections of the substantia nigra. **A:** Efferents. Dopaminergic neurons in the pars compacta send fibers to the striatum, whereas GABAergic neurons in the reticulata act on premotor neurons in the thalamus and the brain stem. **B:** Afferents. Inhibitory (GABAergic) afferents come from the striatum, whereas excitatory (glutamate) fibers come from the subthalamic nucleus and the PPN. Modulatory afferents arise in the raphe nuclei (serotonin) and the locus coeruleus (norepinephrine).

the basal ganglia to participate in control of premotor networks in the brainstem that control eye movements.

The Subthalamic Nucleus Influences all Circuits: Side Effects of Deep Brain Stimulation

All the circuits are influenced by the **subthalamic nucleus** (Figs. 23.4 and 23.11B). Indeed, subdivisions of this small nucleus project with topographic order to the dorsal and ventral pallidum. This might explain why electric stimulation of the subthalamic nucleus (**deep brain stimulation**) aimed at improving motor symptoms in Parkinson's disease can cause side effects such as mood changes (depression or mania), cognitive decline, and personality changes. Affections of circuits involving the prefrontal cortex are especially likely to produce such side effects.

Transmitters and Synaptic Actions in the Cortex–Basal Ganglia–Cortex Loop: Disinhibition

To understand the processing within the basal ganglia and their effects on other parts of the brain, we need to know

which transmitters and what synaptic actions of the neurons are involved. The conditions turn out to be extremely complex. Numerous neuroactive substances have been found in the striatum, although only a few can be correlated with anatomic and physiologic data.

The **corticostriatal** and **thalamostriatal** fibers are excitatory due to release of glutamate (Fig. 23.12). As discussed in the preceding text, the **striatopallidal** and **striatonigral** fibers are GABAergic and have inhibitory effects. The neurons in the globus pallidus are also GABAergic—that is, the **pallidothalamic** fibers from the GP$_i$ and the **pallidosubthalamic** fibers from the GP$_e$ are inhibitory. The **nigrothalamic** fibers, arising in the pars reticulata, are also GABAergic and thus inhibitory. The **thalamocortical** fibers (from the VL and VA, as from other thalamic nuclei) are excitatory (glutamate).

The flow of information from the cerebral cortex through the basal ganglia and back is obviously less straightforward than if all involved synapses were excitatory. Notably, there is a chain of two inhibitory neurons from the striatum to the **premotor** neurons in the thalamus and the brain stem (Fig. 23.12). Increased cortical input to the striatum would lead to decreased activity of

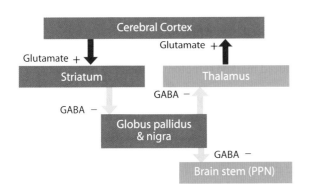

Disinhibition of Premotor Neurons

Disinhibition of premotor neurons.

the pallidal neurons, because excitation of striatal neurons produces increased inhibition in the pallidum. In turn, this would increase the activity of thalamocortical neurons because they would receive less inhibition from the GP_i (Fig. 23.10) Thus, excitatory impulses from the cortex would eventually produce **disinhibition** of the thalamocortical neurons (and other "premotor" neurons in the reticular formation and the superior colliculus receiving fibers from the substantia nigra).

Functional Significance of Disinhibition in Premotor Neuronal Groups

Recordings of **single-cell** activity in the basal ganglia in awake monkeys are compatible with the aforementioned considerations. At rest, most striatal neurons are "silent"—that is, they do not produce action potentials—whereas the pallidal neurons and neurons in the pars reticulata of the substantia nigra fire with a **high, regular frequency.**[7] This presumably keeps the premotor neurons in the thalamus and the brain stem in a state of inhibition when the animal is not moving. Commands from the cortex to the basal ganglia in relation to the preparation or execution of movements release the **premotor neurons** from this inhibition. Indeed, electrophysiologic experiments show that increased striatal activity reduces the activity of many pallidal and nigral neurons, followed by increased firing of thalamocortical neurons.

It has been proposed that the disinhibition of premotor neurons by the basal ganglia is a **gating mechanism** to control the access of other inputs (e.g., sensory) to the motor cortex. As the connections of the basal ganglia are topographically organized at all levels, this would be a specific and focused gating rather than a diffuse one, varying with the nature of the motor task. Such focused effects might serve to reinforce wanted movements while suppressing unwanted ones.

Synchronized Oscillatory Activity Underlies Functional States

It is well known that the connections between the basal ganglia and the cerebral cortex are characterized by **rhythmic** activity. Therefore, considering only the flow of excitatory and inhibitory signals and the rate of neuronal firing in individual nuclei (as we have done so far) offers little insight. We now know that neuronal networks in general are characterized by synchronized, **oscillatory** activity, and this is also so for the basal ganglia. Recordings from humans during **deep brain stimulation** have provided valuable information in this respect. Different functional states are associated with changes is oscillatory rhythms, for example changing from synchronized to desynchronized activity. Further, changes in the oscillatory frequencies are associated with altered behavior. Indeed, symptoms in basal ganglia diseases are probably better characterized by abnormal oscillatory activities than by firing rates in individual nuclei.

The Subthalamic Nucleus Regulates Pallidal and Nigral Activity

While efferents of the internal pallidal segment (GP_i) end primarily in the thalamus and the nigra, the GABAergic fibers from the GP_e are directed toward the subthalamic nucleus (Fig. 23.13). The subthalamic nucleus also receives excitatory afferents from the **motor cortex**, thus constituting a cortical input to the basal ganglia in addition to the major corticostriatal pathway. Most of the **efferents** from the subthalamic nucleus go back to both segments of the pallidum and to the pars reticulata of the substantia nigra. As mentioned, the **subthalamopallidal** fibers exert excitatory actions (glutamate). The efferents of the subthalamic nucleus are **topographically** organized, as shown with axonal transport methods. Thus, different neuronal populations project to the substantia nigra and the pallidum, and

---

7. This is not quite true for the GP_e neurons, however, because they fire with a somewhat lower and more uneven frequency than GP_i neurons and also tend to fire in bursts.

In conclusion, dopamine probably serves to keep the membrane potential in the range where the postsynaptic neuron is apt to fire in **bursts**—that is, in a state suited for efficient signal transmission. Some data suggest that D$_1$ receptor activation enhances the activity of neurons that receive a strong and **focused excitatory input** (from the cerebral cortex) while reducing the activity of neurons receiving weak inputs. This would help in focusing striatal activity, in accordance with other data indicating that the basal ganglia assists in the **selection of behavior**, such as the choice of specific movements.

What Activates the Dopaminergic Neurons?

In light of the dominating effects of dopamine in the striatum, knowing under which conditions the nigrostriatal neurons are activated would be informative. Clues may come from the fact that many of the nuclei sending fibers to the nigra change their activity in relation to **arousal, motivation**, and **emotionally** driven behavior. This concerns the PPN, the locus coeruleus, the raphe nuclei, and the ventral striatum and other cell groups in the basal forebrain. Accordingly, physiologic studies show that striatonigral neurons do not change their firing in relation to movements but in relation to stimuli that are **unexpected** or are judged to be of particular **salience** for the behavior of the animal at the moment. This may concern stimuli signaling reward or punishment, although they must have a fairly high intensity to activate dopaminergic neurons.

In general, dopamine assists in establishing associations between stimuli and their reward value. This kind of **learning** underlies motivated behavior based on prior experience. As mentioned, dopaminergic neurons in the midbrain fire either in bursts or tonically. Selective reduction of burst firing in mice (by genetic manipulations) support the idea that a brief release of dopamine acts as a signal for associative learning, especially related to potentially rewarding or dangerous events.

Habenula Controls Dopaminergic Neurons

The habenula seems to play a particular role in controlling the activity of dopaminergic neurons (and other monoaminergic neurons). It receives afferents from the ventral striatum, other nuclei in the basal forebrain, and the hypothalamus and projects to the substantia nigra pars compacta and the VTA. Signals from the habenula appear to occur especially in situations when an expected reward is not given. It has therefore been suggested to constitute a pivotal link in a "circuit of **disappointment**" (Fritz A. Henn, personal communication). Indeed, the lateral habenula

shows altered activity in **depression** and is the target of **deep brain stimulation** for depressive disorders.

THE VENTRAL STRIATOPALLIDUM

The term **ventral striatum** is used for rather diffusely distributed cell groups in the basal part of the hemispheres (the basal forebrain; see Chapter 31, under "Neuronal Groups in the Basal Parts of the Hemispheres: The Basal Forebrain," for a discussion of its constituting parts). The ventral striatum merges with the dorsal striatum without sharp boundaries. The **nucleus accumbens** represents a fairly distinct part of the ventral striatum and connects the caudate nucleus and the putamen ventrally (Fig. 23.15; see also Fig. 31.10). A similar diffuse cell group, the **ventral pallidum**, merges with the dorsal well-defined parts of the globus pallidus (see Fig. 31.9). The **ventral striatopallidum** is used as a collective term.

Connections of the Ventral Striatum

Although the ventral striatopallidum has no sharp boundaries with other cell groups in the basal forebrain, its relationship to the basal ganglia is witnessed by the similarities of their connections. We mentioned one of the **circuits** through the basal ganglia: from parts of the **prefrontal cortex** and **cingulate gyrus** to the ventral striatum, from there to the ventral pallidum, then to the **MD**, and finally back to the prefrontal cortex. There is probably a further differentiation of connections through the ventral striatum (several circuits). Thus, it receives **afferents** with some topographic localization from the **hippocampal formation**, the **amygdala**, the **orbitofrontal cortex**, and parts of the temporal lobe (all these sources are either parts of the limbic structures or closely connected to them). The nucleus accumbens also send **efferent** fibers to the hypothalamus and the mesencephalic reticular formation (PPN).

Like the dorsal striatum, the ventral striatum receives many **dopaminergic fibers**; those projecting to the ventral striatum are located mainly dorsomedially to the substantia nigra, in the **ventral tegmental area** (VTA). Since the dopaminergic neurons in the VTA project primarily to the ventral striatum, the prefrontal cortex, and other cell groups that are closely linked with limbic structures, the term the **mesolimbic dopaminergic system** is now widely used. To use the word "system" for this is hardly justified, however, as there is little reason to assume that these widespread dopaminergic

Figure 23.15

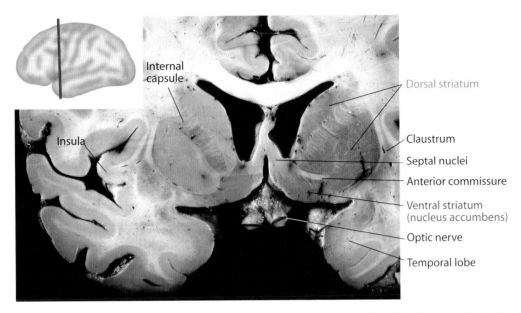

The ventral striatum with the nucleus accumbens. The septal nuclei, which belong to the basal forebrain, are also indicated. Photo of a frontal section through the brain at the level of the anterior commissure (cf. Fig. 6.26).

projections are functionally homogeneous. **Afferents to the VTA** have been traced from the prefrontal cortex, the nucleus accumbens, and the PPN (and other nuclei).

The "Mesolimbic Reward System"

A popular theory suggests that the dopaminergic mesolimbic connections constitute a **"reward pathway"** and that the pleasurable feelings evoked by, for example, narcotic drugs are caused by release of dopamine in the **nucleus accumbens**. Indeed, much evidence points to dopamine as the neurotransmitter most directly involved in the pleasurable effects of drugs of abuse. Nevertheless, many other parts of the brain than the nucleus accumbens are activated by stimuli-evoking reward-motivated behavior, and there are substances that produce reward behavior without activating the mesolimbic dopaminergic neurons. Today, several transmitters other than dopamine are under scrutiny in addiction research—such as glutamate, acetylcholine, serotonin, and several neuropeptides. As said by the American neuropharmacologist Ann Kelley (2002, p. 448) in connection with nicotine addiction: "Thus, repeated exposure of the brain to drugs with abuse potential sets in motion a cascade of activity involving dopamine, glutamate and acetylcholine signaling." Further, opinions on what drives the

mesencephalic dopaminergic neurons has changed from solely focusing on reward to a more general activation by unexpected or highly **salient stimuli** requiring a change of behavior, as discussed earlier.

The Ventral Striatum, Psychosis, and Drug Addiction

The dopaminergic projection to the ventral striatum (especially to the nucleus accumbens) has attracted much interest, because **antipsychotic drugs** appear to bind with particularly high density in the ventral striatum. Such drugs are dopamine antagonists with preferred binding to D_2 receptors. Neurons in the nucleus accumbens of experimental animals change their pattern of activity during development of drug **addiction**, no matter whether the drug is amphetamine, cocaine, or morphine. The addictive behavior is reduced by lesions of the nucleus accumbens or by removing its dopaminergic innervation. Thus, after giving a dopamine antagonist, the experimental animals stop self-administration of cocaine (they could easily obtain an intravenous dose by a movement). Further, dopaminergic activity is increased in paranoid **psychoses** elicited by amphetamines or cocaine (see also Chapter 5, under "GABA Receptors Are Influenced by Drugs, Alcohol, and Anesthetics," "Nicotine Addiction," and "Examples: Drugs Altering Monoamine Activity in the Brain").

However interesting these observations are, they provide only limited insight. By focusing on one transmitter and one part of the brain, we may even gain the impression that there is a simple biologic explanation to complex mental phenomena. Indeed, many parts of the brain other than the nucleus accumbens show altered activity in the conditions discussed here (see Chapter 34 for some comments on mental illness and the cerebral cortex). In

One example is **Tourette's syndrome**, believed to be caused by dysfunction of the basal ganglia. The symptoms can be partially relieved by dopamine antagonists.

Parkinson's Disease: Clinical Features

This disease of unknown etiology usually starts during the fifth or sixth decade of life. The syndrome includes, as mentioned, **akinesia**, **bradykinesia**, **tremor**, and **rigidity**. In addition, there are disturbances of **postural reflexes**. Notably, the body balance during walking is disturbed, so that the patient appears to be "running after his center of gravity." The steps are typically very short, which is due to the bradykinesia (the movements are not only slower than normal but also reduced in amplitude). When being pushed from behind, the patient has difficulty stopping and continues to move forward. The normal pendulum movements of the arms during walking are absent. There is also a conspicuous loss of facial expression (the face becomes like a mask). There are disturbances of the **autonomic nervous system**, such as increased salivation and secretion from sebaceous glands of the skin. We do not know how the basal ganglia influences the autonomic nervous system, and the autonomic symptoms perhaps may be caused by a more general disturbance of monoamine metabolism (not only dopaminergic cell groups are affected in Parkinson's disease).

Tremor is typical, with a frequency of 3 to 6 per second, and it is most pronounced at rest. When the patient uses the hand, the tremor disappears or is reduced in amplitude. The increased muscle tone, or **rigidity**, is different from the spasticity that occurs after lesions of central motor pathways. The resistance to passive movements is equal in extensors and flexors and is independent of whether the muscle is stretched slowly or rapidly. There is no clear-cut increase in the strength of the monosynaptic stretch reflex (such as the patellar reflex), whereas the long-latency stretch reflexes are increased, and this may perhaps contribute to the difficulties with balance and locomotion. The rigidity is apparently not caused by hyperactivity of γ motoneurons but by descending influences that increase the excitability of the α motoneurons so that they fire continuously—perhaps like the situation in a nervous person who is unable to relax his or her muscles. The **plantar reflex** is normal in patients with Parkinson's disease, indicating that there is no damage to the central motor pathways. It is indeed an old clinical observation that the tremor and rigidity disappear if a patient with Parkinson's disease has a **capsular hemiplegia**, and corresponding observations have been made in experimental animals. The last central link in the pathways mediating the tremor and rigidity must therefore be pathways from the cerebral cortex to the motoneurons.

Parkinson's Disease: Structural Changes

The most pronounced structural change in the brain of patients with Parkinson's disease is a profound loss of pigmented (melanin-containing) neurons in the pars compacta of the **substantia nigra** (Fig. 23.8). These are the dopamine-containing neurons. The degeneration of the neurons is accompanied by the accumulation of **Lewy bodies** in the cytoplasm, of which α-**synuclein** makes up the major part. As a consequence of the

loss of dopaminergic nigrostriatal fibers, the dopamine content of the striatum is reduced. Symptoms first appear, however, when the dopamine content of the striatum is reduced by 80% to 90%. Another striking change is loss of 20% to 30% of the **spines** on the medium spiny neurons. As mentioned, this may be due to loss of a possible growth-promoting effect of dopamine. Another possibility is that spine loss is due to glutamatergic overactivity in corticostriatal synapses. The latter explanation is suggested by the observation that loss of dopamine increases activity in glutamatergic synapses and by the close proximity of dopaminergic and glutamatergic synapses on the spines (Fig. 23.9B).

Can We Explain the Symptoms in Parkinson's Disease?

Increased firing of neurons in the subthalamic nucleus is the most striking electrophysiologic finding in Parkinson's disease. As discussed earlier ("The 'Indirect Pathway,' the Subthalamic Nucleus, and Parkinson's Disease"), it is not clear how loss of dopamine in the striatum leads to subthalamic hyperactivity. Even if we ignore that problem, the relationship between the subthalamic hyperactivity and the symptoms is not obvious. It may be a mistake, however, to try to explain the symptoms simply in terms of more or less excitation or inhibition at stations in the cortex–basal ganglia–cortex loop. It seems more likely that abnormal oscillatory activity in parts of the basal ganglia disturb the functions of various, distributed networks. For example, the hyperactivity in the subthalamic nucleus takes the form of **oscillations** in the beta band (10–40 Hz). Interestingly, the oscillations are attenuated by dopaminergic medication and by deep brain stimulation. Thalamic neurons (both in the lateral nucleus and in the intralaminar nuclei) also show various forms of abnormal, oscillatory firing. Further, their activity—in contrast to that in normal persons—shows no modulation in relation to movements. As proposed by Marsden and Obeso (1994), the parkinsonian symptoms may arise mainly because the basal ganglia outputs become "noisy" and thus disrupt the activity of their targets. Some neurons fire rhythmically while others become very difficult to activate. The oscillatory firing of large populations of neurons may be abnormally synchronized. We know that neuronal networks might shift from one functional state to another in milliseconds and, conceivably, such shifts produce the rapid fluctuations in symptoms often observed in Parkinson's disease. The motor system may be better off when the disruptive basal ganglia outputs are removed (be it by thalamotomy, pallidotomy, or deep brain stimulation)—leaving it in "peace" to compensate for the loss of basal ganglia inputs.

Therapeutic Approaches to Parkinson's Disease

The finding of reduced striatal dopamine led to attempts to alleviate the symptoms of Parkinson's disease by giving the patients dopamine, to substitute for the loss of dopaminergic neurons. For various reasons, a precursor of dopamine—**levodopa** (L-dopa)—must be used. This is converted to dopamine in the brain. This treatment has a beneficial effect on the symptoms, particularly on the very troublesome bradykinesia. Even though L-dopa has proved to be a very helpful drug, it does not affect the course of the disease, and the therapeutic effect decreases as the disease progresses. There may be a certain number of remaining dopaminergic neurons in the nigra for L-dopa to be converted to dopamine in the striatal dopaminergic boutons. More profound changes of the striatal neurons and their ability to react to dopamine may also occur. One might think that when the brain is unable to produce enough dopamine itself, it would not be able to produce dopamine from a supplied precursor either. However, enzymes converting L-dopa to dopamine are present not only in dopaminergic neurons in the nigra but also in glial cells and in other types of neurons.

Stereotaxic surgery (pallidotomy, thalamotomy) has now been replaced by **deep brain stimulation** of the subthalamic nucleus or the GP$_i$. Such treatment causes considerable improvement in many patients (the effect appears to be better on positive than on negative symptoms), although it also may produce serious emotional and cognitive side effects. The mechanism underlying the clinical effect of deep brain stimulation is still not clear, however. Intriguingly, both high-frequency stimulation and lesions of the subthalamic nucleus relieve symptoms in Parkinson's disease. Further, while both high- and low-frequency stimulation reduce the subthalamic hyperactivity (in animal studies), low-frequency stimulation has no symptomatic effect in humans.

Replacement of lost dopaminergic neurons by **transplantation** of embryonic cells from aborted fetuses has been tried for some years in patients with Parkinson's disease but for several reasons seems not to be a viable approach. Now efforts are directed at developing dopaminergic neurons for transplantation from human stem cells (thus avoiding ethical and practical problems with the use of human embryos).

Huntington's Disease

This disease is dominantly inherited and usually starts in the fourth decade of life. It is caused by expansion of trinucleotide (CAG) repeats in the **huntingtin** gene (for mechanisms of neuronal death in neurodegenerative diseases, see Chapter 10 under "Common Molecular Mechanisms in Neurodegenerative Diseases"). The disease has a steadily progressing course and is characterized by rapid, jerky, involuntary movements of the face, arms, and legs. In advanced stages, the patient is never at rest. The dance-like quality of the movements led to the terms **chorea** and **choreatic movements** (Greek: *chorea*, dance). The most prominent pathological change involves the **striatum**, with a marked loss of GABAergic projection neurons.

Observations suggest that in **early stages** of the disease, mostly neurons projecting to the GP$_e$ degenerate (the "indirect pathway"; see earlier discussion). This would produce reduced inhibition of GP$_e$ neurons and, by that, increased inhibition of the subthalamic nucleus. (Animal models support that reduced activity of the subthalamic nucleus may be crucial for development of choreatic movements.) This in turn leads to reduced excitation of GP$_i$, and thereby to less inhibition (disinhibition) of thalamocortical neurons in the VL and VA. Thus, the choreatic movements might be causally related to increased excitatory input to motor cortical areas.

In **later stages** of the disease, the striatal neurons projecting to the GP$_i$ also die (as do many neurons in other parts of the brain). This leads to reduced inhibition of GP$_i$, with subsequent increased inhibition of thalamocortical neurons (as in Parkinson's disease). This is taken to explain why bradykinesia develops in later stages of Huntington's disease, while the choreatic movements continue.

This is not obviously logical, however, if the effects of both the direct and indirect pathways are mediated by the GP$_i$. Another explanatory model focuses on dopaminergic hyperactivity in the striatum, caused by loss of GABAergic inhibition in the substantia nigra. Although there are problems also with this model, it fits with the observation that **L-dopa** worsens the choreatic movements of patients with Huntington's disease. The disease also leads to mental deterioration with **dementia**, which is probably best explained by cell loss occurring in the cerebral cortex (particularly the frontal lobes) as well.

The genetic defect is located on the short arm of **chromosome 4**, and this makes it possible to decide whether a person is a carrier of the disease long before the symptoms occur. This becomes important regarding the choice of whether or not to have children. However, to provide individuals with such knowledge as long as there is no effective treatment poses obvious ethical questions.

Tourette's Syndrome

This is a peculiar and multifarious condition with multiple **tics** (quick, involuntary movements that are repetitive at irregular intervals) associated with involuntary vocalization as central manifestations. It has a strong heritable component, but responsible genes have not been identified. The condition is probably caused by a functional disturbance of the basal ganglia and the prefrontal cortex, although the mechanisms are not known. Volumetric studies with MRI indicate that the caudate nucleus is smaller than normal, and fMRI studies show altered activity in the striatum and related cortical regions. It has been postulated that the tics are caused by abnormal activity in small groups of striatal projection neurons (cf. striosomes and matrix discussed in the preceding text). Dopaminergic hyperactivity may play a role in the disease, but other transmitters, such as serotonin and GABA, have also been implicated.

The disease starts during childhood, usually between the ages of 5 and 10 years, and it affects boys more frequently than girls. Often the symptoms diminish before or during adolescence. Many patients have a repertoire of **repetitive behavior**, such as touching others, repeating their own words, or echoing the words or movements of others. Vocalizations (vocal tics) commonly include explosive cursing or compulsive utterance of obscenities, which interrupt normal speech. Many patients describe that an inner tension builds up, and this is temporarily relieved by the tic. Some people with Tourette's syndrome appear to have unusual energy and creativity. As children, they often show hyperactive behavior. This may lead to serious social problems, especially when, as often happens, the disease is misdiagnosed as a behavioral disorder of social origin.

Treatment with **dopamine antagonists** (especially haloperidol, a D$_2$-receptor antagonist) may reduce the involuntary movements and other troublesome symptoms. However, the patient's mental energy and self-perception may be severely affected by the treatment. As vividly described by Oliver Sacks in *The Man Who Mistook His Wife for a Hat*, this may be experienced by some patients as worse than the symptoms. Since 1999, **deep-brain stimulation** has been used in some patients with severe symptoms and poor response to conventional treatments. Beneficial results have been reported with different sites of stimulation (the GP$_i$, the accumbens, and the intralaminar thalamic nuclei).

Figure 24.3

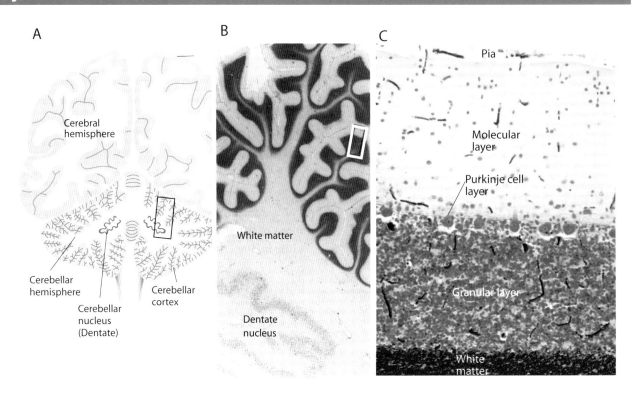

The cerebellum, the cerebellar cortex, and an intracerebellar nucleus. **A:** Frontal section through the cerebrum and the posterior fossa with the cerebellum. Note the folding of the cerebellar surface to form thin folia. (Cf. Fig. 6.32.) **B:** Photomicrograph from the area corresponding to the frame in A. Thionine staining. **C:** Higher magnification of framed area in B, showing the three layers of the cerebellar cortex. Compare Fig. 24.12 showing the structural elements of the cerebellar cortex in detail.

zone on both sides of the midline, and the large lateral parts called the **cerebellar hemispheres.** The medialmost part of the hemispheres, bordering the vermis medially, is called the **intermediate zone** (Fig. 24.4). This zone cannot be distinguished from the rest of the cerebellum on a macroscopic basis but only on the basis of fiber connections. A deep, transversely oriented cleft, the **primary fissure**, divides the corpus cerebelli. The parts of the corpus cerebelli in front of and behind the primary fissure are called the **anterior lobe** and the **posterior lobe**, respectively. The anterior and posterior parts of the vermis constitute the phylogenetically oldest parts of the corpus cerebelli. The midportion of the vermis and the hemispheres are younger and are therefore called the **neocerebellum**. The anterior and posterior portions of the vermis and the adjoining parts of the intermediate zone of the corpus cerebelli receive afferents primarily from the spinal cord and are therefore also termed the **spinocerebellum**. The hemispheres receive their main input from the cerebral cortex (synaptically interrupted in the pontine nuclei) and are therefore termed the **cerebrocerebellum** or the **pontocerebellum**.

With regard to the **efferent connections**, the three main subdivisions of the cerebellum act on the parts of the central nervous system from which they receive their afferents; that is, the vestibulocerebellum sends fibers mainly to the vestibular nuclei, the spinocerebellum influences the spinal cord, and the cerebrocerebellum acts on the cerebral cortex.

Afferents from the Labyrinth and the Vestibular Nuclei

Primary vestibular afferents bring sensory signals from the vestibular apparatus in the inner ear. They enter the cerebellum through the inferior cerebellar peduncle (Fig. 24.1) and end in the flocculonodular lobe and adjoining parts of the vermis (Fig. 24.5). Although most of the primary vestibular afferents end in the **vestibular nuclei**, many neurons in the latter send axons to the cerebellum. In this manner, the cerebellum receives vestibular information also via **secondary vestibular afferents**. The vestibular input provides the cerebellum with

Figure 24.4

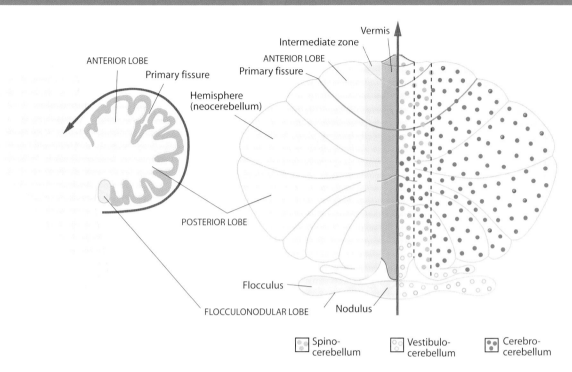

Main cerebellar subdivisions. **Left:** A sagittal section through the cerebellum and the brain stem. **Right:** The human cerebellum unfolded and seen from the dorsal aspect. The left half shows the macroscopic subdivisions of the cerebellum into lobes, as well as the border between the vermis and the hemisphere. Compare Fig. 6.32. The right half shows the terminal regions of the three major afferent contingents to the cerebellum (vestibular, spinal, and cerebrocortical). Because the intermediate zone receives information from both the spinal cord and the cerebral cortex, there is no sharp border between the spinocerebellum and the cerebrocerebellum.

information about the position and movements of the head. **Efferents** from the flocculonodular lobe end in the vestibular nuclei and can thereby influence the body equilibrium (via the vestibulospinal tracts) and eye movements via the medial longitudinal fascicle (Fig. 24.5; see also Fig. 18.7B).

Afferents from the Spinal Cord

Several pathways bring signals from the spinal cord to the cerebellum (Fig. 24.6). Some of these pathways go uninterrupted from the cord to the cerebellum and are called **direct spinocerebellar tracts**, whereas others are synaptically interrupted in brain stem nuclei and are therefore termed **indirect spinocerebellar tracts** (not shown in Fig. 24.6). The spinocerebellar tracts originate from neurons with their cell bodies located in different lamina of the spinal cord (Fig. 24.7). They are therefore influenced by different kinds of **sensory receptors** and spinal **interneurons** and bring different kinds of information to the cerebellum. The spinocerebellar axons end mostly in the spinocerebellum of the same side (as their cell bodies). Some pass uncrossed; other fibers cross twice (first in the spinal cord and then back again in the brain stem). The fibers are located in the **lateral funicle** as they ascend (Fig. 24.7). The tracts are **somatotopically** organized, so that signals from different body parts are kept segregated. The somatotopic pattern is maintained within the cerebellum (Fig. 24.8) so that the leg is represented anteriorly within the anterior lobe, with the arm and the face represented successively more posteriorly. In the posterior lobe, the arrangement is the reverse, with the face represented anteriorly.

Direct Spinocerebellar Tracts

Functionally, the direct spinocerebellar tracts consist of two main groups. One group of tracts conveys information from **muscle spindles, tendon organs,** and **cutaneous low-threshold mechanoreceptors**. Physiologic studies show that many of the neurons of the direct spinocerebellar tracts are activated monosynaptically by primary afferent (sensory) fibers. The tracts conduct very rapidly and appear to give precisely timed information about movements.

Because most of the spinal interneurons are strongly influenced by descending **motor pathways** (e.g., the pyramidal tract), the ascending tract to the lateral reticular nucleus probably informs about their activity as well. The lateral reticular nucleus also receives afferents from sources other than the spinal cord, notably the red nucleus, the vestibular nuclei, and the motor cortex. Many cells, for example, are strongly influenced by tilting of the head, which stimulates **vestibular receptors**.

Finally, information from sensory receptors can reach the cerebellum not only through some of the spinocerebellar tracts but also through fibers sent to the spinocerebellum from the **dorsal column nuclei** and the **trigeminal nuclei**.

Afferent Connections from the Cerebral Cortex

In humans, by far the largest number of cerebellar afferent fibers arises in the **pontine nuclei** (Fig. 24.9; also see Fig. 6.18). The **pontocerebellar tract** ends primarily in the cerebellar hemispheres, which constitute the major part (90%) of the cerebellum in humans. The vast majority of afferents to the pontine nuclei arises in the cerebral cortex and forms the **corticopontine tract** (Fig. 24.8).[1] The main task of the pontine nuclei therefore is to process information from the cerebral cortex and forward it to the cerebellar cortex. The corticopontine tract is uncrossed, whereas most of the pontocerebellar fibers cross; thus, the cerebral cortex of one side acts mainly on the cerebellar hemisphere of the opposite side.

The **corticopontine tract** runs in the internal capsule and then in the crus cerebri (see Fig. 6.20), where it occupies a large part; of the approximately 19 million fibers in the crus of the human brain, the corticopontine fibers constitute the majority (the pyramidal tract, in comparison, contains only about 1 million fibers on each side).

A large fraction of the corticopontine fibers arise in the primary motor cortex (**MI**) and the primary somatosensory cortex (**SI**). There are also substantial contributions from the supplementary motor cortex (**SMA**) and the premotor cortex (**PMA**) and from areas 5 and 7 of the **posterior parietal cortex** (Fig. 24.9). More modest contributions come from parts of the **prefrontal cortex**. In various ways, these areas are active during or before movements.

1. Other **precerebellar nuclei**—that is, brain stem nuclei that send their efferents to the cerebellum—also receive afferents from the cerebral cortex. This concerns mainly the **reticular tegmental nucleus**, located just dorsal to the pontine nuclei (participating in the control of eye movements; see Chapter 25), and the **lateral reticular nucleus**. In quantitative terms, these pathways play minor roles compared with the corticopontocerebellar pathway.

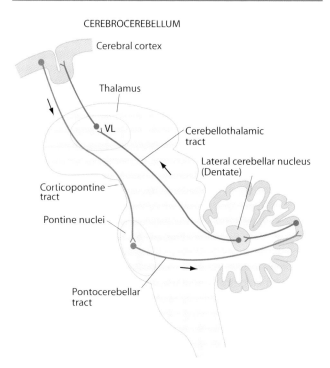

Figure 24.9

Main connections of the cerebrocerebellum. The ascending connections to the cerebral cortex are synaptically interrupted in the dentate nucleus and in the thalamus. The projection from the cerebellar cortex to the cerebellar nuclei is GABAergic and inhibitory, whereas the other links in the cerebrocerebellar pathway are excitatory. Compare Fig. 24.17 showing the crossing of the cerebrocerebellar connections.

Presumably, the cerebellum thus receives information about movement **planning** and about the **motor commands** that are sent out from the cortex; in response, it can modulate the activity of the motor cortex so that the movements are performed smoothly and accurately. The pontine nuclei also receive afferents from the **visual cortex** (mainly extrastriate areas), and physiologic experiments indicate that these fibers inform primarily about moving objects in the visual field. Such connections may be important for the execution of **visually guided movements**.[2] The pontine nuclei also receive connections from parts of the **hypothalamus** and **limbic structures,** notably the **mammillary bodies** and the **cingulate gyrus**. The information conveyed from these regions is probably not directly related to movement. The cingulate gyrus is concerned, for example, with attention and

2. There are modest connections to the pontine nuclei from the **frontal eye field**, involved in control of rapid eye movements, and from area 9 in the dorsolateral part of the prefrontal cortex. Some fibers arise in parts of the **auditory cortex**, whereas few if any pontine fibers come from the rest of the temporal lobe.

with error detection during motor, sensory, and cognitive processes. These connections and those from the prefrontal cortex may form the basis of cerebellar contributions to certain **cognitive tasks** (see "The Cerebellum and Cognitive Functions" later in this chapter). In addition, "limbic" corticopontine connections might contribute to the well-known influence of motivation and emotions on movements.

Topographic Organization of the Cerebrocerebellar Pathway

The corticopontine projection is **topographically organized**, so that different cortical regions project to largely different parts of the pontine nuclei (Fig. 24.10). The fibers coming from the MI and SI are **somatotopically** organized. Further, the pontocerebellar projection shows a topographic organization—for example, upholding the somatotopic pattern in the connections from the MI and SI (Fig. 24.7). The connections from the cerebral cortex to the pontine nuclei exhibit an extreme **divergence**: that is, a small part of, say, the MI influences small clusters of neurons in widespread parts of the pontine nuclei. Presumably, each pontine neuron receives converging inputs from specific combinations of cortical cell groups, thus integrating various kinds of information before forwarding messages to the cerebellum. The next link—the pontocerebellar tract—shows a marked **convergence** (as well as divergence). In this way, the corticopontocerebellar pathway seems to produce numerous specific combinations of cerebrocortical inputs in the cerebellar cortex. These and other data indicate that there is a functional localization within the cerebellar hemispheres, so that smaller parts take care of specific tasks.

The Intermediate Zone Is a Meeting Place for Signals from the Cord and the Cerebral Cortex

The intermediate zone (Fig. 24.4) is mainly defined on the basis of its efferent connections (projecting to the interposed intracerebral nuclei). It also has special features with regard to afferents, however (Fig. 24.11). Whereas the lateral parts of the hemispheres are strongly dominated by inputs from the cerebral cortex, and the vermis is dominated by spinal inputs, the intermediate zone receives connections from both the cerebral cortex and the spinal cord (Fig. 24.4). Animal experiments indicate that the cortical

input to the intermediate zone comes primarily from the MI and SI. Single neurons in the intermediate zone can be activated from both the cerebral cortex and the spinal cord. For example, in the "arm region" of the anterior lobe, intermediate-zone neurons receive converging input from the arm region of the MI and SI and from sensory receptors in the arm. Most likely, the cerebellum in this case **compares** copies of the motor commands sent from the cerebral cortex with the signals from the periphery providing information about the actual movement that was produced by the command (signaled by the spinocerebellar tracts). This may be important to decide whether sensory information is self-generated or caused by external influences and to monitor whether a movement proceeds according to plan.

THE CEREBELLAR CORTEX AND THE MOSSY AND CLIMBING FIBERS

Before discussing the efferent connections of the cerebellum, we need to know something about the cerebellar cortex. Here, the vast amount of information provided by all of the afferents is processed. To some extent, different kinds of information are integrated, and then "answers" are issued to various motor centers of the brain and spinal cord. As mentioned, the cerebellar cortex has the same structure all over (it cannot be subdivided into cytoarchitectonic areas, differing also in this respect from the cerebral cortex), and it lacks association fibers that interconnect different regions. The structural arrangement of the neuronal elements is strictly geometric, so the individual elements can be distinguished fairly easily. This helps explain why the structure and internal connections of the cerebellar cortex are much better known than that of the cerebral cortex.

The Cerebellar Cortex Consists of Three Layers

The superficial, outermost layer is the **molecular layer** (Figs. 24.3 and 24.12). It contains mainly dendrites and axons from cells in the deeper layers and only a few cell bodies. The middle layer is dominated by the large Purkinje cells, arranged in a monolayer, and is called the **Purkinje cell layer**. The deepest, lowermost layer is the **granular layer**, named so because it is packed with tiny **granule cells**. The axons of the granule cells ascend through the Purkinje cell layer into the molecular layer, where they divide at a right

Figure 24.10

A

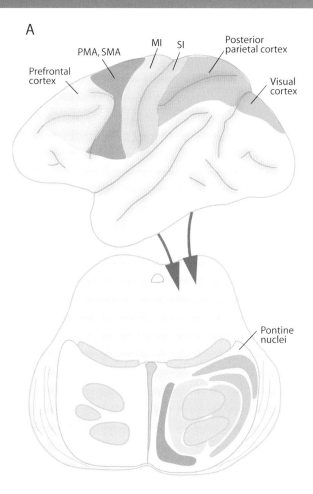

Prefrontal
cortex

PMA, SMA

MI

SI

Posterior
parietal cortex

Visual
cortex

Pontine
nuclei

B

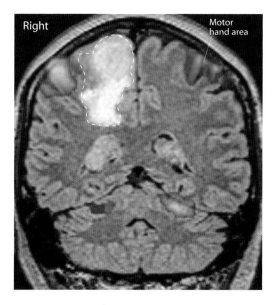

Right

Motor
hand area

Organization of cerebrocerebellar connections. **A:** Areas of the cerebral cortex that are connected with the cerebellar hemispheres by means of the pontine nuclei are shown in different colors. In the pontine nuclei, fibers from each cortical region terminate in its own territory. Note the lamellar arrangement, resembling the skins of an onion. **B:** Frontal plane fMRI. Finger tapping is associated with activation of the motor hand area and, via the cortico-pontocerebellar pathway, activation of the contralateral cerebellar anterior lobe. In the right hemisphere a tumor (glioma) is visible medial to the hand area of the motor cortex (broken line). The investigation was performed to decide if the tumor could be removed surgically without serious functional consequences. (Courtesy of Dr. Baard Nedregaard, Oslo University Hospital, Oslo, Norway.)

Figure 24.11

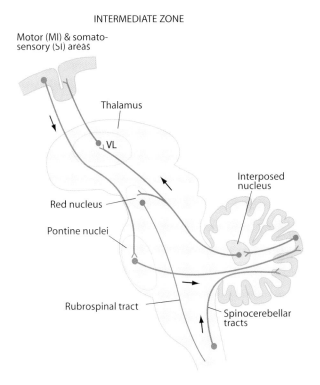

INTERMEDIATE ZONE

Motor (MI) & somato-sensory (SI) areas

Thalamus

VL

Interposed nucleus

Red nucleus

Pontine nuclei

Rubrospinal tract

Spinocerebellar tracts

Main connections of the intermediate zone. Both the spinal cord (via the red nucleus) and the cerebral cortex (via the thalamus) can be influenced by the intermediate zone.

angle into two branches running parallel with the surface of the cortex (Figs. 24.12 and 24.13). These branches are called **parallel fibers** and run in the direction of the long axis of the folia. The parallel fibers form numerous synapses with the Purkinje cell dendrites. The **Purkinje cell dendritic tree** is unusual: first, it has an enormously rich branching pattern; second, the dendritic tree is compressed into one plane, forming an espalier oriented perpendicular to the long axis of the folia and the parallel fibers. This arrangement ensures that each parallel fiber forms synapses with many Purkinje cells (the parallel fibers can be several millimeters long). At the same time, an enormous number of parallel fibers contact each Purkinje cell: it has been estimated that each Purkinje cell receives about 200,000 synapses. Considering that there are approximately 100 billion granule cells but only 30 million Purkinje cells, each Purkinje cell would integrate signals from about 3,000 granule cells.[3]

3. Although older quantitative studies agreed that the number of Purkinje cells in the human cerebellum is about 15 million, a study with an improved stereological method estimated the number to about 30×10^6 million (Andersen et al. 1992). The same study estimated the number of granule cells to about 100×10^9, while the number of neurons in the **dentate nucleus** was 5×10^6.

As mentioned, the **Purkinje cells** are the only ones that send their axons out of the cerebellar cortex and thus constitute the efferent channel. The Purkinje cells contain γ-aminobutyric acid (**GABA**), and they inhibit their target cells, as shown physiologically. The **granule cells** have an excitatory action on the Purkinje cells, releasing **glutamate**.

In addition to granule cells and Purkinje cells, the cerebellar cortex contains **inhibitory interneurons** (Fig. 24.13) that serve to limit the activity of the Purkinje cells and probably increase the spatial precision of the incoming signals (cf. inhibitory interneurons in sensory systems; see Fig. 13.4).

The Cerebellar Cortex Contains Three Kinds of Inhibitory Interneurons

All cerebellar interneurons contain **GABA** (some may also contain glycine, another inhibitory neurotransmitter). One main type of interneuron is the **stellate cell**, located in the molecular layer (Fig. 24.13). It receives afferent excitatory input from the granule cells (parallel fibers), and its axons form synapses with the Purkinje cell dendrites.

Another kind of interneuron, the **basket cell**, is located close to the Purkinje cell layer. Basket cells are also contacted by parallel fibers, whereas their axons end with synapses around the initial segment of the Purkinje cell axons—a location that enables the basket cells to inhibit the Purkinje cells very efficiently. The axonal branches of the basket cells are arranged perpendicular to the long axis of the folia, so that they inhibit Purkinje cells lateral to those that are being activated by parallel fiber excitation. Activation of a group of granule cells would lead to a narrow band of excitation of the Purkinje cells along the folium, flanked by a zone of basket cell–mediated inhibition on each side. Thus, it appears to be a kind of **lateral inhibition**, which is common in sensory systems to increase the spatial precision. Correspondingly, the extent of the cerebellar cortical region activated by each mossy fiber is reduced.

The third kind of inhibitory interneuron, the **Golgi cell**, is located in the granular layer. The dendrites of the Golgi cells extend upward into the molecular layer and are therefore contacted by parallel fibers (like the stellate cells and the basket cells). The axonal branches form synapses with the dendrites of the granule cells and thus reduce the excitation received by the Purkinje cells from the granule cells.

Afferents to the Cerebellar Cortex Are of Two Main Kinds: Mossy and Climbing Fibers

The afferent fibers to the cerebellar cortex fall into two categories, which differ in how the fibers end in the cerebellar cortex. Both kinds have an **excitatory** synaptic action, most likely mediated by glutamate. The **climbing fibers** all come

Figure 24.12

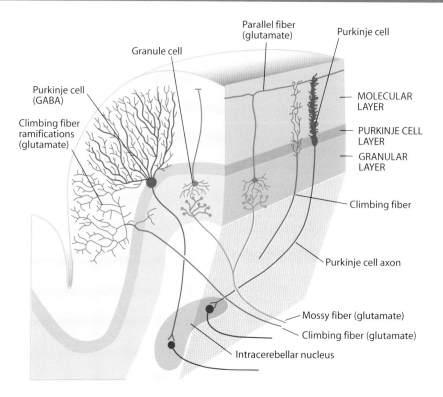

Structure of the cerebellar cortex. The three layers and the main cell types are shown schematically in a piece of cerebellar folium. The Purkinje cell dendrites are arranged perpendicular to the long axis of the folium and the parallel fibers. The two main kinds of afferent fibers (mossy and climbing fibers) are also shown. The mossy fibers end on the granule cells, whereas the climbing fibers enter the molecular layer to end on the Purkinje cell dendrites.

from the **inferior olive**, whereas afferents from nearly all other nuclei end as **mossy fibers** (such as the vestibulocerebellar, the spinocerebellar, and the pontocerebellar fibers).[4]

The **mossy fibers** conduct signals relatively rapidly and end in the granular layer, establishing synapses with the granule cell dendrites (Figs. 24.12 and 24.13). One mossy fiber branches extensively and contacts a large number of granule cells, each of which, in turn, contacts many Purkinje cells (the number of granule cells is much larger than the number of mossy fibers). Thus, each mossy fiber influences many Purkinje cells, but the excitatory effect on each is weak, so that many mossy fibers must be active together to provide sufficient excitation (via the parallel fibers) to fire a Purkinje cell (as mentioned, the parallel fibers excite the

Purkinje cells). A typical feature of the mossy fibers is that they transmit action potentials with a high frequency and make the Purkinje cells fire so-called **simple spikes** with a frequency of 50 to 100 per second.

All the **climbing fibers** cross to the opposite side and end very differently from the mossy fibers: the fibers ascend directly to the molecular layer and divide into several branches, each "climbing" along a Purkinje cell dendrite (Figs. 24.12 and 24.13). As they climb, they form numerous synapses with the dendrites. Each Purkinje cell receives branches from only one climbing fiber (i.e., from only one cell in the inferior olive). Each olivary cell, however, innervates more than one Purkinje cell, as the number of Purkinje cells is higher than the number of olivary cells. Because each climbing fiber forms so many synapses with a Purkinje cell, the total excitatory action is strong. Thus, even a single action potential in a climbing fiber elicits a burst of action potentials in the Purkinje cells—called **complex spikes**. In contrast to mossy fibers, the firing frequency of the climbing fibers is very low under natural conditions (often less than one signal per second). Even maximal stimulation does

4. In addition to the climbing fibers and mossy fibers, demonstrated with the Golgi method a long time ago, a third type of cerebellar afferent has been demonstrated by using the histofluorescence method (visualizing fibers containing catecholamines). Such fibers come from the **raphe nuclei** and from the **locus coeruleus** and contain serotonin and norepinephrine, respectively. They appear to end rather diffusely in both the granular and molecular layers. Direct fibers from the **hypothalamus** also end in this manner.

Figure 24.13

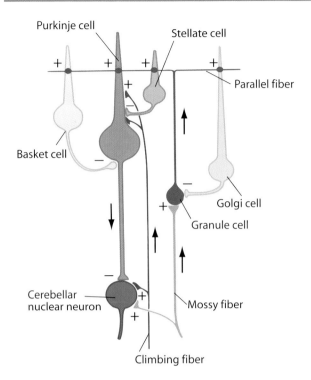

The cerebellar cortex. Schematic of the main cell types and their synaptic arrangements. The three types of GABAergic interneurons are colored green. (Redrawn from Eccles et al. 1967.)

not bring the firing frequency above 10/sec. Accordingly, recordings of Purkinje cell activity in an animal at rest shows continuous firing of simple spikes with high frequency, interrupted now and then by complex spikes.

In conclusion, the Purkinje cells receive excitation from both mossy and climbing fiber afferent inputs but with very different spatial and temporal characteristics of their actions.

The Effects of Climbing Fiber Elimination

Acute **destruction** or inactivation of the inferior olive demonstrates its importance for motor control. Movements become **uncoordinated**, similar to the effect of removing the whole cerebellum. Accordingly, physiologic studies show that inactivation of the olive (by injection of a local anesthetic) produces a marked **disinhibition** of the Purkinje cells. This increases the inhibition of the intracerebellar nuclear cells so that the cerebellar output to other parts of the brain is virtually eliminated.

Connections of the Inferior Olive

As mentioned, the climbing fibers arise in the inferior olive—a large, folded nucleus in the ventral medulla (see Fig. 6.17). The

climbing fibers cross and end in the cerebellar nuclei and the cerebellar cortex in an extremely precise topographic order. One subdivision of the olive receives **afferents** primarily from the **cord** via several precisely organized spino-olivary tracts and project to the spinocerebellum. Another part receives afferents from the **superior colliculus** and project to the midportion of vermis (the "oculomotor vermis"). The superior colliculus receives signals from the retina, the visual cortex, and the SI. These parts of the olive contribute to the control of eye and head movements. A small olivary subdivision receives afferents from the **pretectal nuclei** (see Fig. 27.20) and project to the flocculonodular lobe. The pretectal nuclei receive signals from the retina, and its projection to the olive is of importance for adaptation of the **vestibuloocular reflex** (see Fig. 25.5; see also "Examples of the Role of Cerebellum in Motor Learning" later in this chapter).

The main part of the human inferior olive (the principal nucleus) projects to the cerebellar hemispheres and receives afferents from various **mesencephalic nuclei**, notably the parvocellular **red nucleus**. These mesencephalic nuclei receive afferents from the cerebral cortex (especially the MI, SMA, and PMA) and can therefore mediate cortical information to the cerebellar hemispheres. In addition, the mesencephalic nuclei receive strong connections from the cerebellar nuclei, thereby establishing a **loop**: cerebellum–red nucleus–inferior olive–cerebellum (**dentato-rubro-olivary pathway**; also called the **Guillain–Mollaret triangle**). The functional role of this rather massive pathway is unknown, but functional magnetic resonance imaging (fMRI) studies suggest that it is involved in sensory discriminative tasks, perhaps especially when rhythmic movements are used for sensory exploration.

Finally, the inferior olive receives GABAergic fibers from the cerebellar nuclei (of the opposite side).

Mossy and Climbing Fibers Mediate Different Kinds of Information

The great differences between the mossy and climbing fibers with regard to both structural and physiologic properties strongly suggest that they convey different kinds of information and thus play different parts in cerebellar functions. Because of their ability to vary their signal frequency over a wide range, the **mossy fibers** are presumably well suited for providing precisely graded information about movements (the muscles involved, as well as the direction, speed, and force of movements), localization and characteristics of skin stimuli, details concerning motor commands issued from the cerebral cortex, and so forth. Such assumptions also fit with the physiologic properties of spinocerebellar fibers, known to end as mossy fibers (less is known about the corticopontocerebellar pathway in this respect).

The **climbing fibers**, because of their low range of firing frequency, are less likely to provide precisely graded information. Recordings of the firing of the Purkinje cells in response to climbing fiber activity also suggest that the climbing fibers have a unique functional role. Thus, as mentioned, a single action potential in a climbing fiber is sufficient to trigger a burst of Purkinje cell action potentials (complex spikes). This would suggest an all-or-none action rather than a graded one. Several theories of cerebellar functions postulate that the climbing fibers inform about **errors** in the execution of a movement (giving an "error signal") when the movement does not correspond to what was intended, and there is some experimental support for this hypothesis. Some studies show that the firing frequency of climbing fibers increases in relation to a perturbation of an ongoing movement, whereas the firing frequency is unrelated to, for example, the direction and velocity of the movement. In experiments with walking cats, the firing frequency of climbing fibers leading from the forelimb increases when the foot meets an obstacle, so that the walking pattern must be changed. In monkeys learning a new movement, there is increased climbing-fiber activity from the relevant body parts. When the movement is well rehearsed—that is, the learning phase is over—the climbing fiber firing frequency does not increase during execution of the movement (thus perhaps sending no more error signals).

Climbing Fibers and Motor Learning

These and other kinds of experiments indicate that the climbing fibers play a specific role during **motor learning**. For example, experiments with silencing the olivary activity—and thus eliminating all climbing fiber input to the cerebellum—impair the establishment of the **conditioned blink reflex** (as an example of associative learning).

The climbing fiber input is thought to alter for a long time (days, perhaps years) the responsiveness of the Purkinje cells to mossy fiber inputs. This appears to happen only on simultaneous activation of a Purkinje cell by specific sets of climbing and mossy fibers, leading to a change of Purkinje cell excitability, so that the following mossy fiber signals have less effect than previously. This phenomenon, **long-term depression** (LTD; see Chapter 4, under "Kinds of Synaptic Plasticity") depends on a rise in Ca^{2+} concentration in the Purkinje cell dendrites, which is produced by the binding of glutamate to amino-methylisoxazole propionic acid (AMPA) and metabotropic glutamate receptors. Most likely, however, several cellular mechanisms underlie cerebellar plasticity.[5]

---

5. The hypothesis that LTD is the cellular basis of cerebellar plasticity (and thus learning) is not supported by all available data, however. For example, knockout mice lacking certain glutamate receptors exhibited reduced motor learning in spite of retained ability to produce LTD in the cerebellar cortex.

The Inferior Olive and Rhythmic Movements

A characteristic property of olivary neurons is that their membrane potential shows spontaneous fluctuations that facilitate **rhythmic firing** with a frequency of 5 to 10 Hz. Llinás and Sugimori (1992) propose that the inferior olive functions as a **pacemaker** for movements, by alerting specific combinations of premotor neurons in the cord. Indeed, making the olivary neurons fire rhythmically by systemic administration of the alkaloid **harmaline** produces rhythmic muscular contractions—tremor—in large parts of the body with a frequency of 10 Hz. Further, olivary neurons fire rhythmically in pace with licking movements in the rat, which occur with a frequency of 6 to 8 Hz.

Another peculiarity of olivary neurons is that they are **electrically coupled** (nexus). This enables large assemblies of neurons to fire **synchronously**. The GABAergic fibers from the cerebellar nuclei, mentioned earlier, can switch off the electric coupling so that the synchronously firing neuronal assemblies become much smaller. Conceivably, this relates to how the cerebellum organizes the activation of muscle groups at specific moments during a movement.

The Mossy Fibers and Fractured Somatotopy in the Cerebellar Cortex

The mossy fibers, thought to end with a fairly diffuse somatotopic pattern, were shown by the use of micromapping methods to end in numerous, discrete **patches** in the cortex, each patch defined by its sensory input from a specific minor part of the body (Welker 1987). Each patch is usually less than 1 mm in diameter (in the rat and cat). Thus, the leg region within the posterior lobe consists in reality of a **mosaic** of patches. A salient feature is that adjacent patches can receive inputs from body parts that are widely separated. Further, the same body part is usually represented in several widely separated patches. This arrangement of the mossy fibers was termed **fractured somatotopy** by Welker. It presumably is a means to integrate various inputs sharing relevance for a certain movement. How this pattern of mossy fiber inputs is coordinated with the climbing fiber inputs is not clear, however. As discussed later (Fig. 24.17), the climbing fibers terminate in narrow sagittal strips or zones, and one such strip is often related to one body part only.

EFFERENT CONNECTIONS OF THE CEREBELLUM

As previously mentioned, the three main subdivisions of the cerebellum act largely on the parts of the nervous system from which they receive afferent inputs. The vast majority of the Purkinje cell axons end in the cerebellar nuclei (corticonuclear fibers). The neurons of these nuclei forward the information to the various targets of the cerebellum.

The Cerebellar Nuclei and the Corticonuclear Connections

The cerebellar nuclei are located in the deep white matter of the cerebellum, just above the roof of the fourth ventricle (Figs. 24.3A and 24.14). In humans, there are four nuclei on each side. Close to the midline, under the vermis, lies the **fastigial nucleus** (medial cerebellar nucleus); then follow two small nuclei, and most laterally lies the large, folded **dentate nucleus** (lateral cerebellar nucleus). The two small nuclei have specific names in humans—the **globose** and the **emboliform** nuclei—and correspond to the anterior and posterior **interposed nuclei** in animals.

The **corticonuclear connections** are precisely, topographically organized so that, as a rule, fibers from the anterior parts of the cerebellar cortex end in anterior parts of the nuclei, fibers from medial parts of the cortex end medially, and so forth. There is also a marked **longitudinal localization**, with the vermis sending fibers to the fastigial nucleus, the intermediate zone to the interposed nuclei, and the hemispheres to the dentate nucleus (Fig. 24.15). Somatotopic localization exists within each of the nuclei so that different parts influence movements in different parts of the body. Overall, signals from different parts of the cerebellum are kept segregated through the nuclei and further on to other parts of the brain. Thus, each of the nuclei sends efferent fibers to a separate target region, as shown in a very simplified manner in Figs. 24.6, 24.9, and 24.11.

Direct Projections from the Cerebellum to the Vestibular Nuclei

Parts of the vestibular nuclei correspond in certain respects to the cerebellar nuclei. Thus, the Purkinje cells of the **vestibulocerebellum** (Fig. 24.4) send their axons directly to the vestibular nuclei as **corticovestibular** fibers (Fig. 24.5). These fibers end primarily in vestibular nuclei that send ascending connections to the nuclei of the external ocular muscles (the medial longitudinal fasciculus; see Fig. 18.8B) and, to a lesser extent, in parts of the nuclei sending fibers to the spinal cord. The vestibular nuclei also receive direct projections from Purkinje cells of the vermis of the **anterior** and the **posterior lobes**—that is, outside the vestibulocerebellum as defined here. These fibers end primarily in the lateral vestibular nucleus (nucleus of Deiters; see Figs. 18.7 and 18.8A), which projects to the spinal cord. Therefore, the cerebellar vermis can influence spinal motoneurons via the lateral vestibulospinal tract in addition to its effects mediated by means of the fastigial nucleus to the reticular formation and the lateral vestibular nucleus. The vestibulocerebellum thus contributes to the control of eye movements, whereas the vermis via the vestibular nuclei primarily controls posture and equilibrium.

Cerebellar Nuclear Neurons Are Spontaneously Active

The nuclear cells fire with a high frequency even in an animal sitting quietly. When neurons fire without any obvious excitatory input, they are said to be **spontaneously active**. Indeed, in vitro studies of cerebellar slices show that the nuclear neurons have intrinsic properties that depolarize the membrane even in the absence of an excitatory input (**pacemaker**

Figure 24.14

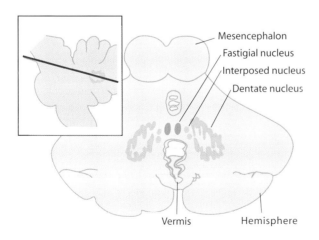 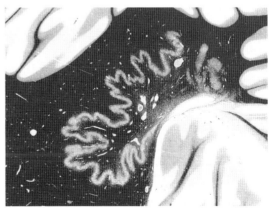

The cerebellar nuclei. **Left:** Drawing of an oblique section through the cerebellum and the brain stem. **Right:** Photomicrograph of a myelin-stained section placed slightly more dorsally than the drawing. Therefore, only the dentate and the interposed nuclei are seen in the photomicrograph.

Figure 24.15

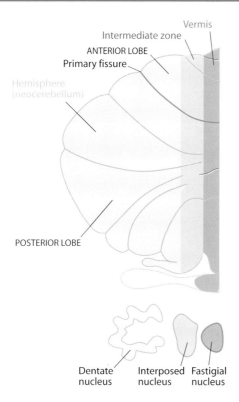

Sagittal arrangement of corticonuclear connections. Purkinje cells in the hemispheres project to the dentate nucleus, whereas Purkinje cells in the intermediate zone and the vermis project to the interposed and fastigial nucleus, respectively. In addition, Purkinje cells in the anterior and posterior vermis project to the vestibular nuclei.

properties). Because all Purkinje cells are inhibitory (GABA), a continuous firing of the nuclear cells is a prerequisite for the information from the cerebellar cortex to be passed on (increased Purkinje cell activity leads to reduced nuclear cell firing). In addition to their tendency for spontaneous depolarization, the nuclear cells receive some excitatory inputs, namely the spinocerebellar and olivocerebellar projections that give off collaterals to the cerebellar nuclei.

Increase or decrease in the firing frequency of the Purkinje cells immediately causes change in the activity of the nuclear cells. A prerequisite for this is synchronous firing of many Purkinje cells with axons converging on a few nuclear cells. Then even minute changes of the activity of each Purkinje cell changes the signals issued from the cerebellum to its target nuclei. Indeed, there is evidence that **synchronous firing** of assemblies of functionally related Purkinje cells is a fundamental feature in cerebellar functioning.

In conclusion, the outputs of the cerebellar nuclei reflect with high temporal precision even very weak inputs to the

cerebellar cortex. This is presumably important for, among other tasks, the cerebellar role in control of rhythm, as we discuss later in this chapter.

Efferent Connections of the Dentate Nucleus

The fibers from the **dentate nucleus** leave the cerebellum through the superior cerebellar peduncle (Fig. 24.2). They cross the midline in the mesencephalon, and some fibers end in the parvocellular part of the **red nucleus** and other mesencephalic nuclei. Fibers also descend to the principal part of the **inferior olive**. Most fibers continue rostrally, however, to end in the thalamus. Here, the dentate fibers end primarily in the **ventrolateral nucleus**; some also reach the ventral anterior nucleus (Fig. 24.16). These nuclei also receive fibers from the basal ganglia, but they end in

Figure 24.16

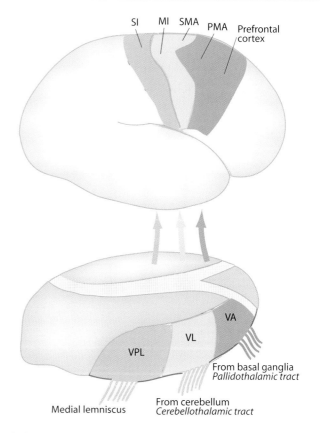

Thalamocortical connections. Schematic of the arrangement within the ventral thalamic nucleus of afferents from the somatosensory pathways, the cerebellum, and the basal ganglia and their further projections to the SI, the MI, and the premotor cortex.

different parts than the cerebellar fibers (as shown schematically in Fig. 24.16), in agreement with physiologic studies showing that the basal ganglia and the cerebellum do not influence identical parts of the cortex. Signals from the cerebellar hemispheres pass primarily to the **MI**, whereas the basal ganglia via the thalamus act mainly on premotor areas and the pre-frontal cortex. In addition, the cerebellum influences parts of the **SMA** and **PMA** that apparently differ from the parts influenced from the basal ganglia. There is also anatomic and physiologic evidence of connections from the dentate nucleus (via the thalamus) to area 9 in the dorsolateral **prefrontal cortex**. Even though such connections most likely are modest compared to those reaching the motor areas, they are thought to be of decisive importance for the cerebellar influence on cognitive tasks.

Efferent Connections of the Interposed and Fastigial Nuclei

As mentioned, the efferents from the intermediate zone reach the **interposed nuclei**. These send their efferents both to the contralateral **thalamus** (to the ventrolateral nucleus mainly, like the dentate) and the **red nucleus** (Fig. 24.11). This enables the interposed nuclei to influence motoneurons via both the rubrospinal tract and the pyramidal tract. Because the rubrospinal tract is crossed, the interposed nucleus (and the intermediate zone) acts on the body half of the same side. The human rubrospinal tract is, however, most likely too small to be of functional significance (see Chapter 22, under "The Red Nucleus and the Rubrospinal Tract").

The **fastigial nucleus** (receiving Purkinje cell axons from the vermis) sends its efferents to both the **vestibular nuclei** and the **reticular formation** (Fig. 24.6). Thus, motoneurons can be influenced via the vestibulospinal and the reticulospinal tracts. On the basis of what we discuss in Chapter 22, the cerebellum via the fastigial nucleus can influence posture and relatively automatic movements such as locomotion. This is supported by the results of animal experiments and by clinical observations. In addition, connections from the fastigial nucleus to the reticular formation mediate cerebellar influences on **autonomic functions**, as shown in animal experiments.

Sagittal Zones and Modules in the Cerebellum

We have so far described that the main subdivisions of the cerebellum—such as the flocculonodular lobe, the vermis, and the hemispheres—differ with regard to connectivity. Further,

we have seen that the lateral parts of the hemispheres, the intermediate zone, and the vermis differ with regard to their efferent connections (Fig. 24.15). This organization of the cerebellum into three longitudinal zones, each projecting to separate parts of the cerebellar nuclei, was first described by the Norwegian neuroanatomists Jan Jansen and Alf Brodal in the 1940s. But the localization within the cerebellum is far more sophisticated than what could be revealed by the fairly primitive methods of 75 years ago. Each of the three **longitudinal zones** of Jansen and Brodal can thus be further subdivided, as shown by the Dutch neuroanatomist J. Voogd and colleagues (Voogd 2014). Figure 24.17 shows the zones of the intermediate zone as an example.

The zonal pattern is especially sharp within the **olivocerebellar** and **corticonuclear** projections. The neurons located within a particular small part of the olive send their fibers to a narrow longitudinal zone, whereas the neighboring zones receive climbing fibers from other parts of the olive (Fig. 24.17). The Purkinje cells of the zones also send their axons to different parts of the cerebellar nuclei. The parcellation of the cortex into sagittal zones in fact goes further than shown in Fig. 24.17. Physiologic studies show that within the anterior lobe each zone consists of several **microzones**, which differ in the information they receive. Apart from the parallel fibers, extending for a few millimeters perpendicular to the longitudinal zones, there are no association fibers interconnecting different parts of the cerebellar cortex. Thus, the cerebellar cortex and the cerebellar nuclei consist of numerous compartments, or **modules**, that function (at least largely) independently of each other. Some data suggest that each module takes care of a specific motor task. As mentioned, in this respect the cerebellar cortex differs from the cerebral cortex, which is characterized by extensive association connections and cooperation among different regions.

CEREBELLAR FUNCTIONS: GENERAL ASPECTS

We have mentioned functional aspects when discussing cerebellar connections and intrinsic organization in the foregoing parts of this chapter. Here we discuss possible cerebellar functions more broadly. It deserves emphasizing, however, that the cerebellum most likely functions as a **node** (or rather several nodes) in distributed, **task-specific networks**, not by acting as an independent unit.[6] When considering the cerebellar connections, it is clear that the quantitatively most important cerebellar connections are with **movement-related networks** (acting on the neuronal groups that give

---

6. The deficits ensuing from removal of the cerebellar contribution to a network may tell us less about what the cerebellum does than what the networks does without the cerebellum. Therefore, the specific contribution of the cerebellum to various tasks may be hard to determine, especially when the cerebellum contributes to networks dominated by many other nodes (e.g. when considering a possible cerebellar contribution to cognitive functions).

origin to the central motor pathways, notably the pyramidal tract, the reticulospinal tracts, and the vestibulospinal tracts). As is discussed later (under "Functions and Symptoms Related to Specific Parts of the Cerebellum"), in animal experiments and in humans the motor symptoms are the most obvious and disturbing after cerebellar lesions. Nevertheless, as we have discussed, some cerebellar connections enable the cerebellum to participate in other kinds of networks, and even with regard to motor functions the cerebellar role is not always clearly understood.

The Timing Theory: Does the Cerebellum Perform a Basic Operation Used in All Its Functions?

Even though the study of cerebellar symptoms provides reasonable insight into the functions of the cerebellum, we are far from understanding how the cerebellum performs its tasks. The striking uniformity and strictly geometric structure of the cerebellar cortex has led to comparison with a **computer**, which can perform the same kinds of computations on various kinds of information. The subdivision of the cerebellum into numerous, apparently independent units or **modules** may fit such a concept. Several theories have been put forward to explain how the cerebellum operates, but none of them has so far been universally accepted.

The German neuroscientist Valentin Braitenberg proposed more than 50 years ago that the cerebellum functions as a kind of **clock,** measuring temporal intervals with great accuracy. The theory was subsequently modified to emphasize the cerebellar role in the control of **movement sequences** and perhaps other sequential behaviors. The theory is based on, among other factors, the regular arrangement of the parallel fibers (Figs. 24.12 and 12.13). Action potentials conducted along the parallel fibers excite the Purkinje cells in a fixed temporal sequence. We mentioned that a timing function might be crucial in the cerebellar contribution to motor control, and recent data suggest that the cerebellar timing function may also be used in **nonmotor tasks**. Thus, patients with cerebellar damage were impaired not only in their ability to reproduce a certain rhythm by tapping their fingers but also in discriminating different sound rhythms—that is, not only impaired execution but also **perception of rhythm**. They had no problems with discriminating sounds of different intensities, however, which suggests that the defect is specific to discrimination of **temporal intervals**. Reduced ability to judge the velocity

of visual stimuli has also been reported in patients with cerebellar lesions.

The **inferior olive** and the climbing fibers may have a crucial role in the timing function of the cerebellum. Thus, the olivary neurons fire rhythmically, and neurons that activate Purkinje cells within a narrow sagittal zone fire synchronously. Further, there is experimental evidence that the firing rhythm of olivary neurons and the rhythm of certain movements is correlated (see also "The Inferior Olive and Rhythmic Movements" earlier in this chapter).

Another aspect of timing is the judgment of **duration**, for example, how much time has passed since we started a particular action (mental or physical). We have, for example,

Figure 24.17

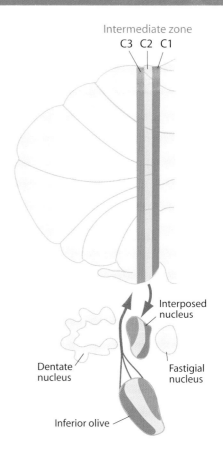

Zonal organization of the cerebellar cortex. Very simplified illustration of the precise topographic pattern of cerebellar efferent and afferent connections. The cortex can be divided into longitudinal zones projecting to different parts of the cerebellar nuclei and receiving afferents from different parts of the inferior olive. Here the intermediate zone is shown as an example. The intermediate zone is divided into three zones termed C1 to C3 differing with regard to olivary afferents and nuclear target region. Each zone, or rather parts of a zone, control certain muscular groups and their coordination in goal-directed movements.

an automatic feeling of when the time from eliciting a PC command to the response is longer than expected. Whether the cerebellum plays a role in this time function as well is not clear.

It should be emphasized that our ability to perceive and estimate time depends not only (or even mainly) on the cerebellum but on a distributed network including the basal ganglia and several parts of the cerebral cortex (see Chapter 23, under "Interval Timing").

The Cerebellum and Learning

Animal experiments indicate that long-lasting changes in synaptic efficacy may take place in the cerebellar cortex during motor learning. Much interest is devoted to theories that consider the cerebellum to be a learning machine. The cerebellum may help **automation** of movements and perhaps also certain **cognitive functions**. There is considerable evidence that **plastic changes** occur in the cerebellum during motor learning. For example, the activation of the cerebellar hemispheres (as measured with fMRI) is higher when a new sequence of movements is learned than when the automated movement is performed afterward. We discussed the possible role of the **climbing fibers** in motor learning and **LTD** as a likely cellular mechanism (see "Mossy and Climbing Fibers Mediate Different Kinds of Information" earlier in this chapter). Recent studies have found that patients with cerebellar lesions have an impaired ability to learn **conditioned responses** (shown for the blink reflex and the withdrawal reflex in the leg).

Because learning takes place in the cerebellum in conditioned responses, it is tempting to assume that corresponding changes occur in the cerebellar hemispheres when humans learn complex **voluntary movements** (such as playing a musical instrument). Indeed, some experiments support this assumption. Thus, patients with cerebellar lesions (or lesions of the inferior olive) show reduced motor learning capacity when wearing prismatic glasses while throwing darts. Both patients and controls missed systematically to one side of the target immediately after putting on the prisms (because the aiming follows the direction of the gaze). During subsequent repetitions, the control persons improved their performance, while no improvement occurred in the cerebellar patients. Conversely, the controls overshot the target after removal of the prisms, although this did not occur in the cerebellar patients.

Although there is a strong case for a cerebellar role in motor learning, this should not be taken to imply that motor learning involves *only* the cerebellum. Indeed, there is good evidence that motor learning involves synaptic changes in distributed networks, including at least motor cortical areas and the basal ganglia (cf. Chapter 22, under "Learning and the Motor Cortex," and Chapter 23, under "Planning and Learning").

Examples of the Role of Cerebellum in Motor Learning

Structural changes of the cerebellum during motor learning have been found in rats that were trained in an **acrobatic task**. After 30 days, the trained rats had significantly more synapses in the molecular layer than the untrained controls. The increase was in both parallel fiber synapses and climbing fiber synapses with Purkinje cells.

A much-studied example of cerebellar plasticity is adaptation of the **vestibulo-ocular reflex** (VOR; see Fig. 25.5), as first shown by the Japanese neurophysiologist Masao Ito. The VOR ensures that when the head moves in one direction, the eyes move in the opposite direction with exactly the same speed. This makes it possible to keep the gaze fixed on a stationary object even though the head moves. The magnitude of the reflex response to a certain head movement (i.e., the gain of the reflex) must be adjusted when, for example, the head grows and alters its proportions. By means of relay stations (see Fig. 25.5), signals from the retina provide information about **retinal slip** (the image is not kept stationary on the retina but moves). Climbing fibers ending in the flocculus provide such signals and thus tell the cerebellum that the velocity of the eye movement is incorrect. Information about head movements from the vestibular apparatus is provided by mossy fibers, which also end in the flocculus. The sensitivity of the VOR can be altered experimentally in a short time, as shown by making experimental animals wear **prismatic glasses** that displace the image on the retina. The most drastic experiment is when the movement of the surroundings appears to be the opposite of the real movement, leading to a complete reversal of the reflex response. Destruction of the **cerebellar flocculus** prevents adaptation of the reflex. (It is disputed, however, whether the change in synaptic efficacy—that is, the learning—is caused by changes in the cerebellum or elsewhere.)

Certain **conditioned responses** are examples of possible cerebellar participation during motor learning. Especially the so-called **nictitating membrane reflex** (a part of the blink reflex) in rabbits has been investigated. When a jet of air hits the eye, the nictitating membrane moves together with the eyelid. This is an unconditioned reflex, in which the trigeminal nerve is the afferent link; the reflex center is in the brain stem involving the sensory trigeminal nucleus, the reticular formation, and the facial nucleus; and the efferent link is the facial nerve to the muscles around the eye. If the jet of air is regularly preceded by a tone (conditioning stimulus), the rabbit will eventually react with a nictitating membrane movement even when the tone is presented alone. The signal pathway for the conditioned response is much more complicated than that for the unconditioned reflex (e.g., the auditory pathways and parts of the cerebral cortex are involved). What is interesting in this connection, however, is that after destruction of the cerebellum, the reflex can no longer be conditioned (i.e., only the unconditioned response occurs, and the animal can no longer be trained to react to the tone only). Damage to the cerebellum after having made the response conditioned abolishes the conditioned (but not the unconditioned) response. It is sufficient to remove a small part of the cerebellar "face area" of the intermediate zone to obtain these effects (this is a further example of the cerebellar functional localization). After establishing the conditioned response, it can be evoked by electric stimulation of pontocerebellar mossy fibers.

The Cerebellum and Cognitive Functions

Many observations now suggest that the cerebellar functions are not restricted to motor ones. While this topic has attracted much interest and numerous neuroimaging studies have been performed in normal persons and cerebellar patients, findings are partly contradictory. It is therefore too early to draw conclusions as to the importance of the cerebellum for mental tasks that are usually considered the domain of the cerebral cortex.

We mentioned that the cerebellum might be important for not only the execution of rhythmic movements but also the **perception of rhythm**. Further, reduced ability to rapidly **shift the attention** from one kind of stimulus to another was found in six patients with lesions of the cerebellar hemispheres. The patients' ability to maintain focused attention was not reduced, and neither was their perception of the stimuli. These and other studies have been taken as evidence that the cerebellum participates in a purely cognitive task—that is, the switching of attention. (An fMRI study of normal persons challenged this interpretation, however. Thus, altered cerebellar activity occurred only when the shift of attention was associated with a motor response.)

Many neuroimaging studies demonstrate (indirectly) that blood flow increases (or decreases) in parts of the cerebellum during the performance of various cognitive tasks. For example, persons trying to solve a **pegboard puzzle** showed increased blood flow in the dentate nucleus. In such studies, one seeks to eliminate the possibility that the increase is caused by the movements alone (e.g., moving the pegs). Another study reported increased blood flow in the cerebellar hemispheres in persons trying to find **verbs** that go with nouns. Further, increased blood flow in the hemispheres was observed in persons playing **imaginary tennis** and in persons **counting silently**. Finally, the cerebellum may also participate in kinds of learning other than learning of movements. Thus, measurements of regional cerebral oxidative metabolism with PET in humans showed that the posterior parts of the cerebellar hemispheres increased their neuronal activity when learning a **tactile recognition task** (more than during just tactile recognition of an object).

Associations between Cerebellar Activity and Cognitive Functions

As mentioned, interpretation of associations between cerebellar change of activity and the performance of cognitive tasks is not straightforward. For example, it is difficult to eliminate the possibility that the cerebellar contribution concerns aspects of execution rather than earlier stages in the processing. When trying to assess the importance of the cerebellum for cognitive functions, we should remember that rather sophisticated tests are required to reveal cognitive defects in cerebellar patients while their motor impairments are obvious and incapacitating. Thus, a study applying a neuropsychological bedside test battery to patients in the chronic stage of cerebellar disease found no clear evidence of cognitive deficits. While cognitive impairments seems to be more prominent in the acute stage of cerebellar disease, even then reports differ with regard to severity of impairment and whether or not specific symptoms depend on the site of the lesion.

The cerebellum has also been implicated in the **development** of cognitive functions. Again, effects might be rather subtle. This point is supported by a study of children who had their cerebellum partly removed before the age of 3 (because of tumors). These children showed no significant signs of disturbed cognitive development, even though their motor acquisition of motor skills was clearly subnormal. The problems with interpreting clinical data become obvious, however, when adding that, among the children, those who had received radiation therapy scored below normal on both cognitive and motor tests.

FUNCTIONS AND SYMPTOMS RELATED TO SPECIFIC PARTS OF THE CEREBELLUM

The separation of the cerebellum into three fairly distinct parts with regard to connectivity (Figs. 24.5, 24.6, and 24.9) is the reason that we discuss these parts separately with regard to function and clinical symptoms. Clinically, one usually distinguishes three cerebellar syndromes:[7] the **flocculonodular syndrome**, the **anterior lobe syndrome**, and the **neocerebellar syndrome**. The existence of three distinct syndromes is most clear-cut in experimental animals, while in humans the neocerebellar syndrome is most often seen. This is not surprising because the hemispheres (the neocerebellum) make up the major part of the human cerebellum.

Because both the ascending fibers from the cerebellum to the cerebral cortex and the descending fibers from the cerebral cortex to the spinal cord are crossed, the cerebellar hemisphere exerts its influence on the body half of the same side (Fig. 24.18). Consequently, with diseases of the cerebellum, the motor **symptoms** occur on the **same side as the lesion**.

---

7. A syndrome is a constellation of symptoms that occur together.

Figure 24.18

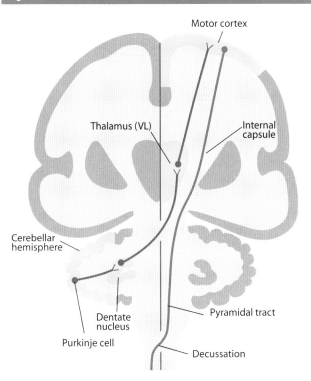

Unilateral lesions of the cerebellum produce symptoms on the same side. Ascending connections from the dentate nucleus cross in the mesencephalon on their way to the thalamus. The next link passes to the motor cortex, where pyramidal tract neurons are influenced. Since the pyramidal tract crosses (in the lower medulla), the cerebellar hemispheres control muscles in the ipsilateral body half.

The Flocculonodular and Anterior Lobe Syndromes

Isolated damage to the **flocculonodular lobe** in monkeys produces disturbances of the **equilibrium**—that is, unsteadiness in standing and walking. When the body is supported, movements of the extremities can be performed normally, however. Sometimes, similar symptoms occur in humans with a special kind of tumor in the posterior cranial fossa, most often called a **medulloblastoma** arising from the nodulus. The animals also exhibit **nystagmus** with the quick phase to the side of the lesion. (Nystagmus is movements in which the eyes move slowly in one direction—as when tracking a moving object with the gaze—and rapidly back.) Eye movements may also be disturbed in humans with cerebellar lesions that affect the vestibulocerebellum.

Damage to the **anterior lobe** in experimental animals primarily produces a change of **muscle tone**. In decerebrate

animals, the decerebrate rigidity increases, as do the postural reflexes. This fits with the observation that electrical stimulation of the anterior lobe reduces the decerebrate rigidity (as mentioned, the Purkinje cells inhibit the cells of the cerebellar nuclei, whereas the nuclear cells have excitatory actions on reticulospinal and vestibulospinal neurons). In addition, some Purkinje cells in the anterior lobe vermis send axons directly to the vestibular nuclei, and removal of this inhibitory action also tends to increase the activity of the vestibulospinal neurons and thus the decerebrate rigidity. In **humans,** it is doubtful whether lesions of the anterior lobe produce increased muscle tone. More marked is **gait ataxia** (unsteadiness of walking) in patients with damage that mainly affects the anterior lobe vermis and the intermediate zone (this occurs in cerebellar degeneration caused by alcohol abuse). The anterior lobe vermis, by means of its efferent connections to the fastigial nucleus and from there to the reticular formation, must therefore be assumed to have a role in coordination of the **half-automatic movements** of walking and postural adjustments. Similarly, selective lesions of the **fastigial nucleus** in monkeys cause difficulties with walking, sitting, and maintaining the **upright position**.

Therapeutic Stimulation of the Cerebellum

Electric stimulation with electrodes surgically implanted at the cerebellar surface has been used in patients with neurological disorders such as **epilepsy** and **cerebral palsy**. The theoretical basis is the inhibitory action of the Purkinje cells with subsequent reduction of abnormally increased neuronal excitability and muscle tone. Even though some report favorable results with such stimulation, it is not quite clear whether the effect is due to the cerebellar stimulation or to some other factor.

Cerebellar Lesions and Eye Movements

As mentioned, lesions of the flocculonodular lobe can cause nystagmus. This may manifest itself as **spontaneous nystagmus** (i.e., nystagmus occurring in a person at rest with no kind of stimulation) or only when the patient tries to keep the gaze in an eccentric position (paralysis of gaze nystagmus). Conceivably, these symptoms are due to the loss of Purkinje cells that normally inhibit the vestibular nuclei (especially the medial nucleus) sending fibers to the nuclei of the extrinsic eye muscles (see Fig. 18.8). In addition, the patients with lesions of the flocculonodular lobe may have difficulties with slow **pursuit movements** (tracking a moving object with the gaze). Pursuit movements may also be impaired after lesions restricted to lateral parts of the **pontine nuclei** or the **cerebellar hemispheres** (impaired to the side of the lesion). Finally, lesions of the cerebellar hemisphere may cause so-called **saccadic dysmetria**—that is, the rapid eye movements overshoot the target and are followed by several correcting movements before the gaze is finally fixed. The role of the cerebellum in the control of eye movements is further discussed in Chapter 25, under "The Cerebellum Controls Both Saccades and Pursuit Movements."

The Cerebellar Hemispheres and the Neocerebellar Syndrome

The neocerebellum plays a different functional role than the phylogenetically older parts of the cerebellum: it is primarily concerned with the coordination of the **least automatic movements**. This stands to reason, since the cerebellar hemispheres send their main output to the MI (via the dentate nucleus and the thalamus) and thus influence the neurons of the pyramidal tract (Figs. 24.9 and 24.18). After removal of one cerebellar hemisphere in a monkey, the voluntary movements become uncertain on the same side of the body: they become **uncoordinated** or **ataxic**. The same effect can be produced by cooling the dentate nucleus (by the use of a cooling electrode) in a monkey that is performing a well-rehearsed movement (as soon as the cooling is reversed, the movements again become normal). Movements that are performed quickly and smoothly become unsteady and jerky by the cooling. The monkey misses repeatedly when trying to grasp an object, even though it knows perfectly well where it is and what is demanded. Sometimes the hand is moved too far in relation to the object and sometimes not far enough. The movements tend to be **decomposed**; that is, instead of occurring simultaneously in several joints, they take place in one joint at a time, and the **velocity** is uneven—sometimes too high and sometimes too low. Selective damage or transient "uncoupling" of the dentate nucleus in monkeys indicates that the cerebellar hemispheres are particularly important when movements must take place in **several joints** at the same time. Picking up a raisin, for example, became impossible because the monkey could no longer coordinate the movements of the joints of the wrist, thumb, and index finger. Precise movements of one finger at the time could be completed normally, however. Difficulties with hitting an object when trying to grasp it with the hand can probably be attributed to the same basic defect, that is, difficulties with coordinating the movements of the wrist, shoulder, and elbow joints.

All the elements of ataxia have been attributed to a **fundamental defect** in control of the force and of the exact timing of the **starting** and **stopping** of movements.[8] As mentioned, the **temporal** aspect appears to be central to the cerebellar contribution to motor control. This is evidenced by patients with cerebellar damage who are unable to perform sequences of finger movements in a particular **rhythm**. The movements are completed by each finger without a fixed temporal relation to movements of the other fingers.

Symptoms in Humans with Lesions of the Cerebellar Hemispheres

Ataxia of this kind is also the most prominent symptom in **humans** with damage to the cerebellar hemispheres. For example, difficulty with the **precision grip** similar to that described in monkeys has been observed in patients with unilateral infarcts of the cerebellar hemispheres. The increase of force when grasping an object is slower than normal, and the adjustment of the grip force is deficient when grasping and lifting at the same time. In clinical neurology, the various elements of ataxia have particular names, such as **dysmetria** (movement is not stopped in time), **asynergia** (decomposition of complex movements), **dysdiadochokinesia** (reduced ability to perform rapidly alternating movements of, e.g., the hand), and **intentional tremor** (tremor arising when trying to perform a movement, such as grasping an object). Speech is also often disturbed in cerebellar diseases. It has been called **speech ataxia** to emphasize that it also appears to be caused by incoordination (in the respiratory muscles, the muscles of the larynx, and others), making the strength and velocity of the speech uneven.

In **acute** damage to the cerebellar hemispheres in humans, the **muscle tone** often appears to be reduced when tested by passive stretch (the symptom is transient). This is called **cerebellar hypotonia**. The underlying mechanism is not clear, although experiments in anesthetized animals suggest that it is caused by reduced γ motoneuron activity. Recent experiments in awake animals and in humans, however, show that the muscle-spindle sensitivity to stretch is not significantly altered by cerebellar lesions (even when they include the dentate and interposed nuclei).

8. It is not certain, however, that this suffices to explain why the symptoms are most marked when movements in two or more joints must be coordinated (such as moving the index finger quickly to the tip of the nose from a position with the arm stretched out).

For the eye to provide useful information to higher visual centers, the picture must be held stationary on the retina. Further, the eyes must be positioned so that the most salient part of a visual scene falls on the central part of the retina with the highest visual acuity. Finally, to sample enough information, the eyes must be moved quickly from one point of salience to another. The control system must therefore be able to move the eyes quickly and precisely to make the image fall on the macula; such movements are called **saccades** (or saccadic movements). In addition, the control system must move the eyes so the retinal image is stationary even if the head or the object is moving. The latter are called **slow-pursuit movements**.

The extraocular muscles responsible for moving the eyes receive their nerve supply from the nuclei of the **third, fourth, and sixth cranial nerves**. The control system coordinates the activity of the α motoneurons in these nuclei. **Premotor networks** interconnecting areas in the cerebral cortex, the brain stem, and the cerebellum carry out this task. To enable coordinated activity, the nuclei of the extraocular muscles are interconnected by numerous fibers forming the **medial longitudinal fascicle**. The control system uses **sensory information** from the retina, which informs about whether the retinal image is stationary or slipping, from the **vestibular apparatus** about the movements of the head, and from **proprioceptors** in the eye muscles about the movements of the eyes in the orbit. All this sensory information is integrated and transformed into a **motor signal** specifying the total activity of the extraocular muscles at any time. For control of **horizontal eye movements**—especially saccades—the most important premotor area, the **paramedian pontine reticular formation** (PPRF), lies close to the abducens nucleus on each side. The PPRF sends fibers to the abducens and oculomotor nuclei and coordinates their activities. A corresponding premotor area for **vertical eye movements** is found in the mesencephalic reticular formation close to the oculomotor nucleus.

There is an important difference between the control of eye muscles and of other muscles subjected to precise voluntary control (e.g., intrinsic hand muscles): the nuclei of the extraocular muscles—in contrast to spinal α motoneurons—receive no direct fibers from the cerebral cortex. The **central control** is exerted via premotor networks in the brain stem. At least two regions of the cerebral cortex are closely involved in the control of eye movements (Fig. 25.8): the **frontal eye field** is primarily related to initiation of saccadic movements, whereas several smaller areas in the **parietotemporal region** are mainly involved in the control of pursuit movements.

The third, fourth, and sixth cranial nerves and their nuclei are discussed in Chapter 27, together with the light reflex and accommodation reflex mediated by the intrinsic eye muscles. Chapter 16 gives a brief account of the structure of the eye.

Horizontal, Vertical, and Rotatory Movements of the Eye

The eye is a sphere, lying in the orbit, surrounded by fat. It can rotate freely in any direction around its center, whereas translatory movements are prevented. To describe the rotatory movements of a sphere, we define **three axes**, passing through the center and oriented perpendicular to each other (Fig. 25.1). For convenience, we describe the movements as taking place in three planes: a **frontal**, a **sagittal**, and a transverse or **horizontal** plane. A movement in the horizontal plane takes place around a vertical axis, and the anterior part of the eye—and therefore the gaze—moves from side to side. We perform **horizontal eye movements** when looking

Figure 25.1

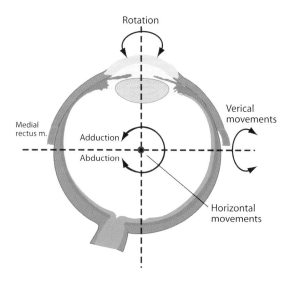

The axes of eye movements. Right eye seen from above. Note that all axes pass through the center of the eye bulb.

Figure 25.2

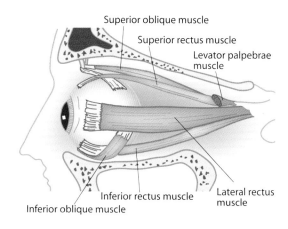

The extraocular muscles seen from the lateral aspect. The lateral wall of the orbit is removed. The straight muscles insert in front of the equatorial plane of the eye, whereas the oblique muscles insert behind it.

to one side; when looking to the left, the left eye rotates laterally and the right eye rotates medially. A movement in the sagittal plane takes place around a transverse axis, and the anterior part of the eye moves up and down. Such movements, directing the gaze up and down, are called **vertical eye movements**. Movements in the frontal plane take place around a sagittal axis, and the eye rotates without any horizontal or vertical movement. For practical reasons only, such movements around a sagittal axis are called **rotatory eye movements** (strictly speaking, all eye movements are rotations around the center of the eyeball).

The Extraocular Muscles and Their Actions

The six extraocular (extrinsic) muscles (Fig. 25.2) ensure that the **visual axes** of the eyes (see Fig. 16.2) can be directed precisely toward any point in the visual field. The scheme in Fig. 25.3 shows the main movements produced by each of the extraocular muscles if they were acting alone (this is a theoretical situation, because in reality they always work in concert). Most of the muscles produce combinations of vertical, horizontal, and rotatory movements. Further, the actions of each of the muscles change with the position of the eye because this changes the position and direction of the line of pull (Fig. 25.4A). The extraocular muscles (Fig. 25.2) all **attach** to the sclera and originate from the wall of the orbit (a brief account of the structure of the eye bulb is given in

Chapter 16). We analyze the **actions** of the extraocular muscles in relation to the previously defined three axes through the center of the eyeball. We then need to know the direction of the force exerted by the muscles in relation to the axis. We must furthermore know whether the muscle insertion in the sclera is anterior or posterior to the **equatorial plane** of the eye, a frontal plane dividing the eye in an anterior and a posterior half.

There are **four straight** and **two oblique extraocular muscles** (Figs. 25.2 and 25.4A, see also Fig. 27.17). We can simplify their functions by stating that two muscles produce predominantly horizontal movements (the medial and lateral rectus muscles), two produce predominantly vertical movements (the superior and inferior rectus muscles), and two produce mainly rotatory movements (the superior and inferior oblique muscles). The straight muscles (the rectus muscles) come from the posterior end of the orbit and run forward to insert in front of the equatorial plane. This means that the **lateral rectus** muscle pulls the front of the eye (the cornea) laterally, whereas the **medial rectus** muscle pulls it medially (these two muscles thus produce pure horizontal movements). Correspondingly, the **superior rectus** muscle pulls the eye (the cornea) upward, whereas the **inferior rectus** muscle pulls it downward. These two therefore produce vertical movements. Because the superior and inferior rectus muscles run anteriorly in a lateral direction (Fig. 25.4A), however, they do not only produce vertical movements but also some horizontal movement (in the medial direction). Thus, when the superior rectus muscle acts alone, it

Figure 25.3

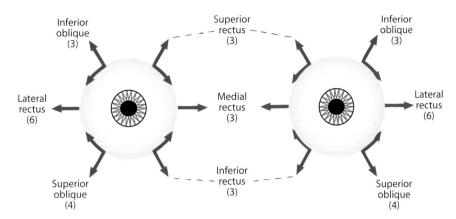

Actions of the extraocular muscles. These are as observed when movements start from a neutral position of the eye. Arrows indicate direction of the action (but not the force). Except for the medial and lateral recti, all muscles rotate the eye, in addition to their other actions. Starting positions away from the neutral may alter the actions of the muscles. For example, the superior rectus is a pure elevator when the eye is 23 degrees abducted (cf. Fig. 25.4).

produces an upward movement combined with a (smaller) medial—that is, an oblique movement. In addition, the muscle produces a small medial rotation of the eye (around the sagittal axis). The **superior oblique** muscle has a more complicated course than the other extraocular muscles (Fig. 25.4A). It originates posteriorly in the orbit and runs forward medially. Just behind the anterior margin of the orbit, it bends sharply around a small hook of connective tissue and continues in a posterolateral direction to insert posterior to the equatorial plane. The muscle acts around all three axes: it rotates the eye around the sagittal axis so that the upper part moves medially and furthermore directs the gaze downward and laterally (Fig. 25.3). The **inferior oblique** muscle originates from the bottom of the orbit in its anteromedial part and runs, like the superior oblique, posterolaterally to insert behind the equator (Fig. 25.2). It directs the gaze laterally and upward and rotates the eye around the sagittal axis with its upper part laterally.

The Eye Muscles Are Built for Precise Control

The structure of the extraocular muscles reflects their use in extremely delicate and precisely controlled movements. The muscle fibers are very thin in comparison with ordinary skeletal muscle fibers, and the **motor units** are among the smallest in the body (only 5–10 muscle fibers per motoneuron). Consequently, the nerves to the extraocular muscles contain many nerve fibers: the abducens nerve in humans (supplying only one muscle) contains around 6,000 axons.

The extraocular muscles are required both to hold a certain tension for a long time (static position holding) and to

produce extremely fast movements. Accordingly, the maximal **speed of contraction** is high in comparison with other skeletal muscle fibers. Further, the maximal **firing frequency** of the motoneurons—occurring during saccadic movements—is unusually high.

The extraocular muscles are composed of a mixture of fibers with fast and slow **twitch** contractions. In addition, there are muscle fibers that do not produce twitches but only a slow **graded contraction** (they receive multiple end plates along the length of the muscle and occur only in eye muscles). Their function is unknown, but, presumably, they contribute to static position holding.

The Actions of Eye Muscles Depend on Eye Position

The aforementioned considerations and the scheme in Fig. 25.3 concern movements starting from a **neutral position** of the eye—that is, when viewing a distant object straight ahead. Changing the position of the eye in the orbit also changes the action of the muscles (for some muscles the change is small, and for others it is quite marked). For example, the superior rectus is a pure elevator when the eye is about 25 degrees abducted (Fig. 25.4A). The oblique muscles perform pure vertical movements when the eye is about 50 degrees adducted (Fig. 25.4A). This is the basis for the simple test of the extraocular muscles in Fig. 25.4B, designed to test each muscle in isolation (as far as possible).

Figure 25.4

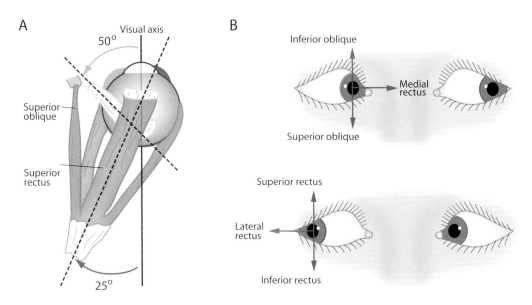

The actions of the eye muscles depend on the position of the eye. **A:** The right eye and eye muscles seen from above. With the eye in a neutral position the direction of force for the superior rectus forms 25 degrees with the visual axis of the eye. Thus, with 25-degree abduction of the eye, the lateral rectus becomes a pure elevator (cf. the position of the eye in B when testing the superior rectus). Furthermore, the figure shows that with about 50-degree adduction, the superior oblique is a pure depressor. **B:** Scheme for testing the eye muscles. Based on testing in extreme positions in which the muscles produce relatively pure vertical or horizontal movements.

Natural Eye Movements Are Conjugated

Virtually every natural eye movement is a combination of the various movement directions described in the preceding text. By combining proper amounts of vertical and horizontal movements, any oblique movement can be produced. Further, all natural eye movements are **conjugated**—that is, the two eyes move together to ensure that the image always falls on corresponding points of the two retinas (see Fig. 16.3). **Double vision** (**diplopia**) results if the eye movements do not occur in conjugation. This is a typical symptom of pareses of the extraocular muscles.

Almost all eye movements require a complicated cooperation of numerous muscles, with activation of synergists and inhibition of antagonists. When, for example, we look to the left, we activate the left lateral rectus and inhibit the left medial rectus, whereas we activate the right medial rectus and inhibit the right lateral rectus. This is the simplest possible example, with a purely horizontal movement. In most other situations, the cooperation between various muscles becomes much more complicated and requires an extensive, sophisticated neural network for control. **Electromyographic** recordings in awake human subjects with their eyes open show that there is some activity in

virtually all of the extraocular muscles. The tension produced by each muscle varies, of course, with the position of the eyes. Patients with a **paralysis** of the **lateral rectus** muscle demonstrate that there is **constant activity** in extraocular muscles. Even though the major muscle for active abduction is paralyzed, a small abduction nevertheless occurs when the patient attempts to look to the affected side. This abduction is caused by the relaxation of muscles that adduct the eye, allowing the tension of the oblique muscles to produce a slight lateral movement.

Eye Muscles, Proprioception, and Efference Copy

There are **muscle spindles** in the extraocular muscles (100–150 altogether in the six human extraocular muscles), but their functional role is not fully understood. Thus, signals from extraocular muscle spindles are apparently not consciously perceived—that is, they do not contribute to the awareness of eye position and movements (in this respect differing from muscle spindles elsewhere). Nor do signals from extraocular muscle spindles evoke stretch reflexes. There is evidence, however, that muscle-spindle signals, providing information about the length and the change of length of the extraocular muscles, are integrated in the cerebral cortex with signals providing information about movements of the head from the labyrinth and with signals from the retina. Experiments in monkeys with transection of the ophthalmic nerve (assumed to contain most of the muscle spindle afferents from the extraocular muscles) did not disturb saccadic and pursuit movements, although they did produce **instability** of the eyes and slow pendular movements in darkness.

It seems that the eye movement control system receives enough information from the **efference copy** (i.e., the copy of the motor commands sent to the extraocular muscles) and does not depend on feedback from proprioceptors. Nevertheless, information from the muscle spindles may contribute to the long-term **calibration** of the efference copy. When there is a mismatch between the command and the feedback (informing about the true movement of the eye), this may be used to change the motor program. Such mismatch arises, for example, when the dimensions of the eye and the eye muscles change as we grow. Thus, proprioceptive information is presumably necessary to ensure **fusion** of the retinal images (avoid strabismus with double vision).

BRAIN STEM AND CEREBELLAR CONTROL OF EYE MOVEMENTS

Kinds of Eye Movement

As mentioned, the control system for eye movements must ensure that the gaze can be moved quickly from one point of fixation to another by **saccadic movements** but also that the gaze can be kept stationary on an object when the object or the head moves by **pursuit movements**. The eye movements may be either **voluntary**, as when we follow a moving object with the eyes, or **reflex**, as when the head moves (a **vestibulo-ocular reflex [VOR]**) or the surroundings move (an **optokinetic reflex**). The VOR and nystagmus are discussed in Chapter 18.

The following is a highly schematic description of eye movements. Different **premotor networks** control each of the kinds of movement, although they all converge on the motoneurons of the extraocular muscles. The separation of the different central networks is less clear-cut than formerly believed, however. Thus, recent studies show that several regions, for example in the cerebral cortex and the cerebellum, participate in the control of both saccadic and pursuit movements.

1. **Saccades** are conjugated movements that change the visual axis of the eyes from one point of fixation to another with maximal speed. Saccades can (at least in a certain sense) be **voluntary**, as when we look at a stationary landscape and fix the gaze at one point for a moment and then move on (with a saccade) to another point of fixation. They can also occur **reflexly**,

as part of vestibular or optokinetic nystagmus. When awake, we perform saccades all the time, often several per second. In this way, we constantly **scan** the visual scene to provide maximal information. Because the visual acuity declines so rapidly outward from the macula, scanning is necessary to use the full analyzing capacity of the visual system.

After a salient (interesting) image has been brought to the macula by a saccade, we need to keep the image stationary long enough for the brain to analyze it (**gaze holding**). What is deemed salient in a visual scene—and thus elicit saccades—is strongly influenced by the task (e.g., driving a car, playing soccer, or moving in a crowded street) and prior expectations.

2. **Smooth-pursuit movements** are performed when we follow a small moving object to keep the image stationary on the central part of the retina. As a rule, we use pursuit movements both of the eyes and of the head when looking at a moving object. One might think that the movements of the head would elicit conjugated eye movements in the opposite direction of the head because of the VOR. This does not occur, however, because the VOR is suppressed during such smooth-pursuit movements. This kind of smooth movement is **voluntary** in the sense that it requires that our attention be directed to something in the visual field; that is, the gaze is voluntarily fixed. Vestibular and optokinetic stimuli can also elicit reflex slow movements that stabilize the retinal image. These are involuntary in the sense that they occur also without paying attention to something in the visual field.

3. **Optokinetic reflex movements** are movements intended to stabilize the retinal image when the whole visual field moves relative to the head. The stimulus is movement of the image on the retina (**retinal slip**). This kind of movement occur. Then a slow movement (following the scene moving outside the window) is interrupted by a quick, opposite movement—resetting the eyes to their original position—when the eyes cannot follow the scene anymore. This movement pattern is called **optokinetic nystagmus**. The optokinetic reflex can be suppressed voluntarily only by fixating on an object that is stationary (or moves with a different speed) in relation to the movement of the rest of the visual scene.

Figure 25.5

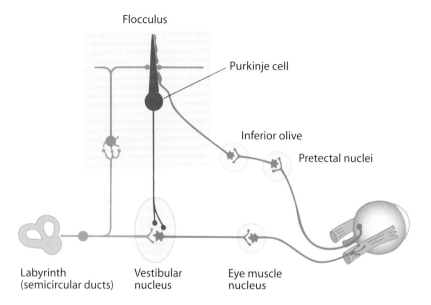

Flocculus

Purkinje cell

Inferior olive

Pretectal nuclei

Labyrinth
(semicircular ducts)

Vestibular
nucleus

Eye muscle
nucleus

Main structural elements of the VOR. Only excitatory connections are shown, even though there are inhibitory neurons in the vestibular nuclei that influence the motoneurons of the antagonists. The reflex arc consists of three neurons from the semicircular duct to the extraocular muscles. The cerebellar flocculus receives signals from the labyrinth and from the retina, and the output of the Purkinje cells can adjust the sensitivity of the vestibular neurons, if necessary, to avoid retinal slip. (Based on Ito 1984.)

4. **Vestibulo-ocular reflex (VOR) movements** are eye movements elicited by movements of the head (Fig. 25.5). The eyes move with the same velocity as the head but in the opposite direction, thereby ensuring that the retinal image is stationary. When the eye cannot move further, a fast movement occurs in the opposite direction, resetting the position of the eye; then the slow movement starts again. These alternate movements are called **vestibular nystagmus**. The quick phase of vestibular nystagmus and saccades share many characteristics but are not identical. The VOR enables us to see an object sharply even when we move around. When the head rotates, the stimulus originates in the semicircular ducts. Even though the VOR has been most studied in relation to rotations in the horizontal plane (Fig. 25.5), the reflex is three-dimensional in the sense that all directions of head rotation elicit specific compensatory eye movements.[1]

5. **Vergence** movements change the visual axes of the eyes in relation to each other when the point of fixation moves away from or toward the eyes. This is necessary to keep the image on corresponding points of the retina. Indeed, **disparity** of the images in the two eyes (not falling on corresponding points, producing diplopia) is the most powerful stimulus to elicit vergence movements, although several other factors also contribute (e.g., blurring of the image, perspective, and change in size). Vergence movements are a prerequisite for fusion of the two images and for stereoscopic vision. **Convergence** of the **visual axes**, which takes place when an object is approaching the eyes, depends primarily on the activity of the medial rectus muscles, with some contribution also from the superior and inferior recti (Fig. 25.3). For use of tools and reading, the convergence movement typically is combined with lowering of the gaze, requiring activity of the inferior rectus muscle in addition to the medial. **Accommodation** and **pupillary constriction** accompany convergence movements. This seems to be ensured by connections between the part of the oculomotor nucleus supplying the medial and inferior rectus muscles and the adjacent parasympathetic Edinger-Westphal nucleus (see Figs. 27.2A and 27.5). The latter contains neurons controlling the ciliary muscle and the pupillary sphincter.

1. The VOR described here—the **rotational VOR**—is not the only VOR. Translatory (linear) accelerations of the head (stimulating the sacculus and utriculus) also elicit compensatory eye movements (**translational VOR, otolith-OR**). In real life both kinds of head movement occur, and the different sensory inputs from the labyrinth must be integrated centrally to yield a motor command that ensures a stable retinal image.

More about Voluntary Saccades and Scanning

When **reading** we fixate a point on the line for an average of 250 msec (60–500) before the gaze is moved on by a saccade. How far the gaze moves before reaching a new point of fixation varies greatly. There is a tendency to fixate on long "content" words rather than on short "functional" words. Native readers of English perceive about 4 letters to the left and 15 to the right of the point of fixation.

A woman with inborn **ophthalmoplegia** (inability to move the eyes) had surprisingly few problems and was able to live a normal life. She apparently used quick head movements to compensate for the lack of saccadic eye movements (Gilchrist 1997) and was thereby able to scan the visual scene with sufficient speed and accuracy.

The Cerebellum Plays a Crucial Role in Adaptations of Eye Movements

We discussed the role of the cerebellum in motor learning in Chapter 24 (under "The Cerebellum and Learning") and used the VOR as an example. It seems obvious that—in order to maintain their accuracy—all kinds of eye movement must adapt to changing internal and external conditions (growth, aging, fatigue, environmental alterations, skill acquisition, and so forth). Such adaptation is a form of motor **learning** that alters behavior to improve goal attainment.

Adaptation of **saccades** depends critically on posterior parts of the cerebellum (the **vermal oculomotor region** or oculomotor vermis) and the fastigial nucleus. For example, transcranial direct current stimulation of this part in humans alters saccadic adaption (to a target that is moved during the saccade). Adaptation of **pursuit movements** also depends on the cerebellum and alterations of Purkinje cell behavior (notably in the flocculus). Such adaptation is an important part of skills learning, for example playing tennis or downhill skiing.

It should be emphasized, however, that plastic changes underlying eye movement adaptation are more widespread and complex than this simplified account may suggest.

The VOR Circuit Adapts to Changing Conditions

The magnitude of the VOR response (not the response itself) to a certain rotational stimulus depends on signals to the vestibular nuclei from the cerebellum (Fig. 25.5). The Purkinje cells of the vestibulocerebellum receive primary vestibular fibers (ending as mossy fibers) that provide information about direction and velocity of the head movement. In addition, the same Purkinje cells receive information, via the inferior olive and climbing

fibers, about whether the image is stationary or slips on the retina. A **retinal slip** indicates that the velocity of the compensatory head movement is too high or too low. The cerebellum is then capable of adjusting the excitability (the gain) of the neurons in the vestibular nuclei—that is, in the reflex center of the VOR. Such adaptive change of **gain of the reflex** is presumably needed continuously during growth and in situations of muscular fatigue. Experiments in which animals wear optic **prisms** that deflect the light so that it appears to come from another direction than it really does show the remarkable capacity for learning in this system.

Brain Stem Centers for Control of Eye Movements

Signals informing about desired eye position, actual position, retinal slip, and position of the head are integrated in the **reticular formation** close to the eye muscle nuclei. From these **premotor** neuronal groups commands are sent to the α motoneurons. By combining anatomic data on the fiber connections with physiologic results (obtained by single-cell recordings, electrical and natural stimulation, and lesions), the **preoculomotor networks** have been described in detail.

A "center" for **horizontal eye movements** has been identified in the **paramedian pontine reticular formation** (**PPRF**). The PPRF lies close to, and sends fibers to, the abducens nucleus (Fig. 25.6). It also sends fibers to the parts of the oculomotor nucleus that contains the motoneurons of the medial rectus muscle. Together with the lateral rectus (innervated by the abducens nucleus), the medial rectus participates in horizontal movements. In addition, there are so-called **internuclear neurons** in the abducens nucleus that send axons to the medial rectus motoneurons of the opposite side (Fig. 25.7). This premotor network ensures simultaneous activation of the lateral rectus on one side and the medial rectus on the other, along with inhibition of the antagonists.

A **lesion** in the region of the **PPRF** reduces horizontal conjugate movements to the side of the lesion. Especially marked is the reduction in saccadic movements. A unilateral lesion of the **medial longitudinal fasciculus** between the abducens and the oculomotor nucleus produces so-called **internuclear ophthalmoplegia** with abolished ability to adduct the eye on the same side (the medial rectus muscle). This may be understood based on the diagram in Fig. 25.7. However, **vergence** movements are possible even though the medial rectus is responsible also in that case. Thus, pathways other than the medial longitudinal fasciculus are responsible for the activation of the medial rectus muscle during vergence movements.

of lobules VI–VII) is particularly concerned with the performance of **saccades**, while the **flocculus** and adjoining parts of the posterior lobe (the **paraflocculus**) seem most important for **pursuit** movements. After cerebellectomy, monkeys are unable to perform pursuit movements, whereas saccades can be performed although with reduced precision and velocity. Clinical observations support the role of the cerebellum in control of pursuit movements also in humans (the deficits observed in patients with cerebellar lesions resemble the dose-dependent effects of alcohol on pursuit movements). The distinction between the vermal oculomotor region and flocculus/paraflocculus is not absolute, however, because both contain neurons related to either saccades or pursuit movements. In accordance with this, animal experiments and observations in humans indicate that the vermal oculomotor region controls both precision of saccades and the velocity of pursuit movements.

Lateral parts of the **pontine nuclei** are necessary for voluntary pursuit movements and for the slow phase of optokinetic nystagmus.[3] This is based on recordings of single-cell activity and lesion experiments in monkeys, as well as in a few patients with small brain-stem infarctions. The relevant parts of the pontine nuclei send efferents to both oculomotor-related cerebellar regions, and they receive afferents from (among other areas) the **middle superior temporal area (MST)**, which is related to visual analysis of moving objects. Parallel pathways seem to exist for the control of pursuit movements, however—for example, the **pontine reticulotegmental nucleus (PRN)**, located immediately dorsal to the pontine nuclei, also relays signals from "cortical oculomotor areas" to the cerebellum. The fact that the PRN is involved also in saccadic movements underscores that the networks controlling different kinds of eye movement are not entirely separate.

CORTICAL CONTROL OF EYE MOVEMENTS

There are no direct connections from the cerebral cortex to the eye muscle nuclei. Activation of the extraocular muscles from the cortex in conjunction with voluntary eye movements is mediated via other brain stem cell groups, among them the premotor "gaze centers" discussed in the preceding text. Recent functional magnetic resonance imaging

(fMRI) and positron emission tomography (PET) studies in humans indicate that a distributed cortical **network** controls eye movements. This network includes discrete regions in the frontal and parietal lobes and at the temporo-occipital junction. While each area appears to be most important for one kind of movement, all areas alter their activity in relation to both saccades and pursuit movements (based on human fMRI studies). Interestingly, cortical areas for control of eye movements (especially saccades) overlap areas related to **shift of attention**. This seems logical because a voluntary saccade is a motor expression of a shift of attentional focus.

Saccades

With regard to specializations among cortical areas, clinical observations indicate that the **frontal eye field** (FEF, or area 8 of Brodmann; Fig. 25.8) is of particular importance for **voluntary saccade**s. Electrical stimulation of the frontal eye field elicits conjugated eye movements to the opposite side. The effect is mediated by fibers descending in the internal capsule to brain stem premotor cell groups, such as the **superior colliculus**, the **pretectal nuclei**, and the **PPRF**, which, in turn, activate motoneurons in the eye muscle nuclei. A unilateral **lesion** of the frontal eye field makes the patient unable to move the gaze voluntarily to the side opposite the lesion (e.g., when asked by the examiner to move the gaze). This is called a **gaze paralysis**. Correspondingly, the activity in the FEF increases more during voluntary than during reflex-evoked saccades. Indeed, the ability to move the gaze laterally is not completely lost after a lesion of the FEF. Thus, smooth-pursuit movements occur when an object is brought into the visual field and then moved slowly laterally—that is, the patient is able to follow the object with his or her gaze. Imaging studies show additional activation of the supplementary motor area (**SMA**), **dorsolateral prefrontal cortex**, and **posterior parietal cortex** (see Fig. 34.4) in relation to voluntary saccades. An area close to the frontal eye field, the **supplementary eye field** is particularly active when saccades are coordinated with hand movements (based on single-unit recording in behaving monkeys). It is also active when saccades are made to a remembered target location—that is, in the absence of visual or other information about the location of the target.

The **superior colliculus** and the **vermal oculomotor area** of the cerebellum both receive information from the frontal eye field and the posterior parietal cortex, and both are necessary for proper execution of saccades. They are not necessary for their initiation, however, because lesions of

3. Voluntary pursuit movements and the slow phase of optokinetic nystagmus appear to be controlled by largely the same neuronal groups because both kinds of movement are disturbed after lesions of the MST, the pontine nuclei, or the flocculus/paraflocculus.

neither the cerebellum nor the superior colliculus abolish saccadic movements.

Pursuit Movements

With regard to cortical control of **smooth-pursuit movements**, several small areas in the parietal lobe and at the temporo-occipital junction are of particular importance (Fig. 25.8; see also Figs. 16.25 and 34.4). This notion is based on, among other data, single-cell recordings. The **middle temporal area** (area **MT**, V5) is important for perception of movement. Neurons in MT respond to **retinal slip** (movement of the image on the retina), which is a strong stimulus to elicit pursuit movements of the eyes. The **middle superior temporal area** (area **MST**) lies close to area MT and is of special interest because it contains many neurons that respond preferentially to moving visual stimuli in a specific direction. The subcortical cell groups intercalated between these cortical regions and the eye muscle nuclei are not fully clarified, however. One important pathway seems to go from the cortex to the **pontine nuclei**, then to the **cerebellum**, further to the **vestibular nuclei** and the **reticular formation**, and thence to the eye muscle nuclei. In addition to in the parietal and temporal areas, neurons with activity related to pursuit movements occur in the frontal eye field and the supplementary eye field. Accordingly, impairment of pursuit movements has been reported in humans with frontal lesions including the supplementary eye field.

Gaze Fixation

The ability to **fix the gaze** is a prerequisite for voluntary slow-pursuit movements. As with most other tasks carried out by the cerebral cortex, the task is solved in a distributed network—a specific fixation center in the cerebral cortex has not been found. In monkeys, single neurons that change their activity in relation to gaze fixation are present in the frontal eye field and in the posterior parietal cortex. PET studies in humans, however, indicate that frontal lobes are particularly important for the ability actively to fix the gaze. This includes the **frontal eye field**, the **anterior cingulate gyrus**, and parts of the **prefrontal cortex**. In general, these regions become active in conjunction with **directed attention**, and lesions in humans produce an impaired ability to fix the gaze.

Often the tendency to fix the gaze on an object is not voluntary (cf. the term "fixation reflex"), at least not in the strict sense (even though fixation depends on the person being conscious). **Optokinetic nystagmus** is an expression of the strong tendency to fix the gaze. When a screen with alternating black and white vertical stripes is moved horizontally in front of a person, nystagmus occurs. The gaze is fixed automatically on one of the stripes and follows it until it leaves the visual field. Then a quick movement resets the eyes to the starting position, and the gaze is fixed again on another stripe. This sequence repeats itself as long as the screen moves.

Miniature Eye Movements

Closer study shows that even during active fixation, the eyes are not completely still. Several kinds of **miniature movement** occur, such as a slow drift of the eyes, **microsaccades**, and tremor. Microsaccades probably serve to avoid **perceptual fading** during fixation (it is a well-known phenomenon that visual targets tend to fade when fixed continuously). The amplitudes of these movements are very small, however, and are not normally perceived. Nevertheless, the phenomenon can be demonstrated by fixating on a square pattern for about 20 sec and then moving the gaze to a white surface. The afterimage of the square pattern is then seen to move, because the eyes are not completely still (Ilg 1997).

PART FIVE

The Brain Stem and the Cranial Nerves

The definition of the term "brain stem" varies. The widest definition—used in Chapter 6—includes the medulla oblongata, the pons, the mesencephalon, and the diencephalon. In this part of the book, and most often in clinical contexts, we restrict it to the **medulla**, the **pons**, and the **mesencephalon**, which together form a macroscopically distinct part of the brain. Which definition is used is of no great importance because the brain stem is a topographically and embryologically defined unit; it does not represent a functional "system." Neuronal groups within the brain stem take part in virtually all the tasks of the central nervous system.

Functionally the brain stem may be said to have two levels of organization. On the one hand, most of the cranial nerves and their nuclei represent "the spinal cord of the head." On the other hand, many neuronal groups in the brain stem represent a superior level of control over the spinal cord and the cranial nerve nuclei. Examples are the vestibular nuclei and various premotor nuclei in the reticular formation. In addition, other neuronal groups—usually included in the reticular formation—exert ascending influences on the thalamus and the cerebral cortex related to consciousness, arousal, and sleep. This section deals with both levels of organization. Chapter 26 discusses the reticular formation, which represents the superior level of control. Chapter 27 describes most of the cranial nerves and their nuclei.

The Reticular Formation: Premotor Networks, Consciousness, and Sleep

The reticular formation extends from the lower end of the medulla to the upper end of the mesencephalon. At all levels, it occupies the central parts and fills the territories not occupied by cranial nerve nuclei and other distinct nuclei and by the large fiber tracts. The **raphe nuclei** (serotonin) and the **locus coeruleus** (norepinephrine) are often included in the reticular formation and are discussed in this chapter. Although the reticular formation consists of many functionally diverse subdivisions, they all share some anatomic features. Thus, the neurons have wide dendritic arborizations and their long axons give off numerous collaterals. The afferent and efferent connections show only a rough topographic order. Efferent connections reach most parts of the central nervous system (CNS, from the cord to the cerebral cortex), while afferents bring all kinds of sensory information. These features show that the reticular formation is built for **integration**. Accordingly, the reticular formation attends primarily to tasks involving the nervous system and the organism as a whole. Subdivisions of the reticular formation form **premotor networks** that organize several complex behaviors. These behaviors include control of body **posture**, **orientation** of the head and body toward external stimuli, control of **eye movements**, and coordination of the activity of the **visceral organs**. These tasks fit with the reticular formation being phylogenetically old and present even in lower vertebrates. In addition, parts of the reticular formation (especially in the upper pons and mesencephalon) send ascending connections to the thalamus and the cerebral cortex. These connections form the **activating system of the brain stem**. The integrity of this system is a prerequisite for **consciousness** and is closely linked to control of **awareness** and **attention**.

Further, parts of the reticular formation, including cholinergic cell groups in the upper pons, are concerned with regulation of **sleep**.

Structure and Subdivisions

The reticular formation extends from the lower end of the medulla to the upper end of the mesencephalon, where it gradually fuses with certain thalamic cell groups (Fig. 26.1).[1] At all levels it occupies the central parts and fills the territories not occupied by cranial nerve nuclei and other distinct nuclei (such as the dorsal column nuclei, the pontine nuclei, and the colliculi) and by the large fiber tracts (such as the medial lemniscus and the pyramidal tract). The reticular formation received its name from the early anatomists because of its network-like appearance in microscopic sections (Figs. 26.2 and 26.3). It is built of cells of various forms and sizes that appear to be rather randomly mixed. Between the cells, there is a wickerwork of fibers passing in many directions (Fig. 26.2). These fibers are partly axons and dendrites of the neurons of the reticular formation and partly afferent axons from other sections of the CNS. The reticular neurons have typically very long and straight **dendrites**, so that they cover a large volume of tissue (Fig. 26.3). This distinguishes the reticular neurons from those found in specific nuclei of the brain stem, such

---

1. Some authors include certain thalamic cell groups—especially the intralaminar nuclei—in the term "reticular formation of the brain stem."

Figure 26.1

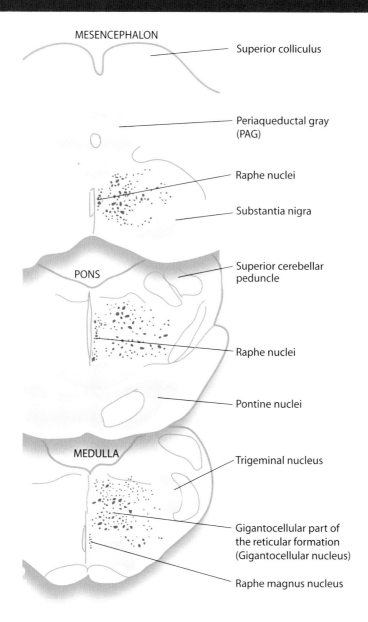

MESENCEPHALON

Superior colliculus

Periaqueductal gray (PAG)

Raphe nuclei

Substantia nigra

PONS

Superior cerebellar peduncle

Raphe nuclei

Pontine nuclei

MEDULLA

Trigeminal nucleus

Gigantocellular part of the reticular formation (Gigantocellular nucleus)

Raphe magnus nucleus

The reticular formation. Transverse sections through various levels of the brain stem (cat) showing the position of the reticular formation. The size of the red dots indicates the size of the neurons, which varies considerably among subdivisions of the reticular formation. (Based on Brodal 1957.)

as the cranial nerve nuclei (see the hypoglossal nucleus in Fig. 26.3).

Medial Parts Are Afferent and Lateral Parts Are Efferent

A more detailed analysis of the reticular formation makes clear, however, that it consists of several **subdivisions**, among which the cells differ in shape, size, and arrangement even though the borders between such subdivisions are not sharp (Fig. 26.1). It is especially important that such cytoarchitectonically defined subdivisions also differ with regard to fiber connections, neurotransmitters, and functions. In the pons and the medulla, approximately the **medial two-thirds** of the reticular formation consists of many large cells, in part so-called giant cells, forming the **gigantocellular reticular nucleus** (Figs. 26.1 and 26.2). The **lateral one-third** contains almost exclusively **small cells**. Tract-tracing methods have shown that the medial part sends out many

Figure 26.2

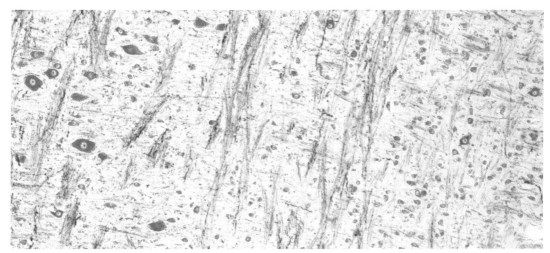

Medial reticular formation   Lateral reticular formation
(Gigantocellular nucleus)

The reticular formation. Photomicrograph of section of the medulla, stained to show myelinated fibers (blue) and cell bodies (red). The cell bodies are distributed diffusely without clear nuclear borders and with small fiber bundles coursing in various directions. The photomicrograph shows the transition between the large-celled medial division and the small-celled lateral division. Magnification, ×300.

Figure 26.3

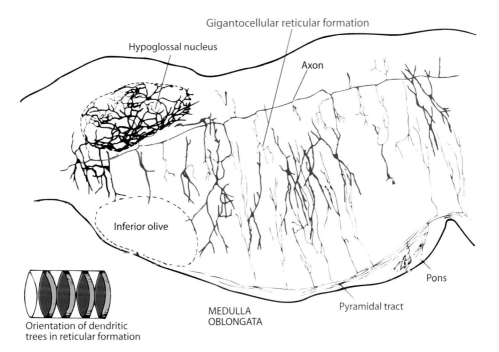

Orientation of dendrites in the reticular formation. Sagittal section through the medulla (rat). The long, straight dendrites are typical of the neurons of the reticular formation, in contrast to the neurons of a cranial nerve nucleus (the hypoglossal) and other specific brain stem nuclei. A long axon with numerous collaterals extending ventrally in the transverse plane is also shown. Collaterals of the pyramidal tract fibers enter the reticular formation. (Modified from Scheibel and Scheibel 1958.)

long, ascending and descending fibers, whereas the lateral small-celled part receives most of the afferents coming to the reticular formation. In general, therefore, we may say that the lateral part is **receiving**, whereas the medial part is **efferent** (executive). The efferents convey the influence of the reticular formation to higher parts, such as the thalamus, and lower parts, such as the spinal cord.

The Reticular Formation Is Built for Integration

Studies with the Golgi method and with intracellular tracers give evidence of how complexly the reticular formation is organized. The long ascending and descending efferent fibers give off numerous **collaterals** on their way through the brain stem (Fig. 26.4). As can be seen in Fig. 26.3, the collaterals run primarily in the transverse plane. Most dendrites of reticular cells have the same preferential orientation, so the reticular formation appears to consist of numerous **transversely oriented disks** (Fig. 26.3). The numerous collaterals of the axons from the cells in the medial parts ensure that signals from each reticular cell reach many functionally diverse cell groups (such as other parts of the reticular formation, cranial nerve nuclei, dorsal column nuclei, colliculi, spinal cord, certain thalamic nuclei, and hypothalamus).

The Raphe Nuclei and the Locus Coeruleus: Common Features

The **raphe nuclei** (*raphe*, seam) together form a narrow, sagittally oriented plate of neurons in the midline of the medulla, pons, and mesencephalon (Figs. 26.1, 26.5, and 26.6). In many ways, these nuclei have similarities with the reticular formation proper and are often considered part of it. The **locus coeruleus** is small group of only about 15,000 strongly pigmented neurons (containing **neuromelanin**) located under the floor of the fourth ventricle (Fig. 26.7). It has clear borders except ventrally where it merges gradually with the adjoining reticular formation, which also contains norepinephric neurons. This is one reason the locus coeruleus is often included in the reticular formation. The locus coeruleus is the largest among several norepinephric (noradrenergic) cell groups spread throughout the brain stem and is the main source of norepinephric nerve terminals in all parts of the CNS.

A characteristic feature of these two nuclei is that they contain only a small number of neurons, while their axons have

Figure 26.4

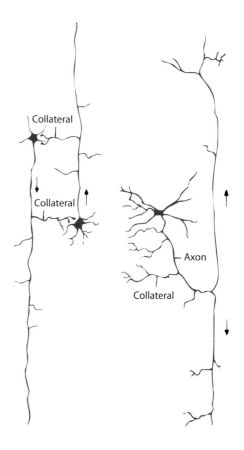

Neurons in the medial part of the reticular formation with long ascending and descending axons. **Right:** Example of a neuron with a bifurcating axon, with one ascending and one descending branch. Both branches give off collaterals as they course through the reticular formation. **Left:** Two neurons with ascending and descending axons, respectively. In this way, neurons with ascending axons can influence the activity of neurons with descending axons.

extremely widespread ramifications, reaching virtually all parts of the brain and the spinal cord. Their synaptic actions are **modulatory**, although the effects vary among different targets due to different distribution of receptors. The raphe nuclei contain mainly **serotonergic** neurons, whereas the locus coeruleus neurons contain **norepinephrine** (cf. Chapter 5, under "Biogenic Amines"). Another special feature is that they send fibers directly to the cerebral cortex, that is, without synaptic interruption in the thalamus, as is typical of most cortical afferent pathways from lower levels. These features are shared with other cell groups, notably the dopaminergic neurons in the mesencephalon and the cholinergic cell groups in the pons and the basal forebrain (cf. Chapter 5, under "Modulatory Transmitter 'Systems'").

Figure 26.5

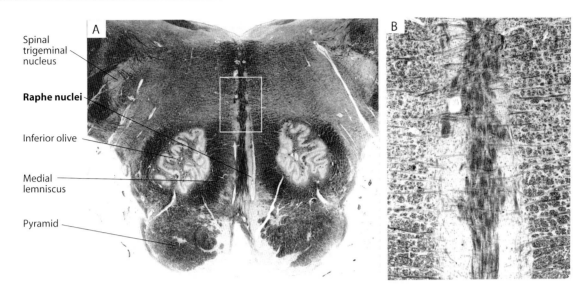

The raphe nuclei. **A:** Transverse section of the upper medulla, stained to visualize neuronal cell bodies and myelinated axons. The raphe nuclei are seen as narrow, light stripes on each side of the midline. **B:** Larger magnification from framed area in A. The cell bodies of raphe neurons are seen as small dots.

Figure 26.6

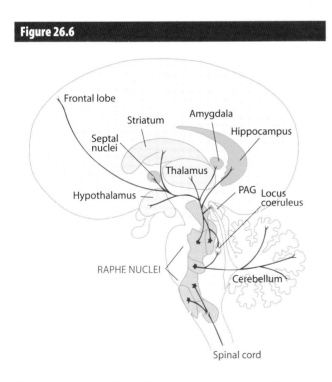

The raphe nuclei and their efferent connections. Schematic midsagittal section through the brain showing the various subdivisions of the raphe nuclei and some main connections. The most rostral nuclei send their fibers rostrally to the thalamus, cortex, and other cell groups, whereas the caudal nuclei project to the spinal cord. Together, the raphe nuclei supply large parts of the CNS with serotonergic fibers.

In other chapters we discuss the effects of the monoamines serotonin and epinephrine on **sensory-information** processing (see Chapter 15, under "Central Control of Transmission from Nociceptors," and Chapter 19, under "Modulation of Taste-Cell Sensitivity") and **on movements** (Chapter 22, under "Monoaminergic Pathways from the Brain Stem to the Spinal Cord"). We give examples of the importance of these monoamines for **emotions** and **motivation** in Chapter 5 (under "Monoamine Metabolism: Implications for Personality, Cognition, and Mental Disorders"). They are of crucial importance for brain **plasticity** and **learning**, and they influence cardiovascular control and other functions governed by the **autonomic nervous system**. Finally, serotonin and norepinephrine participate in regulation of **attention** and **sleep**. The serotonergic raphe neurons and the norepinephric locus coeruleus neurons are both active during wakefulness and less active during sleep (we return to this later, under "Neuronal Groups and Transmitters Controlling Sleep"). They differ, however, in their response to sensory stimuli: only the norepinephric neurons increase their activity in relation to salient stimuli (like the dopaminergic neurons in the substantia nigra).

The Raphe Nuclei

Based on cytoarchitectonic and connectional differences, several raphe nuclei have been identified (Fig. 26.6), even though their

Figure 26.7

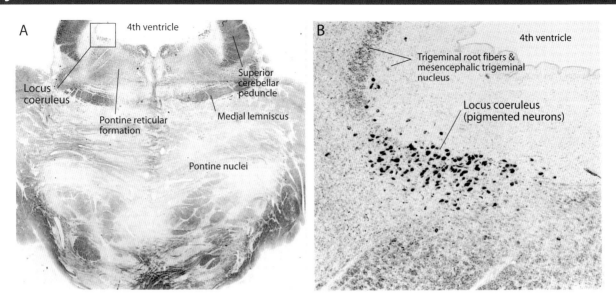

The locus coeruleus. **A:** Transverse section of the upper pons (approximately the same level as in Fig. 3.18). The locus coeruleus is positioned just below the floor of the fourth ventricle. **B:** Larger magnification from framed area in A. The norepinephrine-containing neurons in the locus coeruleus are heavily pigmented. This nucleus and other norepinephric cell groups in the vicinity have neurons with highly branched axons that end rather diffusely in most parts of the CNS.

borders are far from sharp. Together, the raphe nuclei receive **afferents** from many sources, such as the cerebral cortex, the hypothalamus, and other parts of the reticular formation. In spite of the extensive distribution of the **efferent** fibers, the different raphe nuclei have largely different targets. Thus, the caudal raphe nuclei send their efferents to the spinal cord (e.g., the nucleus raphe magnus), whereas the rostral nuclei (the dorsal and median raphe nuclei) send fibers upstream (Fig. 26.6). Further, the rostrally projecting nuclei also differ in their main targets, so that, for example, motor networks and memory networks can be accessed independently.

The actions of **serotonin** depend on the kinds of receptor that are present postsynaptically in the target nuclei (see Chapter 5, under "Monoamine Receptors"). In addition, most raphe neurons contain **neuropeptides** (substance P and thyrotropin-releasing hormone), which presumably contribute to the synaptic effects of efferent fibers from the raphe nuclei. Serotonin also influences the **cerebral circulation**. A final peculiarity of the raphe nuclei is that they send fibers ending in close relation to the **ependymal** cells (which cover the interior aspect of the brain ventricles). Presumably, such fibers contribute to the regulation of transport processes through the ependyma.

Various kinds of behavioral changes have been reported after **lesions** of the raphe nuclei, such as aggression and increased motor activity (to destroy the raphe nuclei in isolation, however, is virtually impossible).

The raphe nuclei and serotonin are of special interest with regard to the pathophysiology of **migraine**. One hypothesis proposes that cortical hyperactivity (that precedes a migraine attack) alters the activity of raphe neurons, which in turn initiate perivascular inflammation (see Chapter 8, under "Sensory Innervation of Brain Vessels"). Migraine patients have reduced serotonin activity, and the most effective migraine drugs are **triptans** that act as serotonin agonists (Maxalt, Zomig, and others). However, the relationship between low serotonin activity and pain is not clear, and neither is the site of action of the triptans.

The Locus Coeruleus

In spite of containing so few neurons, the **efferent** fibers of the locus coeruleus reach virtually all parts of the CNS. It sends, for example, direct fibers to the cerebral cortex, the hypothalamus, the basal ganglia, the hippocampus, and other limbic structures. Direct fibers also reach the spinal cord but only parts of the brain stem (especially sensory nuclei). The dense norepinephric innervation of the reticular formation and the motor nuclei must therefore originate from the scattered norepinephric neurons outside the locus coeruleus.

The **afferent** connections come mainly from a few regions. The locus coeruleus receives direct connections from the **cingulate gyrus** and the **orbitofrontal cortex** (in monkeys and presumably in humans as well). Subcortical afferents seem from recent studies to arise in the medullary part the reticular formation and in the **amygdala**. The medullary connections probably provide the locus coeruleus with integrated sensory information, while fibers from the amygdala might signal the emotional value of sensory information. **Single neurons** in the locus coeruleus respond preferentially to novel, "exciting" sensory stimuli. Because norepinephrine increases the response to specific stimuli and improves the signal-to-noise ratio of postsynaptic neurons, the locus coeruleus is believed to play a particular role in mediating **arousal** and **shifts of behavior** (Fig. 26.8). One example is the facilitatory effect of norepinephrine on **spinal motoneurons** (see Chapter 22,

Figure 26.8

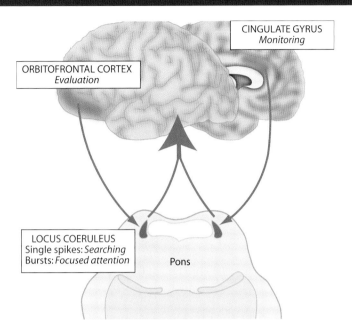

Locus coeruleus and shift of attention. In response to information from the cerebral cortex, the locus coeruleus is thought to initiate a shift of attention. If the ongoing task is judged as not important enough to justify the required effort, or it seems to be unsuccessful, focused attention is replaced by a distributed attention facilitating discovery of more interesting goals.

under "Monoaminergic Pathways from the Brain Stem to the Spinal Cord"). Norepinephrine also has a special role in relation to synaptic **plasticity**. For example, it is especially concentrated in the cerebral cortex during sensitive periods of development.

Possible Tasks of the Raphe Nuclei and the Locus Coeruleus

The modulatory neurotransmitters—including serotonin and norepinephrine—influence virtually all brain functions. This is not surprising, considering the widely branching axons of the neurons containing these neurotransmitters. In view of the small and relatively homogeneous nuclei giving origin to the axons, it seems nevertheless possible that the multifarious actions are subject to a common aim or "plan." However, in spite of several unifying theories, none has obtained general acceptance. Here we present just a few possible unifying concepts.

One of the theories concerning **serotonin** views the raphe nuclei as especially important for **homeostatic control** (another theory tries to collect all serotonin actions under the heading of motor control). One of the facts favoring homeostatic control as a common theme is

that many raphe neurons are **chemosensitive** and measure the CO_2 level in the blood (thus indirectly monitoring the pH of the nervous tissue). Chemosensitive neurons in the medulla participate in control of respiration (normalization of CO_2). Actions of serotonin on spinal motoneurons can perhaps have something to do with the fact that muscular activity is a major source of CO_2 production. Serotonergic actions on pain transmission might be viewed in the perspective of pain as part of a homeostatic response, as discussed in Chapter 15. Further, chemosensitive neurons in the rostral raphe nuclei can increase wakefulness and alter cerebral circulation. They also seem to mediate signals that evoke anxiety associated with high blood CO_2 levels (a single inhalation of air with 35% CO_2 provokes acute anxiety).

An overarching function of the **locus coeruleus** may be to increase **arousal** and **attention** in response to salient sensory information. However, the task may be more specific than this, according to a theory put forward by Aston-Jones and Cohen (2005). During wakefulness, the locus coeruleus neurons alternate between phasic and tonic firing (Fig. 26.8). The phasic state is proposed to optimize ongoing actions (help to maintain the focus on the present task). Tonic activity, on the other hand, allows shift of attention away from the ongoing activity to enable exploratory behavior to select a new (and more reward-ing) behavior. Instruction to **shift behavior** appears to reach the locus coeruleus from parts of the prefrontal cortex (the cingulate and the orbitofrontal cortex). The gyrus cinguli, for example, seems to monitor errors dur-ing execution and helps decide whether actions produce the expected results.

The Efferent Connections of the Reticular Formation

The reticular formation sends fibers to (and thereby acts on) three main regions: the **thalamus**, the **spinal cord**, and **brain stem nuclei**. The cell groups that give off ascending axons are located somewhat more caudally than those that emit descending axons (Fig. 26.9). By means of the numerous col-laterals of both the ascending and descending fibers in the reticular formation (Figs. 26.3 and 26.4), the two kinds of cell groups can influence each other. Further, many interneurons connect different parts of the reticular formation. Thus, a close cooperation is possible between the parts of the reticular for-mation that act on the cerebral cortex and those that act on

Position of efferent reticular cell groups. Drawing of sagittal section through the brain stem (cat). Neurons sending axons to higher levels (the thalamus) are red, while neurons with descending axons are green. The cell groups sending descending fibers are located somewhat more rostrally than the regions sending ascending fibers, providing an opportunity for mutual influences by collaterals (as shown in Fig. 26.4).

the spinal cord. Collaterals of ascending and descending axons mediate actions on brain stem nuclei (Figs. 26.3 and 26.4).

Parts of the reticular formation form **premotor net-works**. Chapter 25 deals with premotor networks in the pons and mesencephalon controlling and coordinating the activity of the **eye muscle nuclei**. Other premotor networks in the reticular formation control **rhythmic movements** such as locomotion (Chapter 22) and breath-ing. Further, premotor networks coordinate the activity of the widely separated motoneurons responsible for **brain stem reflexes**, such as the cough reflex and the vomiting reflex.

Connections to the Spinal Cord: Motor Control

The descending fibers that are related to motor control run in the ventral part of the lateral funicle and in the ventral funicle (Fig. 26.10). Such reticulospinal fibers end primarily on interneurons, which, in turn, can influence motoneurons.

The **ventral reticulospinal tracts** (see also Chapter 22, under "More about Reticulospinal Tracts") are both crossed and uncrossed and mediate both inhibitory and excitatory effects on spinal motoneurons. The reticulospinal neurons are further characterized by their axonal branching pat-tern, with collaterals given off at several levels of the spinal cord. Thus, each neuron can influence muscles in different parts of the body. As discussed in Chapter 22, the ventral reticulospinal tracts are of particular importance for **pos-tural control**, for the **orientation of the head and body** toward external stimuli, and for **voluntary movements of proximal body parts**. Connections from the **superior colliculus**—that mediate sensory information to the reticu-lar formation—are crucial for orienting movements toward **novel stimuli**. Combined anatomic and physiologic studies of single cells have shown the importance of a tectoreticu-lospinal pathway for such movements.

The **dorsal reticulospinal** fibers concern primarily **con-trol of sensory information**. Many of these fibers are mono-aminergic and arise partly in the raphe nuclei and adjoining parts of the reticular formation (see Figs. 15.2 and 15.3).

Ascending Connections to the Thalamus

The majority of the ascending fibers from the reticu-lar formation end in the **intralaminar thalamic nuclei**

Figure 26.10

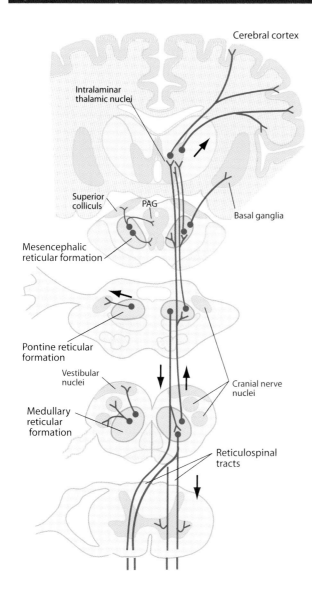

Efferent connections of the reticular formation. Various subdivisions of the reticular formation send fibers to higher levels, such the thalamus, the basal ganglia, and the cerebral cortex. Descending fibers end in the spinal cord. In addition, the reticular formation sends fibers to the cranial nerve nuclei and other brain stem nuclei, such as the PAG, the superior colliculus, and the vestibular nuclei. Most of the long connections are both crossed and uncrossed, although this is not shown in the figure. Numerous shorter fibers interconnecting subdivisions of the reticular formation are not shown.

(Fig. 26.10), unlike the specific sensory tracts that end in the lateral thalamic nucleus. Some fibers also end in the **hypothalamus** and the **substantia nigra** (see Fig. 23.11B). We discuss the functional significance of the ascending reticular connections later in this chapter; suffice it here to say that they are of particular importance for the general level

of activity of the cerebral cortex, which, in turn, concerns consciousness and attention.

The Reticular Formation Receives All Kinds of Sensory Information

Various cell groups send fibers to the reticular formation (Fig. 26.11). **Spinoreticular fibers** are discussed in Chapter 14. These fibers ascend in the ventral part of the lateral funicle together with the spinothalamic tract but diverge in the lower medulla. Among other destinations, the fibers end in the parts of the reticular formation that send long, ascending axons to the thalamus. This provides a **spinoreticulothalamic pathway** that is anatomically and functionally different from the major sensory pathways. Some of the spinoreticular fibers end in areas containing neurons that send axons back to the spinal cord, thus establishing **feedback** loops between the reticular formation and the cord.

In addition to spinal neurons that send their axons only to the reticular formation, many secondary sensory neurons send **collaterals** to the reticular formation. This concerns many of the fibers of the **spinothalamic tract**, which, presumably, mediate **nociceptive** and **thermoceptive** signals to the reticular formation. Collaterals of ascending axons from the sensory (spinal) trigeminal nucleus supply the same kind of information from the face.[2] **Visceral sensory** signals reach the reticular formation by collaterals of ascending fibers from the **solitary nucleus** (which receives afferents from the vagus nerve, for example).

The **superior colliculus** sends fibers to parts of the reticular formation, as mentioned. These connections make it possible for **visual signals** to influence the reticular formation because the superior colliculus receives visual information directly from the retina and from the visual cortex. In addition, the superior colliculus receives somatosensory information from the cortex and integrates visual and somatosensory stimuli enabling orientation toward external stimuli.

Auditory signals reach the reticular formation by collaterals of ascending fibers in the auditory pathways. **Vestibular** signals come from the vestibular nuclei.

The preceding description of afferents indicates that signals from virtually all kinds of receptors can influence neurons of the reticular formation. This is verified by physiologic

---

2. The **medial lemniscus** does not give off collaterals to the reticular formation. Information from low-threshold mechanoreceptors must therefore reach the reticular formation by means of spinoreticular neurons.

Figure 26.11

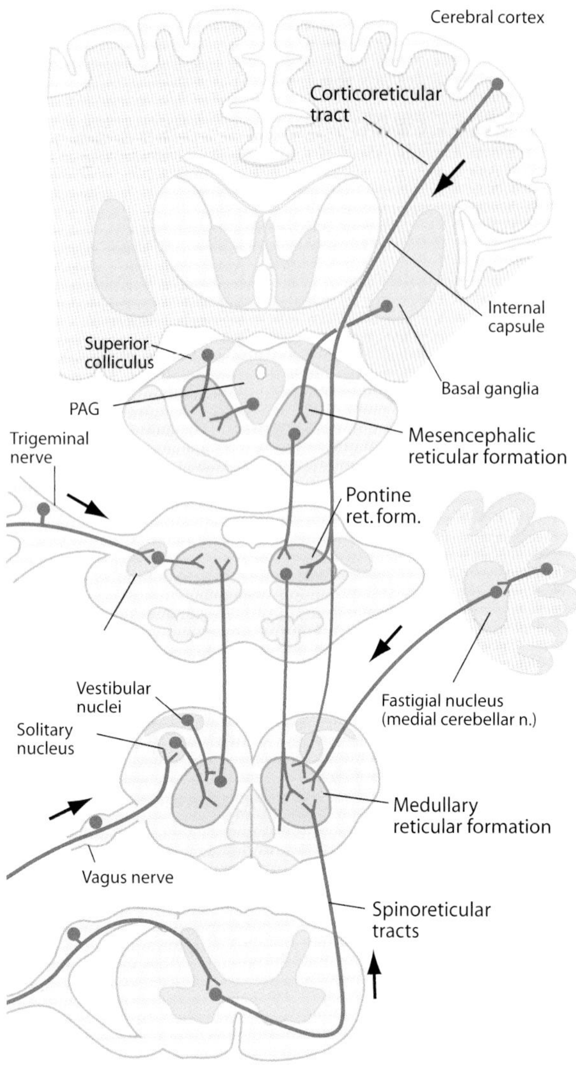

Afferent connections of the reticular formation. Several spinoreticular tracts mediate various kinds of sensory information. In addition, the reticular formation is influenced by sensory cranial nerve nuclei and other brain stem nuclei, such as the PAG, the superior colliculus, and the vestibular nuclei (not shown). The descending fibers from the cerebral cortex are links in indirect corticospinal pathways (cf. Fig. 22.3).

experiments. Electrodes placed in the reticular formation can record potentials evoked by stimulation of receptors for light, sound, smell, and taste. Furthermore, stimulation of peripheral nerves carrying signals from cutaneous receptors and proprioceptors and of visceral nerves evokes activity. Whenever a receptor is stimulated, the signals reach not only the cortical areas important for the perception of the stimulus but also the reticular formation—with possible influence on attention, automatic behavior, and autonomic functions.

Afferents from the Cerebral Cortex and Subcortical Nuclei

Corticoreticular fibers arise mainly in the cortical areas that give origin to the pyramidal tract (Fig. 26.11). They end preponderantly in the regions of the reticular formation that send axons to the spinal cord (Fig. 26.9). As discussed in Chapter 22, the **corticoreticulospinal pathways** cooperate with the pyramidal tract in the control of voluntary and automatic movements.

As discussed in Chapter 23, the **basal ganglia** (the substantia nigra) send efferents to the mesencephalic reticular formation (the locomotor region, or pedunculopontine nucleus [PPN]). Fibers from the **hypothalamus** ending in parts of the reticular formation serve to coordinate the activity of different peripheral parts of the autonomic system. Limbic structures, notably the **amygdala**, also send fibers to the reticular formation. Such connections probably mediate emotional effects on autonomic and somatic motor functions. The periaqueductal gray **(PAG)** is discussed in Chapter 15 in relation to suppression of nociceptive signals, but this mesencephalic complex of smaller nuclei has a wider specter of functions; for example, it helps initiate defensive reactions to external threats or other kinds of stress. This happens by way of its efferent connections to premotor networks in the reticular formation. The reticular formation receives afferents from the **cerebellum** (primarily the fastigial nucleus; see Fig. 24.6). This is an important pathway for the cerebellar influence on alpha (α) and gamma (γ) motoneurons. In addition, this pathway presumably mediates cerebellar influence of the autonomic nervous system. Thus, electric stimulation of the vermis can elicit changes in autonomic functions.

FUNCTIONS OF THE RETICULAR FORMATION

It follows from the preceding discussion that the reticular formation can act on virtually all other parts of the CNS. We considered its effects on the spinal cord in Chapters 14 and 22, and we add more here on this point. In addition, we discuss the effects on the cerebral cortex, which are of particular importance. Parts of the reticular formation that are involved in the control of eye movements are discussed in Chapter 25, whereas the parts involved in the control of autonomic functions are described briefly in Chapter 30 (under " 'Centers' in the Brain Stem for Coordination of Behavior").

The Activating System

Electrical stimulation of parts of the reticular formation alters several functions mediated by the spinal cord, such as muscle tone, respiration, and blood pressure (Fig. 26.12). In addition, the general activity of the cerebral cortex, which is closely related to the level of consciousness, can be altered by stimulation of the reticular formation. The **activating system of the brain stem** was therefore introduced as another name for the reticular formation. It should be emphasized, however, that these widespread effects are not served by the reticular formation as a whole but by relatively specific subregions. Further, stimulation of the reticular formation can also produce **inhibitory** effects on several processes. Therefore, the term "activating system" is not synonymous with "the reticular formation" but pertains to effects obtained from specific subregions only (discussed further later in this chapter).

There is continuous activity in the reticular formation maintained by a constant inflow of signals from various sources. The level of consciousness reflects the tonic activity in specific parts of the reticular formation. In particular, such activity is essential for awareness of sensory stimuli and for adequate behavioral responses to them. When a novel stimulus catches our **attention**, this is mediated by parts of the reticular formation. At the same time, premotor networks in the reticular formation produces the motor responses that ensure automatic orientation of the head and the body toward the source of the stimulus. The motor apparatus is mobilized, together with alterations of respiration and circulation.

Actions on Skeletal Muscles

Animal experiments during the 1940s led to the identification of two regions within the reticular formation that influence muscle tone. Stimulation of a region in the medulla that sends particularly strong connections to the spinal cord (Fig. 26.10) could inhibit stretch reflexes and movements induced by stimulation of the motor cortex. This region was therefore called the **inhibitory region** (Fig. 26.12). A region with opposite effects, the **facilitatory region**, was found rostral to the inhibitory region. It extends rostrally into the mesencephalon and is located somewhat more laterally than the inhibitory region.[3] The actions in the cord concern not

Figure 26.12

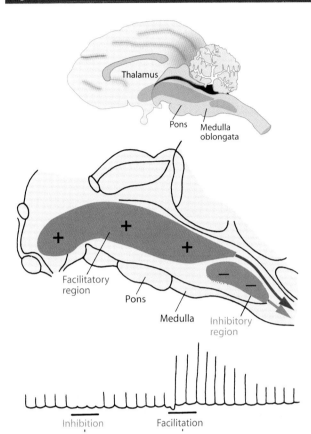

Facilitatory and inhibitory regions of the reticular formation. Schematic sagittal section through the brain stem (cat). The diagram at the bottom shows the amplitude of the patellar reflex (measured with electromyography). In the period marked "Inhibition," the inhibitory region was stimulated electrically, and the reflex response was almost abolished. In the period marked "Facilitation," the facilitatory region was stimulated, and the patellar reflex response was markedly enhanced. (Modified from Kaada 1950.)

---

only α but also γ **motoneurons**, so that the reticular formation can control the sensitivity of the muscle spindles.

Based on the present state of knowledge of the organization of the reticular formation, however, the emphasis is more on its control of specific motor tasks than on diffuse effects on the muscle system as a whole. For example, certain subregions have a particular role in controlling the **rhythmic locomotor movements**, whereas other regions are devoted to controlling **eye movements**, and some are concerned primarily with **orienting movements** of the head and the body in response to optic and vestibular stimuli. In such functions, parts of the reticular formation—consisting of extensive premotor networks—collect the relevant information

---

3. The distinction between inhibitory and facilitatory regions is less sharp than originally believed, however. In several places, single neurons with inhibitory or facilitatory actions on muscles are intermingled.

about, for example, the position of the head and body and ensure through their output signals the coordinated activity of specific muscles to produce a proper response. Common to premotor networks is that they control the activity of many muscles.

Effects on Respiration and Circulation

Microelectrode studies have shown that neurons with respiratory movement–related activity lie in several regions of the reticular formation, even though they are concentrated in the **ventrolateral medullary reticular formation**, which is often termed the **ventral respiratory group (VRG)**. This region contains many premotor neurons that control (monosynaptically and polysynaptically) the rhythmic activity of motoneurons innervating the diaphragm and other respiratory muscles. The **rhythm generator** itself consists most likely of a small neuronal network in the rostral part of the VRG, the so-called **pre-Bötzinger complex** (Fig. 26.13).[4] Thus, animal experiments indicate that this small region is both necessary and sufficient to elicit rhythmic respiratory movements (this network has properties in common with other rhythm generators—e.g., those producing locomotor movements). Normally, however, a much wider network participates in respiratory control, including neurons in the **pontine reticular formation**. The VRG receives sensory signals from the thoracic cage and the **lungs** about the degree of expansion and from **chemoreceptors** about blood pH and CO_2 content. Such information modulates the activity of the rhythm generator, without being necessary for the maintenance of breathing.

The respiratory rhythm generator is unstable shortly after birth in rats (but not in pigs and cats). A theory proposes that similar immaturity—so that the breathing rhythm is easily disturbed or abolished—lies behind **sudden infant death syndrome**.

Parts of the reticular formation also receive all necessary information for **cardiovascular control**. Thus, these regions control blood pressure, the blood volume distribution among the organs, the stroke volume, and the heart rate. Rather extensive networks in the **rostral ventrolateral medulla (RVLM)** are responsible for coordinating the necessary adjustments of vascular resistance and cardiac output. The effects are mediated by reticulospinal fibers acting on preganglionic sympathetic

---

4. Patients suffering from **multiple systems atrophy** can develop breathing problems as part of autonomic failure (among other symptoms). In a group of such patients, postmortem examination revealed cell loss in the pre-Bötzinger complex, while the ambiguus nucleus was normal (the patients swallowed normally).

Figure 26.13

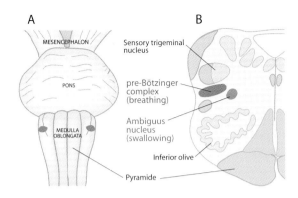

A central part of the network for rhythmic breathing movements (the pre-Bötzinger complex). **A:** The approximate position of the pre-Bötzinger complex projected onto the surface of the medulla. **B:** Transverse section through the upper part of the medulla showing the pre-Bötzinger complex and the ambiguous nucleus; the latter contain motoneurons supplying the pharyngeal muscles. (Based on Schwarzacher et al. 2011.)

neurons and fibers to brain stem preganglionic parasympathetic neurons (with fibers passing in the vagus nerve).

The Reticular Formation and the Relationship between Mental and Bodily Processes

Variations in the activity of the reticular formation are reflected in virtually all aspects of the nervous processes and in the activity of the endocrine organs controlled by the hypothalamus. Such interactions may help explain the intimate correlation of mental and bodily processes. There is much evidence to suggest that our mental state influences the activity of parts of the reticular formation. The thought of a forthcoming, unpleasant event or the memory of an embarrassing or agonizing situation may suddenly make a drowsy person alert and tense (increased muscle tone), produce sweating, increase the heart rate, and so forth. Every doctor who routinely tests reflexes knows that apprehension and anxiousness is accompanied by increased reflex responses and increased muscular tone. An exaggerated patellar reflex at the start of a consultation becomes "normal" as the patient relaxes. Another everyday example is the difficulty in falling asleep when one is preoccupied with distressing thoughts.

All of the these effects can best be explained if mental processes—which are closely linked with activity in the cerebral cortex, limbic structures, and the hypothalamus—influence the activity in parts of the reticular formation. Indeed, stimulation of certain cortical areas can increase the activity of reticular neurons followed by desynchronization of the electroencephalograph (EEG) (unanesthetized animals become attentive). These effects are mediated by direct and indirect connections from the cortex to the brain stem. There are also connections from the hypothalamus and limbic structures (such as the amygdala) to the reticular formation, which may be of particular importance because emotions are most effective in causing activation. That **insomnia** is related to increased activity in the reticular formation is suggested by the fact that most drugs used for sleep-lessness reduce the activity of certain groups of reticular neurons. **General anesthesia** abolishes the transmission through central parts of the reticular formation (resulting in lack of activation of the EEG and unconsciousness), whereas the transmission in the specific sensory pathways is less affected.

We also know that **bodily processes** influence our mental state. For example, a treatment that leads to muscle relaxation usually also reduces mental tension. Again, the effects are prob-ably mediated by a reduction of the activity of the reticular for-mation. At the same time, there are alterations of respiration, blood pressure, heart rate, and other autonomic functions such as sweat secretion, peristaltic movements of the bowel, and secre-tion of gastric juice. There is furthermore evidence that some of the autonomic expressions of anxiety (e.g., palpitations) may by themselves serve to maintain and increase the anxiety.

We return to the interactions between the mind and the body in Chapters 30 (under "The Hypothalamus and Mental Functions") and 31 (under "Is Amygdala Necessary for the Experience of Emotions?").

CONSCIOUSNESS

What Is Consciousness?

"Consciousness" eludes attempts at precise definitions. The British philosopher Kathleen V. Wilkes states: "Perhaps con-sciousness is best seen as a kind of dummy-term like 'thing,' useful for the flexibility that is assured by its lack of specific content" (1984, p. 241). Yet we all "know" what it is to be con-scious. For everyday and clinical use it usually suffices to define consciousness as "the state of being aware of and responsive to one's surroundings" (Oxford Dictionary). When studying the neurobiological basis of consciousness, it is important to distinguish conceptual issues from empirical ones, as empha-sized by Bennett and Hacker (2003) in their book *Philosophical Foundations of Neuroscience*. Only the empirical issues are amenable to scientific study; the conceptual ones must be clarified by conceptual analysis.[5] When the concept is unclear, as indeed is the case with consciousness, "misconceived ques-tions are bound to be asked, and misguided research is likely to ensue. For, to the extent the concepts are unclear, to that extent the questions themselves will be unclear" (Bennett and Hacker, 2003, p. 239). In the following we discuss (rather superficially)

some neural processes that are associated with, or even a neces-sary condition for, a conscious state.

Neurobiological Basis of Consciousness

While no one would deny that consciousness depends on a functioning brain, it probably never will be understood by a **reductionistic** approach, studying in ever more detail the constituent parts of the brain. A "consciousness center" or "module" somewhere in the brain is incompatible with our present knowledge. That unconsciousness follows interruption of the ascending activating system does not imply that the locus of consciousness is somewhere in the mesencephalic reticular formation (similarly, the fact that a car cannot run without a battery does not imply that the battery *is* the car). Indeed, it does not make sense to say that the brain is conscious; only a *person* can be conscious.

For higher mental functions, the cerebral cortex is essential, and the cerebral cortex is certainly necessary for consciousness, although it is not sufficient. Broadly speaking, consciousness depends on coordinated activity in a network comprising the brain stem, the thalamus, and the cerebral cortex. Isolated activity in any one of the parts of the network is not sufficient. For example, activity in specific cortical areas responsible for (con-scious) analysis of sensory information or control of cog-nitive processes cannot produce conscious experience on their own.

In Chapter 16 we discuss whether specific parts of the cor-tex can be linked to visual experiences (under "Integration of Visual Information: One Final Area?"). A "building block theory" of consciousness has some experimental support (e.g., from the study of persons with blindsight) but seems unable to explain important aspects. Much recent research has focused on what has been termed the "hypothesis of unified field consciousness." This implies that conscious-ness might not be separable into different domains—as visual, auditory, somatosensory, emotional, and so forth. Much information now points to **synchronized activity**—binding vast assemblies of neurons in a coherent state as a prerequisite for conscious experience.[6] In particular,

---

5. At the conceptual level, it may be clarifying to distinguish between **intransitive** and **transitive consciousness**. The first denotes simply the state of being conscious or awake, as opposed to being unconscious or asleep. Intransitive consciousness is some-thing one may lose by becoming unconscious and later regain. Transitive consciousness, in contrast, has an object: one is con-scious *of* something.

6. EEG recordings in humans while watching ambiguous pictures support the relevance of synchronization for conscious experience. The picture could be interpreted either as meaningless or represent-ing a face. When persons reported that they saw a face, the EEG showed synchronization of widely separated cortical areas, whereas synchronization did not occur when they saw no meaning in the picture (Rodriguez et al. 1999).

synchronization within an extensive **frontoparietal network** may be characteristic of a conscious state. Indeed, conditions with unconsciousness (such as coma, deep sleep, general anesthesia, and the vegetative state) show reduced metabolic activity in the frontoparietal network.

Many Cognitive Processes Take Place Outside Awareness

Only few of our mental processes—in spite of their dependence on the integrity of the cerebral cortex—take place in "the searchlight of consciousness." There is in fact much experimental evidence suggesting that our "conscious" or "voluntary" behavior often reflects cognitive processes that do not come to full awareness. We mentioned an example in Chapter 16 (under "Subconscious [Implicit] Use of Visual Information") with a woman who had lost awareness of one kind of visual information but nevertheless used the information to guide goal-directed movements. Another example concerns a woman suffering a stroke that damaged the midportion of the corpus callosum who was asked to identify objects with the right and left hand (without vision). The damaged part of the corpus callosum connects the somatosensory areas. Therefore, in this case somatosensory information could not be transferred between the hemispheres. When holding an eraser in her right hand she was able to name it correctly. This is as expected, because the sensory information passes from the right hand to the left hemisphere that is necessary for speech in most people. When she held the rubber in her left hand, however, she did not notice anything or she did not know what it was. In this case, the information went to the "mute" right hemisphere. Nevertheless, she was afterward able to pick out a rubber from a bag with her left hand when asked to find the same object she just held. Thus, processes in the right hemisphere was sufficient to identify the object, store relevant information, and use it afterward in conscious behavior (Gazzaniga 1993).

The Study of Consciousness: Electroencephalography (EEG)

Direct recording from the surface of the cerebral cortex of animals shows that the patterns of electrical waves differ among parts of the hemispheres. In humans, too, direct recordings from the exposed cortex can be done during brain surgery (**electrocorticography**). The electrical waves are conducted through the skull and the soft tissues of the scalp and can therefore be recorded with electrodes placed on the skin of the head. With this method, **electroencephalography (EEG)**, the electrical signals are dispersed and attenuated on their way through the skull and soft tissues, so that the origin of the signals within the hemisphere can be only roughly determined. Nevertheless, the method has

been of great importance both for research and diagnostically since its introduction around 1930.[7]

When analyzing an EEG, one can discern various waveforms and patterns. The α **waves** are relatively slow, with a frequency of 8 to 12/sec (Fig. 26.14). They occur typically in an awake person who is relaxed and resting with his or her eyes closed. When the person opens his or her eyes or starts to think about a mental task (Fig. 26.14), the EEG immediately changes to a pattern with more irregular waves with a higher frequency and lower amplitude. These are called β **waves**. The change of wave pattern from α to β waves is called **desynchronization,** or **activation** of the EEG. During sleep, other waveforms and patterns occur that are typical of specific stages of sleep. Various neurological diseases can be diagnosed because they are associated with characteristic changes of the EEG. To some extent, the EEG can also help localize the disease process. An EEG is particularly important in the diagnosis of **epilepsy**.

The EEG varies considerably with **age**; most marked are the changes during the first couple of years. There are also individual variations. Further, the EEG pattern changes during **sleep** and during **general anesthesia**. **Hyperventilation**, which leads to a reduced carbon dioxide concentration in the blood, changes the excitability of cortical neurons, and this is reflected in the EEG. Finally, several **drugs** affect the EEG.

Thalamocortical Neurons Have Two States of Activity

We do not fully know how the various waveforms in the normal EEG arise, but it is clear that they depend in large measure on different activity states in thalamocortical neurons. Thalamocortical neurons (functioning as relay cells for the transmission of sensory and other signals to the cortex) have unique membrane properties due to the presence of a special kind of Ca^{2+} channel that opens only when the cell is hyperpolarized to a certain level. In addition, massive connections from the cerebral cortex to the thalamus—**corticothalamic** connections—play an important part in the rhythmic firing of thalamocortical neurons.

Thalamocortical neurons generate action potential in two different patterns or modes: they may fire in **bursts** (i.e., they fire two to eight action potentials with a high frequency followed by a pause), or they fire **single spikes** with a varying overall frequency. The bursting pattern is associated with synchronization of the EEG (in states of drowsiness and so-called slow-wave sleep), whereas the single-spike firing occurs together with desynchronization (during attentiveness and during rapid eye movement [REM] sleep). It appears that these different functional states

7. A recent supplement to EEG is the extracranial recording of magnetic fields with **magnetoencephalography (MEG)**. In general, EEG and MEG provide much the same information with regard to timescale and spatial resolution, but MEG is much more expensive. EEG and MEG are also discussed in Chapter 6.

Figure 26.14

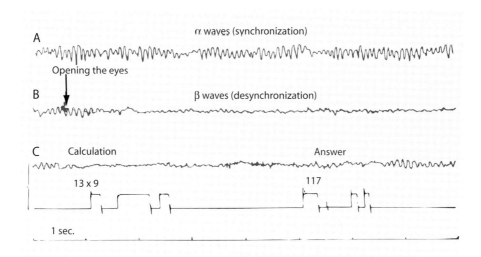

A   α waves (synchronization)

Opening the eyes

B   β waves (desynchronization)

C   Calculation   Answer

13 × 9   117

1 sec.

EEG. Three traces are shown, all of them recorded over the occipital lobes. **A:** The person is in a relaxed state, with his eyes closed. There are α waves typical of synchronization. **B:** At the arrow, the person opens his eyes, and the β waves are replaced by faster, irregular waves with smaller amplitude, called β waves. The EEG is desynchronized. **C:** Desynchronization produced by solving a mental task. The person is asked to make a calculation (13 × 9). After the calculation is completed (at 117), the slower waves return.

of the thalamocortical (relay) neurons determine whether they transmit signals to the cortex. Only in the single-spike mode do the cells transmit to the cortex the information they receive from, for example, peripheral receptors.

Switching between bursting and single-spike firing can be produced by modulatory influences from the reticular formation (see later, "Pathways and Transmitters Responsible for Cortical Activation"). Further, the **reticular thalamic nucleus** (see Fig. 33.10)—consisting of GABAergic neurons with local actions in the thalamus—has a central role in the switching (cf. Chapter 33, under "Inhibition in the Thalamus: Interneurons and the Reticular Thalamic Nuclei").

A Prerequisite for Consciousness: Effects of the Reticular Formation on the Cerebral Cortex

The effect of the reticular formation on the cerebral cortex was brought into focus by a paper published by the neurophysiologists G. Moruzzi (Italian) and H. W Magoun (American) in 1949. Jud– al,, now perspectives were opened on important aspects of brain functioning, especially consciousness, sleep, and wakefulness. Based on their animal experiments, Moruzzi and Magoun formulated a new concept: the **ascending activating system of the brain stem.** Later studies confirmed their hypothesis that (parts of) the reticular formation is necessary for maintenance of normal wakeful consciousness. Neuronal groups in the

reticular formation determine the **level of consciousness**, with its many variations from tense alertness to drowsiness and sleep.

Electrical stimulation of the reticular formation in anesthetized animals produces certain changes of the electrical activity in the cortex, as recorded by EEG. Under **general anesthesia** (without stimulation), relatively slow α waves dominate (Fig. 26.15). On electric stimulation of the reticular formation, the slow waves of the EEG are replaced by beta (β) waves with a faster and more irregular rate and with lower amplitude. Together with this **desynchronization** of the EEG there are signs of increased attention and alertness—that is, an **arousal** is produced. Such an arousal can also be produced in unanesthetized animals with implanted electrodes. For example, a cat lying still with no obvious interest in its surroundings becomes suddenly alert and attentive when the reticular formation is stimulated with a high-frequency train of impulses. Marked reduction of the activity of the reticular formation is associated with unconsciousness as shown experimentally in animals with selective lesions.

As mentioned, the reticular formation can have either activating or inhibiting effects on functions mediated by the spinal cord, depending on which region is stimulated (Fig. 26.12). Similar findings were made with regard to the ascending effects on the cerebral cortex, even though so far we have discussed only the activating effects. It appears that

Figure 26.15

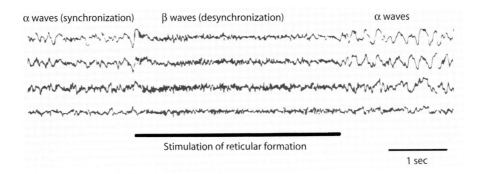

α waves (synchronization)   β waves (desynchronization)   α waves

Stimulation of reticular formation

1 sec

EEG recordings from the classic studies of Moruzzi and Magoun (1949). The four tracings are recorded over different parts of the cerebral cortex of a cat. The thick line at the bottom shows the period of electrical stimulation of the reticular formation. The stimulation produces desynchronization of the EEG (activation), which returns to a synchronized pattern when the stimulation stops.

inhibition—that is, **synchronization** of the EEG—is evoked most easily from the caudal parts, whereas activation or desynchronization is evoked from the rostral parts (corresponding to the effects on skeletal muscles). We return to this later in this chapter when discussing sleep.

In humans with prolonged periods of unconsciousness after **head injuries**, there is often damage of the **mesencephalic reticular formation**. The lesion can be surprisingly small and yet produce deep unconsciousness. This fits with animal experiments showing that interruption of the ascending reticular connections in the mesencephalon produces loss of consciousness, in spite of normal conduction in the large sensory pathways (medial lemniscus, spinothalamic tract, and visual and auditory pathways).

General Anesthesia

In Chapter 5 we mentioned that general anesthetics increase **GABAergic** inhibition ("GABA Receptors Are Influenced by Drugs, Alcohol, and Anesthetics"), and this seems to be common for almost all types of anesthetics. However, other transmitter receptors are targets as well. This concerns, for example, **NMDA receptors**, which are inhibited at least by some anesthetics. This reduces glutamatergic excitation. Experiments with genetically manipulated mice indicate that inhalation anesthetics open a special kind of **K⁺ channel**, thus hyperpolarizing neurons. Other possible targets are **glycine receptors** and special kinds of **voltage-gated Na⁺ channels**. Much research needs to be done before the full picture of molecular actions of general anesthetics is clear, however. In any case, manipulations of ubiquitous molecules like GABA and NMDA receptors are bound to cause widespread and diverse effects on neuronal functioning (at all levels of the CNS).

The next question is how the molecular effects lead to loss of consciousness and the other features of general anesthesia. Although lowering **brain metabolism** is common to all general anesthetics, brain imaging indicates that the effects are due to interference with specific neuronal **networks.** The relative importance of the various networks remains to be determined, however. A common finding is deactivation of the **thalamus** (cf. "Thalamocortical Neurons Have Two States of Activity" earlier in this chapter); in addition brain stem nuclei associated with the **ascending activating system** are influenced by general anesthetics. **Hypothalamic** and **basal forebrain** nuclei involved in attention and arousal are also affected. Finally, functional magnetic resonance imaging (fMRI) studies show marked deactivation of **cortical networks**, notably parietofrontal ones. It is not clear, however, whether this is secondary to thalamic deactivation or due to the direct effects of anesthetics on cortical neurons (or perhaps both). At least the similarity between general anesthesia and sleep is thought to be due in part to thalamic effects.

Control of Sensory Information and Focusing of Attention

The main task of the ascending activating system is probably to **focus our attention** on certain stimuli or internal events rather than to produce a diffuse awareness. To achieve this, it is necessary to prevent irrelevant stimuli from entering consciousness. Together with other mechanisms, inhibition from the reticular formation can ensure that, for example, we do not notice that someone is talking to us while we are absorbed in a book. In Chapters 14 and 15, we discussed how the central transmission of sensory signals is controlled from higher levels of the CNS, usually so that signals from certain kinds of receptors or parts of the body are inhibited. For example, descending connections to the spinal cord from the raphe nuclei and various (other) parts of the reticular formation suppress the central conduction of signals from nociceptors. Further, the central transmission of visual, auditory, and other sensory impulses is controlled by the reticular formation. Thus, even though it is not alone in this capacity, the reticular formation plays an important part in eliminating sensory signals that are considered irrelevant, so that our attention can be focused on salient signals. It should be emphasized, however, that although the reticular formation is instrumental in modulating transmission from sensory receptors, higher levels of CNS are needed to decide what is salient information in a particular situation.

Pathways and Transmitters Responsible for Cortical Activation

What are the pathways used by the reticular formation to influence consciousness, attention, and sleep? All of the major specific sensory pathways (the spinothalamic tract, the medial lemniscus, and the visual and auditory pathways) can be interrupted without affecting consciousness or the activation of the EEG produced by stimulation of the reticular formation. If these sensory pathways are left intact but the ascending connections of the reticular formation are interrupted by a cut in the mesencephalon, the animal becomes unconscious. Electrical stimulation of the reticular formation can no longer activate the EEG, even though stimulation of peripheral receptors evokes potentials in the cortical sensory regions. Thus, the sensory signals reach the cortex, but they are restricted to the sensory regions, and, most important, they are unable to arouse the animal. Pathways other than the major sensory ones must therefore be responsible when the reticular formation activates the EEG over major parts of the cerebral hemisphere and produces behavioral changes indicating increased awareness.

Connections from the reticular formation to the **intralaminar thalamic nuclei** are likely candidates. Thus, electrical stimulation of these nuclei can produce activation of the EEG similar to that seen after stimulation of the reticular formation itself. The intralaminar thalamic nuclei send widespread efferents to the cerebral cortex (cf. Chapter 33, under "The Intralaminar Thalamic Nuclei"). Therefore, a reticulothalamocortical pathway probably is important for the actions of the reticular formation on the cerebral cortex. Many of the reticulothalamic fibers to the intralaminar nuclei are **cholinergic** and come from a few small cell groups at the junction of the mesencephalon and **pons** (Fig. 26.16).[8] In addition

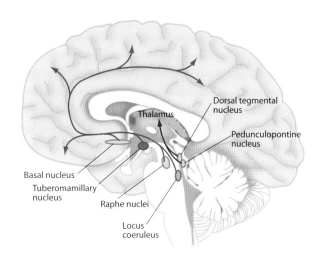

Figure 26.16

Neuronal groups participating in activation of the cerebral cortex.

to this indirect reticulothalamocortical pathway, there are direct projections to the cerebral cortex from **monoaminergic** cell groups in the brain stem—usually considered parts of the reticular formation—such as the **raphe nuclei** (serotonin), the **locus coeruleus** (norepinephrine), and the **ventral tegmental area** in the mesencephalon (dopamine). These nuclei also project to the thalamus, however. Stimulation of each of these cell groups can produce synchronization of the EEG, even though they behave differently in other respects. For example, their activities differ with regard to sleep, as discussed later. Norepinephric neurons increase their firing rate shortly before and during periods with cortical activation and focused attention. Similarly, **serotonergic** raphe neurons and **histaminergic** neurons in the hypothalamus (tuberomammillary nucleus) are more active during wakefulness than during sleep.[9] As with the other modulatory inputs, activation of histaminergic fibers can bring thalamocortical neurons from a state of burst firing to single-spike firing.

Experiments in rats with selective elimination of various neurotransmitter systems suggest the following (very simplified) specializations with regard to tasks requiring focused attention: the **cholinergic** connections increase the precision of the performance, the **norepinephric** ones reduce the effect of distracting stimuli, the **dopaminergic** ones increase the speed of execution, and the **serotonergic** ones limit the frequency of impulsive response errors

---

8. The largest pontine cholinergic cell groups are the **pedunculopontine nucleus** (PPN) and the **lateral dorsal tegmental nucleus**. The PPN consists of several subdivisions, however, and many neurons are glutamatergic; moreover, a part of the PPN has important connections with the basal ganglia and other parts of the brain stem.

9. Histamine-receptor antagonists, commonly used for allergy and motion sickness, block the activating effect of histamine, and this might explain why sleepiness is a side effect.

(see also "Possible Tasks of the Raphe Nuclei and the Locus Coeruleus" earlier in this chapter).

In conclusion, at least five cell groups, using as many transmitters, cooperate in the control of consciousness and attention (Fig. 26.16). They exert their effects partly in the thalamus and partly in the cerebral cortex. Most likely, each of the cell groups and transmitters influence different aspects of wakefulness.

Coma and Vegetative State

For **clinical purposes**, the definition of "consciousness" is practical: a condition of wakefulness in which the person responds appropriately to stimuli and, by his or her behavior, demonstrates awareness of himself or herself and the surroundings. Patients with diseases or damage of the brain can exhibit states of consciousness ranging from full awareness to coma. A person in a **coma** appears to be sleeping but cannot be awakened by any kinds of sensory stimulus. Purely reflex movements may be evoked, however (e.g., the withdrawal reflex). A coma may have several different causes, but it is always a serious condition. The prognosis is poorer the longer a comatose state lasts. After acute head trauma, persistent unconsciousness suggests brain stem involvement, typically of the **mesencephalic reticular formation**.

After a few weeks, some comatose patients enter a **persistent vegetative state** in which they show some signs of wakefulness: they may open their eyes upon strong stimulation and after some time even spontaneously. They may briefly fix the gaze on a person or an object. They show no other signs of being aware of their surroundings, however, and they do not talk. Functional MRI studies in such patients show activity patterns compatible with unconsciousness. For example, in 15 patients noxious stimuli activated expected parts of the brain stem, thalamus, and primary somatosensory cortex but not the rest of the "pain network," including the insula, the cingulate gyrus, and the secondary somatosensory cortex. Nevertheless, doubt exists as to whether some patients in the vegetative state can perceive and respond adequately to external events. Thus, a patient showed activation (measured via fMRI) of relevant motor networks when asked to imagine playing tennis. Further, speech areas were activated when the patient was presented with spoken sentences. It is not clear, however, whether these observations mean that the patient was in fact conscious or whether they just show how much cerebral processing can occur without entering consciousness.

The Locked-In Syndrome

On rare occasions, a patient may appear unconscious yet be fully awake. This occurs typically after brain-stem infarctions that damage the ventral parts of the **pons** with the pyramidal tract and corticobulbar tracts on both sides. The sensory pathways located more dorsally are spared, as is the ascending activating system. This condition is called the **locked-in syndrome**. The patient is unable to move or talk but is otherwise fully conscious and mentally intact. It may also be called a "de-efferented"

condition: everything goes in and is perceived normally, but nothing goes out.

SLEEP

The necessity of sleep and its contribution to mental and physical health may seem self-evident. Yet the more specific functions of sleep and its neurobiological basis are not fully understood. Indeed, control of sleep and its various phases has turned out be very complex, involving many neuronal groups and neurotransmitters. Here we provide only a brief and simplified treatment of this topic.

Sleep Phases

Sleep consists of several phases that can be distinguished based on differences in an EEG. The transition from alertness to drowsiness changes the EEG in the direction of synchronization. When a subject is falling into a deep, quiet sleep, the α **waves** disappear altogether and are replaced by **irregular slow waves** with greater amplitude (**slow-wave sleep**). After an initial light **phase I**, the sleep becomes gradually deeper, until **phase IV**. To waken a person in sleep phase IV requires relatively strong stimuli, whereas only weak stimuli are necessary in phase I. **Phase V** is special because the EEG is desynchronized, and there are conjugated movements of the eyes, much like a person looking at moving objects. Because of these **rapid eye movements**, this phase is called **REM sleep** or **paradoxical sleep**. The eye movements appear to relate to the content of the dream. Thus, patients suffering from neglect of the left visual hemifield (after damage to the right hemisphere) have conjugated eye movements during REM sleep only to the right side, that is, the visual field they attend to when awake. **Muscle tone** is generally reduced, with occasional muscular twitches, and there are changes of **blood pressure** and **heart rate**. Dreaming occurs—at least mainly—during REM sleep.

The various phases of sleep follow each other with the same order throughout the night. Usually, the first REM phase occurs after about 1.5 hours of sleep and lasts for about 10 minutes. Thereafter the REM phases return at intervals of 1 to 2 hours and become gradually longer up to about 30 minutes. When waking up (or being wakened) just after a REM phase, a person remembers the content of the dream vividly.

The cerebral cortex is as active during REM sleep as when awake, but it is partly uncoupled from the **thalamus**, which in the awake state delivers a constant stream of information about the external world. The EEG pattern during sleep is produced by complex interactions between neuronal firing patterns in the thalamus and the cortex. **Inhibitory interneurons** in both places have important roles in producing the synchronized firing of thalamocortical neurons characteristic of sleep.

Why We Sleep—Homeostasis and Learning

There is now much evidence suggesting that sleep has a **homeostatic** function. Indeed, we know that a prolonged period of wakefulness is followed by prolonged sleep; obviously, something must be corrected. In light of the brain's disproportionally large energy consumption, it seems appropriate that its energy demands decrease significantly during sleep (e.g., about 40% reduction in glucose metabolic rate). Also, the energy stores of the brain need rebuilding, the synaptic vesicles need refilling with neurotransmitters, and so forth. Furthermore, animal experiments show that the brain **interstitial space** increases by about 60% during sleep, thus facilitating clearance of potentially **neurotoxic waste products**, such as β amyloid (known to accumulate in Alzheimer's disease).

Other data suggests that sleep is necessary for the sake of **plasticity**. Growth of neurons and establishment (and pruning) of synaptic contacts proceed presumably better when the neurons are not required to participate in task-solving and production of goal-directed behavior. Useful connections need consolidation while others are weakened or removed. The plasticity hypothesis would imply that sleep is important for **learning** and **memory**, a notion that has received experimental support. Thus, there is evidence that brain plasticity is increased during sleep. In agreement with this, even a brief nap immediately after a learning session can improve subsequent performance.[10]

Animal experiments suggest that the **consolidation** of newly learned material takes place predominantly in specific sleep phases. The earliest studies focused on the phases that included dreaming (REM sleep), while more recent evidence emphasize the importance of the phases that include slow-wave sleep.[11] For example, human EEG studies found an increase in slow waves over cortical regions involved in a preceding learning session (e.g., over the posterior parietal cortex after a spatial-task training session). Further, slow-wave increases were associated with improved performance when tested afterward. Consolidation of newly learned material is believed to depend on a **dialog** between the hippocampus and the cortex, and this process appears to go on during slow-wave sleep (but not during REM sleep), as witnessed by correlated firing in the hippocampus and the prefrontal cortex during slow-wave sleep.

Yawning

Most mammals yawn, but we are not sure why. The hypothalamus, the basal ganglia, and the reticular formation have been implicated in the control of yawning (in addition, a number of cranial nerves and spinal nerves are responsible for the execution). One hypothesis proposes that yawning serves to increase **alertness** in situations where we are passive but need to pay attention (lectures may be an example). This assumption is based on the observation that yawning activates parts of the reticular formation and is immediately followed by EEG desynchronization. The yawning movement evokes sensory inputs via (among others) the trigeminal nerve.

"Contagious" yawning—that is, yawning elicited by the sight or the sound of someone else yawning—is an intriguing phenomenon that is not yet explained. Although it is usually thought to occur only in humans and subhuman primates, there is evidence that it also occurs in dogs. It does not occur in children younger than the age of 2, and it is greatly diminished in people with autism and schizophrenia. There is conflicting evidence concerning the theory that contagious yawning is an expression of empathy. An fMRI study showed a change of activity in parts of the parietal cortex and the cingulate gyrus in contagious yawning (regions implicated in empathy but also in several other phenomena).

Pathologic yawning occurs in various diseases, for example in migraine. It also occurs as a side effect of **dopaminergic drugs** and **serotonin-reuptake inhibitors**. The importance of dopamine is supported by the observation that yawning is reduced in patients with Parkinson's disease (with loss of dopamine). Increased yawning has been described as an early sign of infarctions of the upper pons and in patients with **amyotrophic lateral sclerosis (ALS)**. In both cases, it may be due to loss of descending inhibitory control of brain stem "yawning centers."

---

10. Such a beneficial effect of a nap seems to concern primarily learning of declarative tasks—learning a story, traffic rules, and so forth. This kind of learning depends on the integrity of the hippocampus. Learning motor skills, such as a finger-tapping sequence or to ride a bicycle, is less dependent on the hippocampus and does not seem to benefit from of a nap. It should be emphasized, however, that these results relate only to a short nap after a training session, since sleep deprivation impairs all kinds of learning.

11. There is some evidence that REM sleep may be most important for consolidation of emotional and procedural memories, whereas slow-wave sleep is more involved in spatial and declarative memories.

Neuronal Groups and Transmitters Controlling Sleep

As mentioned, the neural basis of sleep and its various phases is not fully understood and is very complex. Several brain regions and neurotransmitters are important. Lesions of the **hypothalamus**, for example, can lead to increased or reduced amounts of sleep (see Chapter 30, under "The Hypothalamus, Sleep, and Hypocretins"), but it is evident from animal experiments that the neuronal groups most directly involved in sleep control are located in the **brain stem**, especially in the **pons**. In agreement with this, fMRI in humans shows increased blood flow in the dorsal pons during REM sleep. Initially, after the discovery of the activating system, it was assumed that sleep was simply the result of reduced activity of the activating system—that is, a purely passive process. Further studies showed, however, that sleep could be induced by electrical stimulation of the lower parts of the reticular formation and that lesions of the same region prevented sleep (insomnia).

For **induction** of sleep, activity in **cholinergic neurons** in the **dorsolateral pons** is crucial (the pedunculopontine nucleus and some smaller cell groups). These neurons project to the thalamus to influence the activity of the large sensory relay nuclei (the geniculate nuclei and the ventral posterior nucleus). In addition, they project to neurons in the nearby reticular formation, which, in turn, project to cholinergic neurons in the hypothalamus and the basal nucleus (among other targets). The effects of acetylcholine in the thalamus are mediated by **muscarinic** receptors. The pontine cholinergic neurons fire in **bursts** (bursting neurons) ahead of the eye movements in REM sleep. Their close relation to REM sleep is further shown by the observation that microinjection of acetylcholine in the dorsolateral pons increases REM sleep for several days.

The roles of **serotonin** and **norepinephrine** in control of sleep are less clear, probably because they are difficult to study in isolation. Thus, cholinergic and monoaminergic neurons lie partly intermingled in the dorsolateral pons (Fig. 26 16). It seems fairly certain, however, that the monoamines exert their main effect on sleep by modulating the activity of the pontine cholinergic neurons. Mostly, the monoamines **inhibit** the **cholinergic neurons**, thus increasing wakefulness. This conclusion is based on the fact that, among other factors, the monoaminergic neurons fire during wakefulness and are "silent" during REM

sleep.[12] Further, microinjection of serotonin hyperpolarizes (inhibits) the bursting neurons in the dorsolateral pons. Finally, **drugs** that enhance the synaptic effect of serotonin (such as reuptake inhibitors) reduce REM sleep in humans.

Spinal **motoneurons** are strongly inhibited from the brain stem during REM sleep. This prevents the execution of movements that are part of the dream (small, "miniature" movements nevertheless occur during dreaming). The inhibition is partly initiated by the pontine cholinergic neurons, although the major control most likely is exerted by **norepinephric** neurons close to the locus coeruleus (the **subcoeruleus nucleus**). Reticulospinal neurons in the medial medullary reticular formation mediate the effects on the motoneurons. After destruction of descending norepinephrine-containing fibers, animals still have REM sleep but behave as if they are acting out their dreams with orienting movements, more complex exploratory behavior, and attack or flight. Similarly, some brain diseases cause disturbed REM sleep (e.g., **REM sleep behavior disorder**), characterized by loss of descending inhibition and the persons acting out their dreams with violent movements. Persons with **narcolepsy** experience sudden, uncontrollable episodes of loss of muscle tone, due to inappropriate activation of the spinal inhibition during wakefulness or during the transition from sleep to wakefulness.

Other neurotransmitters—**GABA**, **dopamine**, and several **neuropeptides**—are involved in control of sleep by influencing the activity of the pontine cholinergic neurons. In addition, **glutamate** and **glycine** act by way of pathways that are more indirect. Thus, many drugs acting on the brain would be expected to influence sleep and wakefulness.

Narcolepsy

Narcolepsy is a genetically linked disease with sudden, irresistible attacks of REM sleep (or components of REM sleep). Starting usually between the ages of 10 and 30, the disease affects men and women equally often. The patients experience increased sleepiness during daytime, whereas night sleep is fragmented. The disease seems to be due to degeneration of a cell group in the lateral **hypothalamus**. The neurons of this group have widespread axonal ramifications and release neuropeptides called

---

12. Raphe neurons increase their activity and serotonin release during wakefulness and reduce their activity during sleep. Yet destruction of the raphe nuclei or blockage of the serotonin synthesis produces insomnia. To reconcile these at least apparently conflicting observations, it has been postulated that serotonin released during waking gradually activates sleep-promoting neurons in the anterior hypothalamus (by acting at the gene level). This might serve as a **homeostatic mechanism** to initiate sleep after some time of wakefulness.

hypocretins (orexins). Hypocretin containing neurons appear especially to target modulatory cell groups, such as the locus coeruleus, raphe nuclei, dopaminergic neurons in the mesencephalon, and the tuberomammillary nucleus (histamine). Because hypocretins seem to be excitatory, they would increase **arousal** by increasing norepinephrine release from the locus coeruleus neurons, as confirmed in animal experiments.

Patients with narcolepsy also have increased concentration of **muscarinic** receptors within the brain stem (cf. the increased REM sleep caused by injection of acetylcholine in the dorsolateral pons, mentioned previously). Further, there is evidence that monoamine metabolism is deficient. Both drugs that block muscarinic receptors and drugs that increase synaptic concentration of monoamines (such as amphetamine and tricyclic antidepressants) are reported to reduce the narcoleptic attacks. Possible connections between the loss of hypocretin neurons in the hypothalamus and the alterations of muscarinic receptors and monoamine metabolism in the brain stem are unknown.

Dreaming

Why we dream has been the subject of much speculation and many theories. REM sleep appears to occur in all mammals; even in the earliest species that developed about 140 million years ago.[13] This fact alone suggests that REM sleep has an important function. Further support for its biological significance comes from other observations. Thus, the proportion of REM sleep increases after a period with REM-sleep deprivation, and it is much more difficult to prevent the occurrence of REM sleep than the other phases of sleep. **Newborn infants** have approximately 8 hours of REM sleep per day and a special sleep rhythm. It consists of periods of 50 to 60 minutes of sleep usually starting with REM sleep rather than slow-wave sleep. By the age of 2, REM sleep lasts only about 3 hours, and the sleep pattern is similar to that in adults. The reason that REM sleep is so dominant during infancy (and before birth) is unknown.[14] One possibility is that REM sleep is necessary for neuronal growth and development of connections, as discussed earlier. The prevailing view today is that dreams contribute to the processing and consolidation of newly learned material, along with the integration of new experiences with older ones. Animal experiments indicate that storage of new material is reduced by prevention of REM sleep during a certain period after a learning situation. During REM sleep in certain animals, a particular pattern of electrical activity—**theta rhythm**—occurs in the hippocampus. Since the hippocampus plays a crucial role in learning, this has been taken to support the relationship between REM sleep and learning.

EEG and fMRI studies in humans suggest that the **default-mode network** (see Fig. 34.2), which is typically most active during mind-wandering and daydreaming, also is active while dreaming. Interestingly, activation of the default mode network is usually associated with deactivation of the executive network (involved in self-control).

The view that dreams are psychologically meaningful, relating in a disguised form to inner conflicts and life events, is the basis for their central place in psychoanalysis since Freud. Rather than emphasizing the role of dreams in learning, psychoanalytic tradition stresses their importance for the elaboration of inner conflicts that are not consciously accessible. These two possibilities might not be mutually exclusive, however. Perhaps a common purpose for all dreams is to help the individual develop **coping strategies**, as this requires the integration of new with old experiences, as well as ensuring that inner conflicts do not block learning and appropriate behavior.

---

13. Whales (Cetacea) appear not to have REM sleep. In these mammals, the two hemispheres alternate to exhibit slow-wave sleep. Perhaps constant vigilance is a necessity for adaptation and survival.

14. It should be noted that the REM sleep of infants differs from that in adults (with regard to EEG and behavioral patterns) and might therefore not necessarily be associated with dreaming.

OVERVIEW

We usually count 12 cranial nerves, even though neither the first (the olfactory nerve) nor the second (the optic nerve) are true nerves. These two, in addition to the cochlear nerve and the vestibular nerve, are discussed in Chapters 16 to 19.

A brief survey of the cranial nerves is given in Chapter 6. The prenatal development of the cranial nerve nuclei is treated in Chapter 9 (under "Cranial Nerves and Visceral Arches").

The cranial nerves connect the brain stem with structures in the head, neck, and thoracic and abdominal cavities. The cranial nerves are not as regularly built as the spinal nerves because some are purely motor, others are purely sensory, and some are mixed (like the spinal nerves). The cranial nerves contain four main fiber types. **Somatic efferent** fibers supply skeletal (striated) muscles, while **visceral efferent** fibers supply smooth muscles and glands and belong to the **parasympathetic** part of the autonomic nervous system. **Somatic afferent** fibers conduct sensory signals from the skin and mucous membranes of the face, from muscles and joints, and from the vestibular apparatus and cochlea, while **visceral afferent** fibers transfer sensory signals from the visceral organs.

In early embryological development, the **cranial nerve nuclei** form longitudinal columns (cf. columnar arrangement of motoneurons in the cord), with each column giving origin to only one of the four kinds of fiber. The columns are arranged so that, in general, motor cranial nuclei (somatic and visceral efferent) lie medially in the brain stem while sensory nuclei (somatic and visceral afferent) lie laterally. Later in development, the columns break up into discrete smaller nuclei, but their mediolateral position and fiber composition remain the same (with some exceptions).

The cranial nerve nuclei and the cranial nerves are links in various **brain stem reflexes** (e.g., the blink reflex and the vomiting reflex). The somatic motor nuclei receive innervation from the motor cortical areas, partly as collaterals of **pyramidal tract** fibers and partly as **corticobulbar** fibers destined only for the brain stem. Somatic sensory nuclei convey signals to the sensory areas of the cerebral cortex by joining the large **ascending sensory tracts** (e.g., the spinothalamic tract and the medial lemniscus).

A fair knowledge of the position of the various cranial nerve nuclei, the course of the nerves, and their main functions serve as a necessary basis for a topographic diagnosis of brain stem lesions.

GENERAL ORGANIZATION OF THE CRANIAL NERVES

Before dealing with specifics for each of the cranial nerves (Fig. 27.1, see also Figs. 6.13 and 6.15), we discuss some features that are common to them all. Like the spinal nerves that connect the spinal cord with the body, the cranial nerves connect the brain stem with the peripheral organs. Several structural features are shared by the spinal cord and the brain stem and thus also by the spinal and cranial nerves. Nevertheless, the brain stem is less regularly built and more complex in its organization than the spinal cord, and the cranial nerves are not as schematic in their composition as are the spinal nerves. Most of the cranial nerves, for example, lack a distinct ventral (motor) root and a dorsal (sensory) root. Some of the cranial nerves are purely sensory, others are purely motor, and others are mixed. Like the spinal nerves, several of the cranial nerves contain autonomic (preganglionic) fibers supplying smooth muscles and glands. Finally, some also contain afferent fibers from visceral organs.

The Cranial Nerves Can Contain Four Different Kinds of Nerve Fibers

The cranial nerves can contain the following kinds of fibers:

Figure 27.1

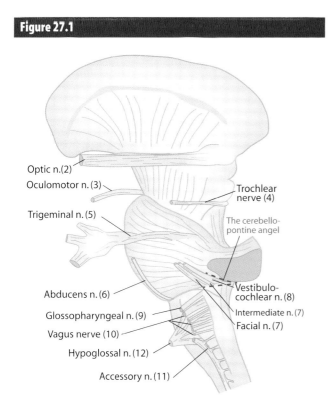

Optic n.(2)
Oculomotor n.(3)
Trochlear nerve (4)
Trigeminal n.(5)
The cerebello-pontine angel
Abducens n.(6)
Vestibulo-cochlear n.(8)
Glossopharyngeal n.(9)
Intermediate n.(7)
Vagus nerve (10)
Facial n.(7)
Hypoglossal n.(12)
Accessory n.(11)

The brain stem and the cranial nerves, as viewed from the left side. See also Figs. 6.14 and 6.15.

1. **Somatic efferent** fibers innervating skeletal (striated) muscles

2. **Visceral efferent** fibers supplying smooth muscles and glands and belonging to the parasympathetic part of the autonomic nervous system

3. **Somatic afferent** fibers with sensory signals from the skin and mucous membranes of the face, from muscles and joints, and from the vestibular apparatus and the cochlea

4. **Visceral afferent** fibers with sensory signals from the visceral organs

The **efferent fibers** of the cranial nerves have their cell bodies in brain stem nuclei corresponding to the columns of spinal motoneurons (see Fig. 21.3) and the intermedio-lateral cell column of the cord. We use the terms **somatic efferent** and **visceral efferent** cranial nerve nuclei of these cell groups (Figs. 27.2 and 27.3). The afferent fibers have their cell bodies in **ganglia** close to the brain stem, corresponding to the spinal ganglia. The central process of the ganglion cells enters the brain stem and ends on neurons in nuclei corresponding to the spinal dorsal horn and the dorsal column nuclei (Figs. 27.3 and 27.4). We use the terms

somatic afferent and **visceral afferent** cranial nerve nuclei for such groups. From such afferent (sensory) nuclei, signals are conducted centrally to the thalamus and the cortex and via brain stem interneurons to the somatic and visceral efferent (motor) cranial nerve nuclei (as links of brain stem reflex arcs; Fig. 27.4).

A Broad View on the Position of the Cranial Nerve Nuclei

In early embryonic life, all neurons giving origin to a particular kind of fiber lie together in one longitudinal column in the brain stem. During further development, these columns break up into smaller groups, and some of them move away from the original column. Nevertheless, the tendency for cranial nerve nuclei of the same category to form **columns** can be recognized also in the adult brain (Fig. 27.2). The demonstration of this regular pattern has been of value in understanding the functions of the cranial nerves. Further, knowledge of this pattern aids us in learning about the cranial nerves and their nuclei.

It is helpful at the outset to remember the following *general rule*, evident from Figs. 27.2 and 27.3: the efferent (motor) nerve nuclei lie medially in the brain stem, whereas the afferent (sensory) nuclei are located laterally. Further, in most cases the nuclei are located at about the same rostro-caudal level as their nerves leave the brain stem. In clinical neurology it is important to know the approximate medio-lateral and rostrocaudal level of each nucleus (Fig. 27.5).

More on the Position of the Cranial Nerve Nuclei

In early embryonic life, the **somatic efferent** nuclei are all arranged in a column close to the midline, but later some move away in a ventrolateral direction (Figs. 27.3 and 27.5). The nuclei remaining in the medialmost column are termed **general somatic efferent** and comprise (from caudal to rostral) the **nucleus of the accessory nerve** (11), the **nucleus of the hypoglossal nerve** (12), the **nucleus of the abducens nerve** (6), and the **nucleus of the oculomotor nerve** (3). (In the following, for practical reasons we use abbreviated names, such as the "accessory nucleus" and the "hypoglossal nucleus".) All of these nuclei innervate **myotome muscles**—the muscles that are developed from the segmentally arranged somites of early embryonic life. The somatic efferent nuclei that have moved away from the medial column all innervate **branchial muscles**—the striated muscles

Figure 27.2

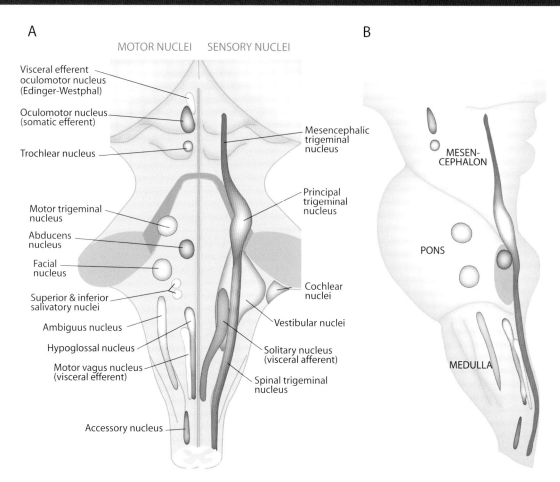

Position of the columns of the cranial nerve nuclei. **A:** Schematic of the brain stem, as viewed from the dorsal side. The nuclei belonging to the same kind (e.g., somatic efferent, visceral afferent) are shown in the same color. They form more or less continuous columns. **B:** The position in the brain stem of some nuclei as seen from the left side. The positions of the various nuclei are only approximate.

developed from the branchial (visceral) arches (facial and masticatory muscles, and muscles of the pharynx and larynx). We call these nuclei **special somatic efferent** (although they most commonly are termed "special visceral efferent").[1]

This group comprises the **ambiguus nucleus** (9, 10), the **facial nucleus** (7), and the **motor trigeminal nucleus** (5).

The **visceral efferent** (parasympathetic) column of cranial nerve nuclei is located immediately lateral to the somatic efferent column (Figs. 27.2, 27.3, and 27.5) and comprises the (**dorsal) motor nucleus of the vagus** (10), the small **inferior** and **superior salivatory nuclei** (9, 7), and the **parasympathetic oculomotor nucleus of Edinger-Westphal** (3). The **visceral afferent fibers** all end in one long nucleus, the **solitary nucleus**, which is located lateral to the visceral afferent column (Figs. 27.2, 27.3, and 27.5).

Most laterally, we find the **somatic afferent nuclei**. This group comprises the **sensory trigeminal nucleus** (5), the **vestibular nuclei** (8), and the **cochlear nuclei** (8). The sensory trigeminal nucleus consists of three functionally different parts (the spinal, the principal, and the mesencephalic

1. Both anatomically and functionally, however, "the special visceral efferent neurons" are more similar to the somatic efferents. First, branchial (visceral) arch striated muscles are among those subject to the most precise voluntary control (the mimetic muscles of the face and the muscles of the larynx) and should therefore not be confused with visceral (smooth) muscles. Second, the neurons are structurally like α motoneurons; that is, they are larger than the preganglionic, parasympathetic neurons. In addition, the visceral arch neurons contain the neuropeptide CGRP that occurs in spinal motoneurons but not in preganglionic parasympathetic neurons. Therefore, we find it preferable to use the term **special somatic efferent**. Otherwise, it is of no great importance which terms are used to group the neurons of the cranial nerves; the important thing is to know where the cell bodies of the various cranial nerves are located, the course of their fibers, and their functions.

Figure 27.3

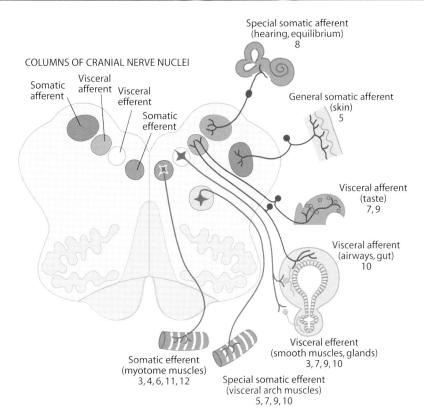

Position of the columns of the cranial nerve nuclei. Schematic cross section of the medulla (cf. Figs. 27.2 and 27.5). As a rule, the motor nuclei are located medial to the sensory nuclei, as shown schematically on the left side. The right half shows how the various kinds of fibers are distributed among the cranial nerves. Note that one kind of fiber usually distributes to several cranial nerves. Some of the peripheral organs innervated by the nerves are also shown to the right.

nuclei). Together, the three parts form one continuous column, which extends from the upper cervical segments of the cord into the mesencephalon (Fig. 27.2).

The fibers of the vestibulocochlear nerve are often classified as **special somatic afferent** because they originate from special sense organs; the trigeminal fibers are then termed **general somatic afferent.**

Figure 27.4 and the discussion here show that fibers of one kind all come from one of the columns of nuclei only, even though the fibers peripherally may follow several of the cranial nerves. Thus, all (general) somatic afferent fibers end in the sensory trigeminal nucleus, whereas the fibers peripherally follow not only the trigeminal nerve but also the glossopharyngeal and the vagus nerves.

Brain Stem Reflexes

Like the spinal nerves that are links in spinal reflex arcs, the cranial nerves constitute afferent and efferent links of reflex arcs with reflex centers in the brain stem (Fig. 27.4). Some brain stem reflexes are simple, such as the monosynaptic stretch reflex—the **masseter reflex**—that can be elicited of the masticatory muscles. Often, however, the reflex centers are more complex, comprising neurons at several levels of the brain stem (for some, even at the cortical level). Thus, the afferent fibers may enter the brain stem at one level, whereas the efferent fibers leave at another. One example is the **corneal reflex** (touching of the cornea elicits an eye wink), in which the afferent fibers of the trigeminal nerve, entering at the midpontine level, descend in the brain stem and form synapses in the lower medulla (the spinal trigeminal nucleus). From the medulla, the signals travel by interneurons to the facial nucleus on both sides, located in the lower pons. The reflex center is in this case rather extensive; consequently, lesions at various levels of the brain stem may produce a weakened or abolished corneal reflex. Depending on the location of the lesion, however, the change of the corneal reflex will be accompanied by various other symptoms, which helps in determining the exact site of the lesion. The

Figure 27.4

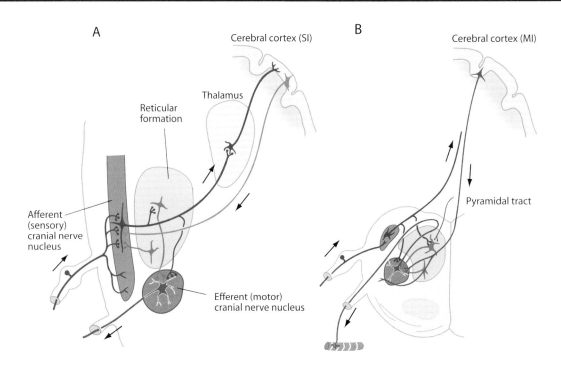

Main features of the organization of the cranial nerve nuclei. **A:** Sensory nucleus (e.g., the trigeminal nucleus). The efferent fibers of the nucleus ascend to the thalamus of the opposite side, and from there the next neuron projects to the cerebral cortex. The fibers destined for the thalamus give off collaterals on their course through the reticular formation and the motor cranial nerve nuclei. Thus, a reflex arc with reflex center in the brain stem is established. Descending fibers from the cerebral cortex influences the sensory nucleus. **B:** Motor nucleus (e.g., the facial nucleus) sending its efferent fibers out of the brain stem to striated muscles. The neurons of the nucleus are influenced by the cerebral cortex, by the reticular formation, and by collaterals of the ascending fibers from the sensory nuclei.

swallowing reflex exemplifies the complex organization of apparently "simple" automatic movements. It is elicited by stimulation of the oral mucosa innervated by the trigeminal, glossopharyngeal, and vagus nerves. From the sensory nuclei, signals are transmitted to premotor networks in the medullary reticular formation, which perform the sensorimotor transformations needed to coordinate the activity of several motor cranial nerve nuclei (5, 7, 9, 10, and 12).

Some other brain stem reflexes are discussed in the following in conjunction with the cranial nerves that mediate them.

The Cranial Nerve Nuclei Are Connected to Central Sensory and Motor Tracts

As mentioned, the cranial nerves and their nuclei are organized in accordance with the same general rules as the spinal nerves (with some exceptions). This means that the cranial nerves are the first links in sensory pathways corresponding to the **dorsal column–medial lemniscus**

system and the **spinothalamic pathway** (Fig. 27.4; see also Figs. 14.2 and 14.4). Further, as the nuclei involved in the sensory pathways conducting from the spinal cord, those of the brain stem are subjected to **descending control** of the sensory transmission. This concerns influences from parts of the reticular formation and from the cerebral cortex.

Several of the somatic efferent (motor) cranial nerve nuclei are influenced by the **pyramidal tract**—that is, by fibers forming the **corticobulbar tract** (Fig. 27.4; see also Fig. 22.1). An important difference between the corticospinal and corticobulbar fibers is that several of the cranial nerve nuclei receive both crossed and uncrossed fibers. Unilateral damage to the descending fibers (e.g., in the internal capsule) produces clear-cut pareses only in some of the muscle groups innervated by the cranial nerves (most marked in the mimetic muscles).[2]

---

2. The part of the facial nucleus supplying the lower part of the face— and often also the motor trigeminal nucleus—receive only crossed fibers, as judged from clinical observations (Monrad-Krohn 1954).

Figure 27.5

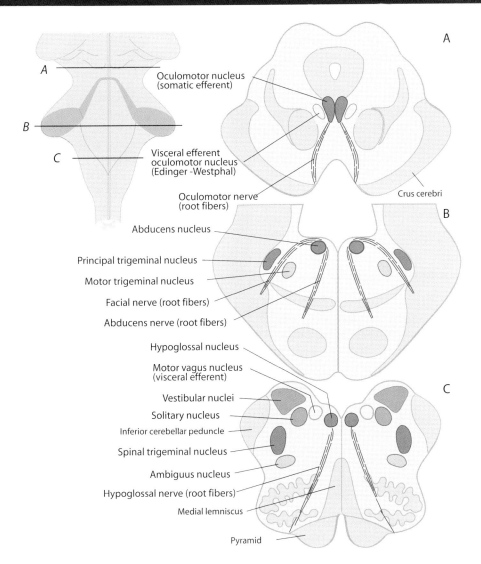

Oculomotor nucleus
(somatic efferent)

A

Visceral efferent
oculomotor nucleus
(Edinger -Westphal)

Crus cerebri

Oculomotor nerve
(root fibers)

B

Abducens nucleus

Principal trigeminal nucleus

Motor trigeminal nucleus

Facial nerve (root fibers)

Abducens nerve (root fibers)

Hypoglossal nucleus

Motor vagus nucleus
(visceral efferent)

C

Vestibular nuclei

Solitary nucleus

Inferior cerebellar peduncle

Spinal trigeminal nucleus

Ambiguus nucleus

Hypoglossal nerve (root fibers)

Medial lemniscus

Pyramid

Position of the cranial nerve nuclei at three levels of the brain stem. **A:** Mesencephalon. **B:** Pons. **C:** Medulla oblongata. Compare with Fig. 27.2.

Clinical Examination of the Cranial Nerves: Anatomic Knowledge a Prerequisite

Examination of the cranial nerves is of great importance in clinical neurology because it can provide exact information about the site of a disease process. A prerequisite is that the examiner has reasonably precise knowledge of where the cranial nerves exit from the brain stem (Fig. 27.1; see also Fig. 6.15) and the position of their nuclei both rostrocaudally and mediolaterally (Figs. 27.2 and 27.5). Further, the functions of the various nerves must be known in sufficient detail as a basis for the necessary tests. On the basis of such

knowledge, together with knowledge of the positions of the long motor and sensory tracts passing through the brain stem, the clinician can make a fairly precise topographical diagnosis in most cases (Fig. 27.6; see also Fig. 14.3).

Figures 6.16–6.18 and 6.20 show the location of the cranial nerve nuclei in cross sections of the brain stem.

Brain Stem Lesions Can Produce Symptoms from Cranial Nerves and Long Tracts

Many disease processes can cause brain stem lesions. Often brain stem symptoms are caused by diseases that produce symptoms also from other parts of the central nervous system (CNS; e.g., multiple sclerosis, amyotrophic lateral sclerosis, metastatic brain disease). Lesions limited to the brain stem are most often due to

Figure 27.6

A

B

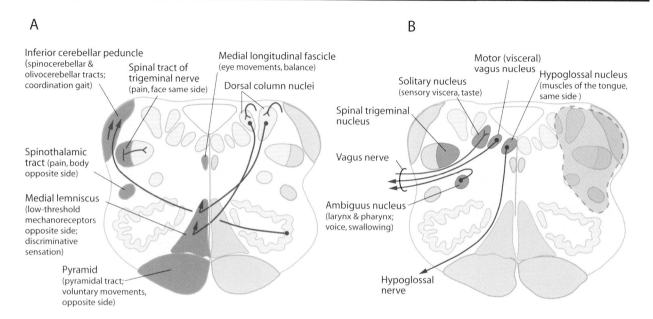

Inferior cerebellar peduncle
(spinocerebellar &
olivocerebellar tracts;
coordination gait)

Spinal tract of
trigeminal nerve
(pain, face same side)

Medial longitudinal fascicle
(eye movements, balance)

Dorsal column nuclei

Spinothalamic
tract (pain, body
opposite side)

Medial lemniscus
(low-threshold
mechanoreceptors
opposite side;
discriminative
sensation)

Pyramid
(pyramidal tract;
voluntary movements,
opposite side)

Motor (visceral)
vagus nucleus

Solitary nucleus
(sensory viscera, taste)

Hypoglossal nucleus
(muscles of the tongue,
same side)

Spinal trigeminal
nucleus

Vagus nerve

Ambiguus nucleus
(larynx & pharynx;
voice, swallowing)

Hypoglossal
nerve

Position of cranial nerve nuclei, some other nuclei, and the main tracts in the medulla. **A:** Major tracts and typical symptoms produced by their interruption. **B:** Cranial nerve nuclei. The area of infarction in a case of Wallenberg's syndrome is indicated with a stippled line. The figure helps identify the symptoms that are likely to occur after lesions of lateral or medial parts of the medulla, respectively.

vascular occlusions of arterial branches causing infarctions (see Figs. 8.3–8.5). Any branch can be affected (although some more often than others), and the resulting symptoms depend on which structures are supplied by the occluded branch. There are, however, large **individual variations** regarding the area supplied by a particular artery and between the right and left side in the same individual. Thus, symptoms will vary after occlusion of a particular artery. Memorizing detailed lists of symptoms typical for each arterial branch has therefore limited value. A fairly precise localization of the lesion can usually be made on the basis of a thorough clinical examination of the cranial nerves and the long ascending and descending tracts (the dorsal column–medial lemniscus, the spinothalamic tract, and the pyramidal tract).

Figure 27.6 gives, as an example, an overview of the structures that can be damaged by lesions in the **medulla**. Most common are lateral infarctions in the area supplied by the **posterior inferior cerebellar artery** (see Fig. 8.3), even though the occlusion often sits in the vertebral artery. The German neurologist Adolf Wallenberg described the clinical picture of such infarctions in 1895, and it has since been known as **Wallenberg's syndrome**. Typical cases present with dizziness and vertigo (vestibular nuclei), gait ataxia (spinocerebellar and olivocerebellar tracts in the inferior cerebellar peduncle), and difficulties with swallowing and hoarseness (ambiguus nucleus and root fibers of the vagus and glossopharyngeal nerves). A characteristic symptom constellation is reduced pain and temperature sensation in the face on the side of the lesion and in the body of the opposite side (face: spinal trigeminal nucleus and descending trigeminal root fibers; body: spinothalamic tract). Most cases also present **Horner's syndrome** (loss of sympathetic innervation of the face on same side as the lesion, see Fig. 28.10) due to interruption of descending fibers to the preganglionic sympathetic neurons in

the cord. Individual cases may present only some of these symptoms or other symptoms as well, depending on the exact site and extension of the lesion.

THE HYPOGLOSSAL NERVE

The **twelfth cranial nerve**, the hypoglossal nerve (Fig. 27.1), is the motor nerve of the tongue. It is composed of only **somatic efferent fibers**. The fibers come from the **hypoglossal nucleus**, which forms a slender, longitudinal column close to the midline in the medulla (Figs. 27.2, 27.3, and 27.5). The nucleus produces an elongated elevation in the floor of the fourth ventricle (the hypoglossal trigone; see Fig. 6.19). The **root fibers** of the nerve pass ventrally and leave the medulla just lateral to the pyramid (Figs. 27.1, 27.5, and 27.6). Several small fiber bundles (rootlets) join to form the nerve, which leaves the skull through the **hypoglossal canal** in the occipital bone. The nerve then forms an arc as it courses downward and forward in the upper neck—external to the carotid artery—to the root of the tongue. The fibers innervate the **striated muscle** cells of the tongue.

The muscles of the tongue are used **voluntarily** during speech and eating. In such activities, the neurons of the hypoglossal nucleus are influenced by fibers of the pyramidal tract coming from the face region of the motor cortex of the opposite hemisphere. Tracing studies in monkeys show, however, that the supplementary motor area, the primary motor area, the primary somatosensory cortex, and the insula also send fibers to the hypoglossal nucleus. The projection is bilateral, as shown in humans with transcranial magnetic stimulation. In subhuman primates about half of the fibers are uncrossed. The fibers that cross do so in the medulla just above the nucleus. A central motor lesion above the nucleus (e.g., in the internal capsule) usually produces only transitory signs of tongue weakness. No clear-cut atrophy of the tongue occurs in cases of central motor lesions.

Reflex movements of the tongue occur in swallowing (and vomiting). The hypoglossal motoneurons are then activated from the brain stem reflex centers located in the reticular formation. Various kinds of stimuli can activate the reflex center for swallowing, notably touch-and pressure receptors at the back of the tongue.

A unilateral **lesion** of the hypoglossal nerve or nucleus produces paralysis of the tongue on the same side. As this is a peripheral paresis, a pronounced atrophy of the tongue muscles ensues. This is witnessed by a wrinkled surface of the tongue because the mucous membrane becomes too big for the reduced volume (Fig. 27.7). When stretching out the tongue, it **deviates** to the paretic side, because of paresis of the **genioglossus muscle**. This muscle passes backward and laterally into the tongue from its origin at the inside of the

Figure 27.7

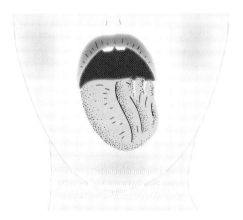

Peripheral paralysis of the hypoglossal nerve on the left side. The tongue deviates to the side of the lesion when the patient tries to stretch it out. Atrophy of the intrinsic muscles of the tongue makes the surface wrinkled.

mandible; its normal action when acting unilaterally is to draw the tongue forward and to the opposite side.

The Ansa Cervicalis

Some of the motor fibers from the first cervical spinal segment join the hypoglossal nerve and follow it for some distance before leaving it and descending in the neck. The descending fibers join other motor fibers from the second and third cervical segments and thereafter form an arc external to the internal jugular vein, called the **ansa cervicalis** (*ansa*, handle). The fibers of the ansa cervicalis innervate the **infrahyoid muscles** and are not related to the hypoglossal nucleus or the muscles of the tongue. Damage to the hypoglossal nucleus or the proximal part of the nerve (before the fibers from C_1 join it) therefore produces no pareses of the infrahyoid muscles.

THE ACCESSORY NERVE

The **eleventh cranial nerve**, the accessory nerve, brings somatic efferent fibers to two muscles in the neck—the **sternocleidomastoid** and the **trapezius**. The accessory **nucleus** is located in a column in the upper part of the **cervical cord** (Fig. 27.2) and contains neurons that are of the ordinary motoneuron type. The root fibers leave the cord and ascend to enter the posterior fossa through the foramen magnum (Fig. 27.8). The nerve then leaves the skull through the **jugular foramen** together with the vagus and the glossopharyngeal nerves. Outside the skull, the nerve passes internal to the sternocleidomastoid muscle and superficially through the upper part of the lateral triangle of the neck before continuing under the upper part of the trapezius muscle.

Some fibers from the **nucleus ambiguus** join the accessory nerve for a short distance intracranially. These fibers leave the nerve just outside the jugular foramen and follow the vagus nerve in their further course. They should therefore be considered a part of the vagus with a somewhat aberrant course rather than as a part of the accessory nerve.

In **central motor lesions** (of the corticobulbar component of the pyramidal tract), pareses of the contralateral sternocleidomastoid and the trapezius are usually observed. Because of its superficial position, the nerve may be damaged in the **lateral triangle** of the neck, producing a **peripheral paresis**. In such a case only the trapezius is paretic because the fibers innervating the sternocleidomastoid leave the nerve higher up. Further, the upper part of the trapezius muscle is usually most basis, all sensory fibers from the pharynx (and the posterior part of the tongue) should be classified as visceral afferent. There is evidence, however, that such fibers end in the somatic afferent trigeminal nucleus and not in the visceral afferent solitary nucleus. Functionally, they may therefore be considered somatic afferent rather than visceral afferent. Vagus may also carry nociceptive signals from parts of the **heart** (see Chapter 29, under "Central Pathways for Visceral Afferent Signals").

Visceral afferent signals in the vagus nerve most likely contribute to **feelings** like hunger or satiety. There is also evidence that signals in the vagus nerve contribute to the feelings associated with infections (loss of appetite, tiredness, somnolence, and so forth) and the induction of **sickness behavior**. Together with other visceral afferent fibers, the vagus contributes to our **general bodily feeling**—also called the "sense of the physiological condition of the body" (Craig, 2002, p. 655). This is discussed further in Chapter 30 under "The Hypothalamus and the Immune System."

Visceral Reflexes

The visceral afferents in the vagus nerve are links in reflex arcs that control **secretion** and **peristaltic movements** of the gastrointestinal tract (and vomiting). Such reflexes also mediate alterations of **airway secretion** and of the **airway resistance** by changing the tone of the bronchial smooth muscles. The **reflex centers** of all these reflexes are located in the medulla, and the efferent links are visceral efferent fibers coming from the dorsal motor nucleus of the vagus.

Visceral afferents from **baroreceptors** in the wall of the large vessels provide information about the blood pressure in the aorta. Increased blood pressure gives rise to increased firing frequency of the afferent fibers. In turn, this produces increased firing of visceral efferent vagus fibers, which reduces the heart rate. The **reflex center** must involve connections from the solitary nucleus to the motor nucleus of the vagus (these two nuclei are close neighbors, as can be seen in Fig. 27.2).

The motor nuclei of the vagus can also be influenced by signals other than those coming from the viscera. For example, the sight, the smell, or even the thought of food can produce increased secretion of gastric juice. These are examples of **conditioned responses**, whereas the stimulation of taste receptors produces an unconditioned (true reflex) response.

Other examples of visceral reflexes are discussed in Chapter 29, under "Visceral Reflexes."

The Vomiting Reflex

Vomiting is usually caused by marked dilatation of the stomach or irritation of its mucosa. The biologic significance of the reflex is presumably to rid the stomach of potentially harmful contents. As we all know, however, vomiting can also be provoked by irritation of the pharynx (putting a finger in the throat) and by foul odors, strong emotions, and travel sickness. Several different afferent links to the reflex center must therefore exist.

The emptying of the stomach is caused by coordinated contractions of the smooth muscles in the stomach wall and striated muscles in the diaphragm and the abdominal wall. In addition, laryngeal muscles (closing the airways) and muscles of the pharynx, the soft palate, and the tongue also participate. Thus, the reflex center must activate visceral efferent neurons and α motoneurons at several levels of the brain stem and the spinal cord in a specific sequence. The **reflex center** is actually quite widespread, but usually matters are simplified by restricting it to the medulla, including the **solitary nucleus**. This receives the visceral afferent fibers from the stomach, forming the afferent link when the reflex is elicited from the stomach itself. From the reflex center in the medulla, signals pass to the motor nuclei via synaptic interruption in the reticular formation and reticulospinal fibers. In addition, there are direct spinal projections from the solitary nucleus to the motoneurons of the diaphragm and abdominal wall.

Substances in the bloodstream cause vomiting by direct action at the **area postrema** of the medulla (see Chapter 8, under "Some Parts of the Brain Lack a Blood–Brain Barrier"). Neurons in the area postrema project to the solitary nucleus. **Apomorphine** and other alkaloids are given orally or subcutaneously to provoke vomiting.

Somatic Efferent Vagus Fibers

The somatic efferent vagus fibers come from the **ambiguus nucleus** (Figs. 27.2 and 27.5), which belongs to the special somatic efferent nuclei. The fibers supply all striated muscles of the **larynx** and parts of the muscles of the **pharynx**. The fibers to the pharynx take off from the vagus as several small branches, whereas most of the fibers to the larynx are collected in the **recurrent laryngeal nerve** (Fig. 27.9). This nerve takes off from the main vagus trunk at the level of the aortic arch on the left side and the subclavian artery on the right. It then arches behind the vessels and ascends in the furrow between the trachea and the esophagus, to reach the larynx. One of the laryngeal muscles located on the outside, the **cricothyroid muscle**, receives motor fibers in the superior laryngeal nerve (which is a predominantly sensory nerve, as mentioned earlier). The vagus also innervates one of the muscles of the soft palate, the **levator veli palatini** muscle.

A **lesion** of the vagus nerve above the exit of the motor branches to the pharynx and the soft palate produces deviation of the uvula and the posterior pharyngeal wall to the normal side (as can be seen, e.g., when a patient is asked to

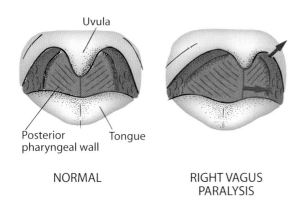

Figure 27.10

Uvula

Posterior pharyngeal wall   Tongue

NORMAL   RIGHT VAGUS PARALYSIS

Paralysis of the right vagus nerve. The uvula and the posterior pharyngeal wall are pulled toward the normal side when the patient says "aah." (Redrawn from Mumenthaler 1979.)

say "aah"; Fig. 27.10). Pareses of the soft palate and the pharynx cause fluid and food to enter the nasal cavity when swallowing (owing to inadequate closure of the nasopharynx). Further, the voice becomes hoarse because the vocal cords cannot be properly adducted. Such a symptom will obviously also occur after a lesion of the recurrent laryngeal nerve anywhere along its course. In case of a unilateral lesion, the voice hoarseness will gradually disappear, because the muscles of the normal side adapt to the changed conditions.

The neurons of the nucleus ambiguus are influenced by, among other sources, the **pyramidal tract** during speech. They can also be activated involuntarily in the **cough reflex** by irritating stimuli of the respiratory tract.

Somatic Afferent Vagus Fibers

This is the smallest contingent of fibers in the vagus nerve. They have their cell bodies in the small **jugular ganglion** and come from a small region of the skin of the external ear—the **auricular ramus** (Fig. 27.9). The fibers terminate in the **trigeminal sensory nucleus**. Touching the innervated area, for example, by an otoscope in the external meatus may evoke a cough reflex and in some individuals even a vomiting reflex. The causes of these phenomena are unknown. They might be due to connections from the trigeminal nucleus to the solitary nucleus or by abnormal signal transmission between sensory fibers of the vagus nerve (ephaptic transmission)

THE GLOSSOPHARYNGEAL NERVE

The **ninth cranial nerve**, the glossopharyngeal, resembles the vagus but is smaller and innervates a more restricted

region. The root fibers leave the medulla immediately rostral to the vagus fibers (Fig. 27.1). The root fibers fuse to form one trunk that leaves the cranial cavity through the **jugular foramen** (together with the vagus and the accessory nerves). The nerve follows an arched course (ventrally) lateral to the pharynx, which it penetrates to reach the base of the tongue. Close to the jugular foramen, the nerve contains two small **sensory ganglia** with pseudounipolar ganglion cells, the **superior** and **petrous ganglia**.

Of the peripheral branches, some innervate the muscles and the mucous membrane of the **pharynx** (together with the vagus, which appears to be the most important quantitatively); other sensory fibers reach the posterior part of the tongue, to innervate **taste buds**, and the mucous membrane (and also the mucous membrane of the soft palate and the tonsillar region). The glossopharyngeal nerve also contains **visceral efferent** (parasympathetic) fibers to the **parotid gland** and to the salivary glands in the posterior part of the tongue (see Fig. 28.11 for the course of the parasympathetic fibers).

The Sinus Nerve and Baroreceptors

A special contingent of visceral afferent fibers in the glossopharyngeal nerve comes from the wall of the **carotid sinus** (the thin-walled, dilated part of the internal carotid artery). The fibers conduct signals from mechanoreceptors recording the tension of the arterial wall; that is, the receptors monitor the blood pressure and are therefore called **baroreceptors** (cf. the same kind of afferents from the aorta running with the vagus nerve). The afferent fibers end in the **solitary nucleus**, and from there the signals are conveyed to a special part of the **ambiguus nucleus** with motoneurons supplying the heart. Increased signal frequency of the cardiac vagus fibers reduces the heart rate, and thereby the blood pressure is reduced. When the blood pressure falls, there is reduced firing of the cardiac vagus fibers, with increased heart rate and blood pressure. This is one of several mechanisms to keep the **blood pressure** within certain limits and ensure that the cerebral blood flow is sufficient at all times.

The Nuclei of the Glossopharyngeal Nerve

The **somatic efferent** fibers to the striated pharynx muscles come from the **ambiguus nucleus**, whereas the **visceral efferent** fibers have their cell bodies in the small **inferior salivatory nucleus** (Fig. 27.2). The signals from this nucleus follow a somewhat complicated course to reach the parotid gland (as cannot present a polite social smile. In **central pareses** (such as capsular hemiplegia), emotional facial expressions are in fact often exaggerated, and the patient cannot suppress a smile or prevent crying. Diseases of the basal ganglia, such as **Parkinson's disease**, present the opposite picture: the emotional, spontaneous expressions are lacking, whereas a voluntary, social smile is possible.

The Facial Nerve and Reflexes

The facial nucleus is also a link in some important reflex arcs. One is the **corneal** or **blink reflex**. It is elicited by touch or irritation of the cornea, and the sensory signals are conducted centrally in the trigeminal nerve to the spinal trigeminal nucleus (Fig. 27.13). From there the signals pass via interneurons in the reticular formation to the facial nucleus of both sides, and a contraction of the muscles of the eyelid is produced. The corneal reflex can be weakened or abolished by a lesion anywhere along the course of the afferent and efferent links or in the rather extensive reflex center.

Another reflex mediated by the facial nerve is the **stapedius reflex**, in which the response is contraction of the tiny **stapedius muscle** in the middle ear. The stimulus is an intense sound conducted centrally in the cochlear (acoustic) nerve to the cochlear nuclei. Most likely, interneurons in the reticular formation transfer the signals to the facial nucleus. The

Figure 27.13

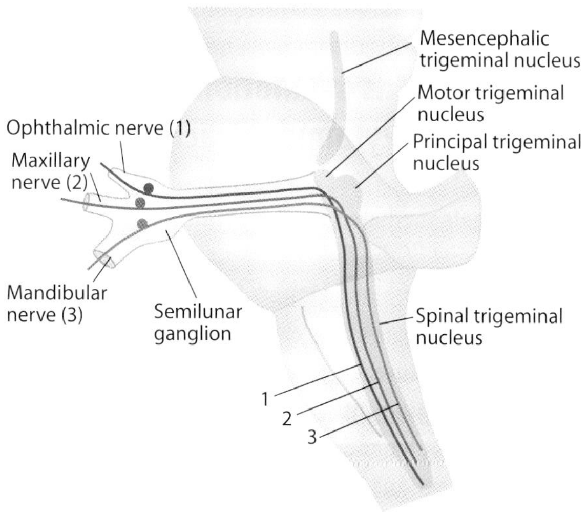

The trigeminal nuclei. In addition, the figure shows the topographic arrangement in the spinal trigeminal nucleus of the fibers from the three main trigeminal branches.

stapedius muscle pulls the stapes a little out of the oval window (see Fig. 17.7) and thereby dampens the transmission of sound waves to the cochlear duct. Accordingly, peripheral facial paresis can produce hypersensitivity to sounds, or **hyperacusis**.

Secretion of Tears and Saliva

The preganglionic parasympathetic fibers of the **intermediate nerve**—acting on the **lacrimal**, the **submandibular**, and the **sublingual glands**—have their cell bodies in the small **superior salivatory nucleus**. This nucleus belongs to the column of visceral efferent nuclei (Fig. 27.2). As mentioned, preganglionic parasympathetic fibers acting on the parotid gland have their cell bodies in the inferior salivatory nucleus and leave the brain stem in the glossopharyngeal nerve.

The **secretion of saliva** is brought about primarily by stimulation of the taste receptors but also by signals from higher levels of the brain (such as the thought of tasty food; it is especially effective to imagine that one is eating a lemon). Strong emotions, for example anxiety before a performance, can inhibit the secretion of saliva, as experienced by mouth dryness. The **secretion of tears**, even more than the salivary secretion, is an example of how visceral functions can be influenced from higher levels of the brain. The continuous secretion of tears is of course primarily a physiologic protection of the eyes and increases in response to any irritation of the cornea or the conjunctiva; nevertheless, the most profuse tear production occurs when we express strong emotions by **crying**. When crying, the signals to the superior salivatory nucleus producing the flow of tears are not mediated by the pyramidal tract or other efferent cortical fibers descending in the internal capsule, in correspondence with the fact that tears cannot be produced voluntarily nor can the secretion of tears be suppressed. Most likely, fibers from the **hypothalamus** are responsible for the activation of the visceral efferent neurons during crying. Nevertheless, the hypothalamus is under the influence of higher levels, such as parts of the cerebral cortex and the limbic structures. Thus, the conscious experience of the emotions (such as sorrow or pity) starts the train of neural events leading to tear secretion.

The Intermediate Nerve

The small **geniculate ganglion**, containing the cell bodies of the sensory fibers of the intermediate nerve, is found where the facial nerve bends posteriorly in the temporal bone. Here a branch of the intermediate nerve, the **greater petrosal nerve**, leaves the main trunk of the facial nerve to course anteriorly. It contains **visceral efferent** (parasympathetic) fibers that end in the small parasympathetic **pterygopalatine ganglion** located behind the orbit. From there postganglionic fibers follow trigeminal branches to the **lacrimal gland** and **glands in the nasal cavity** (see Fig. 28.11). The rest of the intermediate nerve fibers leave the facial nerve as it passes downward posterior to the middle ear. This branch is called the **chorda tympani** because it passes through the middle ear (tympanic cavity) on its way forward to join the **lingual nerve** (a trigeminal branch) outside the skull. The chorda tympani contains **visceral afferent** fibers from **taste buds** in the anterior two-thirds of the tongue. These fibers have their cell bodies in the geniculate ganglion. In addition, the chorda tympani carries **visceral efferent** (parasympathetic) fibers that end in the small **submandibular ganglion**. From this ganglion, postganglionic parasympathetic fibers pass to the submandibular and the sublingual (salivary) glands.

THE TRIGEMINAL NERVE

The **fifth cranial nerve** is primarily the sensory nerve of the face, with mainly **somatic afferent fibers.** In addition, it contains a small portion with **special somatic efferent** fibers to the masticatory muscles. The trigeminal nerve is the nerve of the **first branchial (visceral) arch** and innervates structures that are developed from this arch.

The nerve leaves the brain stem laterally on the pons (Fig. 27.1) with a small (medial) motor root and a large (lateral) sensory root. Shortly after leaving the pons, the nerve expands to form the large **semilunar ganglion**, which contains the cell bodies of the pseudounipolar (sensory) ganglion cells. Three large branches continue anteriorly from the ganglion: the **ophthalmic**, the **maxillary**, and the **mandibular** nerves (Fig. 27.13).

The **ophthalmic nerve** enters the orbit and supplies the eye bulb (including the cornea), the upper eyelid, the back of the nose, and the skin of the forehead with sensory fibers (Fig. 27.14). It also sends fibers to the mucous membranes of the anterior part of the nasal cavity. The **maxillary nerve** runs forward in a sulcus in the bottom of the orbit and sends fibers to the lower eyelid, the skin above the mouth, the upper teeth and gingiva, and the hard palate and posterior (major) part of the nasal cavity. The **mandibular nerve** innervates the lower teeth and gingiva, the tongue, and the skin of the lower jaw and upward, well into the temporal region (Fig. 27.14). The branch of the mandibular nerve supplying the tongue with

Figure 27.14

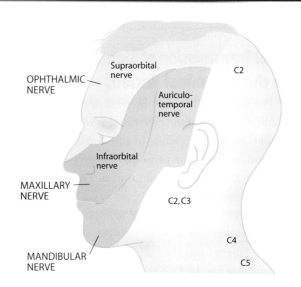

Distribution in the facial skin of the three main trigeminal branches. The names of some further branches and the segmental origins of sensory fibers to the rest of the head and the neck are indicated.

somatic sensory afferent fibers is called the **lingual nerve**. This nerve receives visceral afferent (taste) fibers from the **chorda tympani**, destined for the anterior two-thirds of the tongue.

The **motor fibers** of the trigeminal nerve follow the mandibular nerve but leave this in several smaller twigs to the masticatory muscles (and some other muscles with relation to the lower jaw and the soft palate).

The Sensory Trigeminal Nucleus

With regard to function and fiber composition, the sensory part of the trigeminal nerve corresponds to the spinal dorsal roots. The trigeminal nerve, therefore, belongs to the somatosensory system and conducts signals from **low-threshold mechanoreceptors**, **thermoreceptors**, and **nociceptors** in the face and in the mucous membranes of the face. As with other spinal nerves, fibers leading from different kinds of receptors are intermingled in the nerve but are arranged by receptor type when entering the CNS. Then the fibers distribute to the three subdivisions of the long sensory trigeminal nucleus (Figs. 27.2 and 27.13). Fibers from proprioceptors (muscle spindles, joint receptors) end in the **mesencephalic nucleus**, fibers from low-threshold mechanoreceptors end in

Figure 27.16

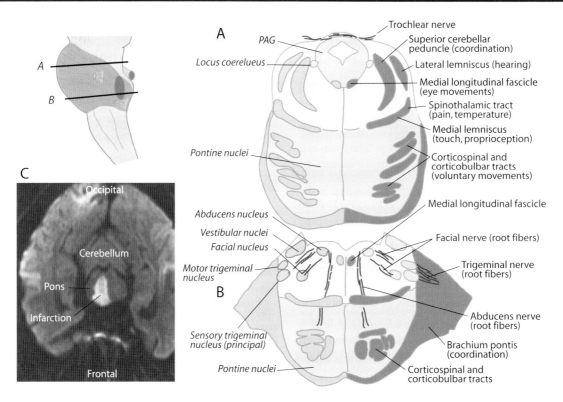

Position in the pons of cranial nerve nuclei, their root fibers, and the clinically most important tracts. **A** and **B**: Drawings of transverse sections through the upper and lower pons, respectively. Tracts are marked and named to the right, while nuclei are shown to the left in the drawings. The figure helps predict the major symptoms that might ensue after lesions in various parts of the pons. **C**: MRI at a level between A and B showing a recent infarction (light) in the pons due to occlusion of the basilar artery. (Courtesy of Dr. S.J. Bakke, Oslo University Hospital, Oslo, Norway.)

these tasks are performed reflexly, and usually eye position, light access, and lens curvature are controlled simultaneously. We discuss the extraocular muscles and the control of eye movements in Chapter 25.

Typical **symptoms** resulting from lesions of the extraocular muscles or their nerves are **strabismus** (squint), **double vision**, and **dizziness** (probably due to double vision). In addition, patients usually keep their heads bent or turned in order to reduce the double vision (i.e., trying to keep a position in which the paretic muscle[s] is used as little as possible). Figure 25.4B shows a simple scheme for examination of the six extraocular muscles.

The Abducens Nerve

The abducens nerve leaves the brain stem close to the midline at the junction of the medulla and the pons (Fig. 27.1; also see Fig. 6.15). Figure 27.11 shows the location of the **abducens nucleus** and its relation to the facial nerve. The abducens nerve runs forward intracranially and passes through the **cavernous sinus** (see Fig. 8.9) before entering the orbit through the superior orbital fissure (Fig. 27.17). It supplies only one muscle, the **lateral rectus**. The muscle pulls the eye so the cornea faces laterally (abducts the eye; see Fig. 25.3). Even though other muscles can abduct the eye somewhat (the superior and the inferior oblique muscles), the lateral rectus is necessary for more than a slight lateral movement (Fig. 27.18). A person with a unilateral lesion of the abducens nerve usually keeps the head turned somewhat to the side of the lesion to compensate for the loss of lateral motion of the eye.

The abducens nerve can be **injured** by expanding processes in the orbit that compresses the nerve, by an aneurysm on the internal carotid artery (Fig. 27.17), meningitis, skull fractures, or thrombosis of the cavernous sinus (see Fig. 8.9).

Figure 27.17

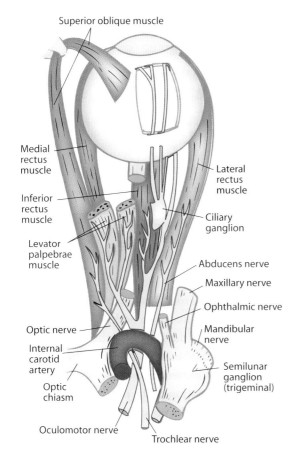

Superior oblique muscle

Medial rectus muscle

Inferior rectus muscle

Levator palpebrae muscle

Lateral rectus muscle

Ciliary ganglion

Abducens nerve

Maxillary nerve

Ophthalmic nerve

Optic nerve

Internal carotid artery

Mandibular nerve

Optic chiasm

Semilunar ganglion (trigeminal)

Oculomotor nerve

Trochlear nerve

The right eye with muscles and nerves, as viewed from above. Three cranial nerves innervate the muscles of the eye. Some of the extraocular muscles and the optic nerve have been cut. The external layers of the eye bulb have been partly removed to expose the postganglionic fibers from the ciliary ganglion on their way to the intrinsic eye muscles. Note the position of the trigeminal ganglion and the internal carotid artery.

The Trochlear Nerve

This is the only one of the cranial nerves to leave the brain stem on the dorsal side (just below the inferior colliculus) (Figs. 27.1 and 27.16; also see Fig. 6.19).[6] The **trochlear nucleus** lies a little ventrally to the aqueduct in the mesencephalon (Fig. 27.2). Like the abducens nerve, the trochlear traverses the cavernous sinus and enters the orbit through the **superior orbital fissure**. It innervates the **superior**

6. Another peculiarity of the trochlear nerve is that it crosses the midline before leaving the brain stem, so that the left trochlear nucleus innervates the right superior oblique muscle and vice versa. Some of the fibers of the oculomotor nerve also cross before leaving the brain stem.

Figure 27.18

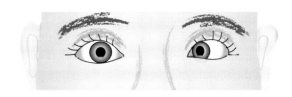

Paresis of the right abducens nerve. When the patient looks to his right, the right eye does not follow the left, because the right rectus muscle is paralyzed.

oblique muscle (Fig. 27.17; also see Fig. 25.1), which directs the gaze downward and laterally (see Fig. 25.3).

The Oculomotor Nerve

The nerve emerges from the ventral aspect of the mesencephalon, in the interpeduncular fossa (Fig. 27.1; also see Fig. 6.20). This is the largest of the three nerves supplying the extraocular muscles; as mentioned, it contains somatic efferent and visceral efferent fibers. The **somatic efferent** fibers come from the large **oculomotor nucleus** (nucleus of the oculomotor nerve) situated close to the midline in the mesencephalon, ventral to the aqueduct (Figs. 27.2 and 27.5). The medial longitudinal fasciculus, with ascending fibers from the vestibular nuclei, lies close to the oculomotor nucleus (and to the abducens and trochlear nuclei as well). The **visceral efferent** (preganglionic parasympathetic) fibers come from the small **Edinger-Westphal nucleus** located near the oculomotor nucleus (Fig. 27.2 and 27.5). Often the term "oculomotor complex" is used for the somatic efferent and visceral efferent nuclei together.

The **oculomotor nerve** passes forward to the orbit through the **cavernous sinus** together with the other nerves to the eye (entering through the superior orbital fissure). The somatic efferent and parasympathetic fibers part in the orbit (Fig. 27.17). The somatic efferent fibers innervate certain extraocular muscles: the **superior** and **inferior rectus**, the **medial rectus**, and the **inferior oblique**. These muscles can move the eye medially, upward, and downward and rotate it around the sagittal axis (see Fig. 25.2). In addition, the oculomotor nerve supplies the **levator palpebrae** muscle (Fig. 27.17), which lifts the upper eyelid.

The **visceral efferent** oculomotor fibers end in the small **ciliary ganglion** situated behind the eye (Fig. 27.17). Here the fibers establish synapses with the postganglionic neurons, which send their axons anteriorly in the wall of the eye to innervate the intrinsic (smooth) muscles of the

PART SIX

The Autonomic Nervous System

The autonomic nervous system (or visceral system) is not a term that can be defined precisely, either anatomically or functionally. The old belief that the somatic and the autonomic parts of the nervous system are completely independent is not tenable. The more we have learned about the nervous system, the clearer it has become that simplistic divisions like this are arbitrary. Some authors therefore maintain that the term "autonomic nervous system" should be abandoned and replaced by simply referring to **visceral neurons**—that is, the neurons that innervate visceral organs. For practical reasons, it is nevertheless helpful to use the term "autonomic nervous system" and to **define** it very broadly as the neuronal groups and fiber connections that control the activity of **visceral organs**, **vessels**, and **glands** (as well as the vessels and glands that are not parts of visceral organs). Visceral organs contain smooth-muscle cells and glandular cells. We can therefore also define the autonomic system as the parts of the nervous system that control the activity of **smooth muscles** and **glands**, regardless of their location in the body (in contrast to the somatic or cerebrospinal system, which controls striated skeletal muscles). Mostly we are not aware of the processes going on in the organs controlled by the autonomic nervous system, and their activities are not subject to voluntary, conscious control.

The autonomic system can be subdivided in different ways. As with the somatic system, we distinguish **peripheral** and **central** parts. Whereas the peripheral parts of the autonomic and somatic systems can be separated fairly well, the division becomes much less clear within the central nervous system (CNS). The peripheral parts of the autonomic system are described in Chapters 28 and 29. Although the nerves to visceral organs contain both efferent (motor) and afferent (sensory) fibers, the anatomic differences between the autonomic and the somatic

Figure 28.1

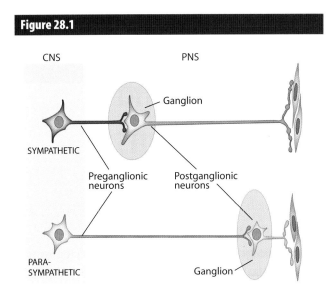

Basic organization of the peripheral part of the autonomic system. Two consecutive neurons conduct the signals from the CNS to the effectors. Note the difference in length between the pre- and postganglionic fibers in the sympathetic and the parasympathetic systems. Effectors may be glandular cells and not only smooth-muscle cells, as shown here.

their axons are called **postganglionic**. The cell bodies of the preganglionic neurons are located in the spinal cord and the brain stem. The **preganglionic neurons**, both the sympathetic and the parasympathetic ones, use **acetylcholine** as a neurotransmitter.

Another typical feature of the visceral efferent neurons is that, as a rule, the postganglionic fibers form extensive **plexuses** around the organs they innervate.

Postganglionic Fibers Do Not Establish Typical Synapses

The thin, unmyelinated postganglionic fibers do not form typical synapses with the effector cells, in contrast to the somatic efferent fibers innervating skeletal muscle cells (see Fig. 21.5). When the postganglionic fibers reach the vicinity of the effector cells, they branch extensively, and there are small swellings—**varicosities**—along the branches (Fig. 28.1). In each varicosity there are vesicles with neurotransmitters. The varicosities do not form synapses but can be located fairly close to the effector cells. In some places, the distance is only 50 nm, thus permitting very direct and precise control of the effector cell. Most often, however, the distance between the varicosities and the effectors is so great that the neurotransmitter, after being released, must diffuse over a considerable distance to reach its target. This means

that the neurotransmitter acts on several effector cells within a certain distance. When the diffusion distance is great, the transmitter acts slowly, with a long latency and a prolonged action (cf. the fast action at the neuromuscular junction). Often, only a few of the smooth-muscle cells in the wall of a hollow organ (such as a vessel) are close enough to the varicosities to be directly influenced by the transmitter. In such cases, the action potential elicited in some smooth-muscle cells is propagated from cell to cell via **gap junctions** (nexus) between them (electric coupling). In general, therefore, the actions of the autonomic nervous system are more **diffusely distributed**, both **spatially** and **temporally**, than is the case in the somatic system. The properties of the **smooth-muscle** cells contribute to increase this difference, because their action potentials last much longer than those of skeletal muscle cells do. Further, smooth-muscle cells (e.g., in the wall of the gastrointestinal tract) can be made to contract by stimuli other than nervous ones, such as by **stretching** and by the actions of **hormones**. The autonomic system therefore contributes to the regulation of the contraction of smooth-muscle cells in the gastrointestinal tract and in the walls of the vessels, but it is not alone in this capacity (again in contrast to the control of skeletal muscle cells by the motoneurons).

Some Organs Are Subject to More Precise Autonomic Control than Others

There are, nevertheless, great differences between different organs with regard to the precision of their autonomic innervation. Some visceral organs require much faster and more accurate control than others. The smooth muscles of the **eye** (the ciliary muscle and the pupillary sphincter, regulating the curvature of the lens and the diameter of the pupil) are subject to very precise control. The same holds for the muscles of the **ductus deferens**, in which the propulsive contractions must be fast and well coordinated. Such demands are not made of the smooth muscles of the gastrointestinal tract and the vessels. Corresponding to different functional requirements, the pattern of autonomic innervation also varies in different organs. The intrinsic eye muscles, for example, receive a large number of nerve fibers so that all muscle cells come in close contact with varicosities of nerve fibers. This is called **multiunit arrangement**, because it is similar to the conditions in the somatic system with many precisely controlled motor units. In places with few nerve fibers to supply a large number of smooth-muscle cells, so that only a few cells are close to nerve varicosities, we use the term **single-unit arrangement**. Thus, numerous

Figure 28.2

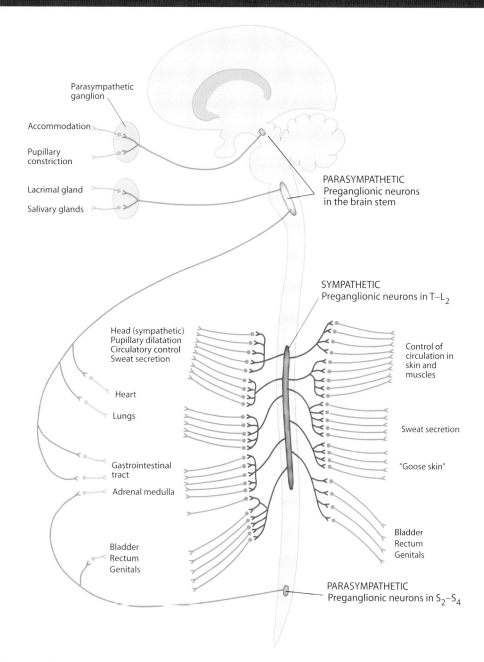

Main anatomic features of the autonomic nervous system. The preganglionic sympathetic neurons have their cell bodies in the inter-mediolateral column, whereas the corresponding parasympathetic neurons are located in the brain stem and the sacral cord. The cell bodies of sympathetic postganglionic neurons in ganglia lie close to the vertebral column (paravertebral and prevertebral ganglia), whereas those of parasympathetic postganglionic neurons lie in ganglia close to the organ. The sympathetic fibers reach all parts of the body, but the parasympathetic fibers have a more restricted distribution. (After Pick 1970.)

muscle cells behave as a unit when one or a few of them are activated.

Autonomic Ganglia and Plexuses

The autonomic ganglia contain **multipolar neurons** of various sizes (Fig. 28.3) with long, branching dendrites.

The axons are mostly unmyelinated and very thin. The cell bodies of the ganglion cells are embedded in a meshwork of fibers consisting of afferent fibers, ganglion cell dendrites, and axons of the ganglion cells. At least some of the ganglia receive **sensory fibers** from visceral organs. There are also **interneurons** in the autonomic ganglia. Such features, and other data, indicate that the ganglia are not just simple

Figure 28.3

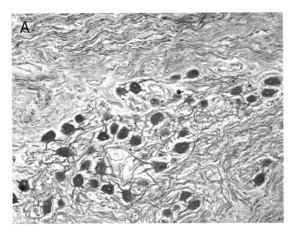 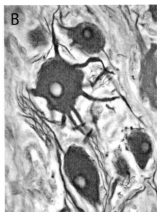

Autonomic ganglion. Photomicrograph of section through the celiac ganglion impregnated with heavy metals to show nerve fibers (black) and neurons (red). **A:** The multipolar postganglionic neurons lie in a wickerwork of preganglionic and postganglionic nerve fibers. Thus, the autonomic ganglia consist of groups of postganglionic neurons embedded in a plexus. **B:** Higher magnification of postganglionic neurons.

synaptic interruptions of purely motor (efferent) pathways but can serve as **reflex centers** for some visceral reflexes.

When an organ is innervated by both sympathetic and parasympathetic fibers, these two components intermingle and form **autonomic plexuses** just outside or in the wall of the organs. At many places, cell bodies of postganglionic cells form small clumps intermingled with the fibers of the plexuses. Thus, ganglia and plexuses often coexist, and the ganglia then have the same prefix as the plexuses. For example, the **cardiac plexus** on the outside of the heart contains both kinds of fibers as well as the cell bodies of the postganglionic parasympathetic neurons. Especially well-developed plexuses are found around the large vessels in the upper abdomen, where ¨parasympathetic vagus fibers intermingle with sympathetic fibers. These **prevertebral plexuses** receive their names from the arteries they surround and follow peripherally: the **celiac plexus**, the **superior** and **inferior mesenteric plexus**, and the **renal plexus**. The prevertebral plexuses continue into the pelvis as the **hypogastric plexus**.

Differences between the Sympathetic and the Parasympathetic Systems

The two systems differ in several respects. The location of **preganglionic neurons** differs: the sympathetic ones are found in the T_1–L_2 spinal segments, whereas the parasympathetic preganglionic neurons lie in the brain stem and the S_2–S_4 spinal segments (Fig. 28.2). Further, the **ganglia** are located differently: sympathetic ones lie close to the CNS, whereas the

parasympathetic ganglia are located close to the target organs. Thus, the sympathetic preganglionic fibers are short, and the parasympathetic ones are long (Figs. 28.1 and 28.2).

Another difference between the two systems is the **neurotransmitters** used by the **postganglionic neurons**: the sympathetic fibers release **norepinephrine**, whereas the parasympathetic fibers release **acetylcholine** from their varicosities.

Finally, the **distribution** of postganglionic fibers is different. Thus, virtually all parts of the body receive sympathetic fibers, whereas the parasympathetic fibers are mostly restricted to the true visceral organs. The body wall and the extremities (skin, muscles, joints) do not receive parasympathetic fibers.

Table 28.1 gives a broad overview of the functions of the two systems; a more comprehensive discussion is provided later in this chapter.

The Parasympathetic Innervation Is Usually More Precise than the Sympathetic

As a rule (with notable exceptions), the sympathetic system is more diffusely organized than the parasympathetic. This is evident, for example, in the relation between the number of preganglionic and postganglionic fibers. In the parasympathetic **ciliary ganglion** (see Fig. 27.17), two postganglionic fibers leave the ganglion for each preganglionic fiber reaching it—that is, a 2:1 relationship (in the cat). For the sympathetic **superior cervical ganglion** (Fig. 28.7), the relationship is 30:1 in the cat and 60 to 190:1 in humans (this ganglion contains more than 1 million neurons in humans). Further, the **parasympathetic** innervation is in several places arranged with **multiunits**—that is, small "motor units" with the possibility of precise control. This concerns, for example, the innervation of the intrinsic eye muscles.

Table 28.1	Summary of Some Main Actions of the Autonomic System	
Organ	**Sympathetic System**	**Parasympathetic System**
Arteries (arterioles)	Vasoconstriction	Vasodilatation in glands and genital organs
Skin	Vasoconstriction; sweat secretion; goose skin	No innervation
Skeletal muscles	Vasoconstriction	No innervation
Heart	Increased rate and stroke volume	Reduced heart rate
Airways	Relaxation of bronchial smooth muscle (reduced airway resistance)	Contraction of bronchial smooth muscle; secretion from mucous glands
Gastrointestinal tract	Reduced blood flow and peristaltic movements	Increased peristaltic movements; secretion of gastric juice, bile, and pancreatic juice
Urinary bladder	Relaxation of muscle for emptying (detrusor)	Contraction of detrusor; relaxation of urethral sphincter
Rectum	Relaxation of muscle for emptying; closure of internal sphincter (smooth muscle)	Contraction of muscle for emptying; relaxation of internal sphincter
Genital organs	Contraction of the ductus deferens (ejaculation)	Erection (penis, clitoris)
Eye	Pupillary dilatation	Pupillary constriction; accommodation; secretion of tears

See Table 28.2 for further details.

The **sympathetic** innervation is often (but not always) arranged with **single units**—that is, a large number of smooth muscle cells are activated from one postganglionic fiber and behave as a functional unit.

Another difference concerns **the topographic arrangement** of the preganglionic neurons. Whereas the sympathetic neurons show only a fairly rough topography within the intermediolateral column in relation to the location of the target (Fig. 28.7; Table 28.2), the parasympathetic neurons are as a rule collected in distinct nuclei (Figs. 28.2 and 28.11) or subdivisions of a nucleus (such as the motor nucleus of the vagus), each related to one target organ.

The difference in innervation precision between the sympathetic and the parasympathetic systems mentioned previously have several **exceptions**, however. One example is the ductus deferens, in which the rhythmic contractions are elicited by sympathetic fibers. A multiunit arrangement is required to ensure the necessary precision and speed of the contractile wave moving the sperm during ejaculation. Another example is that the parasympathetic innervation of the gastrointestinal tract is rather diffuse (single-unit arrangement).

PERIPHERAL PARTS OF THE SYMPATHETIC SYSTEM

Preganglionic Fibers and the Sympathetic Trunk

The peripheral parts of the sympathetic system consist of both neurons conveying signals to visceral organs and sensory fibers leading in the opposite direction. The efferent,

preganglionic sympathetic neurons have their cell bodies in the **intermediolateral column** in the spinal cord (Fig. 28.4). The preganglionic fibers leave the cord (like other efferent fibers) through the ventral roots, but because the intermediolateral column is present in only the T_1–L_2 segments, only the ventral roots of these segments contain preganglionic sympathetic fibers (the sympathetic system is also called the thoracolumbar system). The sympathetic fibers follow the somatic fibers for a short distance, however. Just after the ventral and the dorsal roots fuse, the sympathetic preganglionic fibers leave the spinal nerve to end in a **sympathetic ganglion** (Fig. 28.5). In early embryonic life, one ganglion develops on each side for every spinal segment, but during further development, some ganglia fuse, so the final number is smaller than the number of segments. This reduction is most marked in the cervical region.

The ganglia are located just outside the intervertebral foramen, laterally on the vertebral column (Fig. 28.6). The row of such **paravertebral ganglia** extends from the base of the skull to the coccygeal bone in the pelvis minor. Because fiber bundles interconnect the ganglia, a continuous string called the **sympathetic trunk** is formed (Figs. 28.5 and 28.6). The ganglia form small swellings along the trunk. There is usually one ganglion for each pair of spinal nerves, except in the cervical region, where there are only three: the **superior**, **middle**, and **inferior cervical ganglia**. The middle ganglion can be missing, and the inferior cervical ganglion is usually fused with the uppermost thoracic ganglion

Table 28.2 Principal Features of Autonomic Innervation

Organ	Sympathetic			Parasympathetic		
	Preganglionic Neuron	Postganglionic Neuron	Action	Preganglionic Neuron	Postganglionic Neuron	Action
Eye	T_1–T_2	Superior cervical ganglion	Pupillary dilatation	Parasympathetic oculomotor nucleus (Edinger-Westphal)	Ciliary ganglion	Pupillary constriction, accommodation
Lacrimal gland	T_1–T_2	Superior cervical ganglion	?	Superior salivatory nucleus (7)	Pterygopalatine ganglion	Secretion
Submandibular and sublingual glands	T_1–T_2	Superior cervical ganglion	Vasoconstriction	Superior salivatory nucleus (7)	Submandibular ganglion	Secretion, vasodilatation
Parotid gland	T_1–T_2	Superior cervical ganglion	Vasoconstriction	Inferior salivatory nucleus (9)	Otic ganglion	Secretion, vasodilatation
Heart	T_1–T_{4-5}	Superior, middle, and inferior cervical + upper thoracic ganglia	Increased rate and stroke volume	Motor vagus nucleus (part of ambiguus nucleus) (10)	Cardiac plexus	Reduced heart rate
Bronchi, lungs	T_1–T_{3-4}	Inferior cervical + upper thoracic ganglia	Bronchial dilatation	Motor vagus nucleus (dorsal) (10)	Pulmonary plexus	Bronchial constriction and secretion
Stomach	T_6–T_{10} (greater splanchnic nerve)	Celiac ganglion	Inhibition of peristaltic movement and secretion; contraction of pyloric sphincter	Motor vagus nucleus (dorsal) (10)	Gastric plexus	Increased peristaltic movement and secretion, inhibition pyloric sphincter
Pancreas	T_6–T_{10} (greater splanchnic nerve)	Celiac ganglion	?	Motor vagus nucleus (dorsal) (10)	Periarterial plexus (?)	Secretion
Small intestine, ascending and transverse large intestine	T_6–T_{10}	Celiac ganglion + superior and inferior mesenteric ganglia	Inhibition of peristaltic movement and secretion	Motor vagus nucleus (dorsal) (10)	Myenteric and submucous plexus (ganglion)	Peristaltic movement and secretion
Descending large intestine, sigmoid, and rectum	T_{10}–L_2	Inferior mesenteric, hypogastric, and pelvic ganglia (plexuses)	Inhibition of peristaltic movement and secretion	Sacral cord S_3–S_4	Myenteric and submucous plexus (ganglion)	Peristaltic movement and secretion
Ureter, bladder	T_{10}–L_2	Hypogastric and pelvic ganglia (plexuses)	?	Sacral cord S_3–S_4	Pelvic plexus	Contraction of detrusor
Head and neck (skin and skeletal muscles)	T_1–T_{2-4}	Superior cervical ganglion	Vasoconstriction sweat secretion, and piloerection	—	—	—
Upper extremity	T_3–T_6	Stellate ganglion, upper thoracic	Vasoconstriction sweat secretion, and piloerection	—	—	—
Lower extremity	T_{10}–L_2	Lower lumbar and upper sacral ganglia	Vasoconstriction, sweat secretion, and piloerection	—	—	—

Figure 28.4

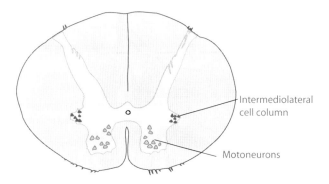

The intermediolateral cell column contains the cell bodies of the preganglionic sympathetic neurons. Cross section of the thoracic cord.

Figure 28.5

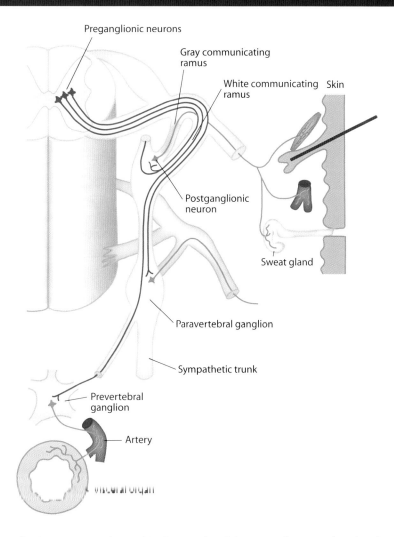

The sympathetic system. Postganglionic neurons are located in the ganglia of the sympathetic trunk and in the prevertebral ganglia. Sympathetic fibers to the trunk and the extremities follow the spinal nerves, whereas fibers to the visceral organs form separate nerves and follow the main vessels to the organs.

Figure 28.10

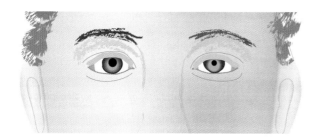

Horner's syndrome. The left half of the face shows the characteristic symptoms of loss of sympathetic innervation: red and dry skin, constricted pupil (miosis), and drooping of the upper eyelid (ptosis).

neurons—release **epinephrine** (and small amounts of norepinephrine) into the bloodstream on sympathetic stimulation.

The visceral organs of the **lower abdomen** and the **pelvis** receive their sympathetic innervation from the intermediolateral column in the lower thoracic and upper two lumbar segments (Table 28.2). These fibers also leave the sympathetic trunk as separate nerves (lumbar splanchnic nerves) to reach prevertebral ganglia. The postganglionic fibers follow the arteries to the organs (Fig. 28.6). The prevertebral ganglia are embedded in a meshwork of fibers, forming **prevertebral plexuses** (Fig. 28.3), with names corresponding to those of the ganglia (Fig. 28.7). The plexuses formed mainly by sympathetic fibers continue from the lower part of the abdominal aorta into the pelvis minor as the **hypogastric plexus**. In the pelvis, the hypogastric plexus mixes with parasympathetic fibers from the pelvic nerves and forms the **pelvic plexus** around the pelvic organs, as mentioned earlier.

PERIPHERAL PARTS OF THE PARASYMPATHETIC SYSTEM

As mentioned, the **preganglionic parasympathetic** (visceral efferent) neurons have their cell bodies in the brain stem and in the sacral cord (Fig. 28.2). The neurons look like the sympathetic preganglionic neurons of the intermediolateral column.

The Cranial Nerves Contain Preganglionic Parasympathetic Fibers

The preganglionic fibers of the **cranial part** of the parasympathetic system follow the **oculomotor**, the **facial** (intermediate), the **glossopharyngeal**, and the **vagus nerves**. The

fibers come from the visceral efferent column of cranial nerve nuclei (see Figs. 27.2 and 27.3). The preganglionic fibers of the cranial nerves supplying structures in the head end in several parasympathetic **ganglia**, located outside the skull close to large cranial nerve trunks (Fig. 28.11). These are the **ciliary**, the **pterygopalatine**, the **otic**, and the **submandibular ganglia**. From these ganglia, the postganglionic fibers pass to the effector organs (the intrinsic muscles of the eye, the lacrimal gland, and the salivary glands).

The preganglionic fibers of the **vagus nerve** do not end in well-defined ganglia but in more diffusely distributed collections of postganglionic neurons in the walls of (or just outside) the thoracic and abdominal organs. These postganglionic neurons have short axons running in the wall of the organ and innervate smooth-muscle cells and glands. As mentioned in Chapter 27, the vagus nerve sends parasympathetic fibers to the heart, the lungs, the gastrointestinal tract down to the descending colon, the gallbladder, the liver, and the pancreas (see Fig. 27.9). With postganglionic sympathetic fibers, the vagus nerve forms the **cardiac plexus**, which lies around the aortal arch and extends down onto the heart. The cardiac plexus also contains scattered groups of postganglionic parasympathetic cell bodies, with the largest group just underneath the aorta. The **sinus node** and the **atrioventricular** node receive the densest innervation of parasympathetic postganglionic (vagus) fibers, whereas the ventricles receive few such fibers (they receive a dense sympathetic postganglionic innervation, however). In the **airways,** the vagus participates in plexuses around the trachea and the bronchi—the **tracheobronchial plexus**—containing scattered postganglionic neurons.

The Sacral Part of the Parasympathetic System Supplies the Genitals, Bladder, and Rectum

The cell bodies of the preganglionic neurons in the sacral cord are located in the $(S_2) S_3$–S_4 segments, with a position corresponding to the intermediolateral column of the sympathetic system (Figs. 28.9, 28.11 and 28.12). The parasympathetic preganglionic fibers leave the cord through the ventral roots and follow the spinal nerves for a short distance. Then they leave the spinal nerves as separate, small **pelvic splanchnic nerves**. In contrast to the sympathetic preganglionic fibers, the parasympathetic ones do not pass to the sympathetic trunk but join postganglionic sympathetic fibers in the **pelvic plexus**, located immediately lateral to the rectum, the bladder, the prostate gland (in the male), and the cervix (in the

Figure 28.11

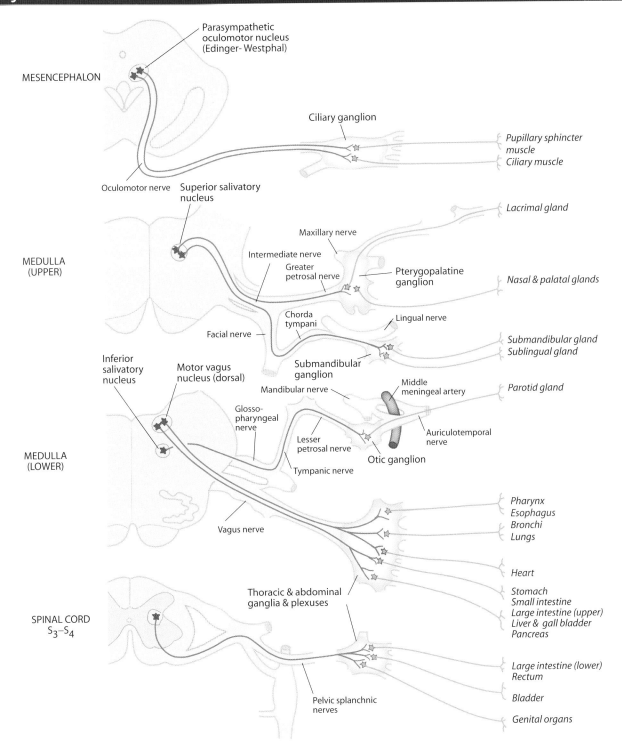

The parasympathetic system. The cell bodies of the preganglionic neurons are located in the brain stem and in the sacral cord. The peripheral course of the parasympathetic fibers is often quite complicated because they "jump" from one cranial nerve to another on their way to the target.

female). Many of the postganglionic parasympathetic neurons are located in the pelvic plexus (the **pelvic ganglion**).

Postganglionic parasympathetic fibers innervate all the **organs of the pelvis** and, in addition, the corpora cavernosa (erectile tissue) of the **penis** and the **clitoris**. The **descending** and **sigmoid colon** and the **rectum** are innervated from the sacral parasympathetic division. Of particular practical importance is the parasympathetic innervation of the rectum and the **bladder**, which is responsible for **emptying** these organs (Fig. 28.12). We treat the emptying reflex of the bladder in Chapter 29, under "Visceral Reflexes".

Figure 28.12

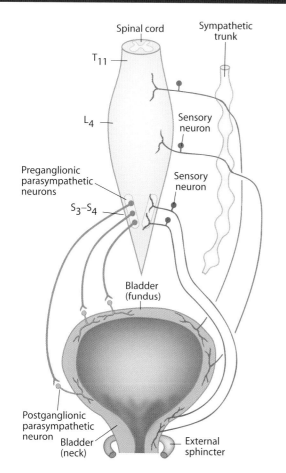

Spinal cord
Sympathetic trunk
T_{11}
L_4
Sensory neuron
Preganglionic parasympathetic neurons
Sensory neuron
S_3–S_4
Bladder (fundus)
Postganglionic parasympathetic neuron
Bladder (neck)
External sphincter

Innervation of the bladder. **Left:** The parasympathetic innervation of the smooth muscles that are responsible for emptying the bladder. The preganglionic neurons are located in the spinal segments S_3–S_4, whereas the postganglionic cell bodies are found just outside or in the wall of the bladder. **Right:** The course of the sensory fibers from the bladder. From the lower part, the sensory fibers follow the efferent parasympathetic fibers, whereas the sensory fibers from the upper part (the fundus) follow the sympathetic fibers (via the sympathetic trunk). The striated, external sphincter muscle is innervated by motoneurons in the sacral segments S_3–S_4 (not shown).

The "Mini-Brain of the Gut"

The digestive tract contains about 500 million neurons embedded in two plexuses in the wall. Largest is the **myenteric plexus**, which is located between the circular and the longitudinal external smooth-muscle layers; the smaller **submucous plexus** is situated below the mucous membrane. The plexuses are formed by the axons of the enteric neurons, together with postganglionic sympathetic fibers (with their cell bodies in the prevertebral ganglia). The neurons of the enteric system monitor the **tension** in the intestinal wall and the **chemical milieu** of the mucosa, and they control the **peristaltic movements** of the bowel, moving the content toward the anus. In addition, they influence blood flow, the secretion from mucosal glands, and the absorption of nutrients. **Immune cells** in the wall of the intestine are also influenced by local cholinergic neurons.

It was formerly believed that the enteric neurons were parasympathetic postganglionic. Only a minority contains acetylcholine, the classic transmitter of postganglionic parasympathetic neurons, however. It has become increasingly clear that these plexuses and ganglia represent a part of the peripheral nervous system that is, to a large extent, independent of the rest of the nervous system. Some even use the term "the mini-brain of the gut." Thus, the neurons in the myenteric and submucous ganglia are able to function even after the sympathetic and parasympathetic nerves to the gastrointestinal tract have been cut.

Broadly speaking, the enteric system integrates information about the local conditions with central commands through sympathetic and parasympathetic postganglionic fibers. However, the importance of central control differs among parts of the gastrointestinal tract. Thus, the CNS has essential roles in the control of the esophagus, the stomach and the sigmoid-rectum, whereas the enteric system operates largely independent of the CNS in the control of the small intestine and the colon.

Neuronal Types and Neurotransmitters

The enteric plexuses contain not only **motor neurons**—innervating smooth-muscle cells and glands—but also **interneurons** and **sensory neurons,** the latter having processes entering the mucosa. Numerous neurotransmitters—in particular, many **neuropeptides**—have been found in the enteric ganglion cells. With few exceptions, however, they are not yet functionally characterized. Different kinds of neurons contain different combinations of neuropeptides and classic transmitters (acetylcholine, GABA, and serotonin). **Excitatory neurons**, sending their axons upward (toward the mouth), ensure constriction of the bowel above a bolus of intestinal contents. Such neurons typically contain **acetylcholine** and **substance P. Inhibitory neurons** send their axons downward (toward the anus) and inhibit the circular muscle layer in front of a bolus, thus easing its propulsion. Such neurons may contain **ATP, vasoactive intestinal peptide (VIP)**, or nitric oxide (**NO**). Neurons acting on epithelial cells to increase the transport of **water** and **electrolytes** may contain either VIP or acetylcholine (with a variety of peptides, such as galanin, neuropeptide Y, cholecystokinin [CCK], or calcitonin gene–related peptid.

A special kind of neuron contains the **gastrin-releasing peptide (GRP)**. A group of such neurons are found in the wall of the stomach and send processes to the gastrin-producing cells in its distal part (the antrum). Stimulation of the vagus causes release of GRP, which then induces release of gastrin to the bloodstream. It affects acid-producing cells (parietal cells) in the upper part of the stomach.

Finally, some enteric neurons send their central process to prevertebral and pelvic ganglia. Thus, there are local **reflex arcs** not involving the CNS. The sensory neurons are activated primarily by gut distension and elicit reflex inhibition via the reflex arc.

FUNCTIONAL ASPECTS OF THE AUTONOMIC NERVOUS SYSTEM

Defense and Maintenance

When the autonomic system is considered as a whole, certain main functional features emerge (Table 28.1). The **parasympathetic system** controls primarily processes that are necessary for the maintenance of the organism over the long term. The parasympathetic system thus activates the digestive processes, ensures that waste products are expelled by contraction of the bladder and rectum, protects the eye against strong light, ensures focused vision, reduces the activity of the heart, reduces the diameter of the air ways, and increases bronchial secretion. The **sympathetic system** as a whole is more concerned with mobilizing the resources of the body when an extra effort is required. In situations of fear and anger, there are usually signs indicating increased sympathetic activity, such as increased blood pressure, increased heart rate, and dilatation of the pupils. At the same time, stored energy is mobilized by epinephrine secreted into the bloodstream from the adrenal medulla (increased blood level of glucose and fatty acids). Epinephrine also activates the heart and dilates the bronchi (relaxation of smooth-muscle cells). The activity of the gastrointestinal tract is inhibited. In general, such responses are adequate in flight-or-fight situations.

A More Nuanced View

The simple dichotomy presented in the preceding text disregards that, in addition, the sympathetic system takes part in daily maintenance and is active not just in stressful situations. For example, the sympathetic system is crucial for the temperature-regulating functions of the skin, and sympathetic activity is required every time we rise from the sitting position to avoid a fall in blood pressure and fainting. Further, the sympathetic system cooperates with the parasympathetic system in control of reproductive functions. Moreover, the sympathetic system is not activated in an **all-or-none** fashion: some parts may be active, while others are not. Thus, the sympathetic output to an organ may be regulated up and down independently of sympathetic outputs to other organs. Finally, both systems may send signals at the same time to an organ (the heart, e.g., receives both kinds of signals at the same time). The traditional scheme with reciprocal autonomic innervation—with autonomic "tone" determined by a point on a continuum from sympathetic to parasympathetic—is therefore not tenable.

Actions of Sympathetic Fibers on the Circulatory Organs

The postganglionic sympathetic fibers innervate vessels in all parts of the body. In general, the sympathetic innervation of the circulatory system ensures that the **cardiac output** can be increased, that the **blood pressure** can be maintained, and that the **blood flow** is directed to the organs needing it the most. Sympathetic effects on the **cerebral circulation** are discussed in Chapter 8, under "Regulation of Cerebral Circulation."

The sympathetic system increases the **heart rate** by acting on pacemaker cells in the sinus node. Further, the **stroke volume** increases. Cardiac muscle cells with a lower spontaneous firing frequency than the cells of the sinus node are the pupil by activating the **pupillary dilatator muscle** and by causing contraction of the radially oriented vessels of the iris (the latter effect is probably most important for pupillary dilation). A small smooth muscle attached to the upper eyelid, the **tarsal muscle**, is also innervated by sympathetic fibers. The tonic activity of this muscle helps to keep the eyelid up while we are awake (the paresis of the tarsal muscle is responsible for the slight drooping of the eyelid occurring in Horner's syndrome).

Orthostatic and Postprandial Hypotension

Some people have poor control of the blood-flow distribution in situations with change of body position from supine to standing (orthostatic hypotension). This is believed to be due to a failure of the sympathetic system. Such persons also often feel limp and uncomfortable after a meal because of a fall in the blood pressure (postprandial hypotension). Microneurographic studies suggest that this is caused by a lack of sympathetic activity. Normally after a meal, the sympathetic signal activity increases in nerves to the lower extremities, whereas in the patients with postprandial hypotension no such increase occurs. (To maintain the blood pressure, the blood flow to the lower part of the body must be reduced when that to the digestive tract increases.)

Function-Specific Sympathetic Control

The preceding discussion shows that various categories of sympathetic fibers can be controlled independently. There is not a uniform "sympathetic tone" for all parts of the sympathetic system. High activity in some parts must coexist with low activity in others if the sympathetic system is to fulfill its tasks in controlling blood pressure and body temperature, reproduction, and so forth. Accordingly, recent anatomic studies show that sympathetic neurons innervating different targets are more clearly segregated than formerly believed. For example, double labeling with retrograde tracers show that, in the intermediolateral column, neurons supplying the **superior cervical ganglion** and the **stellate ganglion** are largely segregated (although they are found mainly in the same spinal segments, with 90% in T_1–T_6). Thus, higher levels of the CNS (such as the hypothalamus) can selectively control subdivisions of the sympathetic system.

Microneurographic observations further support that selective control takes place. During rest, the firing frequency is uniform to different muscles. In this situation, a common signal (probably from the brain stem) commands all sympathetic neurons controlling muscle blood flow. As soon as a muscle starts working, however, the sympathetic signal frequency drops in the nerve to this muscle, while it remains unaltered to the resting muscles. In this situation, the sympathetic

system exerts a differential control of the muscles; that is, the signal frequencies depend on their individual needs.

The specificity of sympathetic control of muscle blood flow can presumably arise in two ways. One possibility is lowered **central drive** (from the brain stem) to the preganglionic neurons that control specific muscles. In turn, this may be due to sensory signals from **ergoreceptors** in the working muscle or because the **motor cortex** informs higher levels of the autonomic system about which muscles are being selected for a motor task (efference copy). The other possibility is that a purely **spinal reflex** inhibits the preganglionic neurons that control blood flow to the working muscles.

The Effects of Parasympathetic Fibers

As mentioned, the sympathetic and the parasympathetic systems have mostly antagonistic effects on the organs innervated by both (Tables 28.1 and 28.2). Because the postganglionic fibers usually contain neuropeptides in addition to acetylcholine, however, their actions may be more complex than either stimulation or inhibition of the organ.

The parasympathetic postganglionic fibers produce **glandular secretion** (e.g., from the lacrimal gland, salivary glands, and glands of the respiratory and gastrointestinal tracts). Parasympathetic fibers are furthermore responsible for increased strength and frequency of **peristaltic contractions** in the gastrointestinal tract and the bladder. The parasympathetic innervation is particularly important for the emptying of the **bladder** (Fig. 28.12) and the **rectum** (control of micturition is treated in Chapter 29 in connection with visceral reflexes).

As mentioned, the **heart** receives parasympathetic preganglionic fibers through the vagus nerve. The **sinus node** and the **atrioventricular node** receive particularly dense innervation of postganglionic (cholinergic) fibers. Lowering of the heart rate—by affecting the sinus node—is the most marked effect of vagus stimulation. In addition, the vagus exerts more complex effects on the ventricles. Most likely, this happens by **presynaptic inhibition** of sympathetic postganglionic fibers, thus reducing the contractile force of the heart muscle. Some effects of vagus stimulation are not mediated by acetylcholine but, most likely, by neuropeptides such as **somatostatin** and **VIP**. In the resting situation the heart receives parasympathetic signals with a low frequency (higher in endurance-trained than in untrained persons). During work, the influence of the vagus diminishes with the need for increased cardiac output. In some situations, however (e.g., when in **pain** and during **diving**), coactivation of sympathetic and parasympathetic nerves to the heart can occur. This may probably ensure more efficient cardiac function, for example by allowing longer filling time for the ventricles. The effect of the vagus on the **coronary arteries** in humans is believed to be constrictive. In the **airways,** the vagus produces bronchial constriction and secretion.

Most of the **vessels** of the body do not receive parasympathetic innervation. Exceptions are vessels of glands and of the external **genitals**, in which parasympathetic signals cause vasodilation (i.e., they inhibit the smooth-muscle cells). Increased activity of the parasympathetic fibers to the penis (and the clitoris) produces **erection** (see Chapter 29, under "The Erection and Ejaculation Reflexes").

In the **eye,** parasympathetic fibers of the oculomotor nerve reduce the diameter of the pupil and produce accommodation of the lens (see Chapter 27, under "The Light Reflex and the Accommodation Reflex").

Emotions and the Autonomic Nervous System

The autonomic system is not independent of higher mental processes, even though its processes are not under conscious control or are, as a rule, not consciously perceived. The activity of sympathetic fibers to the skin, for example, is strongly influenced by emotions, as witnessed by **blushing** when embarrassed and **paleness** when frightened. Further, the effect of emotions on the circulatory system may manifest itself as palpitations, hypertension, or bradycardia and peripheral vasodilatation, leading to a fall in blood pressure and perhaps **fainting**. In fainting, there are marked changes of both sympathetic and parasympathetic activity. The control of the **gastrointestinal tract** may be altered by emotions—for example, with increased peristaltic movements and secretions leading to diarrhea. Also, **bladder emptying** is under emotional influence, as witnessed by the frequent urge to void when nervous—for example, before an exam or an athletic contest. In case of very **strong fear**, involuntary emptying of the bladder and rectum may occur. Emotional influence on **erection** is another example: sensory stimuli and simple reflexes alone do not determine the parasympathetic actions on the vessels in the penis and the clitoris.

Pathways and **nuclei** mediating the effects of emotions on preganglionic autonomic neurons (and thus on visceral organs) involve parts of the cerebral cortex, the hypothalamus, the amygdala, the periaqueductal gray (PAG), and the reticular formation. For example, electrical stimulation of the amygdala can produce emptying of the bladder and rectum in experimental animals. Probably the pathway is via the PAG (also see Chapter 31, under "Amygdala and Conditioned Fear" and "Some Aspects of Cortical Control of Autonomic Functions and Emotions").

NEUROTRANSMITTERS IN THE AUTONOMIC NERVOUS SYSTEM

Preganglionic Neurons

The signal transmission between neurons of the autonomic system is mediated by neurotransmitters, as elsewhere in the nervous system. The preganglionic fibers end with typical synapses on the dendrites of the postganglionic neurons. As mentioned, all (or the vast majority of) **preganglionic** neurons use **acetylcholine**; that is, they are cholinergic. The released acetylcholine binds to **nicotinic receptors** in the membrane of the postganglionic neurons in the autonomic ganglia.

Many (perhaps all) preganglionic neurons also contain **neuropeptides** (enkephalin, somatostatin, neurotensin, and others), as demonstrated with immunocytochemical techniques. The various neuropeptides appear to be expressed differentially in subgroups of autonomic ganglion cells. The functional significance of these neuropeptides, which coexist with acetylcholine in preganglionic neurons, is so far not clear, but the two substances are most likely released together.

Postganglionic Neurons

Most **postganglionic parasympathetic** neurons release **acetylcholine**. In the peripheral organs, acetylcholine binds to **muscarinic receptors** in the membrane of cardiac, smooth-muscle, and glandular cells.

Most **postganglionic sympathetic** neurons release **norepinephrine** and are **noradrenergic** (norepinephric). The effects on the effector cells are mediated by two kinds of receptors, the α- and β-**adrenergic receptors**, which are distributed differently and have different effects on the postsynaptic cells. In the heart, norepinephrine produces increased heart rate by its binding to β **receptors**. By binding to α **receptors**, norepinephrine produces contraction of smooth-muscle cells in most blood vessels, in the ductus deferens, and in the pupillary dilatator muscle of the eye. Binding to β-receptors elicits relaxation of smooth-muscle cells in the wall of the bladder, the uterus, and the airways.

Epinephrine, which is released from the **chromaffin cells** of the **adrenal medulla** by sympathetic stimulation, has largely the same effects as norepinephrine. Thus, epinephrine binds to α- and β-adrenergic receptors of the heart, vessels, and the respiratory tract. In addition, epinephrine stimulates the release of free fatty acids from **adipose tissue** and the breakdown of **glycogen** to glucose. These **metabolic effects** are mediated by β receptors in fat and liver cells.

Subgroups of Adrenergic Receptors

Each of the two main kinds—α- and β-adrenergic receptors—has several subtypes with different distributions and actions. When norepinephrine binds to the α_1 **receptor**, it produces opening of Ca^{2+} **channels**, which leads to depolarization and, in turn, elicits contraction or secretion. The action of the α_1 receptor is not directly on the Ca^{2+} channel but indirectly via intracellular second messengers (diacylglycerol and activation of proteinkinase C). The α_2 **receptor** is mostly localized presynaptically and modulates the transmitter release. The β_1 **receptor** is mostly localized postsynaptically in the heart, on adipose cells, and in the CNS. It acts through cyclic AMP as a second messenger. The β_2 **receptor** has a different distribution than the β_1 receptor and is primarily found in smooth-muscle cells of the **respiratory tract**. Binding of epinephrine (or drugs with similar action) to β_2 receptors relaxes the smooth-muscle cells, notably in the walls of the bronchi. This relaxation produces dilatation of the bronchi and reduces airway resistance.

Noncholinergic and Nonadrenergic Transmission in the Autonomic System

In addition to the classical neurotransmitters acetylcholine and norepinephrine, several other neuroactive substances have been demonstrated in the autonomic nervous system. As mentioned, many preganglionic and postganglionic neurons contain neuropeptides, as well as acetylcholine or norepinephrine. Further, some autonomic neurons—notably in the enteric system—contain neither acetylcholine nor norepinephrine. Such **noncholinergic** and **nonadrenergic** autonomic fibers are also found in the respiratory tract, the gastrointestinal tract, the bladder, and the external genitals. Some of them release **ATP** or **NO** as a neurotransmitter; others contain neuropeptides such as **somatostatin**, **substance P, VIP,** and **CCK.**

The **coexistence** of norepinephrine and other transmitters was first suggested by the observation that blocking the receptors for norepinephrine did not prevent all effects of sympathetic nerve stimulation. In the **ductus deferens**, which receives a very dense sympathetic innervation, stimulation of the nerves produces, first, a fast contraction caused by release of ATP and, subsequently, a slow contraction produced by norepinephrine. In the **salivary glands**, the parasympathetic postganglionic fibers release both acetylcholine and VIP. The acetylcholine produces secretion from the glandular cells, whereas the VIP produces vasodilatation. Another example concerns the arteries of the **penis** and the **clitoris**, which dilate to cause erection. This vasodilatation is caused by parasympathetic postganglionic fibers that release NO (but not acetylcholine).

Some parasympathetic postganglionic fibers in the **heart** release somatostatin and probably VIP. In the **stomach**, vagus stimulation can produce release of VIP in addition to acetylcholine. Stimulation of nerves to the human **airways** can produce bronchial dilatation, although not by release

of norepinephrine or acetylcholine. The effect appears to be mediated by release of **VIP** from postganglionic nerve varicosities.

Presynaptic Receptors Modulate the Transmitter Release from Postganglionic Nerve Terminals

Neurotransmitters released from the postganglionic neurons bind not only to postsynaptic receptors in the membrane of smooth-muscle and glandular cells but also to presynaptic receptors in the membrane of the varicosities along the fibers (see Fig. 5.3). Thus, for example, norepinephrine that is released from sympathetic fibers can bind presynaptically and inhibit further release of norepinephrine or bind to parasympathetic cholinergic terminals in the vicinity. In the **heart**, sympathetic fibers inhibit the release of acetylcholine in this manner, but, as mentioned, also the opposite interaction can occur (presynaptic inhibition of norepinephrine release by acetylcholine). The sympathetic inhibiting effect on the peristaltic contractions of the gastrointestinal tract is mediated, at least partly, by binding of norepinephrine to α receptors on the parasympathetic, cholinergic terminals: that is, the release of acetylcholine is inhibited.

Sensitization

When the postganglionic autonomic fibers to an organ are interrupted, the sensitivity of the organ to the transmitter (which is no longer released) is increased. Epinephrine and norepinephrine in the bloodstream, for example, have a more powerful action after an organ has lost its sympathetic innervation, and the same holds for adrenergic drugs. This phenomenon, called **sensitization**, is not restricted to the autonomic system, however. It occurs, presumably, after denervation of any neuron. For example, skeletal muscle cells have increased sensitivity to acetylcholine after having lost their nerve supply. The underlying mechanism is probably increased postsynaptic density of receptors, as though the neuron attempts to maintain normal synaptic activity.

Drugs with Actions on the Autonomic Nervous System

Several drugs influence the synaptic transmission in the autonomic nervous system. **Atropine** blocks the action of acetylcholine (released from postganglionic parasympathetic fibers) on **muscarinic** receptors. Other drugs have similar **anticholinergic** effects, often as a side effect. This is the case for several psycho-pharmaceuticals. The peripheral actions of the parasympathetic system are inhibited, causing symptoms such as dilated pupils (mydriasis) and reduced accommodation of the lens (causing difficulties in seeing close objects clearly). The heart rate increases, and the secretory activity is reduced in several glands. The reduced salivary secretion causes dryness of the mouth, a very bothersome side effect of anticholinergic drugs. Atropine, for example, is used to reduce secretion of glands in the respiratory tract during surgical anesthesia. The peristaltic contractions of the bowel are reduced, causing constipation. The bladder contractility is reduced, with danger of incomplete emptying (especially in cases of prostatic enlargement causing increased urethral resistance the danger of urinary retention should be kept in mind). Because the sweat glands receive a cholinergic innervation, their secretion may also be reduced (most antiperspirants contain substances with an anticholinergic action).

Pilocarpine is an example of a drug with a **parasympathico-mimetic** action—that is, it is a cholinergic drug. Administration of pilocarpine causes increased salivation and tear flow, reduced heart rate, and increased secretion from, and peristaltic movements of, the gastrointestinal tract. The pupil is small (miotic), causing reduced vision in dim light.

Many drugs activate adrenergic receptors—that is, they have **sympathicomimetic** effects. Some act on both α and β receptors; others act preferentially on one or the other receptor type (or on subtypes). **Isoprenaline** (isoproterenol) acts selectively on β receptors and produces increased heart rate and bronchial dilatation. **Metaraminol** acts preferentially on α receptors and

causes peripheral vasoconstriction and, thereby, increased blood pressure.

Drugs that **block α receptors** (such as **phentolamine**) produce peripheral vasodilatation and a fall in blood pressure, whereas drugs that **block β receptors** mainly cause reduced heart rate and stroke volume, as well as bronchial constriction. The development of more selective β blockers, acting selectively on β_1 receptors present in the heart, has made it possible to treat hypertension without unwanted bronchial constriction (β_2 receptors are found primarily in the lungs). In contrast, the development of adrenergic drugs acting selectively on β_2 receptors (and not on β_1 receptors) has made it possible to treat patients with bronchial obstruction (as asthmatics) without such side effects as increased cardiac activity and hypertension.

Drugs can also influence the signal transmission in the **autonomic ganglia**. As mentioned, acetylcholine is the main transmitter in both sympathetic and parasympathetic ganglia. The nicotinic receptors in the ganglia are nevertheless somewhat different from those present at the neuromuscular junction. This makes it possible to influence one of these targets without affecting the other.

All neurotransmitters present in the peripheral parts of the autonomic system are also found in the CNS, together with adrenergic and cholinergic receptors. Therefore, drugs designed to act on peripheral parts of the autonomic nervous system may produce side effects through actions in the **CNS**—that is, in case they pass the blood–brain barrier. **Beta (β) blockers,** for example, which are used extensively to treat hypertension, can give central side effects, such as dizziness, disturbed sleep, and depression.

Sensory Visceral Neurons and Visceral Reflexes

Afferent fibers conveying sensory information from the viscera to the central nervous system (CNS) go together with the visceral efferent (sympathetic and parasympathetic) fibers. Sensory fibers follow the sympathetic **splanchnic nerves**, leaving the sympathetic trunk at various levels, the **parasympathetic cranial nerves** (the oculomotor, the intermediate, the glossopharyngeal, and the vagus nerves), and, finally, the parasympathetic **pelvic nerves** leaving the sacral spinal nerves to innervate pelvic organs. As a general rule, fibers conducting signals from **visceral nociceptors** follow sympathetic nerves, whereas the parasympathetic nerves contain fibers conducting from other kinds of receptors.

The visceral afferent neurons are structurally indistinguishable from the somatic afferent ones—that is, they have their pseudounipolar cell bodies in ganglia of the spinal and cranial nerves. The peripheral process follows the sympathetic or parasympathetic nerves to the organs, whereas the central process enters the dorsal horn or the brain stem sensory nuclei (the solitary nucleus). The vast majority of the visceral afferent fibers are thin **Aδ** and **C fibers**.

The normal function of the sensory innervation of the internal organs is primarily related to **homeostasis** and mediation of **visceral reflexes**, such as coughing, vomiting, swallowing, circulatory and respiratory reflexes, emptying of the rectum and bladder, and so forth. These reflexes have their **reflex centers** in the spinal cord or in the reticular formation. The control of **micturition** is discussed, including not only the spinal reflex mechanisms involved but also the necessary contributions from the **pontine micturition center** and the cerebral cortex. With regard to homeostasis, "**silent nociceptors**" may be of special relevance by mediating information about the local milieu of the internal organs. Visceral afferents also mediate information from the **immune system** to the brain, evoking fever and other aspects of **sickness behavior** during infections and other inflammatory diseases. With some exceptions, such as taste and fairly diffuse sensations

of hunger, fullness, and so forth, the sensory signals from the viscera are not consciously perceived. Under abnormal conditions sensory signals from the viscera can produce the sensations of intense pain and feeling of sickness. We discuss the special features of **visceral pain** and the phenomenon of **referred pain** in particular.

VISCERAL RECEPTORS AND AFFERENT PATHWAYS

Visceral Receptors

Morphologically, most of the visceral receptors are free nerve endings (see Fig. 13.1).[1] They respond to various kinds of stimuli, even though they are structurally identical. A large group consists of **mechanoreceptors** recording the tension of the tissue in which they are located. Such receptors are found, for example, in the heart, the lungs, and the walls of hollow abdominal organs. They provide information about the degree of filling of hollow organs and can elicit reflex contractions aimed at emptying the organ or moving the content. Some stretch receptors may give rise to sensations of pain by responding to strong **dilatation** of a hollow organ and to forceful **contractions** of the smooth musculature, but most visceral **nociceptors** are believed to be **chemoreceptors** sensitive to substances in the tissue produced by **inflammation** or **ischemia**.

Other chemoreceptors, strategically placed in the vascular system (at the aortic arch and at the bifurcation of the common carotid artery), react to the **carbon dioxide** and **oxygen** concentration in the blood.

Typically, visceral receptors have large **receptive fields**, with a low density of nerve endings. These features fit with

---

1. There are some encapsulated nerve endings in the visceral organs. Thus, **Pacinian corpuscles** are present in the pancreas, the mesenteries, and the vessel walls. Their functional role at these sites is unknown.

the observations that visceral receptors exhibit marked **spatial summation**—that is, the threshold for eliciting action potentials becomes lower as the area of stimulation increases. This may explain why strong but spatially very restricted stimuli (such as knife cuts) usually do not evoke pain from visceral organs.

Peripheral Routes for Nociceptive Signals

As mentioned, most visceral afferents leading from nociceptors follow the sympathetic nerves (Fig. 29.1). Exceptions to this rule are nociceptors in the neck of the **bladder**, the **prostate**, the **cervix uteri**, and the **rectum**. "Pain fibers" from these organs follow the **parasympathetic pelvic nerves**

Figure 29.1

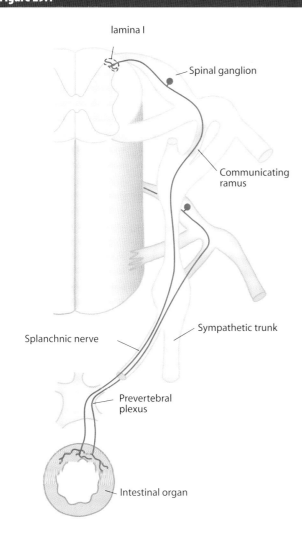

lamina I

Spinal ganglion

Communicating ramus

Sympathetic trunk

Splanchnic nerve

Prevertebral plexus

Intestinal organ

Sensory fibers follow sympathetic nerves to the visceral organs. The fibers pass through the prevertebral plexuses and ganglia before they enter the spinal nerves via the communicating rami.

to the sacral spinal nerves (see Fig. 28.12). Signals from nociceptors in the fundus of the uterus and of the bladder, however, follow the sympathetic nerves of the hypogastric plexus, ending in segments T_{11}–L_2.

Fibers carrying nociceptive signals from the **arteries** in the extremities and the body wall follow the spinal nerves, together with the sympathetic efferent fibers.

Nociceptive Pathways from the Heart

Although nociceptive signals from the **heart** were assumed to follow exclusively the sympathetic nerves, some observations indicate that this may hold only for signals from the anterior wall of the heart, while signals from the posterior wall and the lower surface may be conducted in the vagus nerve. Observations after surgical interventions to relieve pains of **angina** were taken as evidence that all nociceptive fibers from the heart follow the sympathetic nerves. These are the middle and lower **cardiac nerves** arising from the cervical sympathetic trunk and some smaller twigs leaving the sympathetic trunk below the stellate ganglion (4–5 upper thoracic ganglia). Although most patients reported complete relief of angina pains after cutting of the dorsal roots in the upper thoracic and lower cervical segments (or removing the corresponding ganglia), some patients were not helped. However, some patients reported pain relief after cutting of the vagus nerve, and electric stimulation of the vagus nerve has been reported to evoke burning pain deep in the chest. Perhaps these findings may be explained if the nociceptive signals follow different nerves from the anterior and posterior cardiac walls. Indeed, animal experiments indicate that sympathectomy does not relieve pain arising in the posterior cardiac wall.

Central Pathways for Visceral Afferent Signals

The sensory signals from the visceral organs pass through the dorsal roots and end primarily in the dorsalmost parts of the dorsal horn—that is, **lamina I** (Fig. 29.1; also see Fig. 13.16). Notably, the visceral afferents avoid the substantia gelatinosa (lamina II, which receives numerous C fibers from somatic structures). The sensory fibers following the cranial nerves end in the **solitary nucleus** in the medulla (see Fig. 27.2). From these receiving cell groups in the spinal cord and in the brain stem, the signals are transmitted to motor nuclei—especially those consisting of **preganglionic autonomic neurons**—in the reticular formation, and to the **hypothalamus** and the **thalamus**. For the most part, the visceral afferent signals that arrive through the dorsal roots are transmitted centrally through the **spinothalamic** and **spinoreticular tracts** (see Figs. 14.4 and 26.11). Details are not known, however, with regard to the central transmission of visceral afferent signals.

The Dorsal Columns Carry Signals from Visceral Nociceptors

Surprisingly, in addition to constituting a major pathway for signals from somatic low-threshold mechanoreceptors, the dorsal columns have also been shown to carry sensory signals from visceral organs. This concerns **postsynaptic** dorsal column sensory units, many of which are activated by noxious stimuli (see Chapter 14, under "The Dorsal Columns Contain More Than Primary Afferent Fibers"). In the **gracile nucleus**, some neurons receive converging inputs from cutaneous low-threshold mechanoreceptors and high-threshold receptors in the **pelvic viscera**. Corresponding convergence occurs in the next link, in the ventral posterolateral nucleus of the thalamus. Signals from cutaneous low-threshold mechanoreceptors on the arms and chest and from nociceptors in the **heart** converge on neurons in the **cuneate nucleus** and the thalamus. Thus, the dorsal column—medial lemniscus pathway can obviously contribute to signaling from visceral nociceptors, although this is not usually apparent from studies of its functions or the effects of lesions. Nevertheless, there is evidence that signals in the dorsal columns can contribute to the experience of pain in humans. For example, a patient with intense pain due to cancer of the large bowel was made pain-free by bilateral sectioning of the gracile fascicles at the T_{10} level (the effect lasted until his death 3 months later). Animal experiments confirm that nociceptive signals from the lower abdomen and the pelvis cease to activate the cerebral cortex after transection of the gracile fascicle. Finally, the convergence mediated by the dorsal columns may also contribute to **referred pain** (discussed later).

VISCERAL REFLEXES

Many of the visceral reflexes elicited by signals from visceral receptors and receptors in the walls of vessels have their **reflex centers** in the spinal cord. The more complex reflexes, however, requiring coordination of activity in several parts of the body, have reflex centers in the brain stem or in the hypothalamus. We return to this in Chapter 30. **Vasomotor reflexes** were discussed in Chapter 28. Other important visceral reflexes are produced by stimulation of receptors in the **lungs** and the **airways**, such as coughing and respiratory adjustments (see later discussion). The **vomiting reflex** can be elicited by irritation of the mucosa of the stomach but also in various other ways (see Chapter 27, under "The Vomiting Reflex"). The **emptying reflexes** of the rectum and the bladder are elicited by stimulation of stretch receptors in their walls and have reflex centers partly in spinal segments (S_2) S_3–S_4 and partly in the brain stem. These visceral reflexes are unusual because they can be suppressed voluntarily. The emptying reflex of the bladder is discussed further later.

Reflexes Elicited from Receptors of the Lungs

Signals from **stretch receptors** in the bronchial walls contribute to inhibition of inspiratory movements when the lungs have been inflated to a certain extent (the Hering-Breuer reflex). Receptors producing **coughing** are probably free endings between the epithelial cells of the airways, in part located very close to the epithelial surface (irritation receptors). Such free nerve endings contain **substance P** (as do many other sensory neurons), which is released by exposure to irritant gases.

A special kind of receptor—the **juxtapulmonary (J) receptor**—is located close to the lung alveoli. It responds to increased pulmonary capillary pressure. Increased pressure in the left atrium (which receives the blood from the lungs) immediately leads to increased pulmonary capillary pressure, with the danger of developing **lung edema**. Thus, it seems reasonable that the capillary pressure must be monitored closely. Stimulation of the J receptors produces rapid and shallow breathing but may probably also cause bronchial constriction (this is known to occur in patients with heart failure and increased pulmonary capillary pressure).

It is furthermore believed that signals from the J receptors can reach consciousness and cause a feeling of shortness of breath, or **dyspnea**. J receptors are also believed to elicit the dry cough typical of lung edema, as occurring in patients with congestive **heart failure** or persons suffering from **altitude sickness**.

The Emptying Reflex of the Bladder

As mentioned, the bladder-emptying reflex is evoked by stimulation of **stretch receptors** in the wall of the bladder, which record filling. The signals are conducted in myelinated afferent fibers to the lumbosacral cord (Fig. 29.2; see Fig. 28.12). Many sensory units that lead from the bladder are slowly adapting with dynamic sensitivity; that is, they respond more upon rapid than upon slow distension of the bladder. No signals are sent when the bladder is empty, but when urine starts to accumulate the sensory units start firing. Normal adult **bladder capacity** is about 500 mL. The pressure in the human bladder during filling is typically between 5 and 15 mm Hg, whereas emptying is normally elicited at 25 to 30 mm Hg. At night (during **sleep**), the bladder fills to about the double of the daytime volume before evoking an urge to void. This is a prerequisite for 8 hours

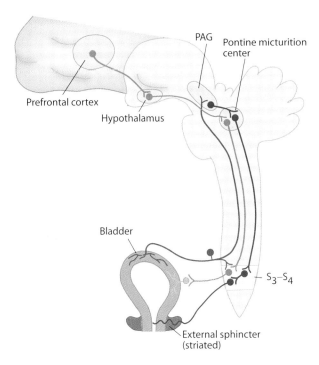

Figure 29.2

Pathways and nuclei involved in control of micturition. The reflex center for the emptying reflex is located in the sacral cord but is controlled by descending connections from the pontine micturition center. This is under control of higher centers, like the PAG, the hypothalamus, and the cerebral cortex.

uninterrupted sleep.[2] Urine does not leak out in the filling phase because the **intraurethral pressure** is kept higher than the **intravesical** pressure. The intraurethral pressure is maintained by several factors, among them smooth muscles and elastic tissue in the urethral wall.

In the filling phase, the smooth muscle of the bladder wall—the **detrusor muscle**—is relaxed, while the striated external sphincter in the pelvic floor is tonically active. When the intravesical pressure reaches the critical level, brisk activity of parasympathetic neurons makes the detrusor muscle contract. In addition, the striated sphincter muscle and other muscles in the pelvic floor must relax. Normal emptying of the bladder thus requires **coordinated control** of parasympathetic preganglionic neurons in the S_3–S_4 segments and of α motoneurons in the S_1–S_3 segments.

2. One or more of the centers of the micturition reflex must therefore be inhibited during sleep. This inhibition develops between the ages of 3 and 5. In children with **enuresis** (bedwetting), this inhibition seems to be lacking, as about the same bladder-filling volume elicits emptying during the night as during the daytime.

The **parasympathetic** control of the detrusor muscle is mediated by **acetylcholine**. In addition, **vasoactive intestinal peptide (VIP)** released from parasympathetic fibers might contribute to inhibition of the smooth muscles surrounding the urethra.

The Role of the Sympathetic System in Bladder Control Is Not Clear

The innervation with norepinephric nerve fibers is generally sparse in the human bladder and urethra, with the exception of the male bladder neck (see "The Erection and Ejaculation Reflexes" below). This is different from the situation in cats and dogs (used for much of the research on bladder control), in which the bladder wall receives a dense norepinephric (noradrenergic) innervation. Further, the few norepinephric fibers in humans seem to be related to blood vessels, based on study of serial sections and the histofluorescence method. Thus, conclusions based on animal experiments—namely that in the filling phase the sympathetic system inhibits the detrusor (via β receptors) and stimulates smooth muscles in the upper part of the urethra (via $α_1$ receptors)—are probably not applicable in humans. Other data also support a minor role of sympathetic innervation in human bladder control. For example, sympathectomy does not alter the filling capacity significantly, and sympathetic stimulation does not seem to inhibit the detrusor in the filling phase.

The dense norepinephric innervation of the male bladder neck seems to play a role mainly during **ejaculation**; the contraction preventing back-flow of semen to the bladder, functioning as a **genital sphincter**. Indeed, drugs acting on $α_1$ adrenergic receptors affect bladder emptying: agonists may worsen urinary retention in patients with an enlarged prostatic gland and, conversely, selective α antagonists are used to improve bladder outflow in such patients.

In the total picture we must also take into account that many norepinephric fibers end in the pelvic plexus and associated small parasympathetic ganglia. Thus, sympathetic influence on bladder control might occur indirectly by acting on postganglionic parasympathetic neurons. Furthermore, α-adrenergic receptors are present at many levels of the reflex pathway—centrally in the cord and at higher levels, in the autonomic ganglia, and in the smooth-muscle cell membrane; further, they are located both pre- and postsynaptically and are activated by both norepinephrine released from postganglionic sympathetic fibers and by circulating epinephrine. Thus, deciding the site of action of a certain adrenergic drug is not straightforward.

Central Control of Micturition

Normal emptying of the bladder requires more than intact spinal reflex arches. This is evident in patients with **transection of the cord** above the sacral level. If the lesion is complete, all descending connections acting on the sacral reflex centers are interrupted. These patients experience great difficulties with emptying the bladder because, among other problems, the activities of the detrusor muscle and the internal sphincter are not coordinated. This is called **dyssynergia**. (In addition, the bladder often becomes hyperactive—i.e., the emptying reflex is elicited at a lower pressure than before.) Patients with lesions of the brain stem above the pons do not have dyssynergia. Further observations show that the **dorsolateral pons** (near the locus coeruleus) contains a neuronal network that coordinate the spinal reflexes involved in micturition—the **pontine micturition center** (Fig. 29.2). Ascending spinoreticular fibers, which inform about the filling pressure, join the spinothalamic tract ventrolaterally in the cord. The fibers end in the **periaqueductal gray (PAG)**, which is assumed to send signals to the micturition center. The marked **emotional** influence on micturition, such as frequent urination in association with nervousness and fear, is probably mediated by connections from the **amygdala** to the PAG (see Fig. 31.6).

More about Disturbed Bladder Control after CNS Lesions

Animal experiments indicate that the descending (reticulospinal) fibers from the pontine micturition center lie dispersed in the lateral funiculus, with the majority in its dorsal part. Clinical observations, however, indicate that in humans the fibers might lie more ventrally, close to the pyramidal tract in the lateral funicle. Thus, damage of the **pyramidal tract** in the spinal cord is often associated with **urge incontinence** (inability to inhibit the emptying reflex) as a sign of impaired central bladder control.

Although lesions above the pons do not disturb the normal emptying of the bladder, patients with such lesions may have problems with controlling of the initiation of micturition (inhibition in particular). The cell groups responsible for the voluntary control of micturition are not known in detail, although medial parts of the **frontal lobe** and the **hypothalamus** appear to be involved (Fig. 29.2). Among other evidence, clinical observations show that damage to the frontal lobes may cause **urge incontinence**.

Cortical Activity and Bladder Control

Positron emission tomography (PET) and functional magnetic resonance imaging studies indicate that neurons in the **dorsolateral pons** and the **prefrontal cortex** increase their activity during **micturition**. The activity is largest on the right side in both men and women. In persons trying to void without succeeding, the activity increases in the frontal lobe but not in the dorsolateral pons. There is sign of increased activity, however, in a slightly more ventral pontine region; in animals, this region controls the pelvic muscles (presumably including the external urethral sphincter) by descending reticulospinal fibers. When trying to **inhibit voiding** when the bladder is full, activity increases in the anterior **cingulate gyrus** and the **insula**. This fits with data showing that the insula receives visceral sensory inputs. Both the insula and the anterior cingulate gyrus are furthermore known to influence the autonomic system. In addition, the anterior cingulate gyrus is active during focused attention and when selecting appropriate behavior. The insula may be responsible for sending descending commands—eventually inhibiting the detrusor—when micturition should be postponed.

The Erection and Ejaculation Reflexes

As mentioned, erection depends on parasympathetic signals to the vessels of the penis or the clitoris, whereas ejaculation is due mainly to sympathetic signals to the smooth muscles of the ductus deferens and the prostate. The preganglionic neurons of these functions have their cell bodies in the lumbosacral cord (see Figs. 28.7 and 28.11). In addition, successful expulsion of the semen requires coordination of smooth muscles closing the upper urethra (the genital sphincter, see "The Role of the Sympathetic System in Bladder Control Is Not Clear" earlier in this chapter) and striated **muscles of the pelvic floor**—that is, sphincter muscles and muscles around the penile cavernous bodies, especially the **bulbospongiosus** (bulbocavernosus) **muscle**. The α motoneurons of the latter muscles are found in the sacral cord. In male rats, these groups of motoneurons are three times larger than in female rats. This **sexual dimorphism** arises early in the prenatal development and depends on the presence of minute amounts of androgens.

Evidently, erection and ejaculation require precise temporal coordination of several muscles. The coordination is carried out in the spinal cord by a complex **premotor network**. For example, the activity of sympathetic preganglionic neurons in the lower thoracic–upper lumbar cord must be coordinated with the activity of parasympathetic preganglionic neurons and α motoneurons in the sacral cord. Cell groups in the **reticular formation** of the **pons**, close to those controlling micturition, and in the **hypothalamus** control the spinal reflex centers for erection and ejaculation. They are not necessary for erection and ejaculation, however. Thus, provided the lesion is above the midthoracic level, both erection and expulsion of the semen can occur after transection of the cord. In such patients, erection is evoked by sensory stimuli from the penis (the patient has no conscious sensations, however, because the ascending sensory tracts are interrupted).

The spinal reflex centers of erection and ejaculation are **inhibited** from an area in the ventral part of the upper medulla by way of descending connections that act on parasympathetic and sympathetic preganglionic neurons and α motoneurons. The lack of such inhibitory connections may explain why some patients with transection of the cord above the sacral level suffer from **priapism**—that is, a hyperactive erection reflex.

The hypothalamic cell groups are influenced, among other areas, by the **cerebral cortex** and the **amygdala**. Normally, of course, descending connections from these higher levels are involved in the induction of erection, more or less independently of the sensory signals that act through the spinal reflex arc.

VISCERAL PAIN

Salient Features

Visceral pain differs in many respects from pain originating in somatic structures; it is usually more diffuse, less precisely graded, and of a different quality than pain arising in the skin. Also, whether or not a visceral disease evokes pain seems less predictable than when somatic structures are affected. For example, myocardial ischemia, while usually causing the typical pain of **angina pectoris**, may sometimes be painless, or just accompanied by vague feelings of fatigue and illness. Even acute myocardial infarction is painless in about 30% of cases.[3]

Visceral disease processes, such as **appendicitis**, initially cause a vague discomfort, with nausea rather than pain. Also, a feeling of fainting may occur, probably due to lowered blood pressure. The initial discomfort or pain is typically felt deep in the midline in the thorax or the abdomen, regardless of the organ involved. This first phase usually lasts for minutes to some hours. Thereafter, the pain moves to sites more specific to the diseased organ but not necessarily where the organ is located. The pain is typically felt in the body wall or the extremities innervated from the same spinal segments as the diseased organ. This **referred pain**—described in more detail later—is easier to localize and describe than the initial discomfort or pain. Skin areas with referred pain may become **hyperesthetic** (increased sensitivity for touch) or **hyperalgesic** (increased pain upon nociceptor activation). The hyperalgesia is usually most marked in muscles and can be accompanied by tonic

contractions. Appendicitis, for example, usually leads to a bandlike hyperesthetic region of the skin corresponding to the dermatomes T_1–T_{11} (see Fig. 13.14) on the right side. In addition, **circulatory changes** may occur in the same area, presumably caused by reflex actions on preganglionic sympathetic neurons. Thus, looking for such sensory and circulatory changes may provide valuable diagnostic clues when suspecting diseases of visceral organs.

Typically, visceral pain is accompanied by **slow pulse**, **lowered blood pressure**, and **cold sweat**—that is, effects mediated by the autonomic nervous system. **Nausea** and vomiting, and a tendency to keep still are also frequent in patients with visceral pains.[4] Many of these effects are probably orchestrated by the **PAG**. The PAG receives nociceptive signals and coordinates a varied specter of autonomic and somatic reactions to stressful stimuli (see Fig. 30.1 and Chapter 15, under "The PAG Coordinates Stress Responses").

Several factors might contribute to the **diffuseness** of visceral pain. As mentioned, the density of sensory innervation is generally low in visceral organs with, consequently, very large **receptive fields** of the sensory units. In addition, the central branches of the visceral spinal ganglion cells run for a long distance, both rostrally and caudally in the cord. Thus, signals entering in one dorsal root can activate spinothalamic cells at many segmental levels.

Stimuli that Activate Visceral Nociceptors

The adequate stimuli for visceral nociceptors differ from those of somatic nociceptors. This may be so because visceral organs are not normally subject to stimuli that are potentially tissue damaging and thus require a change of behavior. In fact, stimuli that harm the visceral tissue may not provoke pain, while apparently innocuous stimuli may cause intense pain. Surgery of visceral organs (e.g., of the abdomen) can be performed without the patient feeling pain as long as the abdominal wall is anesthetized. Pain is felt only when the mesenteries or the peritoneum is pulled. Cutting with a sharp knife, for example, is not painful, and neither is tearing or pinching. Indeed, cancer of the lungs, kidneys, liver, and gut may cause considerable tissue destruction without evoking pain. Still, abnormal **distension** of a hollow organ or forceful **contraction of smooth muscles** in its wall produces intense pain. This occurs when a stone blocks the ureter or the gall ducts or when

---

3. A PET study compared cerebral activation patterns in patients with angina and patients with silent ischemia. Both groups had increased activation of the thalamus, but those with silent ischemia had less extensive cortical activation (Rosen 2012). This suggests that the lack of pain experience in silent ischemia is due to cortical factors.

---

4. However, the bouts of pain due to obstruction of a hollow visceral organ (the ureter or the intestine) are usually accompanied by an intense urge to move.

something obstructs the intestine. The wall of the organ is distended above the obstruction, and forceful contractions of the smooth musculature are produced in an attempt to overcome the obstruction. Such spasmodic contractions usually occur with regular intervals, explaining the typical bouts of pain experienced in such cases.

Another cause of visceral pain is **ischemia**, which can occur when an artery is narrowed by thrombosis or embolism. The most common example is the pain felt when a coronary artery is narrowed (angina pectoris) or occluded (myocardial infarction). Pain may also be felt when viscera are **inflamed** and when **irritating substances** come in contact with the peritoneum, as in cases of perforation of a gastric ulcer or an inflamed gallbladder. The spread of bile, gastric content, or blood to the peritoneal cavity causes extreme pain and shock. Sensory units leading from the **bladder** change their behavior when the mucosa is inflamed. First, mechanoreceptors recording stretching of the wall become more sensitive (lowered thresholds); second, many "silent nociceptors" start firing (see Chapter 13, under "Silent Nociceptors, the Immune System, Homeostasis, and Sickness Behavior"). Under normal conditions, even marked stretching of the wall does not activate such receptors, whereas in inflammation they respond to even moderate distension of the bladder. This may explain the frequent voiding in patients with **cystitis** and the urge to void even when the bladder is almost empty.

The **arteries** are also sensitive to noxious stimuli. An arterial puncture (e.g., to draw a blood sample) is painful, and so is stretching, distension, and electric stimulation (as judged from observations during brain surgery). For example, balloon dilatation of the middle cerebral artery evoked migraine-like headache. (Indeed, the pain of **migraine** has traditionally been explained as due to dilatation of arteries. Nevertheless, there is now much evidence that migraine headache can occur without concomitant vasodilatation.)

Sympathectomy

Knowledge of the special features of visceral pain and of the segmental innervation of visceral organs (see Table 28.2) is of importance for surgical interventions of the autonomic nervous system. Such operations are performed most often on the sympathetic system (sympathectomy). Indications are chronic pain conditions, especially **complex regional pain syndromes** (see Chapter 15, under "CRPS: A Special Type of Pathologic Pain"), but sympathectomies are also performed to reduce excessive sweating (**hyperhidrosis**) and to increase the **blood flow** of the extremities (to interrupt vasoconstrictor fibers). For example, interruption of the lumbar sympathetic trunk interrupts the sympathetic outflow to

the lower extremities (see Fig. 28.9). The use of sympathectomies for these conditions is controversial, however, due to unwanted side effects and lack of convincing documentation of effects.

Sympathectomy or sympathetic block is also performed occasionally to interrupt the pathways for **pain** signals from **visceral organs**. For example, in some patients with intractable pain arising in the upper abdomen (usually because of terminal cancer of the pancreas or the stomach), the transmission of sensory signals can be blocked by alcohol injections into the **celiac plexus**. Because this procedure also blocks the efferent sympathetic signals, the patients experience transitory orthostatic hypotension due to vasodilatation in the abdominal organs.

Referred Pain

As mentioned, pain of visceral origin is often not felt where the organ is located but in some other place, often in the body wall or the extremities (Fig. 29.3). This phenomenon is called **referred pain**. The referred pain—for example, in the left arm in the case of angina and under the right scapula in the case of a gallstone—can be localized fairly precisely by the patient. At the site of the diseased organ, however, there is usually only a diffuse pain, difficult both to localize and to describe. As mentioned, it typically takes some time for referred pain to develop.

The most widely accepted explanation of referred pain is based on the observed **convergence** of signals from somatic structures (especially the skin) and viscera.[5] Such convergence occurs in the dorsal horn, in the dorsal column nuclei, and in the thalamus, as discussed earlier in this chapter and in Chapter 14 (under "Spinothalamic Cells Receive Signals from the Skin, Muscles, and Visceral Organs"). As a rule, the diseased organ and the site of referred pain receive sensory innervation from the same **spinal segments**. Conceivably, the signals coming from the visceral organs are interpreted as arising in the skin and not in the visceral organ because signals from the visceral organs are never consciously perceived under normal circumstances (e.g., nociceptors of the heart are not normally stimulated). As mentioned, the referred pain usually takes some time to develop, and the occurrence of (referred) hyperesthesia and hyperalgesia is presumably explained by **sensitization** of central neurons receiving convergent inputs, leading to hyperexcitability and even spontaneous firing (i.e., independent of signals from the periphery). The importance of central sensitization is supported by the observation that the referred pain is felt even after blocking the sensory nerve fibers that lead from

---

5. That local anesthesia of the diseased organ prevents the development of referred pain proves that it depends on the nervous system.

Processing

University of Nottingham

Customer Number: 34752007	ISBN: 9780190228958
Budget/Fund Code	SCIENCE/TEACH – 2018
Classification	QP370
Site / Location	JCG
Shelfmark	O – size QP370.B7
Order Date	07/27/2017
Order Type	orders

Hand Notes:

Figure 29.3

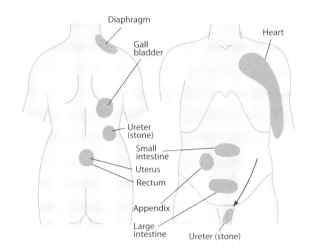

Referred pain. Examples of typical sites of pain in diseases affecting various visceral organs. (Based on Cope 1968.)

the area of referred pain. Further, the **expansion of the painful area** after some time is best explained by central sensitization of propriospinal neurons—transmitting signals to segments above and below those innervating the diseased organ. Indeed, animal experiments show that the receptive fields of dorsal horn neurons expand dramatically when the tissue from which they receive sensory signals is chronically inflamed.

Another peculiarity is that referred pain shows a tendency to localize to parts of the body that previously have been the site of a painful process. For example, a patient felt the pain of angina in a part of the spine that had been fractured many years ago. It seems as if a pain can be "remembered" as a persistent central sensitization (plasticity).

The peripheral axon of some **spinal ganglion cells** divides, with one branch going to the skin and another going to a visceral organ or a muscle. For example, one study found that about one-fifth of the fibers in the splanchnic nerve could be activated by electric stimulation of a somatic nerve. This may also contribute to the occurrence of referred pain. In such instances, an **axon reflex** (see later discussion) may cause cutaneous hyperesthesia and vascular changes, as sensory signals from the visceral organ are conducted not only into the cord but also peripherally in the branch into the skin. There sensory fibers may release **neuropeptides** such as substance P and VIP, which cause changes of blood flow and sensitize sensory nerve endings (see Chapter 13, under "Primary Sensory Neurons: Colocalization of Classical Neurotransmitters and Neuropeptides").

Examples of Referred Pain

The pain arising in the **heart** is usually referred to the ulnar aspect of the left arm or the upper part of the chest (Fig. 29.3). These regions of the skin and the heart both receive sensory innervation from the upper thoracic segments of the cord. The **gallbladder** and the skin in the region of the lower end of the scapula are both innervated from the eighth thoracic segment. The shoulder pain on irritation of the **diaphragm** is explained by the common innervation from the fourth and fifth cervical segments. Pain from the urinary **bladder** can be referred to two areas of the skin: one innervated by the spinal segments S_2-S_3 and one higher up on the back innervated by the lower thoracic and upper lumbar segments (see Fig. 13.15). This fits with the segments of the cord innervating the bladder (see Fig. 28.12).

In patients with **intracranial processes** that affect pain-sensitive parts of the meninges, the pain is referred to other parts of the head than the site of the pathological process (see Chapter 8, under "Headache Arising from Intracranial Structures").

Antidromic Impulses and the Axonal Reflex

Electrical stimulation of dorsal roots can produce vasodilatation in the dermatome of the root concerned. This is caused by impulses (signals) conducted in the peripheral direction by the sensory fibers. Impulses conducted in the direction opposite the normal direction are called **antidromic**. Of course the action potentials are exactly the same as those conducted in the normal—**orthodromic**—direction. Antidromic impulses in **C fibers** can release **substance P** from the peripheral branches. Substance P probably causes the release of **histamine** (presumably from mast cells). Histamine causes vasodilatation, especially of the capillaries, and at the same time the capillaries become leaky. Thus, a local edema is produced.

Various phenomena can probably be explained by this phenomenon. When the skin is stroked with a fairly sharp object, it reddens (vasodilatation) after a few seconds on both sides of the stripe. This can be explained as follows: the stroking of the skin stimulates C fiber nociceptors, and action potentials are conducted to the CNS (and we experience a sharp pain). At the same time, however, the action potential is also conducted peripherally in the branches of the C fiber that do not innervate the stimulated skin stripe. These branches end in the skin outside the stripe, where they liberate substance P and cause vasodilatation. The process is called a reflex, and because it uses only the peripheral process of a pseudounipolar ganglion cell, it is called an **axon reflex**. The reflex cannot be elicited in an area of the skin that has been deprived of its sensory innervation, proving that the phenomenon is mediated by nerve fibers.

Under normal conditions, the antidromic impulses in sensory fibers hardly play any role, but they may help explain certain pathological phenomena. An example from the **airways** can be mentioned. In disposed individuals, irritating gases can produce a marked edema of the mucous membranes. The edema is caused apparently by histamine release, which, in turn, is caused by substance P released by an axon reflex from the sensory fibers that innervate the mucous membrane (partly coming close to the surface of the epithelium).

The Central Autonomic System: The Hypothalamus

Sympathetic and parasympathetic parts cannot be clearly separated in the higher neuronal groups that control autonomic functions. This is not unexpected, as there is a constant need for coordination of the activity of preganglionic sympathetic and parasympathetic neurons. As discussed in Chapter 28, it is not so that *either* the sympathetic *or* the parasympathetic system is active. Further, higher levels can select specific subgroups of preganglionic neurons for a certain task. We have also mentioned regions in the brain stem—in the reticular formation in particular—that initiate various automatic behaviors, such as stereotyped, purposeful movement patterns and effects mediated by the autonomic nervous system. Such brain stem "centers" do not operate independently, however; in most instances their activity is modulated and controlled from higher levels of the brain, among which the hypothalamus has a prominent role. In addition, the hypothalamus plays a unique role—by means of the pituitary gland—in the superior control of the **endocrine system**.

Even though the hypothalamus is the part of the brain most closely linked with control of the autonomic nervous system, its functional role is wider. Thus, a central task of the hypothalamus is to **coordinate** autonomic, endocrine, and somatic motor responses to behavior that is appropriate for the immediate needs of the body, such as feeding, drinking, and reproduction. The overall aim is to maintain bodily **homeostasis** in a broad sense. The hypothalamus is also connected with higher parts of the central nervous system (CNS), however, including the cerebral cortex and the amygdala. These connections are important links in the interactions between **bodily** and **mental processes** (psychosomatic interrelations), which play a role in both health and disease. Interactions between the nervous system and the **immune system** in particular may help explain how mental states influence health and disease and how bodily processes influence our mental states.

The **afferent connections** of the hypothalamus are multifarious, reflecting its integrative role. The hypothalamus receives information about olfactory and taste stimuli; the conditions in the gastrointestinal tract; blood pressure, noxious stimuli, and skin temperature; and the intensity of ambient light. Afferents from limbic structures inform about emotional and motivational aspects. Hypothalamic **efferent connections** are also widespread and have three main targets: the pituitary, autonomic preganglionic neurons; somatic-efferent cell groups; and higher levels of the brain (limbic structures and the cerebral cortex).

The role of the amygdala (and some other nuclei) and the cerebral cortex in the control of autonomic functions is discussed in Chapter 31.

Premotor Networks

Physiologic experiments have localized several regions of the brain stem involved in the control of autonomic processes (see Chapter 26, under "Effects on Circulation and Respiration," and Chapter 29, under "Visceral Reflexes"). Electrical stimulation and lesions of restricted parts of the reticular formation of the pons and medulla produce changes in blood pressure, cardiac activity, respiration, sweat secretion, gastrointestinal activity, and other processes. Such higher-level centers exert control of the lower autonomic reflex centers of the spinal cord and coordinate their activities. The anatomic substrates of the brain stem "centers" are groups of neurons in the medullary and pontine reticular formation; as a rule, the centers are not well-defined nuclei but are formed by extensive **networks** of interconnected neurons. Visceral afferent fibers ending in the **solitary nucleus** inform the networks of the state of the body. From there, signals pass to various **premotor** groups in the reticular formation, which, in turn, send efferents to motor nuclei (autonomic and somatic) in the brain stem and the cord.

Coordination of Segmental Reflexes and Movement Patterns

The task-specific premotor networks ("centers") in the brain stem exert top-down coordinating actions on spinal reflex centers. They ensure, for example, that the segmental vasomotor reflexes operate together to serve the needs of the whole organism, not only its individual parts. We discussed in Chapter 28 how the blood supply of other organs is subordinate to the needs of the brain. In Chapter 29 (under "Central Control of Micturition") we discussed how normal bladder control requires coordination of many spinal cell groups. Further, cell groups in the reticular formation initiate movements and postural adjustments as parts of complex behaviors in response to thirst, hunger, external dangers, sexual arousal, and so forth. Several such behaviors are coordinated from the **superior colliculus** and the **periaqueductal gray (PAG)** in the mesencephalon by way of their efferent connections to the reticular formation. Connections from the PAG initiate coordinated alterations of circulation and respiration, pain perception, and automatic movements in response to threatening or novel stimuli (Fig. 30.1). Pain, for example, might be understood not merely as a signal of tissue damage but also as a signal of the need to change behavior.

Brain Stem Premotor Networks Are Controlled from Higher Levels

A perfect coordination cannot be performed by the brain stem autonomic centers, however. This is witnessed by the poor control of autonomic functions such as blood pressure and body temperature in **decerebrate animals**. Optimal autonomic control, and coordination of autonomic with endocrine and somatic processes, requires that the brain stem and spinal centers be supplied with afferent fibers from higher centers, especially in the hypothalamus but also in the amygdala (which acts on the brain stem partly through the hypothalamus).

The PAG Coordinates Behavior in Response to Threatening Stimuli

The PAG is not a unit, either anatomically or functionally. It consists of several columnar groups of neurons, each differing with

Figure 30.1

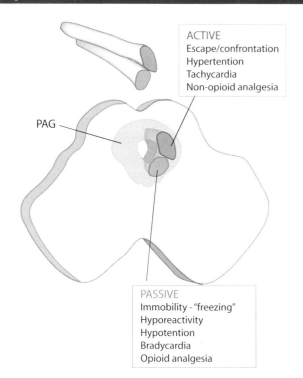

ACTIVE
Escape/confrontation
Hypertention
Tachycardia
Non-opioid analgesia

PAG

PASSIVE
Immobility - "freezing"
Hyporeactivity
Hypotention
Bradycardia
Opioid analgesia

PAG and different responses to stress. Highly simplified. Stimulation of PAG in experimental animals evokes two main adaptive response patterns. A dorsolateral neuronal column (blue) initiates active coping strategies, with an increased autonomic state of readiness and increased somatomotor activity. Stimulation of a ventrolateral column (green) elicits passivity and withdrawal. The first response is appropriate if the animal expects to be able to control the situation (e.g. by flight, attack, or frightening), while the second would be appropriate when there is little hope of control (e.g., extensive physical injuries or repeated social defeats). (Based on Bandler et al. 2000).

regard to connections (Fig. 30.1). Stimulation of a **dorsolateral column** elicits arousal, tachycardia, rise in blood pressure, and increased respiration, and it facilitates orienting responses. At the same time, a **non-opioid** analgesia is produced. The actions are mediated by, among others, connections to the locus coeruleus, the ambiguus nucleus, the solitary nucleus, and parts of the reticular formation but also by ascending connections to the anterior hypothalamus and the intralaminar thalamic nuclei. Together, this part of the PAG initiates **defensive behavior** in response to strong emotions or aversive external stimuli. Stimulation of a **ventrolateral column** in the PAG elicits inhibition of movements, like the **"freezing"** response to sudden fear (e.g., when a rat sees a cat). In addition, the PAG probably mediates the immobility typical of conditions with strong visceral pain. The immobility is accompanied by a fall in blood pressure, bradycardia, and **opioid-dependent** analgesia. These effects are mediated by efferent connections to the nucleus raphe magnus and the reticular formation in the ventrolateral medulla and to the lateral hypothalamus and the basal forebrain.

level of psychic stress is the possibility of obtaining an **outlet for frustration**—for example, with physical exercise. Finally, animal experiments support that **social attachments** reduce psychic stress. Accordingly, a social network is among the factors known to increase a person's **resilience.**

Expectation and Health

The relation between **expectation** and disease has attracted much interest. For example, several studies address how **optimism as a personality trait** influences psychological adaptation, handling of stress (such as major surgery), and self-reported health. Altogether, there are clear positive correlations; that is, an optimistic attitude is associated with better self-reported health, fewer psychiatric symptoms, lower blood pressure, and so forth. While a causal relationship remains to be established, as mentioned, there is solid evidence that our mental state (via the hypothalamus) influences several physiologic processes. Further, studies of the **placebo** and **nocebo** phenomena strongly support the importance of expectations for handling of stressful situations (see Chapter 15).

There are exceptions, however, from a positive correlation between optimism and health (or indirect measures, such as immunity). Thus, some studies find a negative correlation between optimism and immunity when stressors are complex, long lasting, and unpredictable (Segerstrom 2005). Perhaps in such situations inevitable frustrations and disappointments might be less adaptive than resignation (as would be chosen by a less optimistic person).

The Hypothalamus and the Expression of Emotions

It should be emphasized that the concept "emotion" gives meaning only in relation to a person—only a person can have (or feel) emotions, not his or her brain or parts of the brain. An emotion is not a *thing* that can be localized physically. Nevertheless, a functioning cerebral cortex is a prerequisite for the *feeling* of emotion, and the hypothalamus is among the parts of the brain most directly involved in **emotional expressions** (in an experimental context, emotional expressions can be defined as behavior in response to stimuli producing sensations with an emotional coloring). This agrees with the importance of the hypothalamus for control of autonomic processes. Emotions are expressed, as we know from everyday experience, to a large extent through changes of the functions of autonomically innervated organs, such as palpitations, dryness of the mouth, fainting, blushing, paling, alterations of the digestive tract,

sweating, frequent micturition, and so forth. In addition, automatic movements—such as rapid, superficial breathing, facial expressions, and postures—witness emotions. Such movements, organized by brain stem premotor networks, are probably influenced from the hypothalamus (see the discussion of emotional smile and facial palsy in Chapter 27 under "Facial Expressions of Emotion Do Not Depend on the Pyramidal Tract").

The importance of the hypothalamus for emotional expressions is witnessed by observations in humans during brain surgery with local anesthesia. Pressure on or traction of the hypothalamic region can elicit reactions of panic, crying, laughter, or profuse talking. The patients sometimes also report a change of mood, such as depression or euphoria. It thus appears that the activity of the hypothalamus is significant not only for emotional reactions but also for the emotions themselves. Conceivably, the emotions are evoked by feedback connections from the hypothalamus to the limbic structures (e.g., the amygdala) and the cerebral cortex—structures that are necessary for the experience of emotions (as distinct from emotional reactions). The higher regions presumably interpret the hypothalamic activity as evidence of external or internal stimuli that normally evoke strong emotions.

Emotional Expressions in Animals without the Cerebral Cortex

The role of the hypothalamus in emotional reactions has been studied in cats and dogs in which the whole cerebral cortex, the basal ganglia, and large parts of the thalamus have been removed. So-called **sham rage** can be provoked in such animals. Their expression of rage must depend on the hypothalamus, because only the hypothalamus is connected with the brain stem. Such animals react much like normal animals to painful stimuli, with biting, scratching, snarling, and increased ventilation. Because the whole cortex is removed, it is unlikely that true emotions are experienced, however. It seems reasonable to conclude that the hypothalamus contains cell groups that coordinate and put into action the behavior expressing the rage. In contrast to normal animals, the rage of such "hypothalamic" animals is not directed toward anything in particular; they lack the ability to know the nature and the location of the stimulus provoking the pain (as one might expect in an animal lacking the cerebral cortex and most of the thalamus). Further, the expression of the rage dies out very quickly after the stimulus is over, whereas the reactions continue for a while in normal animals (as in humans) This observation suggests that other parts of the brain normally act on the hypothalamus to produce emotional reactions, as we discuss in Chapter 31, under "The Amygdala."

PART SEVEN

Limbic Structures

This part of the book deals with parts of the forebrain that are closely associated with the cerebral cortex with regard to development and connections. The cerebral cortex is divided into two parts (without definite delimitations) on the basis of phylogenetic development: the **neocortex**, which is the most recent part and comprises most of the cortex in higher mammals, and the **allocortex**, which is the oldest part. The neocortex is discussed in Chapters 33 and 34, while Chapters 31 and 32 deal with the allocortex and closely related subcortical nuclei. The nomenclature used for the oldest part of the cortex varies, but usually the term "allocortex" is used for the parts of the cortical mantle with a simple, often only three-layered structure instead of the six layers that are typical of the neocortex. In reptiles, the allocortex constitutes what little cortex there is. The allocortex receives afferents from adjacent subcortical nuclei (in contrast to the neocortex that is closely connected with the thalamus). Together these subcortical nuclei and the allocortex are commonly said to comprise the so-called **limbic system** (gyrus limbicus is another name for the cingulate gyrus). The cell groups comprising the "limbic system" coincide in part with what was formerly called the **rhinencephalon,** although this term, strictly speaking, comprises only the parts of the brain that receive olfactory fibers. There are wide variations among authors, however, with regard to which neuronal groups are included in the "limbic system," indicating that the term lacks reasonable precision. Indeed, the term "system" becomes misleading when used to lump—rather arbitrarily—neuronal groups with major functional differences. In this book we therefore use the neutral term **limbic structures** to avoid giving a misleading impression of functional unity.

The Amygdala and Other Neuronal Groups with Relation to Emotions

OVERVIEW

This chapter deals primarily with structures that are of special importance for emotions, motivation, and affective behavior. We include in the discussion the **cingulate gyrus,** the **septal nuclei,** the **amygdala,** and neuronal groups in the **basal forebrain.** In addition, we discuss neocortical regions involved in emotional processing, notably parts of the **prefrontal cortex** and **the insula.**

The **amygdala** is located in the tip of the temporal lobe and consists of several distinct nuclei with different connections. It plays an important role in social behavior and in emotional learning and memory. In particular, a central task of the amygdala is the establishment of links between stimuli and their emotional value. The amygdala has connections with brain stem nuclei (e.g., the periaqueductal gray [PAG]) and influences somatic and autonomic responses to strong emotions (e.g., mediating conditioned fear responses). It also can influence the endocrine system. Amygdaloid connections with the cingulate gyrus, the prefrontal cortex, and the hippocampus mediate influences on cognitive processes, affective behavior, and memory.

Wide areas of the cerebral cortex influence the activity of the **autonomic nervous system**. This influence is exerted mainly via the amygdala, the hippocampal formation, and the septal nuclei, which, in turn, influence the hypothalamus and brain stem nuclei. In addition, there are some direct connections from the **insula** and the **orbitofrontal cortex** to the hypothalamus. Further, neocortical areas in the frontal and temporal lobes project to the amygdala and can therefore influence the hypothalamus indirectly.

Extensive cortical areas show altered activity in relation to **emotions**. On the other hand, no area is concerned *solely* with emotional processing. One of the important tasks of the **cingulate gyrus** is choosing behavior in response to conflicting stimuli. The orbitofrontal and medial parts of the frontal lobes are also closely linked with processing of emotions and their integration with cognitive processes.

The term the **basal forebrain** (*substantia innominata*) is used with reference to diffuse neuronal populations below and medial to the well-defined basal ganglia. It contains many **cholinergic neurons** and is involved in the regulation of **attention, motivation,** and **memory**.

WHAT IS THE "LIMBIC SYSTEM"?

The structures included in the term the "limbic system" are often regarded as the substrate of emotions and subconscious processes, in contrast with the cognitive, conscious processes that are assumed to be located in the neocortex. Sometimes terms such as "the emotional brain" or even "the reptile brain" have been used to describe these regions. Each of the neuronal groups of the "limbic system" participates in various functional domains, however, and using one term for them all gives a false impression of unity. Indeed, the decision as to which structures should be included in the term the "limbic system" has become more and more arbitrary, as new methods have shown that many more parts of the brain participate in emotional processing than believed when the term was coined.[1] For example, parts of the neocortex (not only the allocortex) are strongly implicated in processing of emotions—the **prefrontal cortex** and the **insula,** in particular. Further, cell groups in the basal parts of the hemispheres—the so-called **basal forebrain** (including the nucleus accumbens, discussed in Chapter 23)—are densely interconnected with both limbic structures and the neocortex, and these cell groups participate in both emotional and cognitive processing. We therefore include a description of the basal forebrain in this chapter, while the prefrontal cortex is

---

1. Some authors include in the "limbic system" the mammillary body, the anterior thalamic nucleus, the ventral striatum, and the hypothalamus. Some even include brain stem cell groups such as the ventral tegmental area, the raphe nuclei, the PAG, and certain cholinergic neuronal groups.

discussed mainly in Chapters 33 and 34 in conjunction with the discussion of parts of the cerebral cortex involved in higher mental functions.

Our present knowledge indicates that all complex behavioral reactions engage the amygdala, the septal nuclei, the hippocampal region, the reticular formation, the hypothalamus, the basal ganglia, and large parts of the cerebral cortex. As witnessed by their numerous interconnections, all of these regions cooperate to exert an integrated influence on the peripheral somatic and autonomic effectors. What the American psychologist S. P. Grossman (1976, p. 361) said about the septal nuclei probably holds for the rest of the limbic structures too: "Just about every behavior and/or psychological function which has been investigated to date has been shown to be affected in some way by septal lesions."

In conclusion, the "limbic system" does not represent a unity that can be defined with a reasonable degree of precision. As stated by the American neurologist Antonio Damasio (1995, p. 20), "the bizarre distinction between cognition and emotion, as if somehow one could have thoughts without emotion, a mind without affect . . . The rift between emotion and cognition acquired a neuroanatomical counterpart in the duality between limbic system and neocortex."

The Circuit of Papez

In 1937 James Papez described what he considered a closed circuit of connections starting and ending in the hippocampus. From the hippocampus, the flow of signals was postulated to pass to the mammillary nucleus, from this nucleus to the anterior thalamic nucleus, from there to the cingulate gyrus, and then finally back to the hippocampus. This circuit of interconnected cell groups was hypothesized to form the anatomic basis of emotional reactions and expressions. These suggestions formed the basis for the concept of the "limbic system," which was introduced in the early 1950s by Paul MacLean.

THE AMYGDALA

Main Anatomic and Functional Subdivisions

The amygdala (the amygdaloid nucleus) is located in the temporal lobe, underneath the uncus (Figs. 31.1, 31.2, and 31.3). In humans, the amygdala is a complex of subnuclei, each with a distinctive internal structure, neurotransmitters, and connections. Here we restrict ourselves to distinguishing between a small **corticomedial** (including a **central nucleus**) and a large **basolateral** nuclear group (including the **lateral**

Figure 31.1

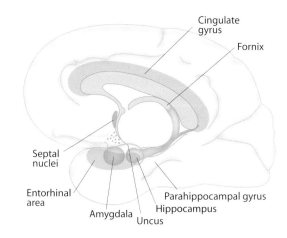

The limbic structures. The right hemisphere, as viewed from the medial aspect. The regions and cell groups indicated in red are usually included in the term "limbic system."

nucleus). The basolateral group increases in size from lower to higher mammals and is particularly well developed in humans. The corticomedial nuclear group lies close to the olfactory cortex (see Fig. 19.3).

To simplify, we may say that the **corticomedial nuclei** are connected primarily with the olfactory bulb, the hypothalamus, and the visceral nuclei of the brain stem, whereas the **basolateral nuclei** are mainly connected with the thalamus and prefrontal cortex. In addition, the basolateral nuclei send fibers to the ventral striatum and the basal nucleus. This would suggest that the corticomedial part of the amygdala is concerned primarily with autonomic functions, whereas the basolateral parts are more involved in conscious processes related to the frontal and temporal lobes. The many intrinsic connections among the various nuclei show that they must cooperate extensively, however.

The amygdala (or its many components) participates in several higher mental functions, each of which is very complex. Its "functions" are correspondingly complex and hard to define. Nevertheless, some salient features are clear. Thus, a central task of the amygdala is the establishment of links between **stimuli** and their **emotional value** (put very simply, whether something is good or bad). Most of our memories have some—often quite strong—emotional coloring, which is crucial for our ability to react appropriately to a stimulus. Think of the importance of being able to judge the facial expressions of other people, the emotional aspects of their speech, and so forth. As we discuss in this chapter, damage to the amygdala in monkeys leads to, among other things, difficulties in **social interactions**.

Figure 31.2

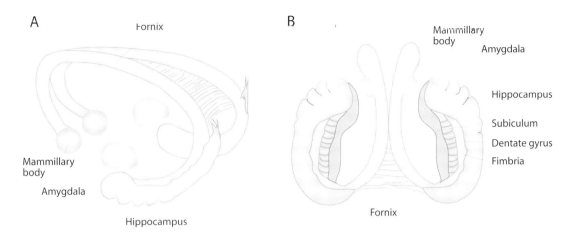

The hippocampus, fornix, mammillary nucleus, and amygdala. **A:** Viewed obliquely from behind. **B:** Viewed from above.

The Amygdala Is Not a Unit

The amygdala as we describe it here is structurally and functionally heterogeneous, and when we lump the various nuclei under one name in this text it is purely for convenience. Indeed, in a critical review Larry Swanson and Gorica Petrovich (1998, p. 330) concluded "it is necessary to ask whether the concept of a structurally and functionally defined amygdala is indeed valid, or whether the concept is hindering attempts to understand general principles of telencephalic architecture by imposing an arbitrary classification on heterogeneous structures that belong to different functional systems." Some conflicting results in the literature may be more apparent than real due to disregard of the amygdala's heterogeneity.

Figure 31.3

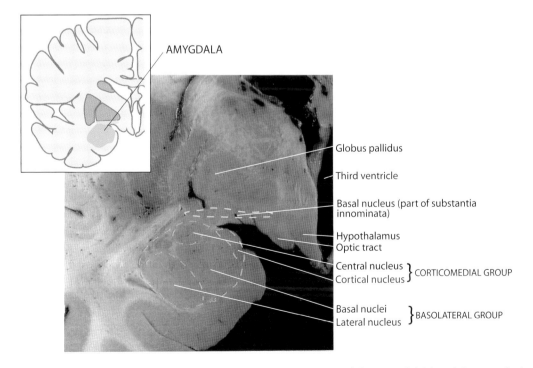

The amygdala. Frontal section through the left hemisphere (cf. Fig. 31.1). Some of the amygdaloid nuclei are marked with orange stippled lines. The basal nucleus is indicated with a green stippled line. The amygdala and the cerebral cortex of the temporal lobe are closely connected. The section is placed more posteriorly than the one in Fig. 31.9.

Afferent Connections of the Amygdala

The **corticomedial** nuclei receive afferents from the **olfactory bulb**, the **hypothalamus**, the **intralaminar thalamic nuclei**, and the **septal nuclei** (Fig. 31.4). They also receive **dopaminergic** fibers from the ventral tegmental area in the mesencephalon, as well as fibers from the **parabrachial area** (in the dorsolateral pons). The latter projection may convey information about taste and painful stimuli. Thus, ascending fibers of spinal **lamina I** nociceptive neurons end in parts of the parabrachial area that project to the central amygdaloid nucleus (among other targets). The sensory units of this pathway have very large receptive fields and receive convergent inputs from the skin and viscera. It seems likely that this lamina I–parabrachial–amygdaloid pathway contributes to the **emotional aspects of pain**.

The **basolateral nuclei** receive fibers from several **thalamic nuclei**, the **prefrontal cortex**, parts of the **temporal lobe**, and the **cingulate gyrus** (Fig. 31.4). Together, the basolateral nuclei—the **lateral nucleus** in particular—receive all kinds of sensory information. This may include emotionally neutral information from cortical association areas or emotionally laden information about unpleasant and threatening stimuli from the reticular formation, the

intralaminar thalamic nuclei, and perhaps parts of the cortex (the insula). Thus, the amygdala receives, for example, information about **fear-provoking stimuli** and their **context**. Efferents from the lateral nucleus reach other amygdaloid nuclei that may influence the cortex (emotions) and brain stem cell groups (behavioral reactions, including autonomic responses associated with emotions).

Efferent Connections of the Amygdala

The efferent connections of the amygdala are mostly reciprocal to the afferent ones. One major efferent pathway goes to the **hypothalamus**. Most of these fibers are collected in the macroscopically visible **stria terminalis**, which arches over the thalamus (Fig. 31.5). The fibers end primarily in the **ventromedial hypothalamic nucleus** (cf. the efferents from the hippocampal formation, which run in the fornix and end in the mammillary nucleus). Other efferents pass to the **thalamus** (especially to the mediodorsal nucleus), enabling signals from the amygdala to reach the **prefrontal cortex** (Fig. 31.5). As mentioned, these connections may be important for the feeling of emotions, such as fear and anxiety. In particular, the amygdala–prefrontal connections might ensure that we spend our limited attentional resources on the most important stimuli (those with emotional coloring)

Figure 31.4

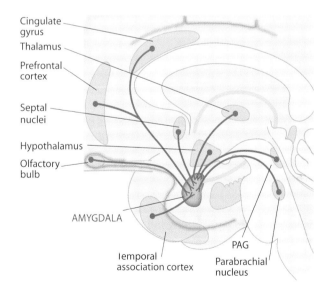

Afferent connections of the amygdala. Note the connections with the hypothalamus, cortical areas in the temporal and the frontal lobes, and brain stem nuclei. Not all known connections are shown.

Figure 31.5

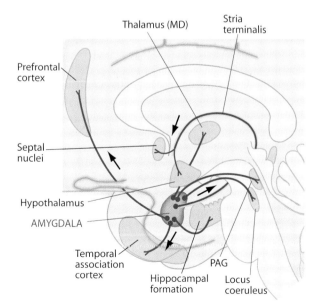

Efferent connections of the amygdala. Note connections to the hypothalamus, the PAG, the hippocampus, and cortical areas in the temporal and frontal lobes. See also Fig. 31.6.

and, further, that emotional and cognitive information is integrated prior to decisions and actions.

Parts of the allocortex receive fibers from the amygdala, especially the **hippocampal formation** (the entorhinal area and the subiculum) and the **septal nuclei.** Fibers to the **ventral striatum** (including the nucleus accumbens; see Fig. 23.15) and the **basal nucleus** (Figs. 31.3 and 31.9; also see Fig. 10.3) arise in the basolateral nuclei of the amygdala. The projections to the basal nucleus can induce **arousal** and increased **attention** (as indicated by activation of the electroencephalogram [EEG]). There is experimental evidence that synaptic learning effects on neurons in the auditory cortex depend on inputs from the amygdala (and the basal nucleus) besides the specific auditory information via the medial geniculate body. It seems likely that this is related to the well-known effects of motivation on **learning**: we remember better the material that has emotional coloring (see Fig. 4.11).

Finally, there are connections from the amygdala (especially from the central nucleus) to various **brain stem nuclei**, such as the **PAG** (Fig. 31.6; also see Fig. 30.1), parts of the **reticular formation**, and **parasympathetic** cranial nerve nuclei. These connections—together with those to the hypothalamus—are important for the autonomic and somatic expressions of emotions. The connections to the PAG are involved in eliciting **conditioned fear behavior**. The PAG sends fibers to various brain stem premotor networks (Fig. 31.6). In rodents, conditioned fear includes so-called **freezing**; that is, the animal becomes completely still. The freezing reaction, which includes suppressed pain transmission, occurs typically when a mouse meets a predator, such as a cat. When exposed to a sudden threat, humans also experience a similar halt of all movements, until an appropriate behavioral response is selected (flight, fight, or continued immobility).

Basic Emotions

Emotions in animals can only be inferred indirectly from their behavior, which may explain why it is not clear how many

---

Figure 31.6

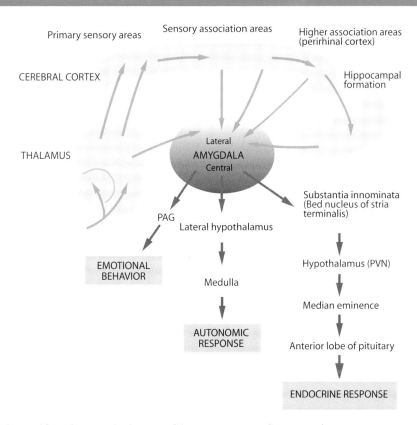

The amygdala and conditioned fear. The neural substrate of the autonomic, endocrine, and somatic responses elicited by a conditioned stimulus (sound) associated with an electric shock to the foot. The connections of the amygdala with the sensory association areas are necessary for discriminative aspects of stimulus analysis, while connections with the hippocampus mediate contextual conditioning. (Based on LeDoux 1995.)

varieties of emotions animals have compared with humans. Commonly, however, three basic emotions are identified in cats, dogs, and monkeys: **rage, fear,** and **pleasure** (love). Even though the emotions of animals certainly are more diverse than this, there is no doubt that the emotions of humans have more variation and nuances. This should be kept in mind when drawing conclusions with regard to emotions and psychosomatic interrelations in humans on the basis of animal experiments. The anthropologist Paul Ekman (1984) identified seven core emotions in humans, based on their relation to culture-independent facial expressions: **happiness, sadness, anger, fear, disgust, surprise,** and **contempt.** This list does not—and is not intended to—capture the rich nuances of human emotions (as witnessed by the large number of words for emotions). Rather, each of the core emotional expressions—for example a smiling face—can express a wide variety of positive emotions, such as amusement, pride, relief, and so forth (Ekman 1993).

Amygdala and Conditioned Fear

As mentioned, the amygdala has a role in a variety of emotions and behaviors influenced or governed by emotions. This, with its anatomic heterogeneity, underscores that the amygdala is not a functional unit. In the search for the biologic substrate of specific behaviors, **conditioned fear** has been intensively studied (Fig. 31.6), and crucial links in the pathways that underlie this phenomenon have been "dissected" out in experimental animals. Such detailed data may help us understand how the amygdala participates in other kinds of tasks.

More about the Circuits for Expression of Fear

Situations with purely mental stress can produce a conditioned-fear reaction in rats as in humans. In rats, the conditioning may be established by repeatedly administering a painful stimulus (e.g., an electric shock to the foot) after sounding a tone. After a while, the tone alone elicits fear-related behavior—that is, behavior that normally occurs in threatening or dangerous situations (such as the sight of a cat). As discussed earlier, the fear reaction of a rat includes autonomic, somatic, and endocrine responses, such as freezing and increased secretion of cortisol. When a tone is the conditioning stimulus, the necessary information about the sound is transmitted directly from the thalamus to the **lateral amygdaloid nucleus.** The auditory **cortex** is necessary for the occurrence of the fear reaction only if the animal must discriminate between two tones with different frequencies. The **hippocampus** is not necessary for the tone conditioning. It is necessary, however, for a weaker **contextual conditioning;** that is, the fear reaction can also be elicited by clues in the environment of the experimental situation (such as objects, sounds, or odors). Signals are relayed (directly and indirectly) from the lateral nucleus to the **central nucleus** (Fig. 31.3). Efferents from the central nucleus to autonomic and somatic cell groups in the brain stem (among them the PAG) probably mediate main

components of the fear reaction. Thus, destruction of the central nucleus abolishes both the freezing and autonomic responses in conditioned fear.

Main Tasks of the Amygdala

The tasks performed by the amygdala have been clarified by lesion and stimulation experiments in animals and recently by numerous functional magnetic resonance imaging (fMRI) studies in humans. Further, important information comes from examination of a few persons who lack the amygdala (usually after surgical treatment of epilepsy). While the connection between the amygdala and emotions is firmly established, much investigation remains to be done before we understand its specific contributions to emotional processing and human behavior.

Effects of Electric Stimulation of the Amygdala

Many behavioral changes have been produced by **electrical stimulation** of the amygdala in animals with **implanted electrodes.** Stimulation produces a varied pattern of somatic and autonomic responses, which appear to be parts of more complex behavioral reactions. As would be expected from the anatomic data discussed in the preceding text, stimulation of medial and lateral parts of the amygdala gives different responses. Stimulation of the **corticomedial nuclear group** produces smacking, salivation, and licking and chewing movements. Emptying of the rectum and the bladder may occur, together with inhibition of voluntary movements. Stimulation of the **basolateral nuclear group** often produces **arousal** and signs of increased attention: the animal lifts its head, its pupils are dilated, and it looks around. Strong stimulation can produce dramatic effects, such as signs of fear or rage.

In **humans,** the amygdala has been stimulated in conjunction with brain surgery of the temporal lobe under local anesthesia. As in animals, a wide spectrum of autonomic and emotional reactions has been produced but most pronounced is a feeling of **anxiety.** Memory-like hallucinations and **déjà vu** experiences (the feeling of having experienced the same situation before) have also been reported. This is called a **dreamy state** and can occur in **epileptic seizures** that start in the temporal lobe. Similar effects—that is, **fear** and various kinds of **hallucinations**—have been produced by stimulation of the anterior portion of the hippocampus and the lateral cortex of the temporal lobe (in the superior temporal gyrus). This can presumably be explained by the close connections between these regions and the amygdala, all parts of a more widespread **network** for handling emotions and memories.

Animal experiments show that a central task of the amygdala is to establish **associations** between sensory stimuli and their affective value. It is crucial that we can decide quickly—before slower conscious deliberations—whether a stimulus (or a situation) is threatening or safe (punishment or reward). Accordingly, fMRI studies in humans show activation of the amygdala when viewing pictures with an emotional content. Further, bilateral lesions of the amygdala in monkeys reduce behavior elicited by emotions. For example, the animals show no fear of snakes (monkeys have an inborn fear of snakes). This can probably be explained by the removal of amygdaloid effects on the hypothalamus and on the brain stem autonomic and somatic motor centers (among them the PAG; Fig. 31.6). Sensory stimuli (such as the sight of a snake), although consciously perceived, would not be able to elicit the normal behavioral reactions.

The sight of **faces** expressing **anger** or **fear** causes a robust activation of the human amygdala, as shown via fMRI. Correspondingly, patients with amygdaloid lesions have difficulties with **recognizing facial expressions**. Interestingly, such patients do not show the normal tendency to remember events or stimuli that have an emotional coloring better than neutral ones. This has been demonstrated, for example, by showing films containing emotionally neutral material and scenes that evoke strong emotions.

Amygdala and Social Interactions

Selective lesions in adult monkeys produce a pattern of behavior characterized by **social disinhibition**.[2] For example, they initiate more physical contact, suggesting "that heightened affiliative social interactions following amygdala lesions stems from a more general inability to properly perceive danger or threat in the environment and use such information to modulate social behavior adaptively" (Machado et al., 2008, p. 263). This would fit with the amygdala working as a sort of **alarm**—it evaluates very rapidly a stimulus for its threatening value and initiates appropriate behavior. However, selective lesions of the amygdala in monkeys produce fewer behavioral changes than reported in early experiments with lesions that included adjoining parts of the temporal lobe (see Chapter 34, under "Symptoms after Lesions of the Temporal Cortex"). For example, no signs of abnormal **social development** were observed the first 6 months after bilateral lesions of the amygdala in infant monkeys in relationships with

either the mother or other infants in the group. However, the infants did not exhibit the normal signs of distress to separation from the mother, presumably due to a reduced ability to perceive danger and threatening situations.

Is the Amygdala Concerned Only with Negative Emotions?

Whereas most studies have focused on a correlation between amygdala activity and negative emotions such as fear and anger, recent studies suggest that the amygdala plays a role for the recognition of positive emotions as well. For example, a meta-analysis of human positron emission tomography (PET) and fMRI studies found that both negative and positive stimuli were associated with higher amygdala activity compared with neutral stimuli. Indeed, single-unit studies in monkeys identified distinct populations of amygdaloid neurons responding to positive and negative stimulus valence, respectively (the two kinds of neuron were not spatially segregated in the basolateral amygdala, however).

Is Amygdala Necessary for the Experience of Emotions?

The finding that the amygdala is necessary for expression of emotions (at least some aspects of them) raises the question of whether the amygdala is necessary also for the **feeling** of emotions (such as fear or anger). A patient with bilateral destruction of the amygdala, described by the British psychiatrist R. Jacobson (1986), illustrates this point. The patient appeared calm and relaxed outwardly and had normal heart rate in situations in which she experienced great anxiety and wanted to run away. Presumably, the coupling between the emotions and the emotional expressions was disrupted in this patient (see Chapter 30, under "The Hypothalamus and the Expression of Emotions"). Further, 20 patients with amygdaloid lesions after epilepsy surgery described their daily emotions—positive and negative—in the same manner as normal controls (Anderson and Phelps 2002). Not all patients with bilateral damage of the amygdala exhibit such a **dissociation** of the experienced emotion and the emotional expressions, however. Indeed, there are surprisingly large **individual variations** in symptoms among patients with amygdaloid lesions. Conceivably, the age at which the lesion occurred plays a decisive part: with early lesions, other parts of the brain

---

2. **Hypersexuality** was one of the behavioral changes reported in the early studies with large bilateral lesions of the amygdala in monkeys. However, this may be related to damage to allocortical areas near the amygdala rather than to the amygdala itself. Nevertheless, it is conspicuous that the amygdala is among the brain regions with the highest density of receptors for **sex hormones.** Conceivably, the level of sex hormones in the blood influences the activity of neurons in parts of the amygdala (the sex hormones are lipid-soluble and pass the blood–brain barrier easily).

would be expected to at least partly take over the tasks of the amygdala. Further, prior experiences and subtle difference in context may strongly influence how different subjects with lesions of the amygdala experience and respond to identical stimuli.

The Amygdala, Learning, and Unlearning

The conditioned-fear reaction discussed previously requires a learning process: the rat learns to associate an innocuous stimulus with something painful. Destruction of the amygdala prevents establishing the conditioned response. Indeed, induction of long-term potentiation occurs in certain parts of the amygdala in conjunction with development of a conditioned fear response. Thus, experiments with monkeys after a lesion restricted as far as possible to the amygdala show that they have difficulties in **learning** the association between objects and their meanings. They can recognize objects but cannot relate them to other kinds of information, such as whether the object is associated with a reward or something unpleasant. Many other observations support that the amygdala, as mentioned, is necessary for the learning of associations between stimuli and their significance in terms of **reward** or **punishment**.

We may say that the amygdala is crucial for the "tagging" of experiences and sensations with emotional feelings and for the remembering of these associations. The amygdala is not alone in this respect, however. Both the amygdala and parts of the prefrontal cortex are necessary in monkeys for the learning and later retrieval of associations between visual stimuli and food rewards. The connections involved are partly direct fibers from the amygdala to the **ventromedial prefrontal cortex** and partly a pathway interrupted in the mediodorsal thalamic nucleus. Experiments in rats suggest that connections between the basolateral amygdala and the **ventral striatum** (nucleus accumbens) are also necessary for establishing stimulus–reward associations.

Connections from **medial prefrontal cortex** appear to be necessary for unlearning—**extinction**—of the conditioned fear response. Extinction occurs when the conditioned stimulus regularly occurs without a subsequent unconditioned stimulus—but not in rats after removal of the medial prefrontal cortex. Other data also indicate that extinction depends on an active **inhibition** of the amygdala from the prefrontal cortex, not on the disappearance of the synaptic changes underlying the associations.

The Amygdala, Anxiety, and Neurotransmitters

The amygdala contains many neurotransmitters, and to sort out the functional role of each is a formidable task. For practical reasons, therefore, scientists concentrate on studying one or a few at a time, with the danger of overlooking the contributions of other transmitters. We restrict ourselves here to the transmitters involved in **conditioned fear** and **psychic stress**. As mentioned, signals pass from the lateral to the central nucleus through both direct and indirect routes.

Electrical stimulation of the **lateral nucleus** evokes primarily γ-aminobutyric acid (**GABA**)-mediated inhibition in the **central nucleus** (acting at both $GABA_A$ and $GABA_B$ receptors). Some inhibition occurs presynaptically by reducing the release of **glutamate**. Drugs that reduce **anxiety** (anxiolytics) may function by interfering at this level. For example, the **benzodiazepines** (Valium and others) bind to specific sites on the GABA receptor (benzodiazepine receptors) and potentiate the effect of GABA. The density of benzodiazepine receptors is high in the amygdala and particularly high in the lateral nucleus (and one other subnucleus of the basolateral complex). Local infusion of benzodiazepines in these nuclei reduces expressions of conditioned fear in experimental animals.

Corticotrophin-releasing hormone (**CRH**) may also be an important transmitter in the amygdala in relation to anxiety and stress. Besides containing CRH-positive cell bodies, the central nucleus receives many CRH-containing fibers (neurons in the **parabrachial area** and the **locus coeruleus** contain CRH, for example). Injection of CRH into the cerebral ventricles increases **stress reactions** and fear-related behavior, presumably by acting in the amygdala (but also in other areas). For example, noradrenergic neurons in the locus coeruleus are activated, which may contribute to arousal as part of a stress reaction. Acute and chronic stress increases CRH in the amygdala; accordingly, microinjections of CRH antagonists in the central nucleus abolish some stress reactions.

The **expectation** of **pain** evokes an endocrine response, as one part of a stress reaction (see Chapter 30, under "Mental Processes Influence the Endocrine Organs"). This may be mediated by neurons in the central nucleus, which project to the paraventricular hypothalamic nucleus. **CRH**-containing neurons in the paraventricular nucleus project to the median eminence. There CRH is released and reaches the anterior pituitary via the portal system (see Fig. 30.8). CRH increases the secretion of ACTH, thus increasing **cortisol** in the bloodstream.

Several transmitters other than CRH show changes in relation to anxiety and stress. **Neuropeptide Y** (NPY) has attracted much interest. Thus, microinjection of NPY in the amygdala evokes largely the opposite effects of CRH on stress and fear-related behavior. NPY is present in many neurons in the amygdala (colocalized with norepinephrine, GABA, or somatostatin) and in terminals of afferent axons. Animal experiments suggest that, whereas CRH is crucial in eliciting a stress reaction, NPY that is released after the reaction has started protects against overshooting.

The Amygdala and Depression

As mentioned, **CRH** is one likely transmitter (among several) for evoking fear-related behavior and stress reactions, and the amygdala is an important site of action. CRH also appears to be related to **mood**. Thus, the concentration of CRH in the cerebrospinal fluid is increased in many deeply **depressed patients** and victims of **suicide**. In the latter group, lowered density of the CRH receptor occurred in the frontal lobe (perhaps because of down-regulation due to a constantly increased level of CRH). A transgenic mouse strain overproducing CRH has increased levels of ACTH and cortisol in the blood as expected. In addition, mice from this strain show behavior indicative of anxiety (e.g., the way they behave in novel situations). This behavioral pattern is normalized by supply of CRH antagonists.

Measurement of **regional cerebral blood flow** supports the fact that the function of the amygdala is altered in seriously depressed patients. Thus, compared with a control group, depressed patients had increased blood flow in the left prefrontal cortex and amygdala. This observation does not tell us how the amygdala is involved in depression, however—for example, whether the blood flow changes are secondary to a change of mood or whether changes in the amygdala come first. Further, depression is associated with alterations in many more parts of the brain than the amygdala—supporting the view that mood and emotions depend on activity in distributed networks connecting subcortical and cortical neuronal groups.

SOME ASPECTS OF CORTICAL CONTROL OF AUTONOMIC FUNCTIONS AND EMOTIONS

Assigning specific functions to cortical regions builds on methods that can provide only indirect answers (functional deficits after lesions, blood flow changes associated with certain behaviors, EEG, single neurons recordings, and so forth). Because distributed networks—not single areas—are responsible for the execution of complex tasks, assigning functions to specific regions must be imprecise and simplistic. Although we need "pigeon holes" and labels to aid our thinking, we should bear in mind that our simplifying concepts have limited explanatory power. All cortical areas we mention here with a focus on autonomic functions and emotions are also involved in other tasks (i.e., participate in other networks). For example, most of the cortical areas regulating autonomic functions also participate in processing of emotions and cognition. This is not unexpected, as the autonomic adjustments are an integral part of complex behavioral responses.

Autonomic Functions

Experimental and clinical data show that wide areas of the cerebral cortex influence the activity of structures innervated by the autonomic nervous system. This influence is mainly exerted via the amygdala, the hippocampal formation, and

the septal nuclei, which in turn, influence the hypothalamus and brain stem nuclei. In addition, there are some direct connections from the **insula** and the **orbitofrontal cortex** to the hypothalamus. Further, neocortical areas in the frontal and temporal lobes project to the amygdala and can therefore influence the hypothalamus indirectly.

The **cingulate gyrus**—one of the limbic structures—appears to be involved in organization and initiation of various kinds of **goal-directed behavior**.[3] It projects to the hippocampal formation, to the septal nuclei, and to the amygdala—all of which have connections to various parts of the hypothalamus (Fig. 31.7). Electrical stimulation of the cingulate gyrus elicits a combination of autonomic (visceral) and somatic effects. Autonomic effects include, for example, alterations of **respiration** and **circulation** (reduced rate of breathing, heart rate, and blood pressure), actions in the **digestive tract** (altered peristaltic movements and secretory activity), and **pupillary dilatation**. Somatic effects are expressed mainly as changes of muscle tone and often inhibition of ongoing movements.

Alterations of functions controlled by the autonomic system can be produced by stimulation of parts of the cortex other than the cingulate gyrus. Stimulation of the **orbitofrontal cortex**, the **insula**, and the **pole of the temporal lobe** produces effects similar to those obtained from the cingulate gyrus—that is, combined behavioral, emotional, and autonomic responses (see Chapter 29, under "Central Control of Micturition," and Chapter 34, under "The Insula"). Stimulation of the aforementioned neocortical regions not only produces effects on autonomic functions; somatic functions are altered as well. In contrast, alterations of autonomic functions can occur after stimulation of cortical regions that one might believe to be purely somatic, such as the motor and the premotor cortical areas. Thus, stimulation of the **motor cortex** produces **vasomotor changes** (i.e., changes of the blood-vessel diameter and, therefore, of blood flow) of the opposite body half. On damage to these cortical areas (as seen in patients with a cerebral **stroke**), vasomotor changes often occur in the paralyzed parts of the body. Even alterations of the heart rate and blood pressure and of the digestive tract can occur. As a final example of combined somatic and autonomic effects, stimulation of the **frontal eye field** (see Fig. 25.8) produces pupillary dilatation in addition to the more obvious conjugated eye movements.

---

3. While minor parts of the cingulate gyrus belong to the allocortex, most of it probably belongs to the oldest parts of the neocortex. The terms **limbic** or **paralimbic cortex** are often used of cortical regions that have intimate connections with limbic structures, such as the amygdala and the hippocampus

Figure 31.7

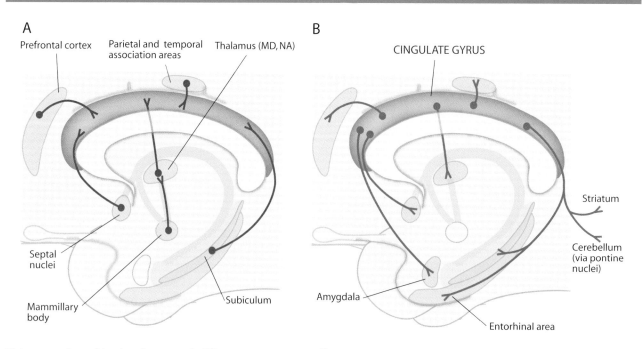

A
Prefrontal cortex
Parietal and temporal association areas
Thalamus (MD, NA)
Septal nuclei
Mammillary body
Subiculum

B
CINGULATE GYRUS
Striatum
Cerebellum (via pontine nuclei)
Amygdala
Entorhinal area

Main connections of the cingulate gyrus. **A:** Afferent connections **B:** Efferent connections. The cingulate gyrus has reciprocal connections with neocortical association areas and with limbic structures and may act as a mediator between them.

Emotions and the Neocortex

As mentioned, cortical areas that show altered activity (as measured with PET and fMRI) in relation to emotions are more extensive that those initially included in the "limbic system" (Fig. 31.8). On the other hand, no area is solely concerned with emotional processing. The **cingulate gyrus** is a pertinent example. Even if it consists of several smaller subdivisions that differ with regard to connections, they all seem to be involved in both cognitive and emotional processing, albeit to a varying degree. The anterior part of the cingulate gyrus (**anterior cingulate cortex [ACC]**) consists of rostral part that is more concerned with affect regulation and a caudal part more concerned with cognitive task. In general, the ACC appears to be important for the choice of behavior in response to **conflicting stimuli**. The ACC also seems to **monitor** mental and bodily processes with a special focus on the detection of errors and conflicts.[4] For this monitoring, emotions

provide important information about values of different signals. Parts of the cingulate gyrus (both anterior and posterior parts) and the anterior **insula** (Fig. 31.8) also alter their activity in relation to emotions such as admiration and **compassion**.

Several parts of the **prefrontal cortex** show altered activity in relation to emotions in humans, and, accordingly, lesions often produce emotional disturbances (see Chapter 34, under "Symptoms after Prefrontal Lesions"). Especially the **orbitofrontal** and **ventromedial parts** seem important for emotional regulation (Fig. 31.8). As mentioned, these parts have reciprocal connections with the amygdala. The orbitofrontal cortex may integrate competing, emotionally colored signals to provide an appropriate response. For example, a study compared the behavior of normal and orbitofrontal-lesioned monkeys in a situation where a snake appeared between the monkey and a piece of food. Presumably, the amygdala informs about the values of the signals (snake and food), whereas the orbitofrontal cortex is necessary for evaluation and appropriate action. Such studies strongly suggest that the orbitofrontal cortex is important for behavioral **flexibility**—that is, the ability to alter behavior when needed and to choose among conflicting choices. Neocortex and emotions are discussed further in Chapter 34.

---

4. Stimulation of the ACC in monkeys produces, for example, **aggressive reactions**, whereas bilateral removal makes the animals tamer. They may also become **socially indifferent**—that is, they appear to have lost interest in other members of their group and do not try to make contact.

Figure 31.8

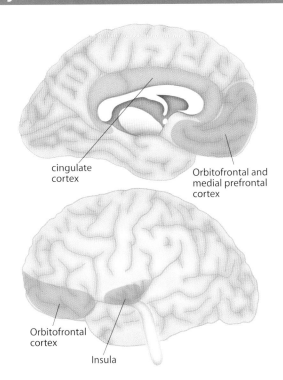

Parts of the cerebral cortex involved in processing of emotions.

Networks for Monitoring Energetic Demands and Fatigue

An interesting hypothesis proposes that a network comprising the amygdala, the nucleus accumbens, the orbitofrontal cortex, the insula, and the ACC monitors the **energetic demands** involved in performing a task (Boksem and Tops 2008). In so doing, the network would need to weigh the potential reward against the energetic cost of a task to reach a decision on whether or not to do it. Presumably, this process would require integration of emotional, motivational, and cognitive signals. The authors furthermore suggest that **mental fatigue** "can best be considered as an adaptive signal that the present behavioural strategy may no longer be the most appropriate . . . fatigue may present the cognitive system with a signal that encourages the organism to lower present goals" (p. 133).

One may speculate whether, regardless of its cause, the feeling of fatigue would be caused by activity in largely the same neuronal network. Figure 31.9 presents this idea, hypothesizing that the feeling of fatigue depends on activity in a distributed network and that this network can be driven by peripheral inputs (caused by inflammation or physical exertion; see Chapter 30, under "Fever" and "Effects of the Immune System on the Nervous System") or by central networks related to evaluation, motivation, and reward. This might resemble closely the situation with the feeling of pain, which we know can be evoked by central as well as peripheral inputs. Fatigue and pain can both be regarded as **alarms**, urging us to change behavior to maintain or reestablish homeostasis.

Below and medial to the well-defined basal ganglia, many neurons are spread out rather diffusely. Unfortunately, the nomenclature for this region is not consistent among authors. Thus, different names are often applied to the region or parts of it without attempting to describe more precisely what is meant. The old anatomists named it the **substantia innominata** (the region without a name), presumably reflecting that nothing was known about its connections and functions. The **basal forebrain** (basal prosencephalon) is usually used synonymously with the substantia innominata. Only recently have its connections, cytochemistry, and functions been clarified, showing that the basal forebrain is not an anatomic or functional unity. It is now commonly accepted to divide the basal forebrain into three overlapping regions, differing regarding neurotransmitters and connections: the **ventral striatopallidum**, the **extended amygdala**, and the **basal nucleus** (Figs. 31.3 and 31.10; also see Fig. 10.3). The ventral striatopallidum was discussed in Chapter 23. We discuss here only certain aspects of the basal forebrain, starting with a large group of cholinergic neurons that are found in the basal nucleus and some adjacent cell groups.

Cholinergic Neurons Projecting to the Cerebral Cortex

Cholinergic neurons of the basal forebrain form a thin disc close to the basal surface of the hemisphere—the **basal nucleus**—and are furthermore found in the **septal nuclei** and the **diagonal band of Broca** that extend dorsally close to the midline (Figs. 31.10 and 31.11). The septal nuclei form the most well-defined anatomic entity among these cell groups and lie just in front of the anterior commissure (Fig. 31.1; also see Fig. 23.15).[5] The diagonal band of Broca forms a transition between the basal nucleus and the septal nuclei.

5. The region containing the septal nuclei is called the precommissural part of the septum (located anterior to the anterior commissure; see Fig. 6.26). The postcommissural part is the **septum pellucidum**, which contains no neurons (see Fig. 6.29).

Figure 31.9

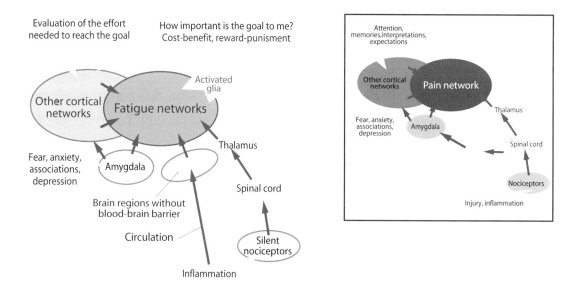

Evaluation of the effort
needed to reach the goal

How important is the goal to me?
Cost-benefit, reward-punisment

Attention,
memories,interpretations,
expectations

Networks responsible for the feeling of fatigue can be driven by peripheral and central inputs. Hypothetical and highly simplified. Inset shows similar diagram for the feeling of pain (cf. Fig. 15.6).

Figure 31.10

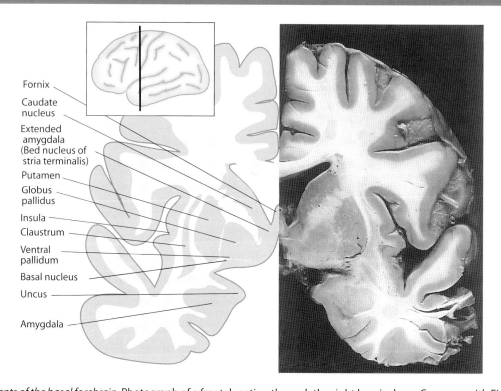

Main components of the basal forebrain. Photograph of a frontal section through the right hemisphere. Compare with Fig. 31.10 showing the nucleus accumbens (ventral striatum) to advantage.

Figure 31.11

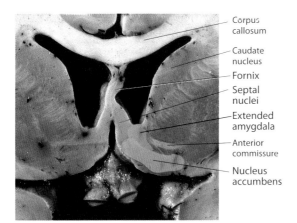

Corpus callosum

Caudate nucleus

Fornix

Septal nuclei

Extended amygdala

Anterior commissure

Nucleus accumbens

The basal forebrain. The positions of three main nuclear components are indicated with different colors in the photograph of a frontal section through the hemisphere (cf. Fig. 23.15).

The Basal Forebrain Also Contains GABAergic Projection Neurons

Not all neurons in the basal forebrain projecting to the cortex are cholinergic. Some neurons, mingled with the cholinergic ones, are **GABAergic.** Some contain the neuropeptide **galanin**, partly colocalized with acetylcholine. In humans the diagonal band of Broca has many **somatostatin**-containing neurons, although it is not known whether they project to the cortex. Thus, although apparently the majority of the neurons in the basal forebrain projecting to the cortex are cholinergic, it is not a transmitter-specific system. This is of relevance when trying to explain the symptoms of diseases with loss of neurons in the basal forebrain (notably **Alzheimer's disease**, discussed in Chapter 10).

The cholinergic (and some GABAergic) neurons of the basal forebrain project to the cerebral cortex (both to the allocortex, including the hippocampus, and the neocortex). The septal nuclei and the diagonal band send fibers mainly to the hippocampal formation, whereas the basal nucleus projects to the neocortex with a rough topographic order.

Although the **afferent** connections of the cholinergic cell groups of the basal forebrain are incompletely known, important inputs arise in the brain stem, notably in the **locus coeruleus** and in cholinergic cell groups in the **dorsolateral pons** (such connections are involved in the ascending activating system discussed in Chapter 26). Further, afferents come from the **hypothalamus**, the **cingulate gyrus**, and the **nucleus accumbens** of the ventral striatum.

The Septal Nuclei

Among the cholinergic cell groups, the **septal nuclei** first attracted interest because early lesion and stimulation experiments showed that they influence autonomic functions, emotions, and behavioral reactions. For example, lesions of the septal nuclei in animals alter sexual and foraging behavior: aggressive behavior appears to be reduced (as stimulation of the septal nuclei can produce aggression). The effects are similar to those produced by lesions of the amygdala and the anterior parts of the cingulate gyrus and presumably can be explained by the connections of the septal nuclei with these parts and the hypothalamus. Symptoms specific to the septal nuclei, constituting the so-called septal syndrome, have not been proved convincingly.

Functional Roles of the Basal Forebrain Cholinergic Neurons

Later studies turned to the role of the cholinergic neurons in **attention** and **memory** mechanisms. Particularly seminal in this respect was the discovery of cell loss in the **basal nucleus** in patients with **Alzheimer's disease**. Some studies in monkeys suggested that the septal nuclei, the diagonal band of Broca, and the basal nucleus all must be destroyed to produce memory impairments. More detailed experimental studies with injection of substances that destroy the cell bodies (but not passing fibers) suggest that the **septal nuclei** and the **diagonal band of Broca** are especially important for **memory** (presumably because of their connections with the hippocampus). Further, there are several clinical reports of patients with small lesions in the anterior parts of the cholinergic cell groups who exhibited clear-cut memory loss (both for recent and past events). One such patient, for example, had a lesion affecting primarily the diagonal band of Broca, as judged via MRI (the difficulties with the exact localization of the damage in such patients warn against firm conclusions, however).

The **basal nucleus** is more concerned with maintaining and perhaps focusing **attention**. Thus, acetylcholine increases the excitability of cortical neurons and enhances the signal/noise ratio, thus improving the precision of specific information processing. Further, many neurons in the basal nucleus increase their firing when an action is rewarded, and other findings also indicate that the basal nucleus' activity is related to **motivation**.

Other Components of the Basal Forebrain: The Ventral Striatopallidum and the Extended Amygdala

The **ventral striatopallidum**—discussed in Chapter 23—consists of the ventral striatum (including the nucleus accumbens) and the ventral pallidum. These parts of the basal forebrain show similarities with the basal ganglia (dorsal striatum and dorsal pallidum) regarding cytoarchitectonics, cytochemistry, and connections (e.g., a dense dopaminergic innervation from the mesencephalon). In contrast to the dorsal striatum (the caudate nucleus and the putamen), which receives the main afferent input from the neocortex, the ventral striatum receives main afferents from the allocortex and the amygdala. A further characteristic of the ventral striatum is that it projects to the hypothalamus and brain stem nuclei, such as the PAG and the motor vagus nuclei. The ventral pallidum projects to the mediodorsal thalamic nucleus that sends fibers to the prefrontal cortex (cf. the projection of the dorsal pallidum to the ventral lateral/ventral anterior thalamic nuclei that project mainly to the premotor areas).

Another rather diffuse cell group in the basal forebrain, continuous with the ventral pallidum, is called the **extended amygdala** because it forms a rostral extension of the medial amygdala (Figs. 31.10 and 31.11). Most of it is made up of the **bed nucleus of the stria terminalis** (Figs. 31.6 and 36.10). The stria terminalis is a bundle of efferent fibers from the amygdala to the septal nuclei and the hypothalamus (Fig. 31.5). The bed nucleus lies medial to the pallidum at the same anteroposterior level and further anterior to the anterior commissure (i.e., close to the septal nuclei). Sometimes this part of the basal forebrain is lumped with the amygdala because they share many transmitters and connections. The anatomic distinction between the extended amygdala and the nucleus accumbens is not sharp, however, and both receive, for example, dopaminergic fibers from the mesencephalon.

The Medial Forebrain Bundle

Many fibers interconnecting the various limbic structures are located in a diffusely delimited, parasagittal fiber mass in the basal part of the hemisphere. This ill-defined structure is called the **medial forebrain bundle** and passes through the lateral parts of the hypothalamus. It extends from the region of the anterior commissure anteriorly and into the mesencephalon posteriorly. Most of the fibers are short, interconnecting nuclei found close to each other, such as the septal nuclei, other nuclei in the basal forebrain, various hypothalamic nuclei, and the PAG in the mesencephalon (see Fig. 31.4). Fibers from the **monoaminergic** cell groups of the brain stem pass through the medial forebrain bundle on their way to forebrain structures, such as the cortex (including the hippocampal formation). Functionally, the medial forebrain bundle is heterogeneous, and lesions of it would affect the function of many neuronal groups and fiber tracts.

The hippocampus and nearby areas in the parahippocampal gyrus (the dentate gyrus and the entorhinal area) comprise the **hippocampal formation**, which plays a crucial role for certain kinds of learning and memory. The quantitatively dominating **afferent inputs** to the dentate gyrus and the hippocampus arise in the **entorhinal area**. The entorhinal area receives afferents from both nearby areas in the temporal lobe and cortical association areas. Thereby, it receives highly processed sensory information—that is, about all important events. The hippocampal projection neurons send signals via intermediaries to several areas, notably back to the entorhinal area and to the mammillary nucleus. Thus, the hippocampus acts largely back onto the areas from which it receives information.

Bilateral damage of the hippocampal formation leads to **amnesia**—impaired memory without intellectual reduction. Lesions restricted to the hippocampus proper also produce amnesia, although it is much less severe than when the whole hippocampal formation has been damaged.

We can roughly distinguish two kinds of memory: one kind concerns the memory of events and facts and is called **declarative** or **explicit** memory; the other concerns skills and habits and is called **nondeclarative** or **implicit** memory. Only declarative memory depends critically on the integrity of medial parts of the temporal lobe. For nondeclarative memory, the basal ganglia, cerebellum, and parts of the neocortex appear to be most important.

Certainly, the hippocampal formation is not the only part of the brain that is important for memory. Parts of the parahippocampal gyrus outside the hippocampal formation appear to play an independent role in memory formation and retrieval. Further, amnesia has also been reported after lesions of the **medial thalamus**, and cholinergic cell groups

of the basal forebrain also have a role (presumably by way of their connections with the hippocampus). Finally, the **amygdala** is crucial for learning of associations between stimuli and their emotional value.

The hippocampal formation appears to be important for memory only for a certain time after an event. Thus, isolated damage of the hippocampal formation does not usually abolish recall of older memories, although it prevents the learning of new material. This is probably because, after a certain time, the memory traces are stored in many parts of the cerebral cortex.

Macroscopic Appearance and Constituent Parts

The **hippocampal formation** consists of the **hippocampus** and nearby regions in the temporal lobe: the **dentate gyrus**, the **subiculum**, and the **entorhinal area** (located in the parahippocampal gyrus; Figs. 32.1 and 32.2, see also Fig. 6.26). Whereas interest formerly was directed mainly to the hippocampus itself, it is now realized that the function of the hippocampus can be understood only in conjunction with the nearby structures in the parahippocampal gyrus, which are closely interconnected with each other and with the hippocampus. Although the hippocampus is included among the limbic structures (see Fig. 31.1), its functional role is distinct from that of the amygdala, the septal nuclei, and the cingulate gyrus. The amygdala and the hippocampal formation are, for example, both crucial for learning and memory but for different kinds.

The **hippocampus** (Figs. 32.1 and 32.3; also see Figs. 6.31 and 31.2) forms an elongated bulge medially in the temporal

Figure 32.1

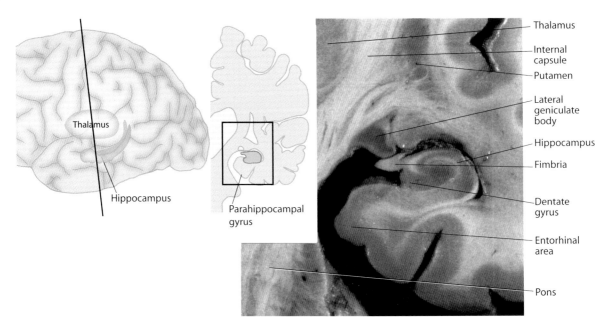

The hippocampus. Photograph of a frontal section through the left hemisphere. The hippocampus forms a continuation of the temporal cortex, as an invagination of the temporal horn of the lateral ventricle. Fig. 22.2 shows the whole section. Compare Figs. 31.1 and 31.2.

Figure 32.2

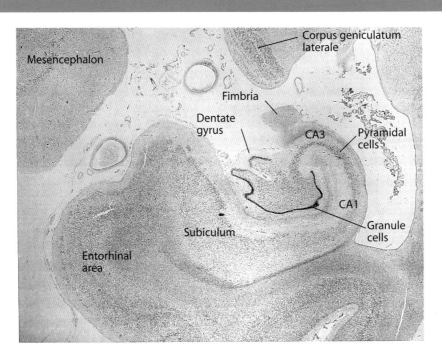

The hippocampal formation. Photomicrograph of thionine-stained frontal section through the human temporal lobe. The temporal horn of the lateral ventricle with some of the choroid plexus is seen above and to the right of the hippocampus. The mesencephalon with the crus and the substantia nigra is seen to the left. Compare with Fig. 32.1.

Figure 32.3

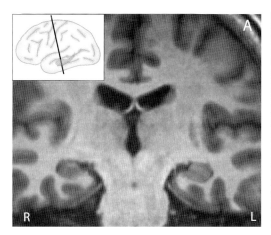
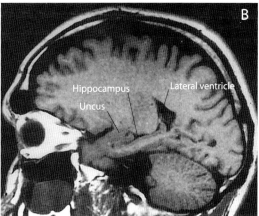

MRIs showing the hippocampus. **A:** Frontal plane. The hippocampus is positioned medially in the temporal lobe (green on the left side). Inset shows approximate position of the hippocampus in the temporal lobe and the plane of sectioning. **B:** Parasagittal plane through the medial part of the temporal lobe. (Courtesy of Dr. S. J. Bakke, Oslo University Hospital, Oslo, Norway.)

horn of the lateral ventricle, produced during early development by invagination of the ventricular wall by the hippocampal sulcus (see Fig. 9.12). The hippocampus is easily recognized in thionine-stained microscopic sections by its conspicuous layer of pyramidal cells (Fig. 32.2). Along the medial aspect of the hippocampus, the **dentate gyrus** forms a narrow, notched band (Fig. 32.1; also see Fig. 31.2). Microscopically, the narrow, dark layer of small granule cells is characteristic (Fig. 32.2). The hippocampus and the dentate gyrus belong to the allocortex and have a simplified laminar pattern compared with the neocortex. Nevertheless, they are far from simply built, with several different cell types and precisely organized, complex patterns of connections. Figure 32.2 shows that the hippocampus (the CA1 field) continues into the **subiculum** but with a marked change in the thickness and organization of layers (both have three neuronal layers). The transition between the subiculum and the **entorhinal cortex** is marked with the appearance of a six-layered cortex.

Two Main Sets of Connections

Two salient features help to simplify the multifarious connections of the hippocampal formation:

1. Dense reciprocal connections with **cortical association areas**

2. Direct and indirect connections with the **amygdala, septal nuclei**, and the **cingulate gyrus**

In interplay with the cerebral cortex, the hippocampal formation obviously handles vast amounts of processed sensory information. That the hippocampus has increased in size in parallel with the cerebral cortex during evolution further supports that its main functions are related to neocortical processes. A large number of **commissural fibers** ensure close cooperation between the hippocampi of the two sides.

Afferent Connections of the Hippocampal Formation

The main afferents to the **dentate gyrus** arise in the entorhinal area Figs. 32.4 and 32.5). Because the dentate gyrus sends its efferents to the hippocampus, the **entorhinal area** is the quantitatively dominating deliverer of information to the hippocampus. Smaller but functionally important contingents to the hippocampal formation come from the **septal nuclei** and **monoaminergic cell groups** in the brain stem (the locus coeruleus and the raphe nuclei). In addition, some fibers come from the **hypothalamus** and several **thalamic nuclei**. Finally, the **amygdala** projects to the subiculum and the entorhinal area. The latter connections most likely contribute to the well-known effect of emotions on learning, as discussed in Chapter 31 (see "The Amygdala, Learning, and Unlearning").

To understand the nature of the information processed by the hippocampus, we must know the afferent connections of the **entorhinal area**. Studies with retrograde transport in monkeys have shown that most **association areas**

Figure 32.4

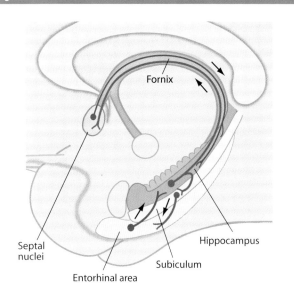

Some main connections of the hippocampus. The connections with the entorhinal area mediate specific, highly processed sensory information, whereas the connections with the septal nuclei are modulatory.

of the neocortex influence the entorhinal area. Signals reach the entorhinal area directly or indirectly by means of fibers to other areas in the parahippocampal gyrus, which, in turn, project to the entorhinal area. Thus, the majority of direct entorhinal afferents arise in adjacent parts of the **parahippocampal gyrus** (see Figs. 6.26 and 31.1) and in the **perirhinal cortex** (located around the rhinal sulcus; see Fig. 19.3). These areas form a continuous cortical region, although different parts are not identical regarding connections. Together, the region receives **visual** information from extrastriate areas in the inferior part of the temporal lobe, **auditory** information from the superior part of the temporal lobe, **somatosensory** information from the posterior parietal cortex, and information from **polysensory** association areas—that is, areas that integrate several sensory modalities. Finally, afferents arrive from the **cingulate gyrus**, the **insula**, and the **prefrontal cortex**. Together, the entorhinal area receives highly processed sensory information. We assume, for example, that information about words comes to the hippocampus regardless of whether we see (read), hear, or read by touch (Braille writing).

Figure 32.5

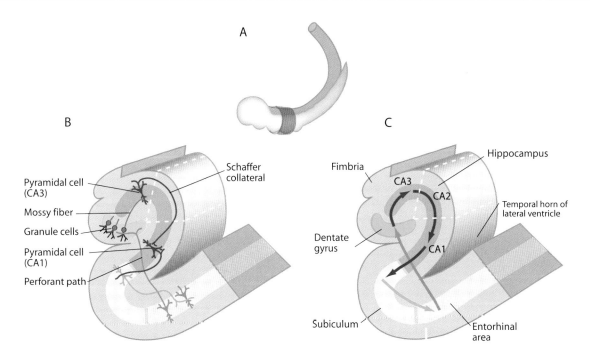

Signal pathways through the hippocampus. Schematics of a frontal slice through the hippocampus, as shown in **A** (cf. Fig. 31.2). **B:** Major kinds of neurons in the hippocampus and the course of their axons (not all collaterals are shown). **C:** The flow of signals through the hippocampal formation. The pathway emanates from and returns to the entorhinal area, which has widespread connections with cortical association areas.

The cortical areas that provide the entorhinal area (and thus the hippocampus) with its main inputs project to other areas as well. For example, both the **perirhinal cortex** and the **subiculum** project to the **mediodorsal thalamic nucleus** (MD), which projects to the prefrontal cortex and parts of the cingulate gyrus. This might explain why **amnesia** (memory loss) is more severe after damage of the perirhinal cortex and the areas neighboring the entorhinal area than after a lesion restricted to the entorhinal area and the hippocampus (we return to this point later).

Modulatory Afferents Increase Hippocampal Plasticity

Although hippocampal afferents from the **septal nuclei** (Fig. 32.4) are not numerous, they have an important functional role. Many of the septohippocampal neurons release **acetylcholine** as a modulatory transmitter, increasing the excitability of the hippocampal pyramidal cells. Further, the hippocampal afferents from the **raphe nuclei** (serotonin) and the **locus coeruleus** (norepinephrine) have modulatory effects on the hippocampal cells. Thus, there is evidence that hippocampal **long-term potentiation** (LTP; see later discussion) is reduced after pharmacologic removal of monoamines from the hippocampus. These modulatory pathways may mediate the effects of attention and motivation, which we know have profound influences on both learning and memory.

Efferent Connections of the Hippocampal Formation

Comparison of the efferent connections with the afferent ones shows that the hippocampal formation has largely **reciprocal** connections with subcortical and cortical areas. Thus, we must assume that whatever the hippocampus is doing, it requires a constant exchange of information with many other areas. Indeed, this is supported by animal experiments and observations in humans showing that the activity in the hippocampal formation and certain parts of the cortex is synchronized in conjunction with aspects of learning and memory.

There are **three parallel pathways** out of the hippocampal formation to cortical areas, but they all eventually reach primarily association areas in the temporal and frontal lobes.

1. The major pathway goes from the entorhinal area to adjacent areas in the **parahippocampal gyrus** and

the **perirhinal cortex** and from there to more distant areas, notably the tip of the temporal lobe, medial and orbital parts of the **prefrontal cortex** (including the cingulate gyrus), and **polysensory areas** in the superior temporal gyrus.

2. A parallel pathway goes directly from the entorhinal area to the same areas that receive the indirect connections.

3. A third pathway goes directly from the **CA1** and the **subiculum** to neocortical areas.

In addition to these neocortical projections, the subiculum sends many fibers to the **mammillary body** (passing in the fornix), which then influences the **cingulate gyrus** via the anterior thalamic nucleus (see Fig. 30.7).[1] Some fibers in the fornix pass to the **nucleus accumbens** and the **ventromedial hypothalamus**. The subiculum also sends fibers to the **amygdala**. Thus, signals from the hippocampus can influence neuronal groups that are closely related to emotions and motivation.

The connections from the hippocampus to the subiculum—and from the subiculum to other areas—are **topographically organized**. For example, a longitudinal subicular zone close to the dentate gyrus projects to the allocortex and nucleus accumbens, whereas a longitudinal zone farther from the dentate gyrus projects to the cingulate gyrus. Thus, as different parts have different connections, symptoms after lesions may be expected to vary with their exact localization within the hippocampal formation. Some controversies among authors regarding the effects of hippocampal lesions on memory are probably due to disregard of such anatomic facts.

Hippocampal Architecture and Intrinsic Connections

Most of the neurons of the dentate gyrus are small **granule cells**, whereas the only well-defined hippocampal cell layer consists of large **pyramidal cells** (Fig. 32.5B). Above and below the pyramidal cell layer are layers that contain the pyramidal cell dendrites and incoming axons. There are also various kinds of

---

1. Until the mid-1970s it was believed that most efferents from the hippocampus were directed to the mammillary body, passing in the fornix (fibers destined for the mammillary body comprise the majority of the fornix fibers). This was based on the erroneous assumption that all axons in the fornix came from hippocampal pyramidal cells. Papez and the postulated circuit interconnecting the limbic structures presumably influenced this view on hippocampal efferents (see Chapter 31 under "The Circuit of Papez"). With the introduction of methods using axonal transport of radioactively labeled amino acids, however, it was shown that the fornix fibers originate in the subiculum.

interneurons, notably the GABAergic **basket cells**, which inhibit the pyramidal cells. The hippocampus can be divided into three **longitudinal zones**, named CA1 to CA3 (Figs. 32.2 and 32.5C). The granule cell axons contact the pyramidal cell dendrites, and the pyramidal cells send axons out of the hippocampus.

Even though the internal architecture of the hippocampus is rather complicated, with several neuronal types with complex interconnections, a relatively simple main transmission route from input to output appears to exist (Fig. 32.5C). This pathway starts in the entorhinal area and has three synaptic interruptions. Neurons in the entorhinal area send their axons, forming the so-called **perforant path**, to the hippocampus, where many end in the dentate gyrus (Fig. 32.5B). The axons of the granule cells of the dentate gyrus, called **mossy fibers**, end primarily on the apical dendrites of the pyramidal cells of CA3. The CA3 pyramidal cells send so-called **Schaffer collaterals** to the apical dendrite of the CA1 pyramidal cells (Fig. 32.5B). From CA1 a significant part of the signal traffic goes to the subiculum and from there to the entorhinal area, thus closing the circuit that passes from the entorhinal area through the hippocampus and back to the entorhinal area. All links in this pathway are excitatory, using **glutamate** as neurotransmitter.

Figure 32.5 gives the impression that signal transmission is confined to a plane perpendicular to the long axis of the hippocampus. Thus, the hippocampus would seem to be organized in numerous **lamellas**, with each lamella presumably representing a functional unit.

While the signal pathway shown in Figure 32.5 appears to be central to hippocampal information processing, the conditions are more complex. For example, the fibers of the perforant path not only contact granule cells of the dentate gyrus but also end directly on the hippocampal pyramidal cells. Thus, several parallel pathways enter the hippocampus. Further, anatomic investigations performed in monkeys show that the efferent fibers from a narrow transverse zone of the entorhinal area extend for a considerable distance longitudinally in the hippocampus. Thus, each entorhinal efferent neuron can presumably contact neurons in many hippocampal lamellas. Further, the collaterals of the hippocampal pyramidal neurons extend not only in the plane of the lamellae (as shown in Fig. 32.5) but also longitudinally. In fact, it is still not clear what should be regarded as a **functional unit** within the hippocampus and the degree of functional localization present.

FUNCTIONAL ASPECTS

Before discussing further the functions of the hippocampal formation, some words about learning and memory may be useful. The following is a very superficial treatment of a large and important field with many controversies. The words "learning" and "memory" have been used numerous times in this book without further discussion of their meaning, assuming (perhaps naïvely) that we all agree on what is meant in the specific context. However, when greater precision is needed, it quickly becomes

evident that neuroscientist do not use terms related to learning and memory in a way that satisfies the philosopher's need of conceptual stringency and clarity (Bennett and Hacker, 2003, pp. 154–171). It should also be emphasized that the different forms of learning and memory are not as independent as this simplified presentation may suggest.

Kinds of Learning

Much of our learning is **associative**: we learn from experience that two phenomena occur together. This holds for **classic conditioning** (learning of a conditioned response), when one stimulus always follows another, and for **operant conditioning,** in which we learn that a certain behavior produces a certain response. An example of operant conditioning is a hungry rat that learns by trial and error to press a lever to obtain food. In the same situation later, the rat knows what the appropriate behavior is. Not all learning is associative, however. With constant exposure to a stimulus, the response is altered—an example is ceasing to notice a loud sound we have heard many times. This is called **habituation**. The response may also increase with repeated exposure, as with painful stimuli (**sensitization**).

Other, more complex kinds of learning are **nonassociative**, such as learning by **imitation** elements of language and movement patterns. Further, **learning by insight**—that is, the realization of a problem's solution without any real-world trial and error—is of crucial importance for humans. Usually, however, learning in real life—as opposed to experimental situations—includes several of these forms at the same time.

Kinds of Memory

One distinction concerns the duration of a memory, and we usually distinguish between **short-term** and **long-term memory** (see Chapter 4, under "Short-Term Plasticity" and "Long-term Plasticity: LTP and LTD"). The former refers to the temporary retaining of information, necessary for its initial manipulation—lasting up to about a minute. The term **working memory** is now preferred for the retaining and early manipulation of information. Another broad classification concerns the memory of **how** (to ride a bicycle, to write, to use a hammer, and so forth) and memory of **that** (e.g., that Mount Everest is 8,848 m high, that I visited my grandmother yesterday, and so forth). In line with this classification, it is customary in the neuroscientific literature to distinguish two main kinds of memory: **explicit** or **declarative** memory and **implicit, procedural,** or **nondeclarative** memory. Declarative memory depends on the integrity of the medial temporal lobe (including the hippocampus)[2], whereas nondeclarative memory depends primarily on the basal ganglia, the cerebellum, and parts of the cerebral cortex (see Chapter 22, under "Learning and the Motor Cortex," Chapter 23, under "What Activates the Dopaminergic Neurons?" and "Functions of the Basal Ganglia," and Chapter 24, under "Mossy and Climbing Fibers Mediate Different Kinds of Information" and "The Cerebellum and Learning").

In contrast, **nondeclarative** memory is needed to learn and perform **skills** (riding a bicycle, dress, use a knife and fork, etc.). **Habits** and **attitudes** also largely fall in this category. The learning leads to altered behavior but not so that the stored material can be subject to a conscious analysis. With skills like playing an instrument or doing arithmetic, the stored information becomes accessible only by performing the skill (memory of *how*). In ordinary teaching situations, much of the learning is implicit—for example, the acquisition of attitudes of which both the teacher and the student are unaware.

In everyday situations and activities, however, the two main kinds of memory are not necessarily distinguishable. For example, in most cases procedural memory requires some aspects of knowledge of facts (memory of *that*) about the activity. The skills of an expert tennis player, for example, are not purely a matter of motor skills but depend also on knowledge-based selection of the right actions, as pointed out by Stanley and Krakauer (2013).

Episodic, Semantic, and Autobiographic Memory

Declarative memory is of two main kinds. **Episodic memory** concerns episodes and events from one's own life ("Where did I put the scissors?"). Afterward we can recall the episode, often

in the form of pictures, which may be described verbally (memory of *what*). **Semantic memory** concerns general knowledge about the world we live in (the capital of Italy, the first president of the United States, the location of the post office, the letters of the alphabet, and so forth). **Autobiographic** memory—that is, the ability to remember events from one's own life—usually combines episodic and semantic memory but also involves memory processes dependent on the amygdala (emotional coloring) and several parts of the cortex (Fig. 32.6). Common to declarative memories is that we, as a rule, must consciously "search our minds" to recall them.

The Hippocampal Formation and Spatial Navigation

One central task of the hippocampal formation—in animals and humans—seems to be **spatial orientation** and **navigation**. Indeed, imaging studies of London taxi drivers suggested correlation between the size of the hippocampus and duration of navigational training (animal experiments have found the same effect). Properties of single hippocampal cells, as first described by O'Keefe and Nadel (1978), are of particular interest in this connection. Thus, the firing of single hippocampal neurons—called **place cells**—changes with the position of the animal in relation to its surroundings: for example, the firing pattern changes with the location of the animal in different corners of the cage. The hippocampal formation obviously receives information

Figure 32.6

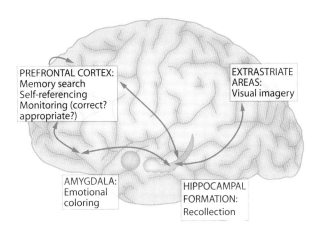

Network serving autobiographical memory. Some of the regions showing increased activity in relation to retrieval of autobiographic memories, as revealed by fMRI. (Based on Cabeza and Jacques 2007.)

---

2. One striking piece of evidence comes from patients with **Alzheimer's disease** (affecting medial parts of the temporal lobe early in the disease process) who have markedly impaired declarative memory whereas the ability to learn new skills is relatively preserved. Also, observations of patients with memory deficits after lesions of the medial temporal lobe (without dementia) indicate that they learn and remember new movements better than new faces, words, places, and so forth.

about starting position, the direction of movement, and the distance moved. Based on such experiments, O'Keefe and Nadel proposed that the hippocampal neurons together form a **cognitive map** of our surroundings. The field was moved further by meticulous studies of the properties of single neurons in the entorhinal cortex, which determine the properties of the hippocampal place cells (for a historical review, see Moser and Moser 2013). Entorhinal neurons are topographically arranged according to their spatial receptive fields. Each neuron fires when the animal occupies specific positions in a field, and these positions forms a **grid pattern**. Different **grid cells** (neurons) have the same grid pattern, but the position and orientation of the grid fields vary from cell to cell. Together, the grid cells produce a systematic map of the surroundings. Indeed, the activity of a few neurons can code for the position of a rat with a few centimeters' accuracy. Other neurons in the entorhinal area are **border cells,** which respond to barriers to movements, and **head-direction cells**, which code for the head direction of the animal. It is not quite clear how the properties of the hippocampal place cells are formed by the input from the entorhinal neurons. Neither is it fully understood how afferents to the entorhinal area form the properties of grid cells. It seems clear, however, that the hippocampus builds a map of the space around us and keeps track as we move around.

In agreement with the single cell studies, **lesions of the hippocampus** in rats severely reduce their ability to find their way back to previous locations. Further, monkeys with lesions of the hippocampal formation have difficulties remembering where an object is located—that is, to associate an object with its location.

How to Combine Spatial Navigation and Declarative Memory

One of the great challenges in understanding the hippocampus is to combine its role in spatial navigation and spatial memory with its undeniable importance for **declarative memory**. Recent animal experiments suggest that both tasks may be carried out simultaneously: neuronal populations may at the same time signal *where* something happens and *what* is going on. Such a double role might—loosely considered—fit with the everyday experience that recall depends strongly on **context**. For example, experiments with divers show that a series of numbers learned under water is better recalled under water than on dry land. Similarly, when unable to recall why we went into a room,

it sometimes helps to go back to the place where we first had the idea.

Relationship between Memory and Long-Term Potentiation

The cellular basis of brain plasticity is discussed in Chapter 4 (under "Synaptic Plasticity"). Because the hippocampus is involved in learning and memory, it is of special interest that the synapses are plastic at several steps in the circuit shown in Fig. 31.4. Thus, their efficacy can be increased for a long time after intensive stimulation. Indeed, **long-term potentiation** (LTP) was first discovered in the hippocampus, although it was later found in many other areas of the brain, among them the cerebral cortex and the amygdala. LTP is produced whenever the hippocampal pyramidal cells are subjected to excitatory inputs—for example, from the Schaffer collaterals (Fig. 32.5B)—while they are in a depolarized state (i.e., caused by another excitatory input). Thus, simultaneous synaptic activation of the cell from two sources can make it "remember," in the sense that the next time the cell is activated by the same fibers, the postsynaptic effects are stronger than before.

To demonstrate a direct relationship between LTP and learning is difficult, however. For example, only specific subsets of synapses in widely distributed networks are likely to show LTP in a natural learning situation. To look for such altered synapses would seem like looking for "a needle in a haystack." Nevertheless, much indirect evidence supports that hippocampal LTP is related to learning and memory. Increased synaptic efficacy has been found in the hippocampus in rats housed in an environment rich in stimuli and challenges (assuming that more learning takes place in such a situation than in a standard cage). LTP-like phenomena have also been observed in the hippocampus after specific training situations. Another piece of evidence is that **N-methyl-D-aspartate (NMDA)-receptor** antagonists both prevent induction of LTP and reduce learning and memory in experimental animals. Gene-technological manipulations have produced strains of mice in which hippocampal LTP cannot be induced, and these animals also show reduced learning ability. Finally, structural synaptic changes have been observed in the hippocampus in conjunction with the induction of LTP. Even more compelling, structural synaptic changes (formation of new synapses and splitting of spines into two) have been reported in the hippocampus in rats at the time they improve their performance in a learning situation.

Making Memory Traces Permanent: The Hippocampal–Cortical Dialogue

In humans, the amnesia after lesions of the hippocampus and surrounding structures is predominantly anterograde, with retrograde amnesia for some years (depending on the size of the lesion). This has been taken as evidence that synaptic changes related to specific events are only temporarily retained in the hippocampus, before permanent changes are established in other parts of the brain. Other clinical observations of patients with damage in various parts of the brain indicate that well-consolidated memories are retained in a distributed fashion. When a memory is consolidated—presumably as long-term synaptic changes—the hippocampal formation may no longer be necessary for recall. The time required to reach this stage is not known, but based on observations of patients with damage to medial parts of the temporal lobe, it probably takes a year or more. During this period, we imagine a gradual consolidation of the synaptic changes in the relevant parts of the cortex and in subcortical structures. It seems unlikely that the information is first held in the hippocampus for a certain period and then transmitted out to the permanent stores in a finally processed form. More likely, the consolidation takes place by a continuous "**dialogue**" between the hippocampus and other parts of the cortex. The special **theta rhythm** (6–10 Hz) in hippocampus is probably related to information encoding and memory recall. For example, coupling between the hippocampus and the prefrontal cortex seems to happen by means of synchronized theta oscillations. Sleep may be of special importance for the dialogue, as witnessed by specific patterns of synchronized activity in the hippocampus and in cortical areas that are particularly active during the learning phase (see Chapter 26, under "Dreaming"). Further, it appears that every time a memory is recalled, it becomes labile and can be modified before renewed consolidation occurs. This is presumably the basis of the well-known modifications of childhood memories that are recalled and retold over and over again. New material and insights are unconsciously put into the story.

Medial Parts of the Temporal Lobe and Amnesia

The belief that the hippocampus is of importance for memory goes back to the end of the nineteenth century and was based on careful examination of patients with **amnesia** (loss of memory) as a result of brain damage (Fig. 32.7).

The Hippocampus Is Not Necessary for Short-Term Memory

Various memory tests are used in experiments with monkeys to study the relationship between brain structures and memory. One common test is the so-called **delayed nonmatching-to-sample** test. The monkey is briefly shown an object. After a

Figure 32.7

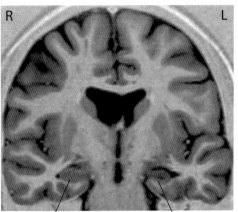

Hippocampus (normal)   Hippocampus (atrophic)

MRI in the frontal plane showing hippocampal atrophy on the left side. A nearby focus of epileptic activity is most likely the cause of hippocampal cell loss, causing so-called mesial temporal sclerosis. (Courtesy of Dr. S.J. Bakke, Oslo University Hospital, Oslo, Norway.)

certain time, the same object is shown along with a new one. To receive a reward (e.g., orange juice), the monkey must move the new object, thus showing that it remembers which one was seen before. The experiment goes on with continually new pairs of items. With a brief interval between the first and second presentation, the performance is independent of the integrity of medial temporal structures. With intervals above 10 sec, however, the frequency of errors increases in monkeys with such lesions as a sign of failing memory. With more than 2-min intervals, the performance is no better than chance, whereas normal monkeys reduce their performance to only about 80% with intervals of 3 min.

It should be emphasized that although short-term memory can be taken care of without the hippocampal formation, this does not rule out the possibility of hippocampal involvement in an intact animal. Thus, brain-imaging data showing hippocampal activation in tests for short-term memory are not necessarily in conflict with the aforementioned experimental findings.

Patients with severe **amnesia** that is not accompanied by intellectual reduction (dementia) typically have lesions that affect the medial parts of the temporal lobe (and often also the medial parts of the thalamus). Such lesions include the hippocampal formation as the most constant finding. The amnesia is **anterograde**—that is, the memory is lost for events that take place after the time of the brain damage (inability to retain newly learned material). There are also varying degrees of **retrograde amnesia**—that is, the patient is unable to recall events that took place before the damage.

"Knowledge Systems of the Brain"

In a wide sense, memories constitute our knowledge of the world and the actions that are necessary to relate successfully to it. Not all this knowledge is accessible for conscious "inspection" and analysis, however. Nevertheless, all memories presumably depend on synaptic changes in specific parts of the central nervous system. Damasio and Tranel (1992) use the term "knowledge systems of the brain" about the widespread networks dedicated to specific tasks.

Examples are knowledge systems dealing with social interactions, faces, objects, language, or ourselves. Although a part of the temporal lobe cortex is particularly important for recognition of faces, this does not necessarily mean that all information about faces is retained there. More likely, this part is unique because it has access to face-related information retained in many other areas. Presumably, the recognition of faces fails after a stroke in the temporal lobe because there is "no one" to activate the relevant networks, not because all synaptic changes pertaining to faces are lost.

PART EIGHT

The Cerebral Cortex

The human cerebral cortex consists of about 20 billion neurons and constitutes more than half of all gray matter of the central nervous system. This gives a rough impression of its functional importance. In lower vertebrates, there are only very modest primordia of the cerebral cortex (allocortex), and it was first in mammals, particularly anthropoid apes and humans, that the cerebral cortex came to dominate the rest of the nervous system quantitatively. This enormous increase in the volume of the cortex necessitated a marked folding of the surface of the hemisphere. The outer layer of the human cerebral cortex is around 0.2 m², but only one-third of this is exposed on the surface. The **neocortex** constitutes most of the cerebral cortex in higher mammals, and this part deals only with the neocortex. In Chapter 33 we deal mainly with the structure and connections of the cerebral cortex from a functional perspective. In Chapter 34 we discuss the complex tasks attended to by the cortical association areas, which make up the bulk of the human cerebral cortex. In previous chapters we treated the role of the cerebral cortex in sensory processes (Chapters 14–19), control of body and eye movements (Chapters 22 and 25), autonomic functions and emotions (Chapter 31), and memory (Chapter 32). The role of the cerebral cortex in relation to sleep and consciousness is briefly discussed in Chapter 26.

The Cerebral Cortex: Intrinsic Organization and Connections

In this chapter we address two levels of organization. The first concerns information processing in a small volume of cortex; the second level concerns the interconnection of functionally different cortical units with long association and commissural fibers. These connections are essential parts of distributed, task-specific cortical networks.

The neurons of the neocortex are arranged in **six layers** parallel to the cortical surface. The layers differ with regard to afferent and efferent connections. In general, layers 2 and 4 are receiving, whereas layers 3 and 5 are mainly efferent. The bulk of afferents from the thalamus end in lamina 4, whereas layer 5 gives origin to subcortical tracts to the cord, brain stem, and basal ganglia. Layers 2 and 3 receive and send out most of the corticocortical fibers, interconnecting various parts of the cortex.

The cortex is divided into numerous **cytoarchitectonic** areas that differ with regard to connections and functional specializations. At a microstructural level, the cortical neurons are arranged in smaller **modules**, often in the form of **columns** perpendicular to the cortical surface. Each column, containing some thousand neurons, represents a computational unit. The neurons of the columns communicate with each other and with neurons in neighboring and distant columns.

There are two main kinds of cortical neuron: the **pyramidal cells** with long axons destined for other parts of the cortex or subcortical targets and **interneurons** (with numerous subtypes) with short axons remaining in the cortical gray matter. The pyramidal cells are **glutamatergic**; whereas all interneurons are **GABAergic** (γ-aminobutyric acid [GABA] is colocalized with different combinations of neuropeptides). In addition, **modulatory transmitters**, such as dopamine and acetylcholine, regulate the cortical excitability level and the signal-to-noise ratio of cortical neurons.

Cortical **connections** fall into four groups. One group of afferents consists of precise, topographically organized connections from the **specific thalamic nuclei**; each thalamic nucleus supplies one particular part of the cortex. Another afferent group consists of diffusely organized connections from the **intralaminar thalamic nuclei** and several other **subcortical nuclei** (releasing modulatory transmitters). The two final groups—making up the majority of all cortical connections—consist of corticocortical fibers, that is, **association fibers** and **commissural fibers**. Association fibers are precisely organized connections linking cortical areas within the same hemisphere, while commissural fibers pass in the corpus callosum and connect areas in the two hemispheres. The **efferent** connections of the cerebral cortex can also be divided into **subcortical** and **corticocortical** ones (association and commissural connections). The subcortical fibers are destined for the thalamus, the striatum, various brain stem nuclei (among them the pontine nuclei projecting to the cerebellum), and the spinal cord. The corticocortical connections are for the most part **reciprocal**—that is, an area receives fibers from the same areas to which it sends fibers.

STRUCTURE OF THE CEREBRAL CORTEX

Levels of Organization

To understand the relationship between the performance of the cerebral cortex and the underlying neural processes, we need to address two levels of organization. The first concerns information processing in a small volume of cortex; we may term this **intracortical** synaptic organization. The second level concerns the interconnection of functionally different cortical units with long association and commissural fibers, which we term **interareal** synaptic organization. How are signals arriving in a small bit of the cortex treated before "answers" are sent to other parts of the cortex or subcortical nuclei? How are the many different cortical areas interconnected to form networks designed for solving specific tasks? The enormous number of neurons and synaptic couplings in the human cerebral cortex explain why we do not have complete answers to such questions. For example, about 100,000 neurons reside below 1 mm^2 of cortical surface (rodent primary somatosensory cortex ([SI], and each neuron receives synaptic contacts from at least some hundred other neurons. Further, the tasks of the cerebral cortex are the most complex of all. To understand the relationship between the "machinery" of the brain and mental functions such as personality, memory, thought, and feelings is indeed the most formidable and exciting challenge of modern neuroscience.

The Neocortex Consists of Six Layers

All parts of the neocortex have a common basic structure, with the neurons arranged in six layers, or **laminae**, oriented parallel to the surface of the cortex (Figs. 33.1 and 33.2). Another general feature is the arrangement of the neurons in rows or **columns** oriented perpendicular to the cortical surface (Figs. 33.2 and 33.3). Both kinds of cellular aggregation relate to functional specializations among the neurons, as we discuss later. Figure 33.1 shows the main features of the layering. It can be seen that the laminar pattern arises because cells of similar shape and size are collected in more or less distinct layers. The density of cell bodies also differs among the layers.

Figure 33.1

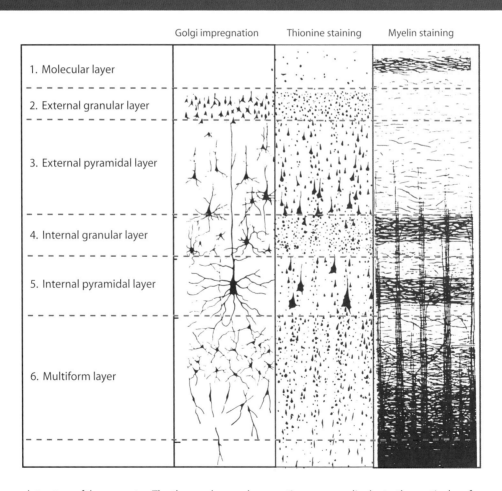

Golgi impregnation   Thionine staining   Myelin staining

1. Molecular layer
2. External granular layer
3. External pyramidal layer
4. Internal granular layer
5. Internal pyramidal layer
6. Multiform layer

The basic six-layered structure of the neocortex. The three columns show sections perpendicular to the cortical surface subjected to different staining methods. **Left:** Appearance in Golgi-impregnated sections, in which the cell bodies and some of the dendrites can be seen. **Middle:** A thionine-stained section in which only the cell bodies are visible. **Right:** Appearance after myelin staining—that is, the main pattern of the myelinated axons is evident, with perpendicular bundles of fibers entering the cortex and horizontal bundles of fibers interconnecting nearby parts of the cortex. Compare Figs. 33.6 and 33.7.

Figure 33.2

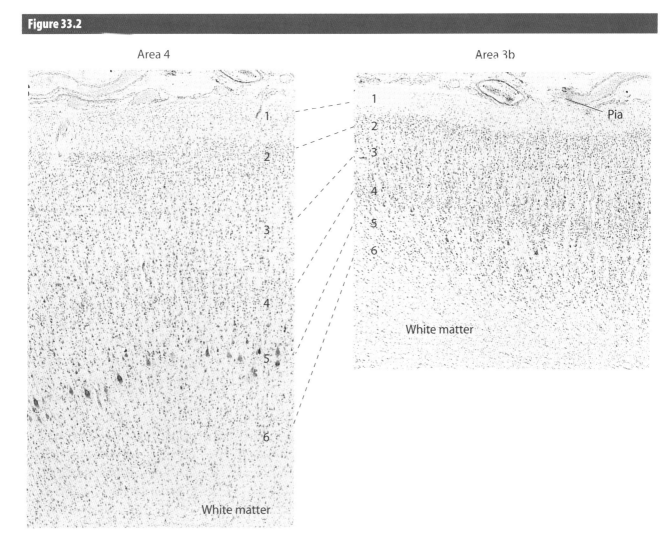

Area 4

Area 3b

Pia

White matter

White matter

Cytoarchitectonics of the cerebral cortex. Photomicrograph of a thionine-stained section through the central region of the human brain. The section is perpendicular to the direction of the central sulcus. The six-layered structure is evident in area 4 (MI) and in area 3b (SI), but development and appearance of the various layers are different in the two areas, especially with regard to layers 4 and 5. The MI in the precentral gyrus is much thicker than the SI. This is not because there are more neurons but because of more extensive dendritic trees, more axonal branches and boutons, and perhaps more glial cells. There is a tendency for the cells to be arranged in vertically oriented rows or columns. See also Fig. 12.3 with a corresponding section from the monkey. Magnification, ×170.

About two-thirds of the neurons are cortical **pyramidal cells** (the name refers to the triangular shape of their cell bodies; Fig. 33.3). A typical pyramidal cell has a long **axon** arising from the base of the pyramid and a long **apical dendrite** that extends toward the cortical surface; it thus extends through several layers superficial to the layer in which the cell body is located. The large pyramidal cells lie in layers 3 and 5, but many of the smaller cells in the other layers are also pyramidal. The large number of **dendritic spines** further characterizes the pyramidal cells (see Fig. 1.1). The rest of the cortical neurons constitute a heterogeneous group with neurons whose cell bodies are not

pyramidal; such neurons are therefore lumped together as **nonpyramidal** cells. Their shape and size vary considerably, but all of them are most likely interneurons. Some of the nonpyramidal cells are multipolar and are called **stellate cells**. Others are called **basket cells** because their axonal branches form a wickerwork around the cell bodies of pyramidal cells. In addition, several other varieties of interneurons are given names that, as a rule, reflect the shape of the neuron.

The most superficial cortical layer, **layer 1**, the **molecular layer**, is rich in fibers but has few neurons (Figs. 33.1 and 33.2). Apart from axons, it contains the apical dendrites of

The Cerebral Cortex Can Be Divided into Cytoarchitectonic Areas

Even though all parts of the neocortex consist of six cell layers, the thickness and structure of the various layers vary from one area to another. This is observed most easily in sections stained to visualize the cell bodies only (Figs. 33.2, 33.5; also see Fig. 22.4). Such **cytoarchitectonic** differences form the basis of the subdivision of the entire cortex into cytoarchitectonic **areas**, as was done around the turn of the twentieth century by Brodmann (1909) and others (Fig. 33.4). This is briefly described in Chapter 6,

and several of the cytoarchitectonic areas are mentioned in previous chapters. The development of cytoarchitectonic areas is briefly discussed in Chapter 9, (under "Specification of Cortical Cytoarchitectonic Areas").

The main importance of the division of the cortex into cytoarchitectonic areas is that these areas have proved in many instances to differ functionally, even though they were initially defined solely on the basis of the size, shape, and arrangement of the neuronal cell bodies. In many cases, a cytoarchitectonically defined area is unique with regard to its afferent and efferent connections and the physiologic properties of its cells.

Figure 33.4

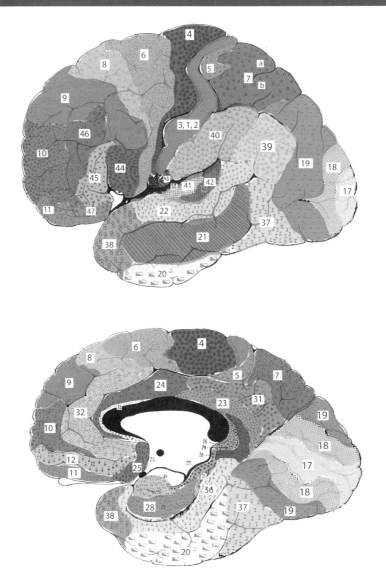

Brodmann's cytoarchitectonic map of the human brain. The various areas are labeled with different symbols and numbers (from Brodmann 1909). Colors have been added to facilitate the distinction of areas.

Although the borders between different cytoarchitectonic areas are sometimes easy to identify, as exemplified in the section of the visual cortex shown in Fig. 33.5, more often the differences are rather subtle. Thus, it should not come as a surprise that authors often disagree with regard to the parcellation of the cortex into areas. Today we try to define a cortical area not only based on cytoarchitectonics but also additional criteria, such as fiber connections, cellular markers, recordings of single-cell activity, and the behavioral effects of stimulation or ablation of the area in question. We return to connections and functions of different cortical areas later in this chapter.

Individual Differences in the Size of Cortical Areas

With regard to **the size of cortical areas**, there are surprisingly large **individual differences**. For example, the volume of the striate area (the most easily identified one) varies by a factor of three among adult humans, and similar differences have been documented for the somatosensory cortex, the auditory cortex, and the prefrontal cortical areas. Because the volume of the hemispheres does not show similar variations, this implies that in a brain with a large striate area, other areas are relatively smaller. Whether such anatomic differences also have functional significance is unknown, but, conceivably, they may contribute to the large differences between humans in mental and other capacities. This idea receives support from comparisons of quantitative

MRI data (measuring gray-matter volume) and people's performance in cognitive tests. For example, the size **of area 10** (at the frontal pole; Fig. 33.4) correlated with the person's **metacognitive ability** (i.e., thinking about one's own thinking). Another example is that the surface area of the anterior **cingulate gyrus** was found to correlate with degree of **cognitive control** (self-regulation). Further, the volume of subdivisions of the posterior parietal cortex was found to correlate with the outcome of tests that are known to depend on the parietal cortex. Interestingly, if one parietal subdivision was larger than average, another was usually smaller.

Intracortical Connectivity: Interneurons and Pyramidal Cell Collaterals

The **pyramidal cells** send their axon toward the white matter to reach other parts of the cortex or subcortical cell groups. Thus, they are the **projection neurons** of the cortex (Figs. 33.3B and 33.6), which most likely constitute more than two-thirds of all cortical neurons. The projection neurons send **recurrent collaterals** before the axon leaves the cortex and can thus influence the level of activity among the cortical neurons in their vicinity. The recurrent collaterals may, for example, excite inhibitory interneurons and thereby limit the activity of the parent cell and other pyramidal cells.

Figure 33.5

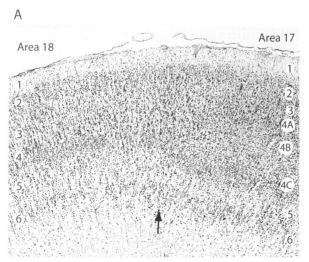
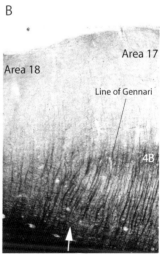

The transition between area 17 (the striate area) and area 18. **A:** Thionine-stained section from the human visual cortex. The various layers change in cell size, cell density, and thickness at the transition between the two cytoarchitectonic areas. Lamina 4 is particularly well developed in area 17 and is subdivided into sublayers (4A–4C). **B:** Section from the same region stained to show myelinated nerve fibers. Note the myelinated fibers running parallel with the cortical surface in lamina 4B (the line of Gennari). See Fig. 16.17, which shows the macroscopic appearance of the line of Gennari. Most areal borders are less clear-cut than the border between areas 17 and 18.

The enormous number of neurons and their complex interconnections within even a small volume of cortical tissue explains why we still do not understand the basic rules underlying intracortical information processing. Promising advances have been made, however, especially in the visual cortex.

Intracortical Signal Traffic in the Visual Cortex

Regarding intracortical signal traffic, detailed studies have been performed in the visual cortex with the use of methods enabling the recording of single-cell activity in relation to specific stimuli and subsequent intracellular injection of horseradish peroxidase. Thus, the dendritic and axonal patterns of individual, functionally characterized neurons can be determined. Successful attempts have also been made to abolish the activity of neurons in specific layers and then study how the properties of neurons in other layers are changed. As expected from the known terminal pattern of axons from the lateral geniculate body, neurons are first activated in **layer 4** after visual stimuli (in addition, neurons in other layers with dendrites extending into layer 4 can be influenced). From layer 4, the excitation is propagated to **layers 2** and **3**, and from there to **layers 5** and **6**. Some cells in layer 6 send axons upward to layer 4. Presumably, at every step in such a pathway through the cortex some processing of the sensory information takes place, such as integration by one neuron of the signals from other, functionally different neurons. In accordance with this assumption, the functional properties of neurons in different layers vary, as shown with microelectrode recordings after natural stimulation of receptors. A projection neuron in layer 5 has quite different properties than a cell in layer 4; for example, the receptive fields of the layer 5 cells are larger (as a sign of convergence of signals from several neurons in layer 4). Other properties of layer 5 neuron also suggest that signals from functionally different layer 4 neurons converge on layer 5 cells (via processing in layers 2 and 3).

Cortical Neurons Are Coincidence Detectors

Many cortical neurons react primarily when information about two events reaches them simultaneously, like cells in the visual cortex that respond poorly to signals from one eye only but vigorously to simultaneous signals from both eyes (binocular cells). Like a good detective who has a special eye for **coincidences** (events occurring simultaneously) and disregards numerous trivial bits of information, the cortical neurons respond preferentially to certain coincidences of stimuli that have a survival value. This is the basis for **association learning**, that is, learning the relationship between cause and effect. We know that a novel or unexpected stimulus, or one occurring in an unusual context, causes arousal and improved retention of new material. Often, synaptic changes occur when a neuron receives simultaneously a specific input about a stimulus or the context and a modulatory input (e.g., acetylcholine from the basal nucleus) signaling the salience of the specific input (see Fig. 4.11).

Glutamatergic **thalamocortical fibers** appear to act through **AMPA** receptors on cortical neurons but not through NMDA receptors (the latter being related to induction of long-term potentiation [LTP]). The recurrent pyramidal cell collaterals, however, act also on **NMDA** receptors. Experimental evidence shows that simultaneous activation of a cortical neuron from the thalamus (AMPA) and from other cortical neurons (NMDA) can induce **LTP**. In the monkey MI, LTP has been established during the learning of new motor skills. Thus, not only are the cortical neurons especially sensitive to coincident inputs, but they may also be the cellular basis of associative learning in the cortex.

Horizontal Integration and Cortical Plasticity

The extensive horizontal intracortical connections appear to be crucial for the working of the cortex. They help explain why the response of so many cortical neurons depends on the **context** of a stimulus (cf. Chapter 16, under "Color Constancy"). As mentioned, horizontal connections ensure that the **receptive fields** of cortical neurons are not static but subject to modification by inputs from their neighbors. For example, single cells in the visual cortex have smaller receptive fields and react more strongly when the **attention** of the animal is directed to the visual stimulus. Horizontal connections most likely also contribute to well-known **psychophysical phenomena**, such as the **filling in** of missing lines in otherwise meaningful visual images (cf. Chapter 16, under "The Blind Spot on the Retina"). When blocking GABA receptors (and thus inhibitory horizontal connections), the receptive fields of cortical neurons enlarge immediately; for example, stimulation of a small peripheral spot activates an area in the SI that is much larger than before. Further, after **amputation** of a finger in monkeys, the area in the SI activated from the neighboring fingers enlarges immediately. These examples show that there must exist excitatory connections in the cortex that are **suppressed** under ordinary conditions. Due to such modifiable connections there is a **dynamic balance** between the cortical representations of various body parts. Presumably, rapid shifts in dynamic balance in cortical networks underlie rapid alterations of the experience of one's own body, such as in **conversion disorders** and **hypnosis**.

Training of a sensory task can alter the cortical representation of the trained part (e.g., training roughness discrimination with the index finger). It seems likely that such examples of **cortical plasticity** are due, at least partly, to changes in the synaptic efficacy of horizontal connections. The same mechanism probably operates during **recovery** after brain damage that affected the cerebral cortex or its connections (see Chapter 11, under "Animal Experiments Elucidating the Mechanisms of Recovery").

CONNECTIONS OF THE CEREBRAL CORTEX

The connections of the cerebral cortex with subcortical structures are described in several of the previous chapters, where we deal with the terminal regions of the major sensory pathways and the areas that give origin to the descending pathways involved in motor control. Here we describe general aspects of connections between the **thalamus** and the cerebral cortex and of the **corticocortical connections** (association and commissural connections). Such knowledge is a necessary basis for the treatment in Chapter 34 of the functional roles of the cortical association areas.

A Brief Survey of Cortical Connections

We can classify the **afferent** connections of the cerebral cortex as follows:

1. Precise, topographically organized connections from the **"specific" thalamic nuclei**; each thalamic nucleus supplies one particular part of the cortex.

2. Diffusely organized connections from the **intralaminar thalamic nuclei** and several other **subcortical nuclei** (the raphe nuclei, the nucleus coeruleus, dopaminergic cell groups in the mesencephalon, and cholinergic cell groups in the basal forebrain); such connections do not respect the cytoarchitectonic borders in contrast to the connections from the specific thalamic nuclei.

3. **Association fibers**—that is, precisely organized connections linking cortical areas within the same hemisphere.

4. **Commissural fibers**—that is, precisely organized connections between areas in the two hemispheres.

The **efferent** connections of the cerebral cortex can also be divided into **subcortical** and **corticocortical** ones (association and commissural connections). The subcortical fibers are destined for the thalamus, the striatum, various brain stem nuclei (among them the pontine nuclei projecting to the cerebellum), and the spinal cord. The corticocortical connections are for the most part **reciprocal**—that is, an area receives fibers from the same areas to which it sends fibers.

Specific Thalamocortical Connections

The thalamus has been mentioned in several contexts (see Chapters 6 and 14 for descriptions of its gross anatomy and main subdivisions). The thalamus supplies all parts of the neocortex with afferents. Each part of the cortex receives fibers primarily from one of the **specific thalamic nuclei**. The main features of this topographic arrangement of the thalamocortical projection are shown in Fig. 33.8 (as we believe it is organized in humans). Figure 33.9 shows the main thalamic subdivisions in a frontal section.

Conditions are more complex than shown in the diagrams, however. First, the topographic arrangement is much more fine-grained. Thus, the projection from one thalamic nucleus is precisely arranged, with subdivisions of the nucleus supplying minor parts only of the large fields shown in Fig. 33.8. As described in Chapters 14 and 16, the thalamocortical connections from the VPL and the lateral geniculate body are somatotopically and retinotopically organized, respectively, with a precision that enables the cortex to extract information about minute spatial details. Further, each thalamic nucleus sends fibers to more than one cortical area. We can take the **mediodorsal nucleus (MD)** as an example. In the scheme, it is depicted as sending fibers to the prefrontal cortex (without any topographic arrangement). In reality, the MD sends fibers to other parts of the cortex too, such as parts of the cingulate gyrus. The MD furthermore consists of several subdivisions, each supplying a different part of the prefrontal cortex. The main point emerging from such knowledge is that the MD is not a functional unit. A small lesion, for example, must be expected to produce quite different effects, depending on its exact location within the MD.

Some of the specific thalamic nuclei are relay stations in the pathways for signals from **sensory receptors** to specific cortical areas (vision, hearing, cutaneous sensation, etc.). The **ventral posterolateral nucleus** (VPL) receives afferents from the somatosensory pathways and projects to

Figure 33.8

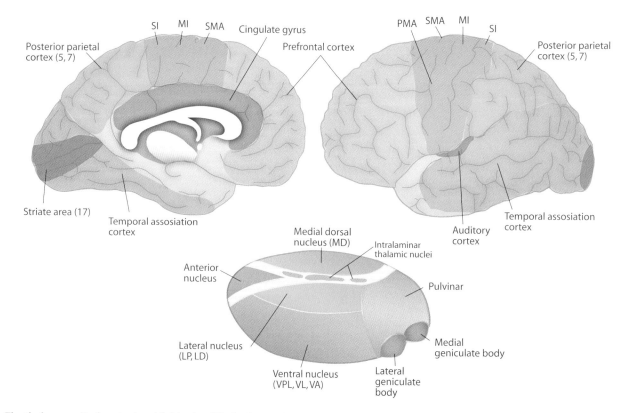

The thalamocortical projection. Highly simplified scheme showing the main features of its topographic organization. Overlap exists between the cortical terminal regions of different thalamic nuclei but is not shown in the figure.

Figure 33.9

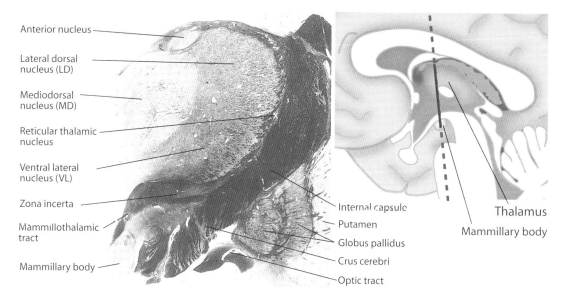

The thalamus. Frontal section through the middle part of the human thalamus. Schematic; myelin stained. (See also Figs. 6.23, 6.27, and 6.30.)

the SI (areas 3, 1, and 2; see Figs. 14.2, 14.4, and 14.6); the **lateral geniculate body** or nucleus receives afferents from the retina and projects to the striate area (see Figs. 16.14 and 16.20); the **medial geniculate body** is the last subcortical station in the auditory pathways, and it sends efferents to the primary auditory area (AI), see Figs. 17.9 and 17.11). Other specific thalamic nuclei, the **ventrolateral nucleus** (VL) and the **ventral anterior nucleus** (VA), are relay stations in the pathways from the cerebellum and the basal ganglia to the motor and premotor cortical areas (see Fig. 24.16). Other thalamic nuclei relay signals from limbic structures: the **anterior thalamic nucleus** receives afferents from the mammillary body (which receives its main input from the hippocampal formation) and projects to the cingulate gyrus; and the MD (Fig. 33.8) can relay signals from the amygdala to the prefrontal cortex (see Fig. 31.5). The posterior parietal cortex (areas 5 and 7) receives fibers from the posterior part of the thalamus, the **lateral posterior nucleus** (LP), and parts of the **pulvinar** (Fig. 33.8). Other parts of the pulvinar projects to the temporal lobe. The LP and the pulvinar receive afferents from nuclei related to vision and eye movements, such as the **superior colliculus** and the **pretectal nuclei**, and may relay such information to the posterior parietal cortex (see also Chapter 25, under "Cortical Control of Eye Movements"). However, the pulvinar is not primarily a relay nucleus but a link in a cortico–thalamic–cortical circuit, as we mention later when discussing corticothalamic connections.

The Corticothalamic Connections

All of the thalamic nuclei receive massive **back-projections** from the cerebral cortex. In fact, the number of corticothalamic fibers is much higher than the number of thalamocortical fibers; for example, the relationship for the VPL has been estimated to 7:1. Yet the corticothalamic connections have until recently received relatively little attention. The largest thalamic nuclei, with weak or no inputs from peripheral sense organs, have reciprocal connections with association areas in the parietal, temporal, and frontal lobes (e.g., the pulvinar and the MD).

In general, the nuclei receive afferents from the cortical areas to which they send their efferents—that is, the thalamocortical and the corticothalamic connections are **reciprocal**. The corticothalamic projections are also precisely, topographically organized. As mentioned, corticothalamic neurons have their cell bodies mainly in **layer 6**, whereas projections to other subcortical nuclei arise mainly in layer 5.

This indicates that the information received by the thalamus is not simply a copy of information sent from the cortex to other regions.

In view of the massive corticothalamic connections, the function of the thalamus cannot be limited to mediating information from subcortical cell groups to the cortex. Even for "relay" nuclei such as VPL, merely quantitative considerations show that crosstalk with the cerebral cortex must be of major importance. All thalamic nuclei receive and presumably process vast amounts of information from the cortex and are therefore intimately involved in processes taking place in the cortex itself. That the corticothalamic fibers really influence the information processing in the thalamus is witnessed by several observations. For example, the receptive fields of neurons in the VPL increase dramatically if their synaptic input from the SI is removed. The same holds true for neurons in the lateral geniculate body and their input from the striate area. Thus, the cerebral cortex exerts strong top-down control of the signals it is going to receive. Equally important, the corticothalamic connections influence the **firing pattern** of the thalamocortical neurons (burst or single-spike firing; see Chapter 26, under "Thalamocortical Neurons Have Two States of Activity"). For example, the feedback from the cortex governs the **synchronization of spindle oscillations** (burst firing) in various parts of the thalamus during early stages of **sleep**.

Higher-Order Thalamic Nuclei

Some authors use the term **first-order thalamic nuclei** for those receiving inputs from peripheral sense organs (e.g., the VPL and the lateral geniculate body), which serve as relay stations in the large sensory pathways. Nuclei not receiving such direct sensory inputs (such as the pulvinar and the MD) are termed **higher-order thalamic nuclei** (Sherman 2005). In spite of constituting the largest part of the human thalamus, their functional roles have attracted less interest than the sensory thalamic nuclei. Due to their massive reciprocal connections with the cerebral cortex, they probably serve as important "dialogue partners" for the cortical association areas. One task of higher-order nuclei may be to coordinate the activity within **cortical networks**. (Cortical afferents from the pulvinar have been found to act preferentially on corticocortical neurons.) Subcortical inputs to higher-order thalamic nuclei from the amygdala and the hippocampus have an important influence on **cognitive functions** related to the prefrontal cortex. Furthermore, inactivation of the pulvinar in monkeys causes impaired eye–hand coordination (in spite of normal vision and motor control). The monkeys also show signs of **neglect** (lack of attention to sensory stimuli without sensory loss). This may perhaps be due to deficient coordination (synchronization) within a **frontoparietal network**.

The Intralaminar Thalamic Nuclei

Modern tracer studies have shown that the cortical projections from each of the intralaminar nuclei end in certain parts of the cortex only; for example, the **contralateral nucleus** sends fibers predominantly to the parietal cortex. Nevertheless, the projections are considerably more widespread and diffuse than those from the specific thalamic nuclei and do not respect areal borders (the intralaminar nuclei were formerly termed the "unspecific thalamic nuclei"). Physiologic studies indicate that the intralaminar nuclei exert general effects on the **excitability** of cortical neurons. Thus, electrical stimulation produces a so-called **recruiting response** in extensive parts of the cortex, which resembles the **EEG** changes associated with **arousal** (desynchronization; see Chapter 26). The coactivation of cortical neurons by signals from the specific thalamic nuclei and the intralaminar nuclei may be important for the binding of specific stimuli with their salience—that is, a form of **coincidence detection** that perhaps may be necessary for awareness of the stimulus.

The tasks of the intralaminar nuclei are related not only to the cerebral cortex; they have even stronger connections with the **striatum** (see Chapter 23, under "Thalamostriatal Connections: Goal-Directed Learning?"). Such connections are precisely organized (another fact speaking against the use of the term "unspecific thalamic nuclei").

Extrathalamic, Modulatory Connections to the Cerebral Cortex

Apart from the major thalamocortical connections, several subcortical nuclei provide sparser cortical inputs without synaptic interruption in the thalamus (the **raphe nuclei**, the **locus coeruleus**, the mesencephalic **ventral tegmental area** [VTA], the **basal nucleus**, and the **tuberomammillary nucleus** in the hypothalamus). These nuclei supply most of the central nervous system with modulatory inputs and are in involved in a number of functions, as discussed in previous chapters. Briefly stated, the fibers from the aforementioned nuclei exert a modulatory control over the **excitability level** of cortical neurons with relation to **wakefulness** and **phases of sleep**. In addition, they probably control more specifically selected cortical neuronal groups when attention is focused on salient stimuli.

All of these transmitter-specific nuclei project to large parts of the cortex with no distinct topographic pattern.

Nevertheless, recent studies in monkeys show that each nucleus (and thus fibers with a particular transmitter) projects with a higher density to some than to other parts of the cortex. For example, **dopaminergic fibers** from the VTA end with the highest density in the prefrontal and temporal neocortex, whereas **noradrenergic** fibers from the locus coeruleus innervate especially the central region (MI, SI). Further, fibers from the various nuclei end in somewhat different cortical layers. A striking feature of the fibers is that, after having entered the cortex, they run **horizontally** for a considerable distance (in contrast to the vertical organization of the afferents from the specific thalamic nuclei). Further, their actions are partly mediated by **volume transmission**. (See Chapter 5, under "Modulatory Transmitter 'Systems,'" and Chapter 26, under "Signal Pathways and Transmitters Responsible for Cortical Activation.")

Inhibition in the Thalamus: Interneurons and the Reticular Thalamic Nuclei

Inhibitory interneurons—the majority **GABAergic**—probably constitute one-fourth or more of all neurons in some of the human thalamic nuclei. In the thalamic sensory relay nuclei, the inhibitory interneurons may contribute to the enhancement of stimulus contrasts (by lateral inhibition) and to selection of certain kinds of stimuli by suppressing other kinds (e.g., in relation to transmission of signals from nociceptors). **Opioid peptides** and other neuropeptides (such as **substance P**) are present in several of the thalamic nuclei, including those relaying nociceptive signals.

The **reticular thalamic nucleus** is unique among the thalamic nuclei because virtually all neurons are **GABAergic**. The nucleus, which forms a thin shell at the lateral aspect of the thalamus (Fig. 33.9), sends its efferent fibers in the medial direction to end in the other thalamic nuclei (and not to the cortex, differing also in this respect from the other thalamic nuclei). Both the corticothalamic and the thalamocortical fibers pass through the reticular nucleus on their way to and from the thalamus and give off numerous collaterals that end in the nucleus (Fig. 33.10). Further, the reticular nucleus receives afferents from the **mesencephalic reticular formation** and has reciprocal connections with the periaqueductal gray (**PAG**), which, among other things, is related to the control of transmission of signals from nociceptors.

The function of the reticular thalamic nucleus is not fully understood, but its connections indicate that it can influence the activity of thalamocortical neurons and thus, indirectly, the activity of the cerebral cortex. Indeed, electrophysiologic studies show that the reticular nucleus can **synchronize** the activity of neurons throughout the thalamus. Further, its activity correlates closely with changes of the **EEG** during sleep and wakefulness. Its relation to **attention** and **control of sensory information**, transfer to the cortex may explain why lesions of the reticular nucleus reduce learning and memory (of spatial tasks).

Figure 33.10

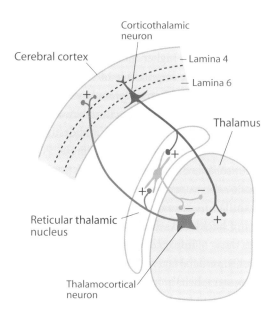

Reciprocal thalamic connections with the cerebral cortex and the reticular thalamic nucleus. Thalamocortical and corticothalamic fibers give off collaterals to the reticular thalamic nucleus. The neurons in this nucleus are GABAergic and influence significantly the functional state of the thalamocortical neurons.

Figure 33.11

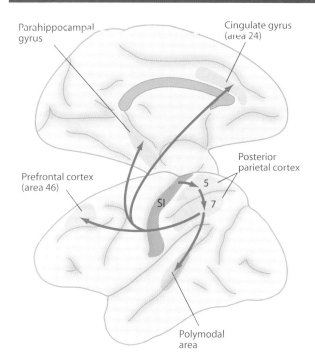

Association connections of the somatosensory cortex (monkey). Only some fiber connections are shown, to illustrate the flow of information progressing from the SI to the posterior parietal cortical areas, and from there to polysensory areas in the temporal lobe, to the prefrontal cortex, and to limbic cortical regions. (Based on Jones and Powell 1970.)

Corticocortical Connections

Vast numbers of corticocortical (association) fibers ensure cooperation among the cortical areas. The *shortest* association fibers connect minor parts within one area (so-called **U fibers**), whereas somewhat longer fibers link together neighboring areas (Fig. 33.3). For example, there are ample connections between the SI and area 5 posteriorly and the MI anteriorly. The MI furthermore receives association fibers from the premotor area and supplementary motor area. The *longest* association fibers interconnect functionally related areas in different lobes: for example, connections from the extrastriate visual areas and the posterior parietal cortex lead to the premotor and prefrontal areas.

When we follow the association connections "outward" from the **primary sensory areas** (SI, VI, and AI), signals first reach **unimodal** association areas—that is, areas that process only on sensory modality (Figs. 33.11 and 33.12). From there, association fibers pass to **polymodal** areas—that is, areas that integrate sensory information of different modalities. One area integrates somatosensory and visual information, another visual and auditory, and so forth. The areas outside the primary sensory areas (such as the areas of the posterior parietal cortex and the extrastriate areas) send their efferent projections not

only to their immediate neighbors but also to distant areas in the frontal lobe (premotor and prefrontal areas) and to "limbic" cortical areas (the cingulate gyrus and the hippocampal gyrus) (Figs. 33.11 and 33.12).

The association areas are densely interconnected. Probably, each association area sends efferent connections to 10 to 20 other areas (although the connections differ in strength). Thus, there is a considerable **divergence** of information. At the same time, there is also considerable **convergence**, as each area receives afferents from several other areas (Figs. 33.11 and 33.12 give very simplified accounts). At the cellular level, the extensive association connections enable neurons to integrate many different pieces of information and to act as **coincidence detectors**, as discussed in the preceding text.

Anatomic and Functional Connectivity

The corticocortical connections provide rich opportunities for communication among cortical neurons at different levels of information processing and constitute the anatomic

34 Functions of the Neocortex

OVERVIEW

This chapter deals primarily with functional aspects of the cortical **association areas**, that is, parts of the cortex that neither receive direct sensory information through the major sensory pathways nor send direct fibers to subcortical motor nuclei. All of the cerebral lobes contain association areas, according to this definition. In Chapter 33 we discuss the connections of the association areas in general. Here we look at the main groups of association areas and their possible functions. It should be realized, however, that the functional roles of a group of association areas, for example, those of the frontal lobe, can be understood only if considered as part of distributed, task-specific networks involving other association areas and subcortical nuclei.

Typically, the association areas receive and **integrate** various kinds of information. Some are specialized for integration of two or more sensory modalities; others integrate highly processed sensory information with information about intentions and goals. The integrative capacity depends on proper use of sensory information and must be learned in early childhood.

The **posterior parietal cortex** integrates visual and somatosensory information and is responsible for, among other functions, the control of **visually guided behavior** and **spatial orientation**. From the parietal areas, signals pass to premotor and motor areas. The posterior parietal cortical areas also have reciprocal connections with the cingulate gyrus and the prefrontal cortex, mediating the influence of emotions, attention, and motivation on behavior produced by somatosensory and visual stimuli.

The **prefrontal cortex**, situated in front of the frontal lobe motor areas, receives information about all sensory modalities and also about the motivational and emotional state of the individual. It is of special importance for planning and initiation of **goal-directed behavior**. More specifically, the prefrontal cortex is important for attention, for selection of a specific behavior among several possible ones, and for suppression of unwanted behavior. These functions are of particular importance for **social behavior**.

The **temporal association areas** are particularly concerned with high-level processing of auditory and visual information. The cortex of the superior temporal gyrus is characterized by its connections with the auditory cortex, whereas the inferior part of the temporal lobe—the **inferotemporal cortex**—is dominated by processed visual information important for object recognition. The **medial parts** of the temporal lobe are of special importance for learning and memory, as discussed in Chapter 32.

The **insula**, hidden in the lateral sulcus, receives all kinds of sensory information and is involved in pain perception, homeostasis, and bodily awareness.

Language and speech depends on a distributed network with two special hubs, one in the frontal lobe (**Broca's area**) and one at the temporoparietal junction (**Wernicke's area**). The anterior (frontal) area is particularly important for the expressive aspects of speech, while the posterior area is more concerned with the sensory aspects.

The left hemisphere is **dominant** for speech in 95% of the population. We also discuss further examples of hemispheric specialization (lateralization). The **corpus callosum** ensures that the two halves of the brain operate as a unit.

Finally, we discuss possible biologic bases of **cognitive gender differences**.

ASSOCIATION AREAS: GENERAL ASPECTS

Functional aspects for several cortical areas are discussed in previous chapters. Here we address primarily functions that can be ascribed to the so-called **association areas** of the cerebral cortex. This term is not precisely defined but is traditionally used for parts of the cortex that neither receive direct sensory information through the major sensory pathways nor send direct fibers to subcortical motor nuclei. All of the cerebral lobes contain association areas, according to this definition.

The connections of the association areas indicate that they are able to integrate information from sensory and "limbic" parts of the cortex (i.e., the cingulate gyrus, parts of the prefrontal cortex, and the hippocampal region) and thereafter issue commands to motor cortical areas and (indirectly) to the hypothalamus.

Comparison of the cerebral hemispheres of humans and monkeys shows that the association areas occupy a much larger fraction of the total in humans. Comparison of monkeys with other mammals, such as cats and dogs, shows again that the main difference between them with regard to the cerebral cortex is the relative size of the association areas. These parts of the cortex are of importance for what we may loosely call **higher mental functions**. The association areas are not "centers" for specific mental faculties, however. First, several areas—often widely separated—participate in one task or function, and one area participates in more than one function. This is witnessed by the high degree of divergence and convergence of the connections of the association areas, as discussed in Chapter 33. Second, the operations of the association areas cannot be understood if considered in isolation; the intimate connections between the association areas and subcortical neuronal groups, such as the thalamus, basal ganglia, amygdala, and hippocampus, are essential for their normal functioning.

Measurements of **regional cerebral blood flow** and metabolism during the performance of various **cognitive tasks** indicate that large parts of the cortex participate in all higher mental functions. When a person is asked to **imagine** that he or she is walking from one place to another in a city he or she knows, the activity increases in the extrastriate visual areas, the posterior parietal cortex, parts of the temporal lobe, and several prefrontal areas. Solving a **mathematical** problem activates many of the same cortical areas but with certain differences, and a **verbal** task activates multiple areas that partly coincide with and partly differ from those activated in the spatial and the mathematical tasks. In Chapter 16 we discussed the cortical substrate of visual imagery under "Visual Awareness and Synchronized Network Activity."

Cognition and Cognitive Functions

The word **cognition** stems from the Latin word *cognitio*, meaning "acknowledge, come to know." According to the *Encyclopedia Britannica*, cognition "includes every mental process that can be described as an experience of knowing as distinguished from an experience of feeling or of willing. It includes, in short, all processes of consciousness by which knowledge is built up, including perceiving, recognizing, conceiving, and reasoning." Among neuroscientists today, the word is often used more broadly to include the **affective** aspects of higher mental functions. For example, the scholarly book *The New Cognitive Neurosciences* (2000) edited by Michael Gazzaniga deals not only with consciousness, language, memory, attention, and similar phenomena but also with emotions. This presumably reflects the realization that there is no sharp distinction between brain structures that govern rational thought and actions on the one hand and those that underlie emotions and subconscious drives on the other.

Task-Specific Networks

The brain receives innumerable pieces of sensory information, which to a large extent are treated in separate systems. For example, separate neuronal populations encode different features of objects, such as color, form, movement, surface texture, heaviness, and so forth. With regard to representation of space, the brain appears to possess several "maps." Yet we experience our surroundings and ourselves as entities, not as isolated fragments. Obviously the activity in numerous specialized neuronal groups, each representing different features of, for example, a visual scene, gives origin to our unitary experiences. To be useful, our experience must furthermore be put into a meaningful context to form the basis for appropriate actions.[1] Imagine, for example, the continuous stream of changing information that must be evaluated and acted upon when driving a car in heavy traffic. No area appears to receive all necessary information, and we have in several chapters mentioned that synchronized oscillations in task-specific networks are the most likely basis of mental phenomena. The vast number of corticocortical fibers are obviously essential in this respect. We have also discussed that although the anatomic connectivity forms the "hardwiring" of the networks, their functioning depends on dynamic, moment-to-moment fluctuations in synchronized activity. Presumably, engagement of specific networks shifts in the timescale of milliseconds. For example, we know from everyday experience how our attention shifts instantaneously. Another example concerns viewing of ambiguous pictures; the experience (e.g., duck or rabbit) changes with no time delay in spite of unchanged sensory input (Fig. 34.1).

---

1. It takes several hundred milliseconds from the arrival of sensory signals at the cortical level to perception, as first shown by Libet (1991) with stimulation experiments in humans. This perhaps reflects that in this situation it takes some time to bring the necessary networks into a state of synchronized activity.

Figure 34.3

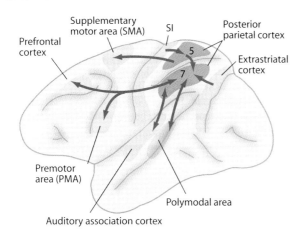

Association connections of the posterior parietal cortex (monkey). Connections with the limbic cortical areas are not shown (see Fig. 33.11). Visual and somatosensory information converge in area 7. Connections are reciprocal.

the proper use of somatosensory information, for goal-directed voluntary movements, and for the manipulation of objects. This fits well with the symptoms that arise in humans after damage to the posterior parietal cortex, as discussed next. Single-cell recordings indicate that **area 7** has an important role in the integration of visual and somatosensory stimuli, which is essential for the coordination of the eye and the hand—that is, for visual guidance of movements. Area 7 is also involved in the control of **eye movements**. Studies in monkeys suggest that certain subregions of the posterior parietal cortex are specialized for reaching movements, grasp, saccades, and smooth-pursuit eye movements (Fig. 34.4). It further appears that activity in these subregions is closely linked with the **intention** to move—that is, the posterior parietal cortex contains a "map of intentions."

Intention and Awareness

Stimulation of parietal and premotor cortical areas in awake patients undergoing surgery corroborates the importance of the parietal cortex for movement intention and awareness of own movements. Stimulation of Brodmann's areas 7, 39, and 40 (Fig. 34.4) provoked an intention to move, and with increasing stimulus strength the patients reported that they had actually performed the movements (although no movement occurred). Stimulation of the premotor cortex, on the other hand, produced overt movements but the patients were not aware of them. Thus, "Conscious intention and motor awareness … arise from increased parietal activity before movement execution." (Desmurget et al., 2009, p. 811).

Figure 34.4

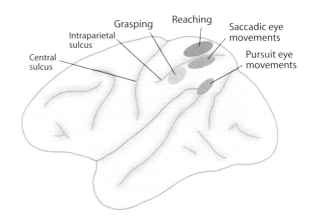

Subregions within the posterior parietal cortex with relation to planning of specific kinds of movement. (Based on Andersen and Buneo 2002.)

Properties of Single Neurons in the Posterior Parietal Cortex

Studies of monkeys with permanently implanted electrodes have demonstrated a wide repertoire of properties among neurons in areas 5 and 7. In general, a task-related increase in firing frequency occurs only when a stimulus is relevant and the **attention** of the animal is directed toward the stimulus. Thus, many neurons are virtually impossible to activate when the animal is drowsy and inattentive. Some cells respond to stimulation of proprioceptors, but their response is much more vigorous when a movement (stimulating the proprioceptors) is **self-initiated** by the monkey than when the joint is passively manipulated by the examiner. In area 5, many neurons change their firing frequency in relation to manipulatory **hand movements**. Other neurons increase their firing in relation to **reaching** movements but only when the hand is moved toward an object the monkey wants to obtain (such as an orange). The increase of firing in such neurons starts at the time the animal discovers the object—that is, before the arm movement starts—and is therefore not a result of proprioceptive stimulation. The American neurophysiologist Vernon B. Mountcastle (1975), who first described such neurons, suggested that they might function as **command neurons** for the target-directed **exploration** of our immediate extrapersonal space. Such neurons appear to respond to the **coincidence** of two events: a sensory stimulus (e.g., the sight of an orange) and a signal that depends on motivation (whether the monkey is hungry and wants the orange; see Fig. 4.10).

Lesions of the Posterior Parietal Cortex

Lesions of the posterior parietal cortex in humans can cause different symptoms, depending on which parts are most affected. Some of the symptoms can be summarized as difficulties with the transformation of sensory stimuli into adequate motor actions. This can probably be explained by lack of parietal influence on the premotor areas (PMAs). The understanding of the **meaning** of sensory stimuli is seriously impaired (but usually not the mere recognition of a stimulus). This **agnosia** concerns especially the recognition of the form and spatial position of objects. A typical symptom after right-sided lesions is a tendency to **neglect** the opposite side of the body and the visual stimuli from the opposite side. Patients may suffer from **apraxia**—that is, they are unable to use well-known tools and objects. They may further have problems with **visually guided movements** (such as stretching out the arm to obtain an object).

Even though the symptoms mentioned here are most often seen after damage of the posterior parietal cortex, most of them have been described after lesions in other parts of the brain too, especially of the prefrontal cortex, the thalamus, and the basal ganglia, all of which have connections with the parietal cortex. These structures take part in a **distributed network** responsible for, among other functions, the control of visually guided behavior and spatial orientation.

The Russian neuropsychologist Aleksandr R. Luria (1987) gives a compelling description of how it is to live with a damaged parietal lobe in the book *The Man with a Shattered World*. The soldier Zasetsky was hit by a bullet that destroyed his left occipito-parietal region. "Ever since I was wounded I haven't been able to see a single object as a whole" (p. 37), he said many years after the injury. He experienced his body as weird; sometimes his head was felt disproportionally large, the torso tiny, and the legs in a wrong place. He experienced not only objects as fragmented but also his own body.

More about Symptoms after Lesions of the Posterior Parietal Cortex

The most marked symptom produced by bilateral parietal lesions is the inability to **grasp** and to **manipulate** objects. Thus, the patient may be unable to move the hand toward an object that is clearly seen, even though there are no pareses and no visual defects. Movements that do not require visual guidance—such as buttoning, bringing an object to the mouth, and so forth—are performed normally. When patients are asked to pour water from a bottle into a glass, they pour the water outside the glass over and over again, even though they can see clearly both the bottle and the glass (**optic ataxia**). Such patients also have severe difficulties with the **appraisal** of **distances** and the **size** of objects. Further, to **fix the gaze** becomes difficult, especially to direct the gaze toward a point in the periphery of the visual field. The combination of **optic ataxia**, **simultanagnosia**, and **oculomotor apraxia** (difficulties with fixating the gaze) is called **Balint's syndrome**.

The **identification of objects** is difficult, because of the inability to attend to more than one detail at a time (such as seeing a cigarette but not the person who smokes it). This may be a fundamental defect after parietal lobe lesions, perhaps also explaining the difficulties mentioned earlier with pouring water into a glass (the patient is unable to locate in space the bottle and the glass at the same time).

Patients with parietal lobe lesions typically have difficulties with **drawing** an object or a scene; again the inability to perceive more than one feature at a time is the probable basic defect. The parts of an object are drawn separately, without the proper spatial relations, or the drawing gives an extremely simplified representation. This symptom occurs most often after damage to the right parietal cortex, in cases of unilateral lesions. The **use of tools** is also difficult or impossible: for example, the patient no longer knows how to use a hammer (**apraxia**).

Unilateral lesions of the right parietal lobe typically produce negligence—**neglect**—of the opposite body half and visual space. These patient behave as if the left part of their bodies does not exist. They dress only the right side, shave only the right half of the face, and so forth. They may deny that the left leg belongs to them and claim that it belongs to the person in the adjacent bed, for example. A similar symptom is denial of the disease and the functional loss, called **anosognosia**. The patient may deny that the limb is paralytic or that he or she is blind. Thus, certain aspects of body knowledge no longer exist in the mind of the patient, but the loss is not consciously perceived. When drawing a face, for example, the right side is drawn normally, whereas the left side is vague or not included in the drawing.

A peculiar constellation of symptoms, the **Gerstmann syndrome**, can occur after lesions of the parietal lobe at the transition to the temporal lobe (usually of the left hemisphere). The symptoms are as follows: **finger agnosia** (the patient cannot recognize and distinguish the various fingers on his or her own or other people's hands), **agraphia** (inability to write), sometimes **alexia** (inability to read), **right–left confusion**, and, **dyscalculia** (reduced ability to perform simple calculations, especially to distinguish categories of numbers such as tens, hundreds, and so forth). The most distinctive feature of the syndrome is the finger agnosia, which can occur in isolation. That finger agnosia can be the only symptom of a parietal lobe lesion indicates that a disproportionally large part of the human parietal cortex is devoted to the hand. Thus, the hand has a unique role as an exploratory sense organ and as a tool, and it has a special place in our inner, mental body image. The British neurologist M. Critchley (1953, p. 210) expressed it as follows: "The hand is largely the organ of the parietal lobe."

FRONTAL ASSOCIATION AREAS

In this context we use the term "association cortex" only about the **prefrontal cortex**—that is, the parts of the frontal lobe in front of areas 6 (premotor area [PMA] and supplementary motor area [SMA]) and 8 (the frontal eye field) (Fig. 34.5; also see Fig. 33.4). The prefrontal cortex consists of several cytoarchitectonic areas, each with a specific set of connections.

Figure 34.5

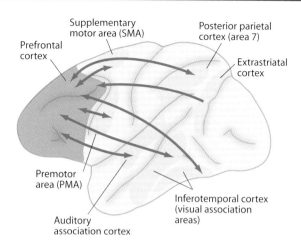

Association connections of the prefrontal cortex (monkey). Note the convergence of all kinds of processed sensory information and the connections with PMA and SMA. Connections with limbic cortical areas are not shown.

Figure 34.6

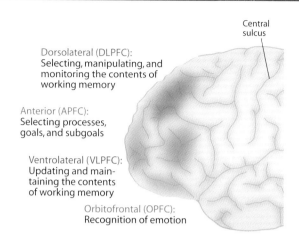

Some functional specializations within the prefrontal cortex. Regions that appear to be related to different aspects of memory, as judged from functional neuroimaging studies (PET and fMRI). The orbitofrontal cortex is activated in association with explicit identification of emotional facial expressions. (Based on Fletcher and Henson 2001 and Adolphs 2002.)

Connections

Together, the prefrontal areas receive strong **afferent** connections from areas in the occipital, parietal, and temporal lobes and, in addition, from the cingulate gyrus (Fig. 34.5). Thalamic afferents come from the **mediodorsal nucleus** (see Fig. 33.8), which, in turn, receives afferents from the **amygdala** and the **ventral pallidum** (among other places). In sum, the prefrontal cortex appears to receive information about all sensory modalities and also about the motivational and emotional state of the individual.

The prefrontal cortex sends **efferents** back to most of the areas from which it receives afferents, among them the SMA and the PMA. In addition, many prefrontal efferents reach the caudate nucleus of the **striatum** (see Fig. 23.7). Finally, some efferents reach the **amygdala** (see Fig. 31.4) and the **hypothalamus** (see Fig. 30.6).

Goal-Directed Behavior

Animal experiments, observations in brain-damaged humans, and brain imaging in normal persons all give a fairly consistent picture of the major tasks of the prefrontal cortex. Figure 34.6 shows some tasks associated with particular prefrontal subdivisions. The prefrontal cortex is obviously of crucial importance for **planning** and **initiation** of **goal-directed behavior**. More specifically, the prefrontal cortex is important for **attention**, **selection** of a specific behavior among several possible, and **suppression** of unwanted behavior. With regard to selection, the prefrontal cortex cooperates with the basal ganglia, as discussed in Chapter 23, under "Functions of the Basal Ganglia."

Working Memory and Learning

The prefrontal cortex is important for certain aspects of **memory**—both for working memory and for the long-term establishment of memory traces (Fig. 34.6). **Working memory** enables us to retain a stimulus long enough for its evaluation and linking with ongoing processes and memory. We discussed in Chapter 32 that medial parts of the temporal lobe, including the hippocampus, are necessary for declarative memory. Functional MRI studies indicate, however, that we remember words or pictures only if their presentation also activates the prefrontal cortex. Presumably, the prefrontal cortex tells the hippocampal region about the emotional coloring and the context of information that is transmitted to the hippocampus from sensory areas.

Learning of rules by association appears to be a central task of the prefrontal cortex. This may be performed by neurons that associate behaviorally relevant but otherwise dissimilar bits of information—such as that a red traffic light means stop. Appropriate behavior requires that we are able to learn such rules, but equally important is that we can replace them quickly with new ones. Both faculties suffer after damage to the prefrontal cortex.

Social Adaptation: "Theory of Mind" and Empathy

In sum, the prefrontal cortex is of crucial importance for our ability to organize our own lives and to function socially. Indeed, the tasks mentioned previously, such as planning and choice of behavior, choosing between signals with different emotional coloring, suppression of unwanted behavior, and so forth, are indispensable for **social adaptation**.

Another important factor in social functioning is our ability to understand—to **mentalize**—another person's beliefs, desires, intentions, and state of mind. This ability is an expression of having what is also termed a "**theory of mind.**" Imaging studies consistently implicate ventromedial parts of the prefrontal cortex in mentalizing as part of a wide network that includes several cortical and subcortical neuronal groups. The distribution of activity varies, however, with the specifics of the situation. **Empathy**, as a special case of mentalizing, exemplifies this point. For example, observing other persons in pain or distress is typically associated with activation of the anterior insula and the anterior cingulate gyrus (parts of the "pain network"), while empathy that is evoked by inferring the other person's pain or distress indirectly is typically associated with activation of ventromedial parts of the prefrontal cortex.

Empathy

Empathy is used with somewhat different meanings. Hein and Singer (2008, p. 154) refer to empathy as "an affective state, caused by sharing the emotions and sensory states of another person." They distinguish empathy from **sympathy**, which they describe as emphatic concern or compassion. By emphasizing that empathy is an affective state, they also distinguish it from the understanding of another person's beliefs, intentions, and desires, which derives from reasoning (i.e., cognitively). Indeed, understanding another person's intentions and feelings is not the same as sharing them.

Symptoms after Prefrontal Lesions

The prefrontal cortex consists of several subregions, which differ with regard to their connections and functional properties. Further, brain imaging shows that the exact position of nodes belonging to networks associated with higher mental functions vary considerably among persons. These facts may explain why the symptoms of prefrontal lesions vary so much and why individual differences are fairly large even after seemingly identically placed lesions. Broadly speaking, however, the symptoms are compatible with the functions discussed earlier.

Prefrontal lesions typically produce changes of **mood** and **personality**, distinguishing them from lesions of other parts of the cortex. Commonly, large lesions produce apathy, indifference, and emotional leveling-off. The patient appears to be uncritical compared with before the damage. For example, he or she may behave in a complacent and boastful manner, which he or she would never have done before. The ability to **alter** the **behavior** on the basis of experience from previous actions appears to be reduced. Clear-cut symptoms occur usually only after bilateral damage to the prefrontal cortex. Occasionally, however, the first signs of a **frontal-lobe tumor** are changes of behavior and personality.

More about Symptoms after Lesions of the Prefrontal Cortex

A striking defect after bilateral lesions of the **dorsolateral prefrontal cortex** is the lack of the so-called **delayed response**. In one experiment a monkey sees that food is put into one of two bowls, then the sight of the bowls is blocked for up to 10 min before the monkey is allowed to choose one of the two. In contrast to normal monkeys, the lesioned ones do not remember which bowl contained the food (even though they do not show reduced performance in other more complicated memory tests). The dorsolateral parts of the prefrontal cortex thus appear to be necessary for the ability to form and retain an inner conception of the existence of an object in time and space when the object is no longer seen. Interestingly, humans manage a similar test first at the age of about 1 year. Before that age, everything that is not seen or felt is presumably nonexistent for the infant.

A characteristic symptom in humans with prefrontal lesions is the inability to **alter the response** when the stimulus changes; they continue to make the same response even though it is no longer adequate. This phenomenon is called **perseveration**. The **Wisconsin card sort test** is often used to reveal such a defect. The person is asked to sort cards in accordance with certain general rules, such as color, number, shape, and so forth. The correct rule to be applied is indicated by the response given by the examiner to the first attempts at sorting the cards. The rules can be changed without warning. Normal persons understand fairly quickly that the rule has been changed and alter their responses accordingly, whereas patients with prefrontal lesions continue sorting in accordance with the first rule, in spite of repeated warnings that they are making mistakes.

Emotional and **personality** changes after frontal lobe lesions are most common when the lesion includes the **orbitofrontal parts**. Such symptoms are difficult to evaluate, and the premorbid personality of the patients appears to play a decisive role. Nevertheless, a general tendency is to become less emotional and to show reduced emotional reactions to events. Such patients also have difficulties in extracting the salient features from a complex situation, making their responses unpredictable and often inappropriate. A test designed for such symptoms uses drawings of complex situations, in part with a dramatic content, such as a man who has fallen through the ice on a lake and is in danger of drowning. Patients with frontal lesions usually attend only to details, saying, for example, "Since there is a sign saying 'Careful!' on the beach, there may be a high-voltage cable nearby." This kind of reduction results in inability to foresee the consequences of one's own actions and poor insight into other people's circumstances. This leads to poor **social adaptation**, with isolation as the final result.

The reduced capacity to retain inner conceptions is most likely the reason such patients have increased **distractibility**, with reduced ability to perform tasks that require continuous activity and attention. Motor hyperactivity, which can be a symptom, may perhaps result from the increased distractibility. Thus, in monkeys with prefrontal lesions, the hyperactivity disappears when they are placed in an environment with few stimuli.

In humans with frontal lobe tumors (e.g., a glioma or a metastasis from a malignant tumor elsewhere), a **depressive disorder** has been observed, but this may be a condition of de-emotionalization and social isolation.

THE TEMPORAL ASSOCIATION CORTEX

A unitary functional role is even less evident for the temporal association areas than for those in the parietal and frontal lobes. Apart from the auditory cortex (areas 41 and 42) (see Fig. 17.11) and the phylogenetically old parts at the medial aspect (see Fig. 31.1), the temporal lobe consists largely of Brodmann's areas 20, 21, and 22, which here are considered the association areas (Fig. 34.4).

Connections

The cortex of the **superior temporal gyrus** is characterized by its connections with the auditory cortex, whereas the inferior part of the temporal lobe—the **inferotemporal cortex**—is dominated by processed visual information from the extrastriate visual areas. In addition, there are strong connections with the **hippocampal formation** and the **amygdala** (see Figs. 31.4 and 31.5). Electrical **stimulation** of the temporal association cortex in humans evokes recall of memories of past events or the experience of dream-like sequences of imagined events (such observations were first made by the Canadian neurosurgeon Wilder Penfield [1950], who stimulated the temporal lobe and other parts of the cortex in patients in whom the cortex was exposed

under local anesthesia for therapeutic reasons). Finally, long association fibers interconnect the temporal association areas with the prefrontal cortex (Fig. 34.5).

Inferotemporal Cortex: Object and Face Recognition

The **inferotemporal cortex** is especially important for the interpretation of **complex visual stimuli**, as judged from experiments in monkeys. Thus, bilateral removal of these regions makes the monkeys unable to recognize and distinguish complex visual patterns (cf. Chapter 16, under "Segregation: Dorsal and Ventral Pathways (Streams) Out of the Striate Area"). These and other observations led to the conclusion that the inferotemporal cortex is of special importance for the **categorization** of visual stimuli. In monkeys, some neurons of the inferotemporal cortex respond only when the monkey sees, for example, a **face** or a **hand**. Some neurons respond preferentially to one particular face, whereas other neurons respond to any face. A neuron that responds briskly when the monkey is shown a drawing of a face may stop firing when important features are removed, such as the mouth or the eyes. Whether monkeys and humans—highly dependent on the ability to recognize faces and interpret facial expressions—have developed a separate system for face recognition is not settled. Selective loss of face recognition—**prosopagnosia**—sometimes occurs after lesions of the temporal lobe and would seem to suggest the existence of a separate "face" system. Further, fMRI studies show that activation in the **fusiform gyrus** in the inferotemporal cortex is associated with face recognition in humans (see Fig. 16.26). Other data, however, are more compatible with a general network for object identification that is used also for face recognition. Thus, objects other than faces can activate the fusiform gyrus, and, conversely, face recognition is associated with activation of several sites outside the fusiform gyrus. Because facial recognition is so important for social interactions and is used intensively from birth, presumably a larger proportion of neurons in temporal association areas become specialized for faces than for identification of other objects.

The Temporal Lobe and Memory

The medial temporal lobe and its importance for learning and declarative memory are discussed in Chapter 32.

In addition, clinical studies of patents with brain damage indicate that **anterolateral parts** of the temporal lobe is necessary for **semantic** memory—that is, our knowledge about facts and objects (i.e., our acquired knowledge about the world). Much of this knowledge is represented symbolically by words and underlies our understanding of their meanings. The temporal lobe is not alone in handling semantic knowledge, however; brain-imaging studies suggest that widespread parts of the association areas participate in semantic processing and memory.

Symptoms after Lesions of the Temporal Cortex

As would be expected, bilateral damage of the temporal lobes produces a syndrome dominated by pronounced **amnesia**. The failure to acquire new knowledge can be ascribed largely to the destruction of the hippocampal formation and neighboring areas in the parahippocampal gyrus, but, as mentioned, lateral parts of the temporal lobe are crucial for semantic knowledge. Therefore, the effects of total temporal lobe lesions also include severe retrograde amnesia. In addition, certain emotional changes are presumably caused by the concomitant destruction of the amygdala located in the tip of the temporal lobe. These aspects are discussed in Chapter 31. In addition, the patients become very **distractible**: they have difficulty maintaining their attention on a certain stimulus or task. Finally, psychic blindness or **visual agnosia** is a typical symptom of temporal lobe lesions that affect the **inferotemporal parts**. Patients are unable to recognize objects and persons they see, even though their vision is normal. As for other association areas, it is the **interpretation** of sensory information that is deficient, not the sensory experience as such. Information about size and shape of objects may nevertheless be available to the posterior parietal cortex to be used in movement control, as discussed in Chapter 16, under "Subconscious (Implicit) Use of Visual Information."

The Klüver-Bucy Syndrome

The constellation of symptoms that occur after bilateral destruction of the temporal lobes is named after the two American neurosurgeons Klüver and Bucy (1937) who first described it in monkeys. Besides amnesia, the animals lack emotional responses and aggressive behavior (increased tameness), and they withdraw from social contact. Furthermore, the syndrome includes visual agnosia, a tendency to examine all objects by mouth, a tendency to pay attention to all visual stimuli, an irresistible urge to touch everything, and hypersexuality. The symptoms are most likely caused by the combined effects of eliminating the amygdala, the hippocampal formation, and most of the neocortex in the temporal lobe.

THE INSULA

The insula, sometimes called the fifth cerebral lobe, is mentioned in several chapters. This is because the insula, as evident from brain-imaging studies, participates in a wide range of cortical networks. Thus, activity changes in the insula occur in relation to somatic and visceral sensory processes, emotional regulation, and aspects of bodily awareness. This part of the neocortex is hidden at the bottom of the lateral fissure (see Figs. 6.29, 6.30, and 14.9). It consists of several cytoarchitectonic subdivisions and receives afferents from several **thalamic nuclei** (ventral anterior, ventral posteromedial, centromedian, and some other nuclei).

The insula resides at the junction of the frontal, parietal, and temporal lobes and has reciprocal connections with all three. This concerns, for example, the orbitofrontal cortex, the cingulate gyrus, the parahippocampal gyrus, the temporal pole, the superior temporal sulcus, premotor areas, secondary somatosensory cortex, and the posterior parietal cortex—that is, regions involved in a wide specter of behaviors and mental processes. The insula also has reciprocal connections with the amygdala and projects to the ventral striatum (nucleus accumbens).

Insula Receives Several Kinds of Sensory Information

We discuss the insula in Chapter 14 because it is connected with the somatosensory cortex (especially the secondary somatosensory cortex) and is among the cortical regions activated by noxious stimuli. It is an essential part of the network responsible for the experience of **pain** (see Figs. 14.9 and 15.5). Also, signals from **low-threshold mechanoreceptors** reach the insula and evoke an emotional response to light cutaneous touch (see Chapter 13, under "Mechanoreceptors of the Skin"). Further, **vestibular signals** reach the insula, where they are integrated with **proprioceptive** information (see Chapter 18, under "Several

Areas Receive Vestibular Signals"). The anterior part of the insula receives **olfactory** and **gustatory** signals and presumably contributes to the integration of these modalities and their further integration with other enteroceptive signals.

The insula not only receives sensory signals from somatic structures but is consistently activated both by nonpainful and painful **enteroceptive stimuli**. For example, nonpainful distension of hollow organs such as the stomach and the esophagus activate the insula associated with the subjective feeling of **fullness**. Further, the awareness of one's own **heartbeats** is associated with activation of the insula. Indeed, the insula may thus play a particular role in our **awareness** of the state of our internal organs.[3] Injection of typhoid vaccine induces **sickness behavior** that is associated with activation of the insula and the anterior cingulate gyrus (Harrison et al. 2009). In agreement with its enteroceptive inputs, electric **stimulation** of the insula evokes abdominal sensations, chewing movements, altered breathing rhythm and intestinal peristaltic movements, and other autonomic phenomena (mediated via the hypothalamus and the amygdala and from there to preganglionic autonomic neurons).

Body Representation and Emotions

The role of the insula does not seem to be limited to monitoring the internal organs and evoking subjective feelings referred to them. Thus, the awareness of voluntary movements, and especially the feeling of **body ownership**, involves a network that probably includes the insula (see Chapter 18). The contribution of the insula in this respect presumably depends on its integration of **proprioceptive**, **vestibular**, and **motor signals**. Further, the anterior insula is activated in conjunction with strong **emotions** (especially **disgust**) and is presumably a part of a network for regulation of affect (see Fig. 31.8).

While there is good evidence that the insula is implicated in emotional processing, it does not seem to be necessary for the **experience of emotions**. This conclusion is based on examination of patients with bilateral damage of the insula (Damasio et al. 2013).

---

3. People differ with regard to how easily they perceive signals from visceral organs (e.g., the heart and the gastrointestinal tract). Such individual differences are associated with differences in the activation of the insula.

Monitoring the State of the Body?

It has been suggested that a common theme for the seemingly disparate functions of the insula may be to detect conflicts between predicted and actual peripheral feedback (cf. inputs from most kinds of sense organs). In this way it may monitor the state of the internal milieu and the individual parts of the body. Its role in pain—setting off an alarm when conflict is detected—would fit such a function, as would insula's participation in the salience network. A similar monitoring role has been suggested with regard to predicted and actual emotions.

LANGUAGE FUNCTIONS OF THE CEREBRAL CORTEX

Clinical observations in the nineteenth century led to the identification of two so-called language or speech areas in the left hemisphere (Fig. 34.7). The anterior area is named after the French physician Paul Broca, who in 1861 described

Figure 34.7

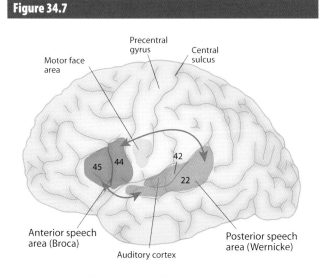

Language (speech) areas of the human brain. Broca's area corresponds to areas 44 and 45 of Brodmann, while Wernicke's area is usually considered to correspond to areas 22 and 42. Long association fibers interconnect the two areas, and these connections explain why a lesion between the two speech areas can produce aphasia (so-called conductance aphasia). Here are shown dorsal and ventral pathways that interconnect different parts of the two speech areas. Additional areas of the cerebral cortex are also involved in networks responsible for language processing. (Based on Friederici 2011.)

loss of speech—*aphasia*—caused by a lesion in the left frontal lobe just in front of the motor face area. The posterior speech area is named after the German neurologist Carl Wernicke, who discovered in 1874 that one of the clinically observed kinds of aphasia was associated with a lesion in the posterior part of the superior temporal gyrus. Aphasia is **defined** as loss (or disturbance) of speech due to a brain lesion. That speech depends almost entirely on only one hemisphere—in most people, the left—is the most marked and best-known example of **lateralization** (of function) or **hemispheric dominance**. We return to the topic of lateralization later.

Language Networks

Brain-imaging studies show that various tests of language functions activate regions corresponding roughly to the areas of Broca and Wernicke but also that several other parts of the cortex participate. This may not be surprising since language depends on several different processes, such as storage of words in short-term memory, **phonologic** (sound) and **semantic** (meaning) processing in relation to the "lexicon" in long-term memory, **syntactic processing** (arranging words into sentences), and the issuing of commands to motor areas about sound production. Further, **prosody** (patterns of stress and intonation of speech) is often crucial for the meaning of spoken sentences. Silent reading or repetition of words activates primarily the anterior region (Fig. 34.6). Specific tests for **semantic** analysis activate extensive areas in the temporal, prefrontal, and inferior parietal cortices, including Broca's and Wernicke's areas (primarily in the left hemisphere). Tests of **phonologic** analysis (such as choosing matching words by sound similarity) activate partly the same and partly different areas than semantic tests. As for other complex mental functions, the main tendency is that extensive regions of the hemisphere participate and that different tasks activate overlapping regions.

Division of Tasks

A division of tasks among nodes in the **network** for language processing were suggested by Shalom and Poeppel (2008, p. 125) as follows: "memorizing (learning new and retrieving stored primitives) in the temporal lobe, analyzing (accessing subparts of stored items) in the parietal lobe, and synthesizing (creating combinations of stored representations) in the frontal lobe." Further, there is evidence of

a specialization within each region. For example, in Broca's area (or region), the superior part (closest to the ventral premotor area) appears to specialize in phonological processing, the midregion in syntactic processing, and the inferior part in semantic processing. A functional subdivision of Broca's area would agree with anatomic data, since it consists of several cytoarchitectonic areas with different connections.

Several Pathways Interconnect the Language Areas

Figure 34.7 shows dorsal and ventral pathways interconnecting Broca's and Wernicke's areas. In reality, there are at least two dorsal and two ventral pathways connecting somewhat different subdivisions of the language areas. Broadly speaking, the **dorsal pathways** serve auditory to motor transformations while the **ventral pathways** support semantic processes. **Syntax** (the arrangement of words and phrases to meaningful sentences) seems to depend on both pathways.

Are There Brain Systems that Are Specific for Language?

A central question is whether language is produced by networks specialized for only this function or by a more general system that also takes part in other cognitive functions. Although rare, over the years many patients have been described with selective loss of language functions without other cognitive defects and vice versa. Such observations have been taken to support the **specificity hypothesis**. Still, positron emission tomography (PET) and fMRI data show considerable overlap among cerebral regions activated by language tasks and by other cognitive tasks. Further, connectionist modeling (computer-based models of neural networks) shows that the **multipurpose hypothesis** is not incompatible with the evidence of selective defects from brain-damaged patients. Models can simulate language learning, such as learning to read words. Although such networks do not have segregated pathways for different functions, partial damage may produce selective visual or semantic defects (somewhat similar to a child with dyslexia). Such modeling experiments challenge "the commonly held assumption that the fractionation of behaviour reflects an underlying fractionation of the brain systems that control such behaviour" (Nobre and Plunkett 1997, p. 263). Thus, a specific impairment after brain damage does not mean that the brain possess a specific module responsible for the lost function.

Lateralization of Language

For most people, even for most left-handers, the left hemisphere is responsible for speech and most (but not all) aspects of language functions. We say that language functions are **lateralized** and that the left hemisphere is **dominant** for language, whereas the right hemisphere is **recessive**. About 95% of right-handers have left-hemisphere language dominance, while the corresponding number for left-handers is about 70% (there is obviously not a strong correlation between the lateralization of speech and hand preference). Several kinds of investigation have confirmed the lateralization of language. Studies of **split-brain** patients (in whom the corpus callosum is cut) are especially instructive in this respect. They confirm, among other concepts, that the right hemisphere when isolated from the left hemisphere is "mute" in most people (even though it can alone be responsible for the expression of single words when strong emotions are aroused). When a split-brain patient is asked to identify with the right hand an object that is not seen, he or she can easily tell the name of the object, what it is used for, and so forth. This is because the tactile information comes to the left, speech-dominant hemisphere. When the left hand is used for the same test, however, the patient is unable to name the object, because the information reaches only the right hemisphere. The patient nevertheless shows signs of appropriate emotional reactions to the object. That the right hemisphere alone is sufficient to analyze the nature of the object is further supported by other experiments in which only the right hemisphere is presented with a picture of, for example, a key. Even though the patient cannot say anything about the object, he or she nevertheless picks out with the left hand a key among several objects (which are not seen). Such data show that a person with only a **right hemisphere** can understand concrete language both in speech and writing but cannot express understanding through language—only through action.

Language Lateralization in Right- and Left-Handers

The numbers concerning language dominance come mainly from studies in which one hemisphere was temporarily anesthetized by injection of a barbiturate into the internal carotid artery. In general, recent brain-imaging studies agree with these data. One fMRI study found that among 50 right-handed persons, 96% had largely left-hemisphere activation when performing a language task (word finding); 4% had bilateral activation, but no one had larger right than left activation. In contrast, 76% of left-handers had left-hemisphere activation with the same test, 14% had bilateral activation, and 10% had right-hemisphere activation. Thus, it appears that only about 10% of left-handers have right-hemisphere dominance for language.

Prosody Depends Mainly on the Right Hemisphere

Not all aspects of language function are localized to the dominant hemisphere. The modulation and melody of the sounds of speech, **prosody**, appear to largely depend on the right hemisphere, as witnessed by several clinical reports. Thus, in some patients who suffer a right-hemisphere stroke, prosody is changed or reduced without concomitant aphasia. Accordingly, brain-imaging studies show activation in the right hemisphere in tests for perception of prosody, notably in the region corresponding to Broca's area and in the superior temporal gyrus (but also some activation of the left hemisphere). Patients with loss of prosody may also be unable to judge the emotional aspects of the speech of other persons; for example, they cannot decide whether the person is sad or happy. Such an **intonational agnosia** may have serious effects on the social life of the patient. The importance of the prosody illustrates that much of what we regard as verbal communication is, in fact, nonverbal.

Asymmetry of the Temporal Plane and Language Lateralization

The most robust anatomic difference between the left and the right hemisphere in humans concerns the upper face of the temporal lobe. **The temporal plane** (*planum temporale*) in the vicinity of the auditory cortex is reported to be more extensive on the left than on the right side in about 70% of the population (see Chapter 17, under "Asymmetrical Organization of the Auditory Cortex in the Temporal Plane"). However, since the language function depends on the left hemisphere in more than 90% of persons, the relationship between speech lateralization and anatomic asymmetry is not absolute. The difference in the temporal plane appears to be present before birth.

Aphasia

There is an enormous literature dealing with the disturbances of speech and language, and there are numerous classifications of aphasias. Very schematically, there are two main types of aphasia. The simplest type is the so-called **motor aphasia**. This occurs most often after destruction of Broca's area (the anterior speech

Figure 34.8

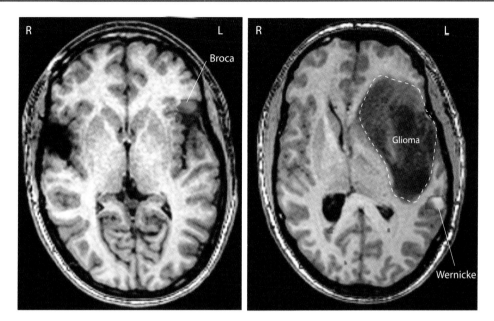

Activation of Broca's area and Wernicke's area as demonstrated with fMRI. An anatomic (T1-weighted) MRI is produced first; thereafter color-coded activity data are superimposed on the brain image. **A:** Broca's area. **B:** Wernicke's area. In this case a large tumor is present in the left hemisphere. The fMRI was done to ensure that the tumor could be removed without causing aphasia. (Courtesy of Dr. B. Nedregaard, Oslo University Hospital, Oslo, Norway.)

area). The patient more or less completely loses the ability to speak and typically produces only single words in a sort of telegraphic style. The few words used may also be applied incorrectly. Other names used for this type are **nonfluent** aphasia (because the speech becomes stuttering) and **expressive** aphasia. The understanding of language is usually preserved, whereas the production of speech is deficient. Nevertheless, there are no signs of pareses of the muscles involved in speech production. Often, motor aphasia is combined with **agraphia**—the inability to express language in writing.

In patients with **sensory** or **receptive** aphasia, the lesion usually affects more posterior parts of the hemisphere at the junction between the parietal, temporal, and occipital lobes—that is, in or close to Wernicke's or the posterior speech area (Fig. 33.7). Typically, the comprehension of language is most severely affected. The various elementary sounds are not properly put together to form meaningful words and sentences. Words that are heard cannot be repeated. In contrast to motor aphasia, spontaneous speech is fluent, but sounds are often put together into meaningless words, and proper words lack relation to each other ("word-salad"). Usually, sensory aphasia is combined with **alexia**—the inability to read.

In reality, the pure forms of aphasia are very seldom encountered; in most patients there is a mixture of motor and sensory symptoms, with one or the other dominating. Often there are other symptoms as well, since lesions of the hemispheres are rarely confined to the speech areas.

The relationship between specific aphasic symptoms and the anatomic location of a brain lesion is not absolute. Virtually all forms of aphasia have been described after lesions in unexpected parts of the brain. Thus, we can only say that the probability of speech disturbances is highest when the lesion affects one or both of the areas depicted in Fig. 33.7 (or the association fibers interconnecting the anterior and posterior speech areas).

Music—The Language of Emotions

Music is an integral part of human culture, and the ability to respond to music (e.g., with rhythmic movements and to differentiate consonant and dissonant intervals) occurs in early infancy. Music is a puzzling phenomenon in an evolutionary perspective, since it has no obvious survival or adaptive function. A basic feature of music is its ability to evoke emotions and induce moods. Accordingly, brain-imaging studies show that listening to music typically activates networks related to emotions and reward in addition to the auditory cortex. These networks include, among other areas, the **ventral striatum** (nucleus accumbens), the **amygdala**, the **insula**, and the **orbitofrontal cortex**. Perhaps somewhat unexpectedly, listening to music, regardless of whether it induced sadness or joy, has been found to activate the **hippocampal formation**. This may be related to a hippocampal role in **stress regulation** (partly via the hypothalamus) and perhaps also to the ability of music to improve memory of an associated text. The **supplementary motor area (SMA)**—which is important for rhythmic and sequential movements—is activated when **imagining** tunes, perhaps because there is a motor element in music imagination. In addition, music perception and expression obviously depend on the proper functioning of executive, salience, and attentional networks.

Acquired **amusia** most often occurs together with aphasia, but it has also been reported to occur in isolation. This suggests that language and music use largely separate parts of the cortex, although they appear to lie close together. This is supported by PET studies of musicians practicing sight-reading (i.e., reading and playing an unfamiliar score at the same time). Impaired music recognition has been observed in patients with lesions of the hippocampal formation and the amygdala.

Lateralization of Music

With regard to the ability to appreciate and express music, there is no simple division of labor between the hemispheres, although it has been assumed that the right hemisphere is most important. Indeed, that the perception of a **melody** depends mainly on the right hemisphere was supported by a study using the Doppler technique to measure changes of total blood flow to the hemispheres during various tasks. The right-sided dominance was true only for nonmusicians, however: professional musicians showed left-hemisphere dominance for the same task that was presented to the nonmusicians. Listening to **rhythm** activated the left hemisphere most strongly in both groups. Furthermore, left-hemisphere activation was relatively more significant when the person listened attentively, trying to discriminate musical elements, rather than having the music as a background. **Imagining** a familiar tune was found to activate association areas around the right auditory cortex and frontal regions on both sides.

FUNCTION OF THE COMMISSURAL CONNECTIONS: THE CORPUS CALLOSUM

In general, by ensuring swift and reliable signal transfer between the two hemispheres, the commissures enable the hemispheres to be specialized and yet function as a unit. Here we mention just a few examples of the significance of the commissural connections.

Visual System

When the optic nerve fibers that cross in the optic chiasm are cut (see Fig. 16.16), signals from one eye reach only the hemisphere of the same side. After such an operation, monkeys are trained in a **visual discrimination task** (to distinguish a triangle and a circle to obtain a fruit reward) with a patch that occludes vision in the left eye. The learning must depend on processes taking place in the right hemisphere, which receives visual information from the right eye. When the monkey has learned the task with use of the right eye, the occlusion is reversed. Nevertheless, even when using the left eye, the monkey solves the task as well as when using the right eye. Thus, the left hemisphere also has "learned" the task. This depends on an effective transmission of visual information from one hemisphere to the other and can be verified by cutting the corpus callosum (and the anterior commissure) before the discrimination training starts. Then the animal learns the task only with the right hemisphere when the left eye is occluded. The transmission of visual information from one hemisphere to the other in this experiment therefore must depend on commissural connections between the extrastriate and probably the inferotemporal areas, since the striate area lacks commissural fibers (Fig. 33.13).

Somatosensory System

Experiments corresponding to those in the visual system have shown that **tactile** and **kinesthetic** signals are also transferred through the corpus callosum. In one experiment a monkey with transection of the corpus callosum (and the anterior commissure) is trained to open a box with the right hand only (without being allowed to see the box). After some training, the opening is performed swiftly. If the monkey is then prevented from using the right hand, the task must be learned over again with the left hand—no learning has taken place in the right hemisphere (which controls the left hand). A monkey with an intact corpus callosum uses both hands with identical dexterity to solve this task, even though only one hand was used during the training period.

Topographic Arrangement

There is a certain **topographic arrangement** of the commissural fibers within the corpus callosum. As one might expect, the posterior parts are necessary for the transfer of visual information, whereas the anterior and middle parts are necessary for transfer of somatosensory signals. (See Chapter 26, under "Neurobiological Basis of Consciousness," which includes a description of a patient with damage of the middle part of the corpus callosum and abolished transfer of tactile information.) The posterior part of the corpus callosum is responsible for transfer of signals related to auditory linguistic processes (e.g., with regard to emotional salience).

LATERALIZATION: THE DIVISION OF TASKS BETWEEN THE HEMISPHERES

As mentioned, the ample commissural connections make it possible for the two hemispheres to **specialize** and still operate as a unit. Specialization must obviously provide advantages, especially with regard to higher cognitive functions. The most clear-cut example of lateralization of function is language, as discussed previously. Broadly speaking, many studies show that the **left hemisphere** is most important for **analytical** and **logical thinking** as expressed verbally and in numbers, while the **right hemisphere** is most important for **spatial abilities**, the comprehension of complicated **patterns**, and **drawing**.

"Dichotomania"

The discovery of hemispheric specializations—especially as revealed by studies of split-brain patients—led to many simplistic and erroneous statements about the functions of the right and the left hemispheres—as if a person has two brains that operate more or less independently. Complex functions are always carried out by cooperation of the two hemispheres, however. In fact, both hemispheres take part in most functions; the differences concern mainly how efficiently they carry out individual processes, such as elements of language functions, emotional processing, visual object recognition, and so forth. A specialist in the field of cerebral lateralization said some years ago that the time has come to put the brain back together again. Another scientist launched the expression "dichotomania" about the urge to equate the many examples of duality in human nature with the two halves of the brain (left–right): scientist–artist, conscious–subconscious, rationalism–mysticism, masculine–feminine, and so forth.

Studies of Split-Brain Patients

A wealth of information on the topic of hemispheric specializations (lateralization) has been provided by the study of so-called **split-brain** patients—patients in whom the **corpus callosum** has been transected (this is done in severe cases of epilepsy to prevent spread of the abnormal discharges from one hemisphere to

the other). The American Roger Sperry was awarded the Nobel Prize in 1981 for his pioneering studies of split-brain patients. Even though lateralization is probably most marked in humans, there is much evidence that it also occurs in animals (e.g., the ability to sing depends on cell groups in the left side of the brain in birds).

Split-brain patients manage well in everyday life, mainly because visual information reaches both hemispheres (because we move the gaze constantly) and there are some bilateral sensory and motor pathways. These patients get into trouble, however, if, for example, somatosensory information is not supplemented with visual information. The preceding example of the commissurotomized monkey and tactile learning is relevant for split-brain patients too. In some situations, conflicts may arise between commands issued from the two hemispheres; for example, the left hemisphere may command the right hand to start dressing, whereas the left hand is ordered to undress.

Lateralization of Hand Function

With regard to lateralization of hand functions, the hemispheric differences are less clear-cut than for language. It is not a question of the ability to use the hand but a matter of preference of one hand for most or all tasks. Even though hand preference is inheritable, strong social factors also contribute to the final outcome of hand preference—for example, in writing. There is most likely a gradual transition with regard to the strength of hand preference, from those with a strong tendency to use the right hand for all tasks if possible (writing, drawing, use of tools, eating, etc.) to those with an equally strong tendency to use the left hand. The latter group probably constitutes 2% to 3% of the total population. Hand preference starts to become expressed from the second year of life and is usually finally established at the age of 5 or 6.

Ear and Visual Field Dominance

A certain degree of "ear dominance" exists in most people, corresponding to speech lateralization—that is, the right ear is dominant for most people. This phenomenon can be studied by use of so-called **dichotic listening**. Two words are presented at the same time, one to each ear. Afterward, most people say that they heard the word presented to the right ear. **Visual field dominance** has been described in studies in which different visual stimuli are presented to the two hemispheres simultaneously. With regard to written words and letters, there is a tendency to prefer those presented in the right visual field (i.e., those transferred to the left hemisphere). For **face recognition**, the reverse situation appears to exist for most people, as can be demonstrated by the presentation of so-called **chimeric portraits** composed of two left halves and two right halves, respectively. The person is asked which of the chimeric portraits most resembles the original (authentic) portrait. Most people claim that the chimeric portrait consisting of two right facial halves most resembles the original. This is taken to suggest that the right hemisphere dominates in the analysis of faces and other complex visual patterns. Another indication of this is that, when the **shape of letters** is made sufficiently ornate, the right hemisphere appears to become necessary for their interpretation.

Lateralization of Emotions

Early observations of split-brain patients suggest that the **right hemisphere** is dominant for the expression of emotions, but further studies show that the right hemisphere does not dominate all aspects of emotional behavior. Thus, the two hemispheres appear to be specialized for specific aspects of emotions. We mentioned **prosody** as an example of right-hemisphere dominance. Overall, the right hemisphere appears to be most important for perception of emotional expressions, whereas both hemispheres are involved in the experience and expression of emotions. The left hemisphere may be most important for judgment of certain kinds of emotional expressions, however. Some data have been interpreted to show that the right hemisphere is dominant for the experience of strongly **negative feelings** (and the left for positive feelings). Patients with **strokes** affecting the **left** hemisphere tend to have more depressive reactions than patients with corresponding right-sided lesions (the right hemisphere is thus perhaps most important for analyzing the total situation). **Right**-hemisphere lesions, especially when they affect the frontal lobe, appear to have a stronger tendency to produce a somewhat inadequate elevation of mood.

Further Examples of Hemispheric Specializations

Studies with detailed analyses of specific aspects of broader categories of cerebral functions reveal that the division of labor between right and left is more differentiated than is apparent from the first split-brain observations. Sophisticated studies of visual perception show that the right hemisphere gives the most important contribution to perception and memory of **specific characteristics** of objects (e.g., the face of a person), whereas the left contributes most to identification of **categories** (e.g., a face versus other kinds of objects). A different picture emerged in a study comparing patients with lesions in the superior temporal gyrus regarding their ability to **identify letters**. Those with right-hemisphere lesions had difficulties with identification of a big letter when it was composed of many small ones, but they easily perceived the small letters. Those with a left-hemisphere lesion had difficulties with identification of the small letters, but they easily identified the big one. Thus, the right hemisphere seems to be most important for identifying the **overall shape**, whereas the left is most important for perceiving the **details**. It may seem paradoxical that the left hemisphere is specialized both for identification of broad categories and details (and that the right hemisphere is specialized for identification of specific properties and the overall shape). Most likely, however, this

reflects that different principles govern lateralization of visual and semantic memory.

Another lateralization of a specific function does not fit with the usual right–left dichotomy of functions. Thus, the right hemisphere is best at **measuring distance** (e.g., the distance between a dot and a line), whereas the left hemisphere excels at judging **mutual positions** (whether the dot is above or below the line).

GENDER DIFFERENCES AND THE CEREBRAL CORTEX

Cognitive Gender Differences

This is a field abundant with bold generalizations, often based on studies with too small a sample size. Even the common notions that men show better spatial and mathematical abilities while women show better verbal abilities need qualifications according to recent meta-analyses. Thus, although the most robust cognitive gender difference is found in **mental rotation** of a 3D figure, no difference was (surprisingly) found in mentally folding a sheet of paper into a 3D figure. With regard to **mathematical** abilities, recent large-scale US studies find no gender differences at any school level. Intriguingly, comparison with older studies indicates that girls have improved their abilities compared with boys (suggesting that gender differences found in older studies cannot be explained biologically). With regard to **verbal** abilities, women perform on average slightly better than men on verbal-fluency tests, whereas no difference seems to exist when testing vocabulary, reading comprehension, or essay writing. Well-documented differences in some other psychological treats are generally small. This concerns, for example, **temperament**, which shows some gender differences but not with regard to negative affectivity (perhaps surprisingly in view of the higher prevalence of depression among women). Reported gender differences with regard to the "Big Five" **personality traits** may be better explained by gender stereotypies rather than by biology. Thus, some differences are found in the United States but not in some other societies. The common notion that women are more **emotional** than men is not fully substantiated by recent meta-analyses: "data, from both children and adults, indicate that gender differences in emotional experience are small, or in many cases trivial." (Hyde 2014, p. 385). Gender differences in **aggression** are found consistently from early age but are not large. Furthermore, the differences seem to be strongly context dependent, judged from experiments in which gender stereotypies are eliminated.

Many other cognitive gender differences have been reported, but data from different researchers are often conflicting. Further, the effect of **gender stereotypies** seems to be considerable and makes it difficult to determine the impact of biological factors. Thus, while gender differences may have a genetic basis, environmental influences interact with genetic predispositions to produce the final cognitive makeup of the individual.

It should finally be emphasized that the average cognitive sex differences, whatever their causes, are generally much smaller than the variability among individuals of the same sex. As noted by the Canadian psychologist Doreen Kimura (1996, p. 259): "In the larger comparative context, the similarities between human males and females far outweigh the differences."

Gender: Cortical Structure and Activation

With regard to neuroanatomic sex differences, the most obvious is the difference in **brain volume**: the brain is on average 10% heavier in men than in women. Most, but not all, of this difference can be accounted for by different body weights. One well-documented difference seems to be that women on average have a slightly higher **gray matter–white matter ratio** than men. The **temporal plane** (involved in language processing) has been reported to be larger in women than in men. Whether this is causally related to sex differences in verbal fluency is so far unknown, however. There are also many reports (most of them unconfirmed) of volume differences in many parts of the cortex. Studies at a more detailed level offer many data, but, unfortunately, conflicting results make it difficult to draw conclusions. One study reported higher synaptic density in men than in women. A morphometric study found no difference in cortical thickness but that men had on average somewhat higher **cortical neuronal density** than women (117,000 ± 31,000 and 101,000 ± 26,000 per mm², respectively). Even if this finding is confirmed, the large individual variation within each sex makes any inferences about causal relationships doubtful.

PET and fMRI studies have investigated sex differences in brain **activation patterns**. For example, one study found that men and women activated somewhat different parts of the brain when they were trying to find their way out of a (virtual) labyrinth. Apart from many regions activated in both sexes, men activated the left hippocampus, whereas women activated the right frontoparietal region. Other studies also point to gender differences in activation

patterns, but the interpretation of such findings is far from straightforward.

Gender Differences and Lateralization

Cognitive gender differences have been speculatively linked with more or less convincingly demonstrated differences in **lateralization** and brain structure. Some observations suggest, for example, that men have stronger lateralization of, for example, visuospatial abilities, whereas women to a higher degree use both hemispheres. (It is not obvious, however, that a strong lateralization gives a higher visuospatial ability; the reverse might just as well be the case.) It was then studied whether there might be sex differences in the cross-sectional area of the **corpus callosum**, which would correlate with differences in lateralization; that is, a corpus callosum with relatively few fibers was expected to correlate with a high degree of lateralization. Indeed, some studies report that the corpus callosum is relatively larger in cross section in women than in men. These speculations have not been confirmed by further and more comprehensive studies, however. First, the reported differences regarding visuospatial abilities constitute merely a few percentages of the individual variations among members of the same gender. Furthermore, the notion that men have more marked lateralization than women cannot be accepted as generally valid. Finally, several studies have not been able to confirm the gender differences in the size of the corpus callosum. They are at best small, whereas the individual variations again are surprisingly large; in monkeys the number of axons in the corpus callosum varies among individuals by a factor of 2. In fact, an inverse relationship between **brain weight** and cross-sectional area of the corpus callosum has been reported: smaller brains, regardless of gender, would be expected to have relatively larger corpus callosum. To complicate matters, one report claimed that the corpus callosum is about 10% larger in left-handers (and persons using both hands equally) than in right-handers. This does not support a correlation between superior visuospatial abilities, strong lateralization, and a small corpus callosum.

In conclusion, the available data do not support that sex differences in cognitive and other abilities can be explained by differences in lateralization.

Nature and Nurture: How We Become Who We Are

The final performance of the brain is a product of genetic and environmental influences, as discussed in Chapter 9. Environmental challenges induce structural and neurochemical adaptations in the nervous system expressed through altered behavior. In humans the environment influences behavior and psychology much more than in animals. Thus, learning explains a large part of human interindividual variability as well as group-level differences. We mentioned gender stereotypes as a confounding factor when interpreting gender studies, but the same problem applies when studying differences between social groups. There is now an intense search for genes that influence **social behavior**. Such genes would be expected to participate in the establishment and refinement of the many task-specific networks discussed in this book. It is striking, however, that the search for genes with decisive influence on human behavior has not been successful. Rather, it appears that personality as well as cognition and emotions are under the influence of numerous genes, each providing a very small contribution to the final phenotype. For example, while cognitive abilities (IQ) are among the most genetically controlled traits (40%–80% of the variability can be explained by heritage), it has proved very hard to find a connection between specific genes and IQ. Considering that, presumably, each of the many contributing genes is under epigenetic influence, the number of variables that determine our final behavior becomes astounding. Indeed, as stated by Story Landis and Thomas Insel in an editorial in *Science* (2008, p. 821): "Genes code for proteins, not for behaviors." They also note that "genomics is not destiny. Indeed, if genomic sequence 'determines' anything behaviorally, it determines diversity. It is important that we be wary about extrapolating from model organisms to humans. We must also avoid using small statistical associations to make grand claims about human nature."

In conclusion, all development—whether genetically determined or not—involves synaptic changes, and from the time of birth there is a dynamic interplay between genes and the environment in the establishment, maintenance, and functional regulation of billions of synapses. A genetically determined disposition—for example, a certain temperament—evokes a certain kind of response from other people. The response induces synaptic and neurochemical changes in the brain as a basis for behavior adaptations. To sort out the mutual roles of nature and nurture in the formation of a person's psychology and behavior then becomes virtually impossible.

Literature

Textbooks and Reference Works

Blinkov, S.M., Glezer, I.I. *The human brain in figures and tables: a quantitative handbook.* New York: Plenum Press, 1968.

Brodal, A. *Neurological anatomy in relation to clinical medicine,* 3rd ed. Oxford: Oxford University Press, 1981.

Cooper, J.R., et al. *The biochemical basis of neuropharmacology,* 8th ed. New York: Oxford University Press, 2002.

Fain, G.L. *Molecular and cellular physiology of neurons.* Cambridge, MA: Harvard University Press, 1999.

Federative Committee on Anatomical Nomenclature. *Terminologia Anatomica: International anatomical terminology.* New York: Thieme, 1998.

Gazzaniga, M., Mangun, G.R. (Eds.) *The cognitive neurosciences,* 5th ed. Cambridge, MA: MIT Press, 2014.

Kandel, E., et al. *Principles of neural science,* 5th ed. New York: McGraw-Hill, 2012.

Levitan, I.B., Kaczmarek, L.K. *The neuron: cell and molecular biology,* 3rd ed. New York: Oxford University Press, 2002.

Lockard, I. *Desk reference of neuroanatomy: a guide to essential terms.* New York: Springer-Verlag, 1977.

Love, S., et al. (Eds.) *Greenfield's neuropathology,* 9th ed. London: CRP Press, 2015.

Luria, A.R. *Higher cortical functions in man.* 2nd ed. New York: Consultants Bureau, 1980.

Mai, J., Paxinos, G. (Eds.) *The human nervous system,* 3rd ed. San Diego: Elsevier Academic Press, 2012.

Nicholls, J.G., et al. *From neuron to brain,* 5th ed. Sunderland, MA: Sinauer Associates, 2011.

Parent, A., Carpenter, M.B. *Carpenter's human neuroanatomy,* 9th ed. Philadelphia: Lippincott, Williams & Wilkins, 1995.

Paxinos, G. *The rat nervous system,* 3rd ed. Philadelphia: Elsevier, 2004.

Rauber, A., Kopsch, F. *Anatomie des Menschen.* Vol. 3: *Nervensystem. Sinnesorgane.* Stuttgart: Georg Thieme Verlag, 1987.

Ropper, A., et al. *Adams and Victor's principles of neurology,* 10th ed. New York: McGraw Hill Education, 2014.

Shallice, T., Cooper, R.P. *The organisation of mind.* Oxford: Oxford University Press, 2011.

Shepherd, G.M. *Neurobiology,* 3rd ed. New York: Oxford University Press, 1997.

Squire, L.R. (Editor in chief.) *Encyclopedia of neuroscience,* 3rd ed. Philadelphia: Elsevier, 2009.

Squire, L.R., et al. *Fundamental neuroscience.* San Diego: Academic Press, 2002.

Atlases

DeArmond, S.J., et al. *Structure of the human brain: a photographic atlas,* 3rd ed. Oxford: Oxford University Press, 1989.

Gouaze, A., Salomon, G. *Brain anatomy and magnetic resonance imaging.* New York: Springer-Verlag, 1988.

Haines, D.E. *Neuroanatomy in clinical context: an atlas of structures, sections, systems, and syndromes,* 9th ed. Philadelphia: Wolters Kluwer Health, 2015.

Mai, J.K., et al. *Atlas of the human brain,* 3rd ed. Philadelphia: Academic Press, 2007.

Miller, R.A., Burack, E. *Atlas of the central nervous system in man,* 3rd ed. Baltimore: Williams & Wilkins, 1983.

Nieuwenhuys, R. *Chemoarchitecture of the brain.* New York: Springer-Verlag, 1985.

Nieuwenhuys, R., et al. *The human central nervous system: a synopsis and atlas,* 3rd ed. New York: Springer-Verlag, 1988.

Olszewski, J. *Cytoarchitecture of the human brain stem.* Basel: Karger, 1954.

O'Rahilly, R.R. *The embryonic human brain: an atlas of developmental stages,* 2nd ed. New York: John Wiley & Sons, 1999.

Roberts, M.P. *Atlas of the human brain in section.* Philadelphia: Lea & Febiger, 1987.

Review Journals

Annual Review of Neuroscience. Annual Reviews

Annual. Contains about 20 or more reviews by leading neuroscientists. Covers a wide range of topics. Requires background knowledge.

Current Opinion in Neurobiology. Current Biology

Six issues annually. Concise reviews of the development in the past few years within a special subfield. Contains comprehensive reference lists. Key references are supplied with brief, focused abstracts.

Nature Reviews Neuroscience. Nature Publishing Group

Monthly. Review articles by leading scientists, and neuroscience news in brief. The Web version features many useful links.

Neuron. Cell Press

Monthly. Each issue usually features one review article (basic neuroscience) and several mini-reviews of high standard, in addition to many research articles.

Scientific American. Scientific American Inc.

Monthly. Regularly one or more articles on various aspects of neuroscience. Requires less prior knowledge than the specialized neuroscience review journals. Well-written, easy-to-follow articles with often superb illustrations.

The Neuroscientist. Williams & Wilkins

Bimonthly. Multidisciplinary reviews, aiming at bridging the gap between basic and clinical neuroscience.

Trends in Cognitive Sciences. Elsevier

Monthly. High-quality reviews covering cognitive neuroscience and neuropsychology.

Trends in Neurosciences. Elsevier

Monthly. Brief reviews of neurobiological topics in rapid development. Written by leading scientists. Requires fairly broad prior knowledge of neuroscience.

Clinical Examples

These books vivify the workings of the human brain in health and disease. They present accurate descriptions of case stories, insightful analysis of symptoms and findings, and—perhaps most important— lively descriptions of how it feels to lose important functions of the brain.

Bruner, J., Luria, A.R. *The mind of a mnemonist: a little book about a vast memory.* Cambridge, MA: Harvard University Press, 1988.

Damasio, A. *Descarte's error: emotion, reason, and the human brain.* New York: Avon Books, 1995.

Kapur, N. *Injured brains of medical minds: views from within.* Oxford: Oxford University Press, 1997.

Klawans, H.L. *Toscanini's fumble and other tales of clinical neurology.* London: Headline, 1988.

Klawans, H.L. *Why Michael couldn't hit: and other tales of the neurology of sports.* New York: W.H. Freeman, 1996.

Luria, A.R., Bruner, J.S. *The man with a shattered world: the history of a brain wound.* Cambridge, MA: Harvard University Press, 1987.

Ramachandran, V.S., Blakeslee, S. *Phantoms in the brain: probing the mysteries of the human mind.* New York: William Morrow, 1998.

Sacks, O. *The man who mistook his wife for a hat.* New York: Picador, 1986.

Sacks, O. *Awakenings.* New York: Picador, 1990.

Sacks, O. *A leg to stand on.* New York: Picador, 1991.

Sacks, O. *An anthropologist on Mars: seven paradoxical tales.* New York: Picador, 1995.

Sacks, O. *The mind's eye.* New York: Picador, 2010.

Introduction

Bennett, M.R., Hacker, P.M.S. *Philosophical foundations of neuroscience.* Oxford: Blackwell Publishing, 2003.

Changeux, J.-P. *Neuronal man: the biology of mind.* New York: Oxford University Press, 1985.

Changeux, J.-P., Chavallion, J. *Origins of the human brain.* New York: Oxford University Press, 1996.

Coltheart, M. How can functional neuroimaging inform cognitive theories? *Perspectiv. Psychol. Sci.* 8:98–103, 2013.

Davis, K., et al. Neuroethical issues related to the use of brain imaging: can we and should we use brain imaging as a biomarker to diagnose chronic pain? *Pain* 153: 1555–1559, 2012.

Davis, N.J. Transcranial stimulation of the developing brain: a plea for extreme caution. *Front. Hum. Neurosci.* 8:600. doi:10.3389/fnhum.2014.00600, 2014.

Della Chiesa, B., et al. How many brains does it take to build a new light: knowledge management challenges of a transdisciplinary project. *Mind Brain Educ.* 3:17–26, 2009.

Dowling, J.E. *Creating mind: how the brain works.* New York: W.W. Norton, 1998.

Farah, M.J. Neuroethics: the ethical, legal, and societal impact of neuroscience. *Annu. Rev. Neurosci.* 63:571–591, 2011.

Farah, M.J. An ethics toolbox for neurotechnology. *Neuron* 86:34–37, 2015.

Gabrieli, J.D.E., et al. Prediction as a humanitarian and pragmatic contribution from human cognitive neuroscience. *Neuron* 85:11–26, 2015.

Glannon, W. Our brains are not us. *Bioethics* 23:321–329, 2010.

Gordon, E. (Ed.) *Integrative neuroscience: bringing together biological, psychological and clinical models of the human brain.* Newark, NJ: Harwood Academic Publishers, 2000.

Greene, J., Cohen, J. For the law, neuroscience changes nothing and everything. *Philos. Trans. R. Soc. Lond. B Biol. Sci.* 359, 1775–1785, 2004.

Ioannidis, J.P.A. Publication and other reporting biases in cognitive sciences: detection, prevalence, and prevention. *Trends Cogn. Sci.* 18:235–241, 2014.

Johnson, J.G., et al. Mind and motion: surveying successes and stumbles in looking ahead. *Progr. Brain Res.* 174:319–325, 2009.

Jones, O.D., et al. Neuroscientists in court. *Nature Rev. Neurosci.* 14:730–736, 2013.

Karten, H., Lumsden, A. Evolution of the nervous system. *Curr. Opin. Neurobiol.* 9:579–581, 1999.

Naquet, R. Ethical and moral considerations in the design of experiments. *Neuroscience* 57:183–189, 1993.

Peart, S. Is discovery worth the pain? *Conquest* 177:1–10, 1988.

Poldrack, R.A. The role of fMRI in cognitive neuroscience: where do we stand? *Curr. Opin. Neurosci.* 18:223–227, 2008.

Ruscioni, E., Mitchener-Nissen, T. The role of expectations, hype and ethics in neuroimaging and neuromodulation. *Front. Syst. Neurosci.* 8:214. doi:10.3389/fnsys.2014.00214, 2014.

Singer, W. The significance of alternative methods for the reduction of animal experiments in the neurosciences. *Neuroscience* 57: 191–200, 1993.

Steitzer, J., et al. Deficient approaches to human neuroimaging. *Front. Hum. Neurosci.* 8:462. doi:10.3389/ fnhum.2014.00462, 2014.

Stevens, C.W. Alternatives to the use of mammals in pain research. *Life Sci.* 50:901–912, 1992.

Striedter, G.F.P. Progress in the study of brain evolution: from speculative theories to testable hypotheses. *Anat. Rec. (New Anat.)* 53:105–112, 1998.

Temel, Y., Jahanshahi, A. Treating brain disorders with neuromodulation. *Science* 347:1418–1419, 2015.

Tye, K.M. Neural circuit reprogramming: a new paradigm for treating neuropsychiatric disease? *Neuron* 83:1259–1261, 2014.

Weiskrantz, L. *Consciousness lost and found. A neuropsychological exploration* (p. 195). New York: Oxford University Press, 1997.

Worden, F.G., et al. (Eds.) *The neurosciences: paths of discovery.* Cambridge, MA: MIT Press, 1975.

Chapter 1: Structure of the Neuron and Organization of Nervous Tissue

Bernard, A., et al. Shifting the paradigm: new approaches for characterizing and classifying neurons. *Curr. Opin. Neurobiol.* 19:530–536, 2009.

Bressler, S.L., Menon, V. Large-scale cortical networks in cognition. *Trends Cogn.Sci.* 14:277–299, 2010.

Cajal, R.Y. *Histologie du systeme nerveux.* Vols. 1–2. Instituto Ramon y Cajal, 1952.

Dunaevsky A., et al. Spine motility with synaptic contact. *Nat. Neurosci.* 4:685–686, 2001.

Ehlers, M.D. Molecular morphogens for dendritic spines. *Trends Neurosci.* 25:64–67, 2002.

Gahr, M. How should brain nuclei be delineated? Consequences for developmental mechanisms and for correlations of area size, neuron numbers and functions of brain nuclei. *Trends Neurosci.* 20:58–62, 1997.

Gardiol, A., et al. Dendritic and postsynaptic protein synthetic machinery. *J. Neurosci.* 19:168–179, 1999.

Harris, K.M., Kater, S.B. Dendritic spines: cellular specializations imparting both stability and flexibility to synaptic function. *Annu. Rev. Neurosci.* 17:341–371, 1994.

Jones, E.G. The nervous tissue. In: Weiss, L. (Ed.), *Cell and tissue biology* (pp. 279–350). Baltimore: Urban & Schwarzenberg, 1988.

Kennedy, M.B., et al. Integration of biochemical signalling in spines. *Nat. Rev. Neurosci.* 6:423–434, 2005.

Kuhl, D., Skehel, P. Dendritic localization of mRNAs. *Curr. Opin. Neurobiol.* 8:600–606, 1998.

Lau, P.-M., Guo-Qiang, B. Synaptic mechanisms of persistent reverberatory activity in neuronal networks. *Proc. Natl. Acad. Sci. USA* 102:10333–103338, 2005.

Major, G., Tank, D. Persistent neural activity: prevalence and mechanisms. *Curr. Opin. Neurobiol.* 14:675–684, 2004.

Park, H.-J., Friston, K. Structural and functional brain networks: from connections to cognition. *Science* 342:579–587, 2013.

Park, M.K., et al. The endoplasmic reticulum as an integrator of multiple dendritic events. *Neuroscientist* 14:68–77, 2008.

Peters, A., et al. *The fine structure of the nervous system: neurons and their supporting cells*, 3rd ed. Philadelphia: W.B. Saunders, 1991.

Segev, I. Single neurone models: oversimple, complex and reduced. *Trends Neurosci.* 15:414–421, 1992.

Singer, W. Dynamic formation of functional networks by synchronization. *Neuron* 69:191–193, 2011.

Sporns, O., et al. Organization, development and function of complex brain networks. *Trends Cogn. Sci.* 8:418–425, 2004.

Cytoskeleton and Axonal Transport

Goldstein, L.S.B. Axonal transport and neurodegenerative disease: Can we see the elephant? *Progr. Neurobiol.* 99:186–190, 2012.

Goldstein, L.S.B., Yang, Z. Microtubule-based transport systems in neurons: the roles of kinesins and dyneins. *Annu. Rev. Neurosci.* 23:39–71, 2000.

Hirokawa, N., Takemura, R. Molecular motors and mechanisms of directional transport in neurons. *Nat. Rev. Neurosci.* 6:201–214, 2005.

Lamprecht, R. The actin cytoskeleton in memory formation. *Progr. Neurobiol.* 117:1–19, 2014.

Matus, A. Microtubule-associated proteins: their potential role in determining neuronal morphology. *Annu. Rev. Neurosci.* 11: 29–44, 1988.

Neukirchen, D., Bradke, F. Neuronal polarization and the cytoskeleton. *Semin. Cell. Develop. Biol.* 22:825–833, 2011.

Pak, C.W., et al. Actin-binding proteins take the reins in growth cones. *Nat. Rev. Neurosci.* 9:136–147, 2008.

Pekny, M., Lane, E.B. Intermediate filaments and stress. *Exp. Cell. Res.* 313:2244–2254, 2007.

Yuan, A., et al. Neurofilaments at a glance. *J. Cell. Sci.* 125:3257–3263, 2012.

Zweifel, L.S., et al. Functions and mechanisms of retrograde neurotrophin signalling. *Nat. Rev. Neurosci.* 6:615–625, 2005.

Chapter 2: Glia

Allen, N.J., Barres, B.A. Signaling between glia and neurons: focus on synaptic plasticity. *Curr. Opin. Neurobiol.* 15:542–548, 2005.

Barnett, S.C. Olfactory ensheathing cells: unique glial cell types? *J. Neurotrauma* 21:375–383, 2004.

Kettenmann, H., Ransom, B.R. *Neuroglia*. 2nd ed. Oxford: Oxford University Press, 2004.

Lemke, G. Glial control of neuronal development. *Annu. Rev. Neurosci.* 24:87–105, 2001.

Tolbert, L.P., Oland, L.A. A role for glia in the development of organized neuropilar structures. *Trends Neurosci.* 12:70–75, 1989.

Astrocytes

Agulhon, C., et al. What is the role of astrocytic calcium in neurophysiology? *Neuron* 59:932–946, 2008.

Allaman, I., et al. Astrocyte-neuron metabolic relationships: for better and for worse. *Trends Neurosci.* 34:76–87, 2011.

Amiry-Moghaddam, M., Ottersen, O.P. The molecular basis of water transport in the brain. *Nat. Rev. Neurosci.* 4:991–1001, 2003.

Araque, A., et al. Synaptically released acetylcholine evokes Ca^{2+} elevations in astrocytes in hippocampal slices. *J. Neurosci.* 22: 2443–2450, 2002.

Barros, L.F., Deitmer, J.W. Glucose and lactate supply to the synapse. *Brain Res. Rev.* 63:149–159, 2010.

Chih, C.-P., Roberts, E.L. Jr. Energy substrates for neurons during neural activity: a critical review of the astrocyte-neuron lactate shuttle hypothesis. *J. Cereb. Blood Flow Metab.* 23:1263–1281, 2003.

Giaume, C., et al. Astroglial networks: a step further in neuroglial and gliovascular interactions. *Nature Rev. Neurosci.* 11:87–99, 2010.

Lundgaard, I., et al. White matter astrocytes in health and disease. *Neuroscience* 276:161–173, 2014.

Nagelhus, E. Water and volume homeostasis in the central nervous system: role of glial cells. Dissertation, Department of Anatomy, University of Oslo, 1998.

Nagelhus, E., Ottersen, O.P. Physiological roles of aquaporin-4 in the brain. *Physiol. Rev.* 93:1543–1562, 2013.

Papadopoulos, M., Verkman, A.S. Aquaporin water channels in the nervous system. *Nature Rev. Neurosci.* 14:265–277, 2013.

Paukert, M., et al. Norepinephrine controls astroglial responsiveness to local circuit activity. *Neuron* 82:1263–1270, 2014.

Perea, G., et al. Neuron-glia networks: integral gear of brain function. *Front. Cell. Neurosci.* 8:378. doi:10.3389/fncel.2014.00378, 2014.

Piet, R., et al. Physiological contribution of the astrocytic environment of neurons to intersynaptic crosstalk. *Proc. NY Acad. Sci.* 101:2151–2155, 2004.

Schummers, J., et al. Tuned responses of astrocytes and their influence on hemodynamic signals in the visual cortex. *Science* 320:1638–1643, 2008.

Sofroniew, M.V., Vinters, H.V. Astrocytes: biology and pathology. *Acta Neuropathol.* 119: 7–35, 2010.

Ventura, R., Harris, K.M. Three-dimensional relationships between hippocampal synapses and astrocytes. *J. Neurosci.* 19:6897–6906, 1999.

Volterra, A., Meldolesi, J. Astrocytes, from brain glue to communication elements: the revolution continues. *Nat. Rev. Neurosci.* 6:626–640, 2005.

Pinheiro, P.S., Mulle, C. Presynaptic glutamate receptors: physiological functions and mechanisms of action. *Nat. Rev. Neurosci.* 9:423–436, 2008.

Repressa, A., Ben-Ari, Y. Trophic actions of GABA on neuronal development. *Trends Neurosci.* 28:278–283, 2005.

Rodriguez, M., et al. The role of non-synaptic extracellular glutamate. *Brain Res. Bull.* 93:17–26, 2013.

Takumi, Y., et al. Different modes of expression of AMPA and NMDA receptors in hippocampal synapses. *Nat. Neurosci.* 2:618–624, 1999.

Tan, K.R., et al. Hooked on benzodiazepines: GABA$_A$ receptor subtypes and addiction. *Trends Neurosci.* 34:188–197, 2011.

Tzingounis, A., Wadiche, J.I. Glutamate transporters: confining runaway excitation by shaping synaptic transmission. *Nat. Rev. Neurosci.* 8:935–947, 2007.

Vanderklish, P.W., Edelman, G.M. Dendritic spines elongate after stimulation of group 1 metabotropic glutamate receptors in cultured hippocampal neurons. *Proc. Natl. Acad. Sci. USA* 99:1639–1644, 2002.

Zarate, J., Manji, H.K. The role of AMPA receptor modulation in the treatment of neuropsychiatric diseases. *Exp. Neurol.* 211:7–10, 2008.

Acetylcholine and Biogenic Amines

Baudry, A., et al. New views on antidepressant action. *Curr. Opin. Neurobiol.* 21:858–865, 2011.

Bentley, P., et al. Cholinergic modulation of cognition: insights from human pharmacological functional neuroimaging. *Prog. Neurobiol.* 94:360–388, 2011.

Bjorklund, A., Dunnett, S.B. Dopamine neuron systems in the brain: an update. *Trends Neurosci.* 30:194–202, 2007.

Briand, L.A., et al. Modulators in concert for cognition: modular interactions in the prefrontal cortex. *Prog. Neurobiol.* 83:69–91, 2007.

Buckholtz, J.W., et al. Genetic variation in MAOA modulates ventro-medial prefrontal circuitry mediating individual differences in human personality. *Mol. Psychiatry* 13:313–324, 2008.

Buhot, M.-C. Serotonin receptors and cognitive behaviors. *Curr. Opin. Neurobiol.* 7:243–254, 1997.

Canli, T., et al. Beyond affect: a role for genetic variation of the serotonin transporter in neural activation during a cognitive attention task. *Proc. Natl. Acad. Sci. USA* 102:1224–12229, 2005.

Caspi, A., et al. Influence of life stress on depression: moderation by a polymorphism in the 5-HTT gene. *Science* 301:386–389, 2003.

Caspi, A., et al. Genetic sensitivity to the environment: the case of the serotonin transporter gene and its implications for studying complex diseases and traits. *Am. J. Psychiat.* 167:509–527, 2010.

Changeux, J.-P., et al. Brain nicotinic receptors: structure and regulation, role in learning and reinforcement. *Brain Res. Rev.* 26: 198–216, 1998.

Descarries, L., Umbriaco, D. Ultrastructural basis of monamine and acetylcholine functions in CNS. *Semin. Neurosci.* 7:309–318, 1995.

Geula, C., Mesulam, M.M. Brainstem cholinergic systems. In: Mai, J.K., Paxinos, G. (Eds.), *The human nervous system*, 3rd ed. (pp. 456–470). San Diego: Elsevier Academic Press, 2012.

Haas, H., Panula, P. The role of histamine and the tuberomammillary nucleus in the nervous system. *Nat. Rev. Neurosci.* 4:121–130, 2003.

Hariri, A.R., Holmes, A. Genetics of emotional regulation: the role of the serotonin transporter in neural function. *Trends Cogn. Sci.* 10:182–191, 2006.

Hasselmo, M.E. The role of acetylcholine in learning and memory. *Curr. Opin. Neurobiol.* 16:710–715, 2006.

Holmberg, J.R., van den Hove, D.L.A. The serotonin transporter gene and functional and pathological adaptation to environmental variation across the life span. *Progr. Neurobiol.* 99:117–127, 2012.

Hurst, R., et al. Nicotinic acetylcholine receptors: from basic science to therapeutics. *Pharmacol. Therap.* 137:22–54, 2013.

Jones, S., et al. Nicotinic receptors in the brain: correlating physiology with function. *Trends Neurosci.* 22:555–561, 1999.

Laviolette, S.R., van der Kooy, D. The neurobiology of nicotine addiction: bridging the gap from molecules to behaviour. *Nat. Rev. Neurosci.* 5:55–65, 2004.

Mesulam, M.-M. The cholinergic contribution to neuromodulation in the cerebral cortex. *Semin. Neurosci.* 7:297–307, 1995.

Miwa, J., et al. Neural systems governed by nicotinic acetylcholine receptors: emerging hypotheses. *Neuron* 70:20–33, 2011.

Mongeau, R., et al. The serotonergic and noradrenergic systems of the hippocampus: their interactions and the effects of antidepressant treatments. *Brain Res. Rev.* 23:145–195, 1997.

Murphy, D.L., Lesch, K.-L. Targeting the murine serotonin transporter: insights into human neurobiology. *Nat. Rev. Neurosci.* 9:85–96, 2008.

Naqvi, N.H. Damage to the insula disrupts addiction to cigarette smoking. *Science* 315:531–534, 2007.

Nees, F. The nicotinic cholinergic system function in the human brain. *Neuropharmacol.* doi:10.1016/j.neuropharm.2014.10.021, 2015.

Nicoll, R.A., Schmitz, D. Synaptic plasticity at hippocampal mossy fibre terminals. *Nat. Rev. Neurosci.* 6:863–876, 2005.

Noudoost, B., Moore, T. The role of neuromodulators in selective attention. *Trends Cogn. Sci.* 15:585–591, 2011.

Panula, P., Nuutinen, S. The histaminergic network in the brain: basic organization and role in disease. *Nature Rev. Neurosci.* 14:474–487, 2013.

Paspalas, C.D., Goldman-Rakic, P.S. Microdomains for dopamine volume transmission in primate prefrontal cortex. *J. Neurosci.* 24:5292–5300, 2004.

Perry, E., et al. Acetylcholine in mind: a neurotransmitter correlate of consciousness? *Trends Neurosci.* 22:273–280, 1999.

Portugal, G.S., Gould, T.J. Genetic variability in nicotinic acetylcholine receptors and nicotine addiction: converging evidence from human and animal research. *Behav. Brain Res.* 193:1–16, 2008.

Reif, A., et al. Nature and nurture predispose to violent behavior: serotonergic genes and adverse childhood environment. *Neuropsychopharmacology* 32:2375–2383, 2007.

Sarter, M., et al. Phasic acetylcholine release and the volume transmission hypothesis: time to move on. *Nat. Rev. Neurosci.* 10:383–390, 2009.

Schloesser, R.J., et al. Mood-stabilizing drugs: mechanisms of action. *Trends Neurosci.* 35:36–46, 2012.

Sharpley, C.F., et al. An update on the interaction between the serotonin transporter promoter variant (5-HTTLPR), stress and depression, plus an exploration of non-confirming findings. *Behav. Brain Res.* 273:89–105, 2014.

Shih, J.C., et al. Monoamine oxidase: from genes to behavior. *Annu. Rev. Neurosci.* 22:197–217, 1999.

Thiele, A. Muscarinic signaling in the brain. *Annu. Rev. Neurosci.* 36:271–294, 2013.

Torres, G.E., et al. Plasma membrane monoamine transporters: structure, regulation and function. *Nat. Rev. Neurosci.* 4:13–25, 2003.

Tully, K., Bolshakov, V. Emotional enhancement of memory: how norepinephrine eables synaptic plasticity. *Mol. Brain* 3:15, 2010.

Tunbridge, E.M., et al. Catechol-o-methyltransferase, cognition and psychosis: Val[158]Met and beyond. *Biol. Psychiat.* 60:141–151, 2006.

Watson, K.K., et al. Serotonin transporter genotype modulates social reward and punishment in rhesus macaques. *PLoS ONE* 4.1:e4156, 2009.

Wise, R.A. Dopamine, learning and motivation. *Nat. Rev. Neurosci.* 5:483–494, 2004.

Witte, A.V., Flöel, A. Effects of COMT polymorphisms on brain function and behavior in health and disease. *Brain Res. Bull.* 88:418–428, 2012.

Purines, NO, and Neuropeptides

Abbracchio, M.P., et al. Purinergic signalling in the nervous system: an overview. *Trends Neurosci.* 32:19–29, 2009.

Burnstock, G. Historical review: ATP as a neurotransmitter. *Trends Pharmacol. Sci.* 27:166–176, 2006.

Burnstock, G., et al. Purinergic signaling: From normal behavior to pathological brain function. *Progr. Neurobiol.* 95:229–274, 2011.

Caldwell, H.K., et al. Vasopressin: behavioral roles of an "original" neuropeptide. *Prog. Neurobiol.* 84:1–24, 2008.

Cudeiro, J., Rivadulla, C. Sight and insight—on the physiological role of nitric oxide in the visual system. *Trends Neurosci.* 22:109–116, 1999.

Darlison, M.G., Richter, D. Multiple genes for neuropeptides and their receptors: co-evolution and physiology. *Trends Neurosci.* 22:81–88, 1999.

Dawson, T., et al. Nitric oxide: diverse actions in the central and peripheral nervous system. *Neuroscientist* 4:96–112, 1998.

Dias, R.B., et al. Adenosine: setting the stage for plasticity. *Trends Neurosci.* 36:248–257, 2013.

Edwards, F.A. ATP receptors. *Curr. Opin. Neurobiol.* 4:313–323, 1994.

Fields, R.D., Burnstock, G. Purinergic signaling in neuron-glia interactions. *Nat. Rev. Neurosci.* 7:423–436, 2006.

Fredholm, B.B., et al. Aspects of the general biology of adenosine A2A signaling. *Prog. Neurobiol.* 83:263–276, 2007.

Garthwaite, J. Concepts of neural nitric oxide-mediated transmission. *Eur. J. Neurosci.* 27:2783–2802, 2008.

Hökfelt, T., et al. Galanin and NPY, two peptides with multiple putative roles in the nervous system. *Horm. Metab. Res.* 31:330–334, 1999.

Hökfelt, T., et al. Neuropeptides—an overview. *Neuropharmacology* 39:1337–1356, 2000.

Jo, Y.-H., Schlichter, R. Synaptic corelease of ATP and GABA in cultured spinal neurons. *Nat. Rev. Neurosci.* 2:241–245, 1999.

Ludwig, M., Leng, G. Dendritic peptide release and peptide-dependent behaviors. *Nat. Rev. Neurosci.* 7:127–136, 2006.

Mansour, A., et al. Anatomy of CNS opioid receptors. *Trends Neurosci.* 11:308–314, 1988.

North, R.A., Verkhratsky, A. Purinergic transmission in the central nervous system. *Pflügers Arch Eur. J. Physiol. (Lond.)* 452:479–485, 2006.

Salter, M.W., et al. Physiological roles for adenosine and ATP in synaptic transmission in the spinal dorsal horn. *Prog. Neurobiol.* 41:125–156, 1993.

Strand, F.L. *Neuropeptides: regulators of physiological processes.* Cambridge, MA: MIT Press, 1999.

Terusama, N., Jianguo, G.G. P2X purinoceptors and sensory transmission. *Pflügers Arch. Eur. J. Physiol.* 452:598–607, 2006.

Chapter 6: Parts of the Nervous System

Brown, A.G. *Organization in the spinal cord: the anatomy and physiology of identified neurons.* New York: Springer-Verlag, 1981.

Cassone, V.M. Effects of melatonin on vertebrate circadian systems. *Trends Neurosci.* 13:457–464, 1990.

Crick, F.C., Koch, C. What is the function of the claustrum? *Philos. Trans. R. Soc. Lond. B Biol. Sci.* 360:1271–1279, 2005.

Erlich, S.S., Apuzzo, M.L.J. The pineal gland: anatomy, physiology, and clinical significance. *J. Neurosurg.* 63:321–341, 1985.

Fernández-Miranda, J.C., et al. The claustrum and its projection system in the human brain: a microsurgical and tractographic anatomical study. *J. Neurosurg.* 108:764–774, 2008.

Hamilton, W.J., et al. *Human embryology: prenatal development of form and function*, 4th ed. Philadelphia: Williams & Wilkins, 1972.

Heimer, L. *The human brain and spinal cord: functional neuroanatomy and dissection guide.* New York: Springer-Verlag, 1995.

Hikosaka, O. The habenula: From stress-evasion to value-based decision making. *Nature Rev. Neurosci.* 11:503–513, 2010.

Kimura, M., et al. What does the habenula tell dopamine neurons? *Nat. Neurosci.* 10:677–678, 2007.

Landon, D.N. *The peripheral nerve.* New York: Chapman & Hall, 1976.

Rexed, B. The cytoarchitectonic organization of the spinal cord in the cat. *J. Comp. Neurol.* 96:415–495, 1952.

Scheibel, M.E., Scheibel, A.B. Terminal axonal patterns in the spinal cord. I. The lateral corticospinal tract. *Brain Res.* 2:333–350, 1966.

Shelton, L., et al. Unmasking the mysteries of the habenula in pain and analgesia. *Progr. Neurobiol.* 96:2012:208–219, 2012.

Swanson, L.W. What is the brain? *Trends Neurosci.* 23:519–527, 2000.

Terminologia anatomica: International anatomical terminology. Federative Committee on Anatomical Terminology. New York: Thieme, 1998.

Torgerson, C.M., Van Horn, J.D. A case study in connectomics: the history, mapping, and connectivity of the claustrum. *Front. Neuroinform.* 8:83. doi:10.3389/fninf.2014.00083, 2014.

Brain Imaging Methods

Buracas, G.T., et al. The relationship between task performance and functional magnetic resonance imaging response. *J. Neurosci.* 25:3023–3031. 2005.

Coltheart, M. How can functional neuroimaging inform cognitive theories? *Perspectiv. Psychol. Sci.* 8:98–103, 2013.

Devor, A., et al. Coupling of the cortical hemodynamic response to cortical and thalamic neuronal activity. *Proc. Natl. Acad. Sci. USA* 102:3822–3827, 2005.

Dolan, R.J. Neuroimaging of cognition: past, present, and future. *Neuron* 60:496–502, 2008.

Lee, M.W.L., et al. An evidence-based approach to human dermatomes. *Clin. Anat.* 21:363–373, 2008.

Levine, J.D., et al. Peptides and the primary afferent nociceptor. *J. Neurosci.* 13:2273–2286, 1993.

Liguori, R., et al. Determination of the segmental sensory and motor innervation of the lumbosacral spinal nerves: an electrophysiological study. *Brain* 115:915–934, 1992.

Nakatsuka, T., Gu, J.G. P2X purinoceptors and sensory transmission. *Pflügers Arch. Eur. J. Physiol. (Lond.)* 452:598–607, 2006.

Sherrington, C.S. Experiments in examination of the peripheral distribution of the fibres of the posterior roots of some spinal nerves: part II. *Philos. Trans. R. Soc. Lond. B Biol. Sci.* 190:45–186, 1898.

Su, J., et al. Phenotypic changes in dorsal root ganglion and spinal cord in the collagen antibody-induced arthritis mouse model. *J. Comp. Neurol.* 523:1505–1528, 2015.

Szucs, P., et al. Axon diversity of lamina I local-circuit neurons in the lumbar spinal cord. *J. Comp. Neurol.* 521:2719-2741, 2013.

Wiesenfeld-Hallin, Z., Xu, X.J. Galanin in somatosensory function. *Ann. NY Acad. Sci.* 863:383–389, 1998.

Zhang, X., Bao L. The development and modulation of nociceptive circuitry. *Curr. Opin. Neurobiol.* 16:460–466, 2006.

Chapter 14: Central Parts of the Somatosensory System

The Spinal Cord and Sensory Pathways

Al-Chaer, E.D., et al. Comparative study of viscerosomatic input onto postsynaptic dorsal column and spinothalamic tract neurons in the primate. *J. Neurophysiol.* 82:1876–1882, 1999.

Andrew, D., Craig, A.D. Spinothalamic lamina I neurons selectively sensitive to histamine: a central neural pathway for itch. *Nat. Rev. Neurosci.* 4:72–77, 2001.

Apkarian, A.V., Hodges, C.J. Primate spinothalamic pathways: I. A quantitative study of the cells of origin of the spinothalamic pathway. *J. Comp.Neurol.* 288:447–473, 1989.

Apkarian, A.V., Hodges, C.J. Primate spinothalamic pathways: III. Thalamic terminations of the dorsolateral and ventral spinotha-lamic pathways. *J. Comp. Neurol.* 288:493–511, 1989.

Bagley, C.A., et al. Psychophysics of CNS pain-related activity: binary and analog channels and memory encoding. *Neuroscientist* 12:29–42, 2006.

Berkley, K., Hubscher, C.H. Are there separate central nervous system pathways for touch and pain? *Nat. Med.* 1:766–773, 1995.

Bester, H., et al. Physiological properties of the lamina I spinoparabra-chial neurons in the rat. *J. Neurophysiol.* 83:2239–2259, 2000.

Blomqvist, A., et al. Cytoarchitectonic and immunohistochemical characterization of a specific pain and temperature relay, the posterior portion of the ventral medial nucleus, in the human thalamus. *Brain* 123:601–619, 2000.

Bourgeais, L., et al. Projections from the nociceptive area of the central nucleus of the amygdala to the forebrain: a PHA-L study in the rat. *Eur. J. Neurosci.* 14:229–255, 2001.

Cohen, L.G., Starr, A. Localization, timing and specificity of gating of somatosensory evoked potentials during active movement in man. *Brain* 110:451–467, 1987.

Cooper, B.Y., et al. Finger movement deficits in the stumptail macaque following lesions if the fasciculus cuneatus. *Somatosens. Mot. Res.* 10:17–29, 1993.

Cullen, K.E. Sensory signals during active versus passive movement. *Curr. Opin. Neurobiol.* 14:698–706, 2004.

Danziger, N., et al. A clinical and neurophysiological study of a patient with an extensive transection of the spinal cord sparing only a part of the anterolateral quadrant. *Brain* 119:1835–1848, 1996.

Davidson, S., et al. Termination zones of functionally characterized spinothalamic tract neurons within the primate posterior thalamus. *J. Neurophysiol.* 100:2026–237, 2008.

Dougherty, P.M., et al. Combined application of excitatory amino acids and substance P produces long-lasting changes in responses of primate spinothalamic tract neurons. *Brain Res. Rev.* 18:227–246, 1993.

Fanselow, E.A., Nicolelis, M.A.L. Behavioral modulation of tactile responses in the rat somatosensory system. *J. Neurosci.* 19:7603–7616, 1999.

Giesler, G.J., et al. Direct spinal pathways to the limbic system for nociceptive information. *Trends Neurosci.* 17:244–250, 1994.

Glendenning, D.S., Vierck, C.J. Jr. Lack of proprioceptive deficit after dorsal column lesions in monkeys. *Neurology* 43:363–366, 1993.

Gordon, G. *Active touch: the mechanism of recognition of objects by manipulation—a multi-disciplinary approach.* Oxford: Pergamon Press, 1978.

Graziano, A., Jones, E.G. Widespread thalamic terminations of fibers arising in the superficial medullary dorsal horn of monkeys and their relation to calbindin immunoreactivity. *J. Neurosci.* 24:248–256, 2004.

Groenewegen, H.J., Berendse, H.W. The specificity of the "nonspecific" midline and intralaminar thalamic nuclei. *Trends Neurosci.* 17:52–57, 1994.

Han, Z.-S., et al. Nociceptive and thermoceptive lamina I neurons are anatomically distinct. *Nat. Rev. Neurosci.* 1:218–224, 1998.

Jola, C., et al. Proprioceptive integration and body representation: insights into dancers' expertise. *Exp. Brain Res.* 213: 257–265, 2011.

Klop, E.M., et al. In cat four times as many lamina I neurons project to the parabrachial nuclei and twice as many to the periaqueductal gray as to the thalamus. *Neuroscience* 134:189–197, 2005.

Kohama, I., et al. Synaptic reorganization in the substantia gelatinosa after peripheral nerve neuroma formation: aberrant innervation of lamina II neurons by Aβ afferents. *J. Neurosci.* 20:1538–1539, 2000.

Lenz, F.A., et al. Stimulation in the human somatosensory thalamus can reproduce both the affective and sensory dimensions of previously experienced pain. *Nat. Med.* 1:910–913, 1995.

Macchi, G., et al. *Somatosensory integration in the thalamus.* Philadelphia: Elsevier, 1990.

Marple-Horvath, D.E., Armstrong, D.M. Central regulation of motor cortex neuronal responses to forelimb nerve inputs during precision walking in the cat. *J. Physiol.* 519:279–299, 1999.

Mayer, D.J., et al. Neurophysiological characterization of the antero-lateral spinal cord neurons contributing to pain perception in man. *Pain* 1:51–58, 1975.

Monconduit, L., et al. Convergence of cutaneous, muscular and visceral noxious inputs onto ventromedial thalamic neurons in the rat. *Pain* 103:83–91, 2003.

Nathan, P.W., et al. Sensory effects in man of lesions of the posterior columns and of some other afferent pathways. *Brain* 109:1003–1041, 1986.

Ralston, H.J., Ralston, D.D. Medial lemniscal and spinal projections to the macaque thalamus: an electron microscopic study of differing GABAergic circuitry serving thalamic somatosensory mechanisms. *J. Neurosci.* 14:2485–2502, 1994.

Seki, K., et al. Sensory input to primate spinal cord is presynaptically inhibited during voluntary movement. *Nat. Rev. Neurosci.* 6:1309–1316, 2003.

Todd, A.J., Spike, R.C. The localization of classical transmitters and neuropeptides within neurons in laminae I–III of the mammalian spinal dorsal horn. *Prog. Neurobiol.* 41:609–645, 1993.

Urban, L., et al. Modulation of spinal excitability: co-operation between neurokinin and excitatory amino acid neurotransmitters. *Trends Neurosci.* 17:432–438, 1994.

Vierck, C.J. Jr., Cooper, B.Y. Cutaneous texture discrimination following transection of the dorsal spinal column in monkeys. *Somatosens. Mot. Res.* 15:309–315, 1998.

Voss, M., et al. Sensorimotor attenuation by central motor command signals in the absence of movement. *Nat. Rev. Neurosci.* 9:26–227, 2006.

Willis, W.D., et al. A visceral pain pathway in the dorsal column of the spinal cord. *Proc. Natl. Acad. Sci. USA* 96:7675–7679, 1999.

Windhorst, U. Muscle proprioceptive feedback and spinal networks. *Brain Res. Bull.* 73:155–202, 2007.

Somatosensory Cortical Areas

Afif, A., et al. Middle short gyrus of the insula implicated in pain processing. *Pain* 138:546–555, 2008.

Arnal, L.H., Giraud, A.-L. Cortical oscillations and sensory predictions. *Trends Cogn. Neurosci.* 16:390–398, 2012.

Blakemore, S.-J., et al. Central cancellation of self-produced tickle sensation. *Nat. Rev. Neurosci.* 1:635–640, 1998.

Bourgeais, L., et al. Parabrachial internal lateral neurons convey nociceptive messages from the deep laminas of the dorsal horn to the intralaminar thalamus. *J. Neurosci.* 21:2159–2165, 2001.

Burton, H., et al. Cortical areas within the lateral sulcus connected to cutaneous representations in areas 3b and 1: a revised interpretation of the second somatosensory area in macaque monkeys. *J. Comp. Neurol.* 355:539–562, 1995.

Bushnell, M.C., et al. Pain perception: is there a role for primary somatosensory cortex? *Proc. Natl. Acad. Sci. USA* 96:7705–7709, 1999.

Caselli, R. Ventrolateral and dorsomedial somatosensory association cortex damage produces distinct somesthetic syndromes in humans. *Neurology* 43:762–771, 1993.

Cauda, F. et al. Massive modulation of brain areas after mechanical pain stimulation. *Cereb. Cortex* 24:2991–3005, 2014.

Craig, A.D. How do you feel? Interoception: the sense of the physiological condition of the body. *Nat. Rev. Neurosci.* 3:655–666, 2002.

Darian-Smith, D., et al. Ipsilateral cortical projections to area 3a, 3b, and 4 in the macaque monkey. *J. Comp. Neurol.* 335:200–213, 1993.

Dum, R.P., et al. The spinothalamic system targets motor and sensory areas in the cerebral cortex of monkeys. *J. Neurosci.* 29:14223–14235, 2009.

Garcia-Larrea, L., et al. Operculo-insular pain (parasylvian pain): a distinct central pain syndrome. *Brain* 133:2528–2539, 2010.

Gehring, W.J., Taylor, S.F. When the going gets tough, the cingulated gets going. *Nat. Rev. Neurosci.* 7:1285–1287, 2004.

Hari, R., et al. Functional organization of the human first and second somatosensory cortices: a neuromagnetic study. *Eur. J. Neurosci.* 5:724–734, 1993.

Hashmi, J.A., et al. Shape shifting pain: chronification of back pain shifts representation from nociceptive to emotional circuits. *Brain* 136:2751–2768, 2013.

Henderson, L.A., et al. Somatotopic organization of processing of muscle and cutaneous pain in the left right insula cortex: a single-trial fMRI study. *Pain* 128:20–30, 2007.

Kell, C.A., et al. The sensory cortical representation of the human penis: revisiting somatotopy in the male homunculus. *J. Neurosci.* 25:5984–5987, 2005.

Lee, S.-H., et al. Motor modulation of afferent somatosensory circuits. *Nat. Rev. Neurosci.* 11:1430–1438, 2008.

Lötsch, J., et al. The human operculo-insular cortex is pain-preferentially but not pain-exclusively activated by trigeminal and olfactory stimuli. *PLoS ONE* 7:e34798, 2012.

Mazzola, L., et al. Stimulation of the human cortex and the experience of pain: Wilder Penfield's observations revisited. *Brain* 135: 631–640, 2012.

Mouraux, A., et al. A multisensory investigation of the functional significance of the "pain matrix." *NeuroImage* 54:2237–2249, 2011.

Nicolelis, M.A.L., et al. Simultaneous encoding of tactile information by three primate cortical areas. *Nat. Med.* 1:621–630, 1998.

Pavlides, C., et al. Projection from the sensory to the motor cortex is important in learning motor skills in the monkey. *J. Neurophysiol.* 70:733–741, 1993.

Penfield, W., Rasmussen, T. *The cerebral cortex of man*. New York: Macmillan, 1950.

Peyron, R. et al. Functional imaging of brain responses to pain: a review and meta-analysis. *Neurophysiol. Clin.* 30:263–288, 2000.

Ploner, M., et al. Differential organization of touch and pain in human primary somatosensory cortex. *J. Neurophysiol.* 83:1770–1776, 2000.

Ploner, M., et al. Cortical representation of first and second pain sensations in humans. *Proc. Natl. Acad. Sci. USA* 99:12444–12448, 2002.

Rainville, P., et al. Pain affect encoded in human anterior cingulate but not somatosensory cortex. *Science* 277:968–971, 1997.

Reed, J.L., et al. Widespread spatial integration in primary somatosensory cortex. *Proc. NY Acad. Sci.* 105:10233–10237, 2008.

Rosetti, Y., et al. Visually guided reaching: bilateral posterior parietal lesions cause a switch from fast visuomotor to slow cognitive control. *Neuropsychologia* 43:162–173, 2005.

Sanchez-Panchuelo, R.M., et al. Mapping human somatosensory cortex in individual subjects with 7T functional MRI. *J. Neurophysiol.* 103:2544–2556, 2010.

Schneider, R.J. A modality-specific somatosensory area within the insula of the rhesus monkey. *Brain Res.* 621:116–120, 1993.

Tracey, I., Mantyh, P.W. The cerebral signature for pain perception and its modulation. *Neuron* 55:377–391, 2007.

Van Buren, J.M. Sensory responses from stimulation of the inferior Rolandic and Sylvian regions in man. *J. Neurosurg.* 59:119–130, 1983.

Wang, Z., et al. The relationship of anatomical and functional connectivity to resting-state connectivity in primate somatosensory cortex. *Neuron* 78:1116–1126, 2013.

Woolsey, C.N. Organization of somatic sensory and motor areas of the cerebral cortex. In: Harlow, H.F., Woolsey, C.N. (Eds.), *Biological and biochemical bases of behavior* (pp. 63–81). Madison: University of Wisconsin Press, 1958.

Pecina, M., Zubieta, J.K. Molecular mechanisms of placebo responses in humans. *Mol. Psychiat.* doi:10.1038/mp.2014.164, 2014.

Petrovic, P., et al. Placebo and opioid analgesia: imaging a shared neuronal network. *Science* 106:71–76, 2002.

Petrovic, P., et al. Placebo in emotional processing-induced expectations of anxiety relief activate a generalized modulatory network. *Neuron* 46:957–969, 2005.

Porro, C.A., et al. Does anticipation of pain affect cortical nociceptive systems? *J. Neurosci.* 22:3206–3214, 2002.

Price, D.D. The inner experience and neurobiology of placebo analgesia: can these perspectives be integrated? *Pain* 154:328–329, 2013.

Price, D.D., et al. A comprehensive review of the placebo effect: recent advances and current thoughts. *Annu. Rev. Psychol.* 59:565–590, 2008.

Scott, D.J., et al. Placebo and nocebo effects are defined by opposite opioid and dopaminergic responses. *Arch. Gen. Psychiatry* 65:220–231, 2008.

Turner, J.A., et al. The importance of placebo effects in pain treatment and research. *JAMA* 271:1609–1614, 1994.

Wager, T., et al. Placebo-induced changes in fMRI in the anticipation and experience of pain. *Science* 303:1162–1167, 2004.

Wager, T.D., et al. Placebo effects on human μ-opioid activity during pain. *Proc. Natl. Acad. Sci. USA* 104:11056–11061, 2007.

Wall, P.D. Pain and the placebo response. *Ciba Found. Symp.* 174:187–211, 1993.

Chapter 16: The Visual System

Retina

Bair, W. Spike timing in the mammalian visual system. *Curr. Opin. Neurobiol.* 9:447–453, 1999.

Demb, J.B. Functional circuitry of visual adaptation in the retina. *J. Physiol.* 586:4377–4384, 2008.

DeVries, S.H., Baylor, D.A. Synaptic circuitry of the retina and olfactory bulb. *Neuron* 10(Suppl.):139–149, 1993.

Dowling, J. *The retina: an approachable part of the brain.* Cambridge, MA: Harvard University Press, 1987.

Euler, T., et al. Retinal bipolar cells: elementary building blocks of vision. *Nature Rev. Neurosci.* 15:507–519, 2014.

Goldsmith, E., Jacobsen, N. Genetic and environmental effects on myopia development and progression. *Eye* 28:126–133, 2014.

Hung, L-F., et al. Spectacle lenses alter eye growth and the refractive status of young monkeys. *Nature Med.* 1:761–765, 1995.

Kuffler, S.W., et al. *From neuron to brain: a cellular approach to the function of the nervous system*, 2nd ed. Sunderland, MA: Sinauer Associates, 1984.

Lee, B.B. Paths to color in the retina. *Clin. Exp. Optom.* 87:239–248, 2004.

Masland, R H. The neuronal organization of the retina. *Neuron* 76:266–280, 2012.

Meister, M., Berry, M.J. II. The neural code of the retina. *Neuron* 22:435–450, 1999.

Nickle, B., Robinson, P.R. The opsins of the vertebrate retina: insights from structural, biochemical, and evolutionary studies. *Cell Mol. Life Sci.* 64:2917–2932, 2007.

Nierenberg, S., Latham, P.E. Population coding in the retina. *Curr. Opin. Neurobiol.* 8:488–493, 1998.

Schiller, P.H. The on and off channels of the visual system. *Trends Neurosci.* 15:86–92, 1992.

Schulte, D., Bumsted-O'Brien, K.M. Molecular mechanisms of vertebrate retina development: implications for ganglion cell and photoreceptor patterning. *Brain Res.* 1192:151–164, 2008.

Shapley, R., Perry, V.H. Cat and monkey retinal ganglion cells and their visual functional roles. *Trends Neurosci.* 9:229–235, 1986.

Vanleeuwen, M.T., et al. The contribution of the outer retina to color constancy: a general model for color constancy synthesized from primate and fish data. *Vis. Neurosci.* 24:277–290, 2007.

Wong, K.Y. Non-photoreceptor photoreception. In: Squire, L.R. (Ed.), *Encyclopedia of neuroscience*, Vol. 10 (pp. 1205–1211). Oxford: Academic Press 2009.

Zhou, Z.J., Lee, S. Synaptic physiology of direction selectivity in the retina. *J. Physiol.* 586:4371–4376, 2008.

Zrenner, E. Will retinal implants restore vision? *Science* 295:1022–1025, 2002.

Visual Pathways and Visual Cortex

Aine, C.J., et al. Retinotopic organization of human visual cortex: departures from the classical model. *Cereb. Cortex* 6:354–361, 1996.

Allison, T., et al. Face recognition in human extrastriate cortex. *J. Neurophysiol.* 71:821–825, 1994.

Bar, M. Visual objects in context. *Nat. Rev. Neurosci.* 5:617–628, 2004.

Barbur, J.L., et al. Insights into the different exploits of colour in the visual cortex. *Proc. R. Soc. Lond. B Biol. Sci.* 258:327–334, 1994.

Baluch, F., Itti, L. Mechanisms of top-down attention. *Trends Neurosci.* 34:210–224, 2011.

Barnes, G.R., et al. The cortical deficit in humans with strabismic amblyopia. *J. Physiol.* 533:281–297, 2001.

Berman, R.A., Wurtz, R.H. Exploring the pulvinar path to visual cortex. *Prog. Brain Res.* 171:467–473, 2008.

Blasdel, G., Campbell, D. Functional retinotopy of monkey visual cortex. *J. Neurosci.* 21:8286–8301, 2001.

Boussaoud, D., et al. Pathways for motion analysis: cortical connections of the medial superior temporal and fundus of the superior temporal visual areas in the macaque. *J. Comp. Neurol.* 296:462–495, 1990.

Bridge, H., Cumming, B.G. Representation of binocular surfaces by cortical neurons. *Curr. Opin. Neurobiol.* 18:425–430, 2008.

Buchtel, H., et al. Behavioural and electrophysiological analysis of strabismus in cats: modern context. *Exp. Brain Res.* 192:359–367, 2009.

Bui Quoc, E., Milleret, C. Origins of strabismus and loss of binocular vision. *Front. Integr. Neurosci.* 8:71. doi:10.3389/fnint.2014.00071, 2014.

Callaway, E.M. Local circuits in primary visual cortex of the macaque monkey. *Annu. Rev. Neurosci.* 21:47–74, 1998.

Cant, J., et al. fMRI-adaptation reveals separate processing regions for the perception of form and texture in the human ventral stream. *Exp. Brain Res.* 192:391–405, 2009.

Cohen, M.R., Newsome, W.T. Context-dependent changes in functional circuitry in visual area MT. *Neuron* 60:162–173, 2008.

Courtney, S.M., Ungerleider, L.G. What fMRI has taught us about human vision. *Curr. Opin. Neurobiol.* 7:554–561, 1997.

Cowey, A. The blindsight saga. *Exp. Brain Res.* 200:3–24, 2010.

Cumming, B.G., DeAngelis, G.C. The physiology of stereopsis. *Annu. Rev. Neurosci.* 24:203–208, 2001.

Das, A. Orientation in visual cortex: a simple mechanism emerges. *Neuron* 16:477–480, 1996.

DeAngelis, G.C. Seeing in three dimensions: the neurophysiology of stereopsis. *Trends Cogn. Sci.* 4:80–90, 2000.

Deco, G., Rolls, E.T. Attention, short term memory, and action selection: a unifying theory. *Prog. Neurobiol.* 76:236–256, 2005.

de Haan, E.F., Cowey, A. On the usefulness of "what" and "where" pathways in vision. *Trends Cogn. Sci.* 15:460–466, 2011.

Desimone, R., Duncan, J. Neural mechanisms of selective visual attention. *Annu. Rev. Neurosci.* 18:193–222, 1995.

Downing, P.E., et al. A cortical area selective for visual processing of the human body. *Science* 293:2470–2473, 2001.

Dupont, P., et al. The kinetic occipital region in human visual cortex. *Cereb. Cortex* 7:283–292, 1997.

Eagleman, D.M. Visual illusions and neurobiology. *Nat. Rev. Neurosci.* 2:920–926, 2002.

Fang, F., He, S. Cortical responsens to invisible objects in the human dorsal and ventral pathways. *Nat. Rev. Neurosci.* 8:1380–1385, 2005.

Gonzales, F., Perez, R. Neural mechanisms underlying stereoscopic vision. *Prog. Neurobiol.* 55:191–224, 1998.

Goodale, M.A., Milner, A.D. Separate visual pathways for perception and action. *Trends Neurosci.* 15:20–25, 1992.

Grill-Spector, K., Weiner, K.S. The functional architecture of the ventral temporal cortex and its role in categorization. *Nature Rev. Neurosci.* 15:536–548, 2014.

Gulyás, B., Roland, P.E. Processing and analysis of form, colour and binocular disparity in the human brain: functional anatomy by positron emission tomography. *Eur. J. Neurosci.* 6:1811–1828, 1994.

Haxby, J.V., et al. Distributed and overlapping representations of faces and objects in ventral temporal cortex. *Science* 293:2425–2430, 2001.

Holmes, G. Disturbances of vision by cerebral lesions. In: Phillips, C.G. (Ed.), *Selected papers of Gordon Holmes* (pp. 337–367). Oxford: Oxford University Press, 1979.

Hubel, D., Wiesel, T. Receptive fields, binocular interaction and functional architecture in the cat's visual cortex. *J. Physiol.* 160:106–154, 1962.

Ishai, A. Seeing faces and objects with the "mind's eye." *Arch. Ital. Biol.* 148:1–9, 2010.

Jeannerod, M., Jacob, P. Visual cognition: a new look at the two-visual systems model. *Neuropsychologia* 43:301–312, 2005.

Kaas, J.H. Why does the brain have so many visual areas? *J. Cogn. Neurosci.* 1:121–135, 1989.

Komatsu, H. The neural mechanism of perceptual filling-in. *Nat. Rev. Neurosci.* 7:220–231, 2006.

Kreiman, G. Single unit approaches to human vision and memory. *Curr. Opin. Neurobiol.* 17:471–475, 2007.

Lamme, V.A.F., Roelfsema, P.R. The distinct modes of vision offered by feedforward and recurrent processing. *Trends Neurosci.* 23:571–579, 2000.

Leopold, D.A. Primary visual cortex: awareness and blindsight. *Annu. Rev. Neurosci.* 35:91–109, 2012.

Livingston, M.S., Hubel, D.H. Psychophysical evidence for separate channels for the perception of form, color, movement, and depth. *J. Neurosci.* 7:3416–3468, 1987.

Logothetis, N.K., Sheinberg, D.L. Visual object recognition. *Annu. Rev. Neurosci.* 19:577–621, 1996.

Löwel, S. Ocular dominance column development: strabismus changes the spacing of adjacent columns in cat visual cortex. *J. Neurosci.* 14:7451–7468, 1994.

Malach, R., et al. Relationship between intrinsic connections and functional architecture revealed by optical imaging and *in vivo* targeted biocytin injections in primate striate cortex. *Proc. Natl. Acad. Sci. USA* 90:10469–10473, 1993.

Menon, R.S. Ocular dominance in human V1 demonstrated by functional magnetic resonance imaging. *J. Neurophysiol.* 77:2780–2787, 1997.

Moutoussis, K., Zeki, S. Motion processing, directional selectivity, and conscious visual perception in the human brain. *Proc. Natl. Acad. Sci. USA* 105:16362–16367, 2008.

Murphey, D.K., et al. Perceiving electrical stimulation of identified human visual areas. *Proc. Nat. Acad. Sci.* 106:5389–5393, 2009.

Nealey, T.A., Maunsell, J.H.R. Magnocellular and parvocellular contributions to the responses of neurons in macaque striate cortex. *J. Neurosci.* 14:2069–2079, 1994.

Parker, A.J. Binocular depth perception and the cerebral cortex. *Nat. Rev. Neurosci.* 8:379–391, 2007.

Pasupathy, A. Neural basis of shape representation in the primate brain. *Prog. Brain Res.* 154:293–313, 2006.

Poghosyan, V., et al. Effects of attention and arousal on early responses in striate cortex. *Eur. J. Neurosci.* 22:225–234, 2005.

Pollen, D.A. On the neural correlates of visual perception. *Cereb. Cortex* 9:4–19, 1999.

Reddy, L., Kanwisher, N. Coding of visual objects in the ventral stream. *Curr. Opin. Neurobiol.* 16:408–414, 2006.

Roe, A.W., et al. Toward a unified theory of visual area V4. *Neuron* 74:12–29, 2012.

Roland, P.E., Gulyás, B. Visual imagery and visual representation. *Trends Neurosci.* 17:281–287, 1994.

Salminen-Vaparanta, N., et al. Subjective characteristics of TMS-induced phosphenes originating in human V1 and V2. *Cereb. Cortex* 24:2751–2760, 2014.

Schwarzlose, R.F., et al. Separate face and body selectivity on the fusiform gyrus. *J. Neurosci.* 23:11055–11059, 2005.

Self, M.W., Zeki, S. The integration of colour and motion by the human visual brain. *Cereb. Cortex* 15:1270–1279, 2005.

Silver, M.A., Kastner, S. Topographic maps in human frontal and parietal cortex. *Trends Cogn. Sci.* 13:488–495, 2009.

True, S., Maunsell, J.H. Effects of attention on the processing of motion in macaque middle temporal and medial superior temporal visual cortical areas. *J. Neurosci.* 19:7591–7602, 1999.

Vaina, L.M., et al. Functional neuroanatomy of biological motion perception in humans. *Proc. Natl. Acad. Sci. USA* 98:11656–11661, 2001.

Van Essen, D.C., Gallant, J.L. Neural mechanisms of form and motion processing in the primate visual system. *Neuron* 13:1–10, 1994.

Wandell, B.A., et al. Visual cortex in humans. In: Squire, L.R. (Ed.), *Encyclopedia of neuroscience*, Vol. 10 (pp. 251–257). Oxford: Academic Press, 2009.

Weigelt, S., et al. Cross-category adaptation reveals toght coupling of face and body perception. *J. Neurophysiol.* 104:581–583, 2010.

Weiner, K.S., Grill-Spector, K. The improbable simplicity of the fusiform face area. *Trends Cogn. Sci.* 16:251–254, 2012.

Zeki, S. *A vision of the brain.* Oxford: Blackwell Scientific, 1993.

Zeman, A. Theories of visual awareness. *Prog. Brain Res.* 144:321–329, 2004.

Color Vision

Barbur, J.L., et al. Insights into the different exploits of colour in the visual cortex. *Proc. R. Soc. Lond. B Biol. Sci.* 258:327–334, 1994.

Conway, B.R. Color vision, cones, and color-coding in the cortex. *Neuroscientist* 15:274–290, 2009.

Foster, D.H. Does color constancy exist? *Trends Cogn. Sci.* 7:439–443, 2003.

Gegenfurter, K.R. Cortical mechanisms of colour vision. *Nat. Rev. Neurosci.* 4:563–572, 2003.

Gulyás, B., Roland, P.E. Processing and analysis of form, colour and binocular disparity in the human brain: functional anatomy by positron emission tomography. *Eur. J. Neurosci.* 6:1811–1828, 1994.

Heywood, C., Cowey, A. With color in mind. *Nat. Rev. Neurosci.* 1:171–173, 1998.

Hofer, H., et al. Organization of the human trichromatic cone mosaic. *J. Neurosci.* 25:9669–9679, 2005.

Komatsu, H. Mechanisms of central color vision. *Curr. Opin. Neurobiol.* 8:503–408, 1998.

Solomon, S.G., Lennie, P. The machinery of colour vision. *Nat. Rev. Neurosci.* 8:276–286, 2007.

Chapter 17: The Auditory System

Moore, J.K., Linthicum, F.H. Jr. Auditory system. In: Paxinos, G., Mai, J.K. (Eds.), *The human nervous system*, 2nd ed. (pp. 1241–1279). Philadelphia: Elsevier Academic Press, 2004.

Cochlea

Ashmore, J.F., Kolston, P.J. Hair cell based amplification in the cochlea. *Curr. Opin. Neurobiol.* 4:503–508, 1994.

Dallos, P. Cochlear amplification, outer hair cells and prestin. *Curr. Opin. Neurobiol.* 18:370–376, 2008.

Eatock, R.A. Adaptation in hair cells. *Annu. Rev. Neurosci.* 23:285–314, 2000.

Fettiplace, R., Hackney, C.M. The sensory and motor roles of auditory hair cells. *Nat. Rev. Neurosci.* 7:19–29, 2006.

Flock, Å., et al. Supporting cells contribute to control of hearing sensitivity. *J. Neurosci.* 19:4498–4507, 1999.

Géléoc, G.S.G., Holt, J.R. Sound strategies for hearing restoration. *Science* 344:1241062. doi:10.1126/science.1241062, 2014

Gillespie, P.G., et al. Have we found the tip link, transduction channel and gating spring of the hair cell? *Curr. Opin. Neurobiol.* 15:389–396, 2005.

Glowatzki, E., et al. Hair cell afferent synapses. *Curr. Opin. Neurobiol.* 18:389–395, 2008.

Hudspeth, A.J. Integrating the active process of hair cells with cochlear function. *Nature Rev. Neurosci.* 15:600–614, 2014.

Kozlov, A.S., et al. Coherent motion of stereocilia assures the concerted gating of hair-cell transduction channels. *Nat. Neurosci.* 10:87–92, 2007.

Kral, A., Sharma, A. Developmental neuroplasticity after cochlear implantation. *Trends Neurosci.* 35:111–122, 2012.

Legan, P.K., et al. A deafness mutation isolates a second role for the tectorial membrane in hearing. *Nat. Neurosci.* 8:1035–1042, 2005.

Maison, S.E., et al. Efferent feedback minimizes cochlear neuropathy from moderate noise exposure. *J. Neurosci.* 33:5542–5552, 2013.

Manley, G.A., Köppl, C. Phylogenetic development of the cochlea and its innervation. *Curr. Opin. Neurobiol.* 8:468–474, 1998.

Middlebrooks, J.C., et al. Cochlear implants: the view from the brain. *Curr. Opin. Neurobiol.* 15:488–493, 2005.

Nelson, E.G., Hinojosa, R. Presbyacusis: a human temporal bone study of individuals with downward sloping audiometric patterns of hearing loss and review of the literature. *Laryngoscope* 116:1–12, 2006.

Nilsen, K.E., Russel, I.J. Timing of cochlear feedback: spatial and temporal representation of a tone across the basilar membrane. *Nat. Neurosci.* 2:642–647, 1999.

Nobili, R., et al. How well do we understand the cochlea? *Trends Neurosci.* 21:159–167, 1998.

Ohlemiller, K.K., et al. Strial microvascular pathology and age-associated endocochlear potential decline in NOD congenic mice. *Hear. Res.* 244:85–97, 2008.

Pauler, M., et al. Atrophy of the stria vascularis as a cause of sensorineural hearing loss. *Laryngoscope* 98:754–759, 1988.

Prakash, R., Ricci, A.J. Hair bundles teaming up to tune the mammalian cochlea. *Proc. Natl. Acad. Sci. USA* 105:18651–18652, 2008.

Ren, T., Gillespie, P.G. A mechanism for active hearing. *Curr. Opin. Neurobiol.* 17:498–503, 2007.

Rubinstein, J.T., Miller, C.A. How do cochlear prosthesis work? *Curr. Opin. Neurobiol.* 9:399–404, 1999.

Sainz, M., et al. Assessment of auditory skills in 140 cochlear implant children using the EARS protocol. *J. Otorhinolaryngol. Relat. Spec.* 65:91–96, 2003.

Takeuchi, S., et al. Mechanism generating endocochlear potential: role played by intermediate cells in the stria vascularis. *Biophys. J.* 79:2572–2582, 2000.

Auditory Pathways and Auditory Cortex

Ahveninen, J., et al. Task modulated "what" and "where" pathways in human auditory cortex. *Proc. Natl. Acad. Sci. USA* 103:14608–14613, 2006.

Alain, C., et al. A distributed network for auditory sensory memory in humans. *Brain Res.* 812:23–37, 1998.

Arnott, S.E., et al. Assessing the auditory dual-pathway model in humans. *NeuroImage* 22:401–408, 2004.

Bamiou, D.E., et al. The insula (Island of Reil) and its role in auditory processing. *Brain Res. Rev.* 42:143–154, 2003.

Bavelier, D., et al. Do deaf individuals see better? *Trends Cogn. Sci.* 10:512–518, 2006.

Bisiach, E., et al. Disorders of perceived auditory lateralization after lesions of the right hemisphere. *Brain* 107:37–52, 1984.

Brainard, M.S. Neural substrates of sound localization. *Curr. Opin. Neurobiol.* 4:557–562, 1994.

Carlyon, R.P. How the brain separates sounds. *Trends Cogn. Sci.* 8:465–471, 2004.

Carney, L.H. Temporal response properties of neurons in the auditory pathway. *Curr. Opin. Neurobiol.* 9:442–446, 1999.

Creutzfeldt, O., et al. Neuronal activity in the human temporal lobe: II. Responses to the subject's own voice. *Exp. Brain Res* 77: 476 489, 1989.

Dahmen, J.C., King, A.J. Learning to hear: plasticity of audotiroy cortex processing. *Curr. Opin. Neurobiol.* 17:456–464, 2007.

Edelman, G.M., et al. *Auditory function: neurobiological bases of hearing*. New York: John Wiley & Sons, 1988.

Ehret, G., Romand, R. *The central auditory system*. New York: Oxford University Press, 1997.

Friederici, A.D. Three cortical language circuit: from auditory perception to sentence comprehension. *Trends Cogn. Sci.* 16:262–268, 2012.

Galuske, R.A.W., et al. Interhemispheric asymmetries of the modular structure in human temporal cortex. *Science* 289:1946–1949, 2000.

Giraud, A.L., et al. Functional plasticity of language-related brain areas after cochlear implantation. *Brain* 124:1307–1316, 2001.

Howard, M.A., et al. Auditory cortex on the human posterior superior temporal gyrus. *J. Comp. Neurol.* 416:79–92, 2000.

Issa, J.B., et al. Multiscale optical Ca²⁺ imaging of tonal organization in mouse auditory cortex. *Neuron* 83:944–958, 2014.

Kanold, P.O., et al. Local versus global scales of organization in auditory cortex. *Trends Neurosci.* 37:502–510, 2014.

Knudsen, E.I., Brainard, M.S. Creating a unified representation of visual and auditory space in the brain. *Annu. Rev. Neurosci.* 18:19–43, 1995.

Lewald, J., et al. Processing of sound location in human cortex. *Eur. J. Neurosci.* 27:1261–1270, 2008.

Lomber, S., Malhorta, S. Double dissociation of "what" and "where" processing in auditory cortex. *Nat. Neurosci.* 11:609–616, 2008.

Magnusson, A.K., et al. Retrograde GABA signaling adjusts sound localization by balancing excitation and inhibition in the brainstem. *Neuron* 59:125–137, 2008.

Masterton, R.B. Role of the central auditory system in hearing: the new direction. *Trends Neurosci.* 15:280–285, 1992.

McGettigan, C., Scott, S.K. Cortical asymmetries in speech perception: what's wrong, what's right and what's left? *Trends Cogn. Sci.* 16:269–276, 2012.

Mesgarani, N., et al. Phonetic feature encoding in human superior temporal gyrus. *Science* 343:1006–1010, 2014.

Nelken, I., Bar-Yosef, O. Neurons and objects: the case of auditory cortex. *Front. Neurosci.* 2:107–113, 2008.

Noreña, A.J., Farley, B.J. Tinnitus-related activity: theories of generation, propagation, and centralization. *Hearing Res.* 295:161–171, 2013.

Oertel, D. Encoding of timing in the brain stem auditory nuclei of vertebrates. *Neuron* 19:959–962, 1997.

Penfield, W., Perot, P. The brain's record of auditory and visual experience. *Brain* 86:596–696, 1963.

Peretz, I., et al. Functional dissociations following bilateral lesions of auditory cortex. *Brain* 117:1283–1301, 1994.

Pickles, J.O., Corey, D.P. Mechanoelectrical transduction by hair cells. *Trends Neurosci.* 15:254–259, 1992.

Poulet, J.F.A., Hedwig, B. A corollary discharge maintains auditory sensitivity during sound production. *Nature* 418:872–876, 2002.

Rauschecker, J.P., Shannon, R.V. Sending sound to the brain. *Science* 295:1025–1029, 2002.

Romanski, L.M., et al. Dual streams of auditory afferents target multiple domains in the primate prefrontal cortex. *Nat. Neurosci.* 2:1131–1136, 1999.

Rutkowski, R.G., Weinberger, N.M. Encoding of learned importance of sound by magnitude of representational area in primary auditory cortex. *Proc. Natl. Acad. Sci. USA* 102:13664–13669, 2005.

Schneider, P., et al. Morphology of Heschl's gyrus reflects enhanced activation in the auditory cortex of musicians. *Nat. Neurosci.* 5:688–694, 2002.

Schreiner, C.E., et al. Modular organization of frequency integration in primary auditory cortex. *Annu. Rev. Neurosci.* 23:501–529, 2000.

Scott, S.K. Auditory processing—speech, space and auditory objects. *Curr. Opin. Neurobiol.* 15:197–201, 2005.

Syka, J. Plastic changes in the central auditory system after hearing loss, restoration of function, and during learning. *Physiol. Rev.* 82:601–636, 2002.

Tanaka, Y., et al: "So-called" cortical deafness. *Brain* 114:2385–2401, 1991.

Warren, J.E., et al. Sounds do-able: auditory-motor transformations and the posterior temporal plane. *Trends Neurosci.* 28:636–643, 2005.

Winer, J.A., et al. Auditory thalamocortical transformation: structure and function. *Trends Neurosci.* 28:255–263, 2005.

Winkler, I., et al. Object representation in the human auditory system. *Eur. J. Neurosci.* 24:625–634, 2006.

Zahorik, P., Wightman, F.L. Loudness constancy with varying sound distance. *Nat. Rev. Neurosci.* 4:78–83, 2001.

Zatorre, R.J., et al. Structure and function of auditory cortex: music and speech. *Trends Cogn. Sci.* 6:37–45, 2002.

Chapter 18: The Sense of Equilibrium

Vestibular Apparatus and Vestibular Nuclei

Büttner-Ennever, J.A. *Neuroanatomy of the oculomotor system.* Philadelphia: Elsevier, 1988.

Büttner-Ennever, J.A. A review of otolith pathways to brainstem and cerebellum. *Ann. NY Acad. Sci.* 871:51–64, 1999.

Büttner-Ennever, J.A, Gerrits, N.M. Vestibular system. In: Paxinos, G., Mai, J.K. (Eds.), *The human nervous system*, 2nd ed. (pp. 1212–1240). Philadelphia: Elsevier Academic Press, 2004.

de Waele, C., et al. Vestibular projections in the human cortex. *Exp. Brain Res.* 141:541–551, 2001.

Eatock, R.A., Songer, J.E. Vestibular hair cells and afferents: Two channels for head motion signals. *Annu. Rev. Neurosci.* 34:501–534, 2011.

Kalluri, R., et al. Ion channels set spike timing regularity of mammalian vestibular afferent neurons. *J. Neurophysiol.* 104: 2034–2051, 2010.

Lindeman, H.H. Anatomy of the otolith organs. *Adv. Oto-Rhino-Laryngol.* 20:405–433, 1973.

Lopez, C., Blanke, O. The thalamocortical vestibular system in animals and humans. *Brain Res. Rev.* 67:119–146, 2011.

Manzoni, D. The cerebellum may implement the appropriate coupling of sensory inputs and motor responses: evidence from vestibular physiology. *Cerebellum* 4:178–188, 2005.

Meng, H., et al. Vestibular signals in primate thalamus: properties and origin. *J. Neurosci.* 27:13590–13602, 2007.

Nathan, P.W., et al. Vestibulospinal, reticulospinal and descending propriospinal nerve fibres in man. *Brain* 119:1809–1833, 1996.

Parker, D.E. The relative roles of the otolith organs and semicircular canals in producing space motion sickness. *J. Vestib. Res.* 8:57–59, 1998.

Rabbitt, R.D., et al. Mechanical amplification by hair cells in the semicircular canals. *Proc. Nat. Acad. Sci. USA* 107: 3864–3869, 2010.

Rinne, T., et al. Bilateral loss of vestibular function. *Acta Otolaryngol. (Stockh)* Suppl. 520:247–250, 1997.

Sadeghi, S.G., et al. Efferent mediated responses in vestibular nerve afferents of the alert macaque, *J. Neurophysiol.* 101:988–1001, 2009.

Stein, B.M., Carpenter, M.B. Central projections of portions of the vestibular ganglia innervating specific parts of the labyrinth in rhesus monkeys. *Am. J. Anat.* 120: 281–317, 1967.

Strupp. M., Brandt, T. Peripheral vestibular disorderes. *Curr. Opin. Neurol.* 26:81–89, 2013.

Sugiyama, Y., et al. Role of rostral ventrolateral medulla (RVLM) in the patterning of vestibular system influences on sympathetic nervous system outflow to the upper and lower body. *Exp. Brain Res.* 210: 515–527, 2010.

Uchino, Y., et al. Otolith and canal integration on single vestibular neurons in cats. *Exp. Brain Res.* 164:271–285, 2005.

Wersäll, J. Studies on the structure and innervation of the sensory epithelium of the cristae ampullaris of the guinea pig. A light and electron microscopic investigation. *Acta Otolaryng. (Stockh.)* Suppl. 126:1–85, 1956.

Wilson, V.J., Melvill Jones, G. *Mammalian vestibular physiology.* New York: Plenum Press, 1979.

Wilson, V.J., et al. Cortical influences on the vestibular nuclei of the cat. *Exp. Brain Res.* 125:1–13, 1999.

Zwergal, A., et al. An ipsilateral vestibulothalamic tract adjacent to the medial lemniscus in humans- *Brain* 131:2928–2935, 2008.

Vestibular Reflexes and Postural Control

Allum, J.H.J., Honegger, F. Interactions between vestibular and proprioceptive inputs triggering and modulating human balance-correcting responses differ across muscles. *Exp. Brain Res.* 121:478–494, 1998.

Balasubramaniam, R., Wing, A.M. The dynamics of standing balance. *Trends Cogn. Sci.* 6:531–536, 2002.

Barbieri, G., et al. Does proprioception contribute to the sense of verticality? *Exp. Brain. Res.* 185:545–552, 2008.

Bloem, B.R., et al. Is lower leg proprioception essential for triggering human automatic postural responses? *Exp. Brain Res.* 130: 375–391, 2000.

Boulinguez, P., Rouhana, J.I. Flexibility and individual differences in visuo-proprioceptive integration: evidence from a morphokinetic control task. *Exp. Brain Res.* 185:137–149, 2008.

Bronstein, A.M., Hood, D. The cervico-ocular reflex in normal subjects and patients with absent vestibular function. *Brain Res.* 373:399–408, 1986.

Deliagini, T.G., et al. Spinal and supraspinal postural networks. *Brain Res. Rev.* 57:212–221, 2008.

Denise, P., Darlot, C. The cerebellum as a predictor of neural messages. II. Role in motor control and motion sickness. *Neuroscience* 56:647–655, 1993.

Finley, J.E., et al. Contributions of feed-forward and feedback strategies at the human ankle during control of unstable loads. *Exp. Brain Res.* 217: 53–66, 2012.

Goldberg, J., Cullen, K. Vestibular control of the head: possible functions of the vestibulocollic reflex. *Exp. Brain Res.* 210: 331–345, 2011.

Kaufmann, H., et al. Vestibular control of sympathetic activity. An otolith-sympathetic reflex in humans. *Exp. Brain Res.* 143:463–469, 2002.

Labuguen, R.H. Initial evaluation of vertigo. *Am. Family Phys.* 73:244–251, 2006.

Lekhel, H., et al. Postural responses to vibration of neck muscles in patients with idiopathic torticollis. *Brain* 120:583–591, 1997.

Lisberger, S.G. Physiologic basis for motor learning in the vestibulo-ocular reflex. *Otolaryngol. Head Neck Surg.* 119:43–48, 1998.

Nashner, L.M. Balance and posture control. In: Squire, L. (Ed.), *Encyclopedia of neuroscience* (pp. 21–29). Philadelphia: Elsevier, 2009.

Shelhamer, M.J. Nystagmus. In: Squire, L. (Ed.), *Encyclopedia of neuroscience* (pp. 1313–1317). Philadelphia: Elsevier, 2009.

Strupp, M., et al. Perceptual and oculomotor effects of neck muscle vibration in vestibular neuritis. Ipsilateral somatosensory substitution of vestibular function. *Brain* 121:677–685, 1998.

Weerdesteyn, V., et al. Automated postural responses are modified in a functional manner by instruction. *Exp. Brain Res.* 186:571–580, 2008.

Wilson, V.J., Schor, R.H. The neural substrate of the vestibulocollic reflex: what needs to be learned. *Exp. Brain Res.* 129:483–493, 1999.

Wu, G., Chiang, J.-H. The significance of somatosensory stimulations to the human foot in the control of postural reflexes. *Exp. Brain Res.* 114:163–169, 1997.

Cortical Level

Anastasopoulus, D., et al. The role of somatosensory input for the perception of verticality. *Ann. NY Acad. Sci.* 871:379–383, 1999.

Angelaki, D.E., Cullen, K.E. Vestibular system: the many facets of a multimodal system. *Annu. Rev. Neurosci.* 31:125–150, 2008.

Astafiev, S.V., et al. Extrastriate body area in human occipital cortex responds to the performance of motor actions. *Nat. Neurosci.* 7:542–548, 2004.

Berlucchi, G., Aglioti, S. The body in the brain: neural bases of corporeal awareness. *Trends Neurosci.* 20:560–564, 1997.

Berlucchi, G., Aglioti, S. The body in the brain revisited. *Exp. Brain Res.* 200: 25–35, 2010.

Berthoz, A., Viaud-Delmond, I. Multisensory integration in spatial orientation. *Curr. Opin. Neurobiol.* 9:708–712, 1999.

Blake, R., Shiffrar, M. Perception of human motion. *Annu. Rev. Psychol.* 58:47–73, 2007.

Blanke, O., Mohr, C. Out-of-body experience, heautoscopy, and autoscopic hallucination of neurological origin. Implications for neurocognitive mechanisms of corporeal awareness and self consciousness. *Brain Res. Rev.* 50:184–199, 2005.

Bos, E., van den, M. Jeannerod. Sense of body and sense of action both contribute to self-recognition. *Cognition* 85:177–188, 2002.

Bosbach, S., et al. Inferring another's expectation from action: the role of peripheral sensation. *Nat. Neurosci.* 8:1295–1297, 2005.

Bottini, G., et al. Cerebral representations for egocentric space. Functional-anatomical evidence from caloric vestibular stimulation and neck vibration. *Brain* 124:1182–1196, 2001.

Brandt, T., Dieterich, M. The vestibular cortex: its location, functions, and disorders. *Ann. NY Acad. Sci.* 871:293–312, 1999.

Carpenter, M.G., et al. The influence of postural threat on the control of upright stance. *Exp. Brain Res.* 138:210–218, 2001.

Cazzato, V., et al. Distinct contributions of extrastriate body area and temporoparietal junction in perceiving one's own and others' body. *Cogn. Affect. Biobehav. Neurosci.* 15:211–228, 2015.

Dieterich, M., Brandt, T. Functional brain imaging of peripheral and central vestibular disorders. *Brain* 131:2538–2552, 2008.

Eulenburg, P., et al. Meta-analytical definition and functional connectivity of the human vestibular cortex. *NeuroImage* 60:162–169, 2012.

Fasold, O., et al. Proprioceptive head posture-related processing in human polysensory areas. *NeuroImage* 40:1232–1242, 2008.

Gallagher, S. Philosophical conceptions of the self: Implications for cognitive science. *Trends Cogn. Sci.* 4:14–21, 2000.

Jeannerod, M. Being oneself. *J. Physiol. Paris* 101:161–168, 2007.

Kavounoudias, A., et al. From balance regulation to body orientation: two goals for muscle proprioceptive information processing? *Exp. Brain Res.* 124:80–88, 1999.

Lackner, J.R., DiZio, P.A. Aspects of body self calibration. *Trends Cogn. Sci.* 4:279–289, 2000.

Lopez, C., et al. Body ownership and embodiment: vestibular and mul-tisensory mechanisms. *Clin. Neurophysiol.* 38:148–161, 2008.

Mehling, W.E., et al. Body awareness: construct and self-report measures. *PLoS ONE* 4:e5614. doi:10.1371/journal.pone.0005614, 2009.

Moro, V., et al. The neural basis of body form and body action agnosia. *Neuron* 60:235–246, 2008.

Moseley, G.L., et al. Bodily illusions in health and disease: Physiological and clinical perspectives and the concept of a cortical 'body matrix'. *Neurosci. Biobehav. Rev.* 36:34–46, 2012.

Pérennou, D.A., et al. The polymodal sensory cortex is crucial for controlling lateral postural stability. Evidence from stroke patients. *Brain Res. Bull.* 53:359–365, 2000.

Reschke, M.F., et al. Posture, locomotion, spatial orientation, and motion sickness as a function of space flight. *Brain Res. Rev.* 28:102–117, 1998.

Schwoebel, J., Coslett, H.B. Evidence for multiple, distinct representations of the human body. *J. Cogn. Neurosci.* 17:543–553, 2005.

Shenton, J.T., et al. Mental motor imagery and the body schema: evidence for proprioceptive dominance. *Neurosci. Lett.* 370: 19–24, 2004.

Shinder, M.E., Newlands, S.D. Sensory convergence in the parieto-insular vestibular cortex. *J. Neurophysiol.* 111:2445–2464, 2014.

Singer, W. Dynamic formation of functional networks by synchronization. *Neuron* 69:191–193, 2011.

Sperduti, M., et al. Different brain structures related to self- and external-agency attribution: a brief review and a meta-analysis. *Brain Struct. Funct.* 216: 151–157, 2011.

Strother, L., Obhi, S. The conscious experience of action and intention. *Exp. Brain Res.* 198: 535–539, 2009.

Strupp, M., et al. Perceptual and oculomotor effects of neck muscle vibration in vestibular neuritis: ipsilateral somatosensory substitution of vestibular function. *Brain* 121:677–685, 1998.

Sundermier, L., et al. The development of balance control in children: comparisons of EMG and kinetic variables and chronological and developmental groupings. *Exp. Brain Res.* 136:340–350, 2001.

Tsakiris, M., et al. On agency and body-ownership: phenomenological and neurocognitive reflections. *Conscious. Cogn.* 16:645–660, 2007.

Tsakiris, M., et al. The role of the right temporo-parietal junction in maintaining a coherent sense of one's body. *Neuropsychologia* 46:3014–3018, 2008.

Urgesi, C., et al. Representation of body identity and body actions in extrastriate body area and ventral premotor cortex. *Nat. Neurosci.* 10:30–31, 2007.

Warren, W.H. Perception of heading is a brain in the neck. *Nat. Neurosci.* 1:647–649, 1998.

Dizziness and Motion Sickness

Balaban, C.D. Vestibular autonomic regulation (including motion sickness and the mechanism of vomiting). *Curr. Opin. Neurol.* 12:29–33, 1999.

Berthoz, A., Viaud-Delmond, I. Multisensory integration in spatial orientation. *Curr. Opin. Neurobiol.* 9:708–712, 1999.

Bles, W. et al. Motion sickness: one provocative conflict? *Brain Res. Bull.* 15:481–487, 1998.

Kalueff, A.V., et al. Anxiety and otovestibular disorders: linking behavioral phenotypes in men and mice. *Behav. Brain. Res.* 186:1–11, 2008.

Karatas, M. Central vertigo and dizziness: epidemiology, differential diagnosis, and common causes. *Neurologist* 14:355–364, 2008.

Kerber, K.A., et al. Disequilibrium in older people—a prospective study. *Neurology* 51:574–580, 1998.

Labuguen, R.H. Initial evaluation of vertigo. *Am. Family Phys.* 73:244–251, 2006.

Lackner, J.R. Motion sickness: more than nausea and vomiting. *Exp. Brain Res.* 232:2493–2510, 2014.

Parker, D.E. The relative roles of the otolith organs and semicircular canals in producing space motion sickness. *J. Vestib. Res.* 8:57–59, 1998.

Reschke, M.F., et al. Posture, locomotion, spatial orientation, and motion sickness as a function of space flight. *Brain Res. Rev.* 28:102–117, 1998.

Rinne, T. et al. Bilateral loss of vestibular function. *Acta Otolaryngol.* Suppl. 520:247–250, 1997.

Rubin, D.I., Cheshire, W. Evaluation of "dizziness" in the neurology office. *Semin. Neurol.* 31:29–41, 2011.

Yates, B.J. et al. Physiological basis and pharmacology of motion sickness: an update. *Brain Res. Bull.* 15:395–406, 1998.

Yates, B.J., et al. Integration of vestibular and emetic gastrointestinal signals that produce nausea and vomiting: potential contributions to motion sickness. *Exp. Brain Res.* 232:2455–2469, 2014.

Chapter 19: Olfaction and Taste

Finger, T.E., et al. (Eds.) *The neurobiology of taste and smell.* New York: John Wiley & Sons, 2001.

Rolls, E.T. Taste, olfactory, and food reward value processing in the brain. *Progr. Neurobiol.* 127-128:64–90, 2015.

Olfaction

Ache, B.W., Young J.M. Olfaction: diverse species, conserved principles. *Neuron* 48:417–430, 2005.

Barbas, H. Organization of cortical afferent input to orbitofrontal areas in the rhesus monkey. *Neuroscience* 56:841–864, 1993.

Buck, L.B. Information coding in the vertebrate olfactory system. *Annu. Rev. Neurosci.* 19:517–544, 1996.

Croy, I., et al. Olfactory disorders and quality of life—an updated review. *Chem. Sens.* 39:185–194, 2014.

de Groot, J.H.B., et al. Chemosignals communicate human emotions. *Physiol. Sci.* 23:1717–1427, 2012.

Firestein, S. How the olfactory system makes sense of scents. *Nature* 413:211–218, 2001.

Gelstein, S., et al. Human tears contain a chemosignal. *Science* 331:226–230, 2011.

Ghosh, S., et al. Sensory maps in the olfactory cortex defined by long-range viral tracing single neurons. *Nature* 472:217–220, 2011.

Gottfried, J.A. Function follows form: ecological constraints on odor codes and olfactory percepts. *Curr. Opin. Neurobiol.* 19:422–429, 2009.

Haberly, L.B., Bower, J.M. Olfactory cortex: model circuit for study of associative memory. *Trends Neurosci.* 12:258–264, 1989.

Hudson, R. Olfactory imprinting. *Curr. Opin. Neurobiol.* 3:548–552, 1993.

Jones-Gotman, M., et al. Contribution of medial versus lateral temporal-lobe structures to human odour identification. *Brain* 120:1845–1856, 1997.

Kay, L.M., Sherman, S.M. An argument for an olfactory thalamus. *Trends Neurosci.* 30:47–53, 2007

Laurent, G., et al. Odor encoding as an active, dynamical process. *Annu. Rev. Neurosci.* 24:263–297, 2001.

Leopold, D.A., et al. Anterior distribution of human olfactory epithelium. *Laryngoscope* 110:417–421, 2000.

Mainland, J., Sobel, N. The sniff is part of the olfactory percept. *Chem. Sens.* 31:181–196, 2006.

Matt, W. All in a sniff: olfaction as a model for active sensing. *Neuron* 71:962–973, 2011.

Mombaerts, P. Targeting olfaction. *Curr. Opin. Neurobiol.* 6:481–486, 1996.

Mombaerts, P. Molecular biology of odorant receptors in vertebrates. *Annu. Rev. Neurosci.* 22:487–509, 1999.

Mori, K. (Ed.) *The olfactory system. From odor molecules to motivational behaviors.* Tokyo: Springer, 2014.

Miyamichi, K., et al. Cortical representations of olfactory input by trans-synaptic tracing. *Nature* 472: 191–196, 2011.

Murthy, V.N. Olfactory maps in the brain *Annu. Rev. Neurosci.* 34:233–258, 2011.

Nakashima, T., et al. Structure of human fetal and adult olfactory neuroepithelium. *Arch. Otolaryngol.* 110:641–646, 1984.

Paik, S.I., et al. Human olfactory biopsy: the influence of age and receptor distribution. *Arch. Otolaryngol. Head Neck Surg.* 118:731–738, 1992.

Price, J.L. Olfaction. In: Paxinos, G., Mai, J.K. (Eds.), *The human nervous system*, 2nd ed. (pp. 1197–1211). Philadelphia: Elsevier Academic Press, 2004.

Ressler, K.J., et al. A molecular dissection of spatial patterning in the olfactory system. *Curr. Opin. Neurobiol.* 4:588–596, 1994.

Richardson, J.T.E., Zucco, G.M. Cognition and olfaction: a review. *Psychol. Bull.* 105:352–360, 1989.

Sanchez-Andrade, G., Kendrick, K.M. The main olfactory system and social learning in mammals. *Behav. Brain Res.* 200:323–335, 2009.

Semin, G.R., de Groot, J.H.B. The chemical bases of human sociality. *Trends Cogn. Sci.* 17:427–429, 2013.

Shepherd, G.M. Discrimination of molecular signals by the olfactory receptor neuron. *Neuron* 13:771–790, 1994.

Trombley, P.Q., Shepherd, G.M. Synaptic transmission and modulation in the olfactory bulb. *Curr. Opin. Neurobiol.* 3:540–547, 1993.

Uchida, N., et al. Coding and transformations in the olfactory system. *Annu. Rev. Neurosci.* 37:363–385, 2014.

Wilson, R.I., Mainen, Z.F. Early events in olfactory processing. *Annu. Rev. Neurosci.* 29:163–201, 2006.

Zatorre, R.J., et al. Functional localization and lateralization of human olfactory cortex. *Nature* 360:339–340, 1992.

Zelano, C., Sobel N. Humans as an animal model for systems-level organization of olfaction. *Neuron* 48:431–454, 2005.

Zou, D.J., et al. Postnatal refinement of peripheral olfactory projections. *Science* 304:1976–1979, 2004.

Zozulya, S., et al. The human olfactory receptor repertoire. *Genome Biol.* 2:1–12, 2001.

Zufall, F., Leinders-Zufall, T. Calcium imaging in the olfactory system: new tools for visualizing odor recognition. *Neuroscientist* 5:4–7, 1999.

Pheromones

Baxi, K.N., et al. Is the vomeronasal system really specialized for detecting pheromones? *Trends Neurosci.* 29:1–7, 2006.

Brennan, P.A., Zufall, F. Pheromonal communication in vertebrates. *Nature* 444:308–315, 2006.

Dulac, C., Torello, A.T. Molecular detection of pheromone signals in mammals: from genes to behaviour. *Nat. Rev. Neurosci.* 4:551–562, 2003.

Karlson, P., Lüscher M. "Pheromones": a new term for a class of biologically active substances. *Nature* 183:55–56, 1959.

Keller, M., et al. The main and the accessory olfactory systems interact in the control of mate recognition and sexual behavior. *Behav. Brain Res.* 200:268–276, 2009.

Swaney, W.T., Keverne, E.B. The evolution of pheromonal communication. *Behav. Brain Res.* 200:239–247, 2009.

Wysocki, C.J., Preti, G. Facts, fallacies, fears, and frustrations with human pheromones. *Anat. Rec. A* 281A:1201–1211, 2004.

Zufall, F., Leinders-Zufall, T. Mammalian pheromone sensing. *Curr. Opin. Neurobiol.* 17:483–489, 2007.

Taste

Acolla, R., Carleton, A. Internal body state influences topographical plasticity of sensory representations in the rat gustatory cortex. *Proc. Natl. Acad. Sci. USA* 105:4010–4015, 2008.

Acolla, R., et al. Differential spatial representation of taste modalities in the rat gustatory cortex. *J. Neurosci.* 27:1396–1404, 2007.

Barretto, R.P.J., et al. The neural representation of taste quality at the periphery. *Nature* 517:373–376, 2014.

Bermúdez-Rattoni, F. Molecular mechanisms of taste-recognition memory. *Nat. Rev. Neurosci.* 5:209–217, 2004.

Boughter, J.D., Gilbertson, T.A. From channels to behavior: an integrative model of NaCl taste. *Neuron* 22:213–215, 1999.

Chandrashekar, J., et al. The receptors and cells for mammalian taste. *Nature* 444:288–294, 2006.

Chen, X., et al. A gustotopic map of taste qualities in the mammalian brain. *Science* 333:1262–1266, 2011.

Duffy, V.B., Bartoshuk, L.M. Food acceptance and genetic variation in taste. *J. Am. Diet. Assoc.* 100:647–655, 2000.

Essick, G.K., et al. Lingual tactile acuity, taste perception, and the density and diameter of fungiform papillae in female subjects. *Physiol. Behav.* 80:289–302, 2003.

Finger, T.E., et al. ATP signaling is crucial for communication from taste buds to gustatory nerves. *Science* 310:1495–1499, 2005.

Frank, M.E., et al. Cracking taste codes by tapping into sensory neuron impulse traffic. *Prog. Neurobiol.* 86:245–263, 2008.

Gilbertson, T.A. Gustatory mechanisms for the detection of fat. *Curr. Opin. Neurobiol.* 8:447–452, 1998.

Heath, T.P., et al. Human taste thresholds are modulated by serotonin and noradrenaline. *J. Neurosci.* 26:12664–12671, 2006.

Huang, Y.J., et al. Mouse taste buds use serotonin as a neurotransmitter. *J. Neurosci.* 25:843–847, 2005.

Hoon, M.A., et al. Putative mammalian taste receptors: a class of taste-specific GCPRs with distinct topographic sensitvity. *Cell* 96:541–551, 1999.

Kinnamon, S.C., Finger, T.E. A taste for ATP: neurotransmission in taste buds. *Front. Cell. Neurosci.* 7:264. doi:10.3389/fncel.2013.00264, 2013.

Liman, E.R., et al. Peripheral coding of taste. *Neuron* 81:984–1000, 2014.

Margolskee, R.F. The biochemistry and molecular biology of taste transduction. *Curr. Opin. Neurobiol.* 3:526–531, 1993.

McCormack, D.N., et al. Detection of free fatty acids following a conditioned taste aversion in rats. *Physiol. Behav.* 87:582–594, 2006.

Mizushige, T., et al. Why is fat so tasty? Chemical reception of fatty acid on the tongue. *J. Nutr. Sci. Vitaminol.* 53:1–4, 2007.

Nelson, G., et al. An amino-acid taste receptor. *Nature* 416:199–202, 2002.

Pritchard, T.C., Norgren, R. Gustatory system. In: Paxinos, G., Mai, J.K. (Eds.), *The human nervous system*, 2nd ed. (pp. 1171–1196). Philadelphia: Elsevier Academic Press, 2004.

Reilly, S. The role of the gustatory thalamus in taste-guided behavior. *Neurosci. Biobehav. Rev.* 22:883–901, 1998.

Roper, S.D. Cell communication in taste buds. *Cell. Mol. Life. Sci.* 63:1494–1500, 2006.

Schoenfeld, M.A., et al. Functional magnetic resonance tomography correlates of taste perception in the human primary taste cortex. *Neuroscience* 127:347–353, 2004.

Scott, K. Taste recognition: food for thought. *Neuron* 48:455–464, 2005.

Shepherd, G.M. Smell images and the flavour system in the brain. *Nature* 444:316–321, 2006.

Simon, S.A., et al. The neural mechanisms of gustation: a distributed processing code. *Nat. Rev. Neurosci.* 7:890–901, 2006.

Small, D.M., Prescott, J. Odor/taste integration and the perception of flavor. *Exp. Brain Res.* 166:345–357, 2005.

Smith, D.V., St. John, S.J. Neural coding of gustatory information. *Curr. Opin. Neurobiol.* 9:427–435, 1999.

Spector, A.C., Travers, S.P. The representation of taste quality in the mammalian nervous system. *Behav. Cogn. Neurosci. Rev.* 4:143–191, 2005.

Sugita, M., Shiba, Y. Genetic tracing shows segregation of taste neuronal circuitries for bitter and sweet. *Science* 309:781–785, 2005.

Wise, P.M., et al. Twin study of the heritability of recognition thresholds for sour and salty taste. *Chem. Senses* 32:749–754, 2007.

Zelano, C., Gottfried, J. A taste of what to expect: top-down modulation of neural coding in rodent gustatory cortex. *Neuron* 74:217–219, 2012.

Chapter 20: Motor Systems and Movements in General

Ahissar, E. And motion changes it all. *Nat. Neurosci.* 11:1369–1370, 2008.

d'Avella, A., Bizzi, E. Shared and specific muscle synergies in natural motor behaviors. *Proc. Natl. Acad. Sci. USA* 102:3076–3081, 2005.

Gallese, V., Lakoff, G. The brains's concepts: the role of the sensory-motor system in conceptual knowledge. *Cogn. Neuropsychol.* 22:455–479, 2005.

Grillner, S., Wallén, P. Innate versus learned movements—a false dichotomy? *Brain Res.* 143:297–309, 2004.

Johansson, R.S., Flanagan, J.R. Coding and use of tactile signals from the fingertips in object manipulation tasks. *Nat. Rev. Neurosci.* 10:345–259, 2009.

Mendoza, G., Merchant, H. Motor system evolution and the emergence of high cognitive functions. *Progr. Neurobiol.* 122:73–93, 2014.

Morillon, B., et al. Predictive motor control of sensory dynamics in auditory active sensing. *Curr. Opin. Neurobiol* 31:230–238, 2015.

Pearson, K. Motor systems. *Curr. Opin. Neurobiol.* 10:649–654, 2000.

Prochazka, A., Ellaway, P. Sensory systems in the control of movement. *Compr. Physiol.* 2:2615–2627, 2012.

Schroeder, C.E., et al. Dynamics of active sensing and perceptual selection. *Curr. Opin. Neurobiol.* 20:172–176, 2010.

Schütz-Bosbach, S., et al. Self and other in the human motor system. *Curr. Biol.* 16:1830–1834, 2006.

Scott, S.H. Optimal strategies for movement: success with variability. *Nature Neurosci.* 5:1110–1111, 2002.

Stanley, J., Krakauer, J.W. Motor skill depends on knowledge of facts. *Front. Hum. Neurosci.* 7:503. doi:10.3389/fnhum.2013.00503, 2013.

Synofzik, M., et al. I move, therefore I am: a new theoretical framework to investigate agency and ownership. *Conscious. Cogn.* 17:411–424, 2008.

Tytell, E.D., et al. Spikes alone do not behavior make: why neuroscience needs biomechanics. *Curr. Opin. Neurosci.* 21:816–822, 2011.

Wolpert, D.M., et al. An internal model for sensorimotor integration. *Science* 269:1880–1882, 1995.

Chapter 21: The Peripheral Motor Neurons and Reflexes

Muscles, Motoneurons, and Motor Units

Aquilonius, S.-M., et al. Topographical location of motor endplates in cryosections of whole human muscles. *Muscle Nerve* 7:287–293, 1984.

Basmajian, J.V., De Luca, C. *Muscles alive: their functions revealed by electromyography*, 5th ed. Baltimore: Williams & Wilkins, 1985.

Bawa, P., Jones, K.E. Do lengthening contractions represent a case of reversal in recruitment order? *Prog. Brain Res.* 123:215–220, 1999.

Berchicci, M., et al. The neurophysiology of central and peripheral fatigue during sub-maximal lower limb isometric contractions. *Front. Hum. Neurosci.* 7:135. doi:10.3389/fnhum.2013.00135, 2013.

Bigland-Ritchie, B., et al. Contractile properties of human motor units: is man a cat? *Neuroscientist* 4:240–249, 1998.

Bizzi, E., et al. Combining modules for movement. *Brain Res. Rev.* 57:125–133, 2008.

Burke, R.E. Revisiting the notion of "motor unit types." *Prog. Brain Res.* 123:167–175, 1999.

Carson, S., Riek, S. Changes in muscle recruitment patterns during skill acquisition. *Exp. Brain Res.* 138:71–87, 2001.

Collins, D.F., et al. Sustained contractions produced by plateau-like behavior in human motoneurons. *J. Physiol.* 538:289–301, 2002.

Dasen. J.S., et al. Hox repertoires for motor neuron diversity and connectivity gated by a single accessory factor, FoxP1. *Cell* 134:304–316, 2008.

De Luca, C.J., Hostage, E.C. Relationship between firing rate and recruitment threshold of motoneurons in voluntary isometric contractions. *J. Neurophysiol.* 104: 1034–1046, 2010.

Deshpande, S., et al. Muscle finer orientation in muscles commonly injected with botulinum toxin: an anatomical pilot study. *Neurotox. Res.* 9:115–120, 2006.

Dong, M., et al. SV2 is the protein receptor for botulinum neurotoxin A. *Science* 312:592–596, 2006.

Enoka, R.M., Fuglevand, A.J. Motor unit physiology: some unresolved issues. *Muscle Nerve* 24:4–17, 2001.

Fallentin, N., et al. Motor unit recruitment during prolonged isometric contractions. *Eur. J. Appl. Physiol.* 67:335–341, 1993.

Gardiner, P., et al. Motoneurones "learn" and "forget" physical activity. *Can. J. Appl. Physiol.* 30:352–370, 2005.

Granit, R. *The basis of motor control: integrating the activity of muscles, α and γ motoneurons and their leading control systems.* New York: Academic Press, 1970.

Henneman, E., et al. Functional significance of cell size in spinal motoneurons. *J. Neurophysiol.* 28:560-580, 1965.

Henneman, E., et al. Rank order of motoneurons within a pool: law of combination. *J. Neurophysiol.* 37:1338–1349, 1974.

Howell, J.N., et al. Motor unit activity during isometric and concentric-eccentric contractions of the human first dorsal interosseus muscle. *J. Neurophysiol.* 74:901–904, 1995.

Jenny, A.B., Inukai, J. Principles of motor organization of the monkey cervical spinal cord. *J. Neurosci.* 3:567–575, 1983.

Jessel, T., et al. Motor neurons and the sense of place. *Neuron* 72:419–424, 2011.

Johnson, M.A., et al. Data on the distribution of fibre types in thirty-six human muscles: an autopsy study. *J. Neurol. Sci.* 18:111–129, 1973.

Kandel, E., Schwartz, J.H. *Principles of neural science.* Philadelphia: Elsevier, 1985.

Khan, S.I., Burne, J.A. Reflex inhibition of normal cramp following electrical stimulation of the muscle tendon. *J. Neurosphysiol.* 98:1102–1107, 2007.

Kiehn, O., Eken, T. Functional role of plateau potentials in vertebrate motor neurons. *Curr. Opin. Neurobiol.* 8:746–752, 1998.

Magnusson, S.P., et al. A mechanism for altered flexibility in human skeletal muscle. *J. Physiol.* 497:291–298, 1996.

McComas, A.J. Motor unit estimation: anxieties and achievements. *Muscle Nerve* 18:369–379, 1995.

Miller, K.J., et al. Motor-unit behavior in humans during fatiguing arm movements. *J. Neurophysiol.* 75:1629–1636, 1996.

Monti, R.J., et al. Role of motor unit structure in defining function. *Muscle Nerve* 24:848–866, 2001.

Navarrete, R., Vrbová, G. Activity-dependent interactions between motoneurones and muscles: their role in the development of the motor unit. *Progr. Neurobiol.* 41:93–124, 1993.

Piehl, F., et al. Calcitonin gene-related peptide-like immunoreactivity in motoneuron pools innervating different hind limb muscles in the rat. *Exp. Brain Res.* 96:291–303, 1993.

Taylor, J.L., Gandevia, S.C. Transcranial magnetic stimulation and human muscle fatigue. *Muscle Nerve* 24:18–29, 2001.

Wang, Y., et al. Motor learning changes GABAergic terminals on spinal motoneurons in normal rats. *Eur. J. Neurosci.* 23:141–150, 2006.

Whitford, M., Kukulka, C.G. Task-related variations in the surface EMG of the human first dorsal interosseous muscle. *Exp. Brain Res.* 215:101–113, 2011.

Reflexes and Spinal Interneurons

Aminoff, M.J., Goodin, D.S. Studies of the human stretch reflex. *Muscle Nerve* (Suppl.) 9:S3–S6, 2000.

Andersen, O.K., et al. Interaction between cutaneous and muscle afferent activity in polysynaptic reflex pathways: a human experimental study. *Pain* 84:29–36, 2000.

Bennett, D.J. Stretch reflex responses in the human elbow joint during a voluntary movement. *J. Physiol.* 474:339–351, 1994.

Brown, D.A., Kukulka, C.G. Human flexor reflex modulation during cycling. *J. Neurophysiol.* 69:1212–1224, 1993.

Capaday, C., et al. A re-examination of the effects of instruction on the long-latency stretch reflex response of the flexor pollicis longus muscle. *Exp. Brain Res.* 100:515–521, 1994.

Cody, F.J.W., et al. Observations on the genesis of the stretch reflex in Parkinson's disease. *Brain* 109:229–249, 1986.

Cody, F.J.W., et al. Stretch and vibration reflexes of wrist flexor muscles in spasticity. *Brain* 110:433–450, 1987.

Dietz, V., et al. Task-dependent modulation of short- and long-latency electromyographic responses in upper limb muscles. *Electroencephalogr. Clin. Neurophysiol.* 93:49–56, 1994.

Edgerton, R., et al. Does motor learning occur in the spinal cord? *Neuroscientist* 3:287–294, 1997.

Fellows, S.J., et al. Changes in the short- and long-latency stretch reflex components of the triceps surae muscle during ischaemia in man. *J. Physiol.* 472:737–748, 1993.

Glendenning, D.S. The effect of fasciculus cuneatus lesions on finger positioning and long-latency reflexes in monkeys. *Exp. Brain Res.* 93:104–116, 1993.

Gregory, J.E., et al. An investigation into mechanisms of reflex reinforcement by the Jendrassik manoeuvre. *Exp. Brain Res.* 138:366–374, 2001.

Hultborn, H. Spinal reflexes, mechanisms and concepts: from Eccles to Lundberg and beyond. *Prog. Neurobiol.* 78:215–232, 2006.

Hultborn, H. State-dependent modulation of sensory feedback. *J. Physiol.* 533:5–13, 2001.

Iles, J.F. Evidence for cutaneous and corticospinal modulation of presynaptic inhibition of Ia afferents from the human lower limb. *J. Physiol.* 481:197–207, 1996.

Jackson, J.H. Evolution and dissolution of the nervous system (the Croonian Lectures). *BMJ* 1:591–754, 1884.

Katz, R., Pierrot-Deseilligny, E. Recurrent inhibition in humans. *Prog. Neurobiol.* 57:325–355, 1999.

Kimura, T., et al. Transcranial magnetic stimulation over sensorimotor cortex disrupts anticipatory reflex gain modulation for skilled action. *J. Neurosci.* 26:9272–9281, 2006.

Krutky, M.A., et al. Interactions between limb and environmental mechanics influence stretch reflex sensitivity in humans. *J. Neurophysiol.* 103:429–440, 2010.

Kurtzer, I.L. Long-latency reflexes account for limb biomechanics through several supraspinal pathways. *Front. Integr. Neurosci.* 8:99. doi:0.3389/fnint.2014.00099, 2015.

Lacquaniti, F., et al. Transient reversal of the stretch reflex in human arm muscles. *J. Neurophysiol.* 66:939–954, 1991.

Lewis, G.N., et al. Proposed cortical and sub-cortical contributions to the long-latency stretch reflex in the forearm. *Exp. Brain Res.* 156: 72–79, 2006.

Liddell, E.G.T. *The discovery of reflexes.* New York: Oxford University Press, 1960.

Manning, C.D., et al. Proprioceptive reaction time and long-latency reflexes in humans. *Exp. Brain Res.* 221:155–166, 2012.

Marsden, C.D., et al. Stretch reflex and servo action in a variety of human muscles. *J. Physiol. (Lond.)* 259:531–560, 1976.

Matthews, P.B.C. Restoring balance to the reflex actions of the muscle spindle: the secondary endings also matter. *J. Physiol.* 572: 309–310, 2006.

Matthews, P.B.C. The human stretch reflex and the motor cortex. *Trends Neurosci.* 14:87–91, 1991.

Mazzocchio, R., et al. Depression of Renshaw recurrent inhibition by activation of corticospinal fibres in human upper and lower limb. *J. Physiol.* 481:487–498, 1994.

McCrea, D.A. Can sense be made of spinal interneuron circuits? *Behav. Brain Sci.* 15:633–643, 1992.

Nakazawa, K., et al. Short- and long-latency reflex responses during different motor tasks in elbow flexor muscles. *Exp. Brain Res.* 116:20–28, 1997.

Prochazka, A., et al. What do *reflex* and *voluntary* mean? Modern views on an ancient debate. *Exp. Brain Res.* 130:417–432, 2000.

Pruszynski, J.A., et al. The long-latency reflex is composed of at least two functionally independent processes. *J. Neurophysiol.* 106:449–459, 2011.

Ribot-Ciscar, E., et al. Increased muscle spindle sensitivity to movement during reinforcement maneuvers in relaxed human subjects. *J. Physiol. (Lond.)* 523:271–282, 2000.

Rossi, A., Decchi, B. Flexibility of lower limb reflex responses to painful cutaneous stimulation in standing humans: evidence of load-dependent modulation. *J. Physiol.* 481:521–532, 1994.

Sandrini, G., et al. The lower limb flexion reflex in humans. *Progr. Neurobiol.* 77:353–395, 2005.

Schemmel, J., et al. Stretch sensitive reflexes as an adaptive mechanism for maintaining limb stability. *Clin. Neurophysiol.* 121:1680–1689, 2010.

Scott, S.H., et al. Feedback control during voluntary motor actions. *Curr. Opin. Neurobiol.* 33:85–94, 2015.

Sherrington, C.S. *The integrative action of the brain.* Cambridge, UK: Cambridge University Press, 1947.

Witney, A.G., et al. The cutaneous contribution to adaptive precision grip. *Trends Neurosci.* 27:637–643, 2004.

Wolpaw, J.R. The complex structure of a simple memory. *Trends Neurosci.* 20:588–594, 1997.

Zehr, E.P., Stein, R.B. Interaction of the Jendrássik maneuver with segmental presynaptic inhibition. *Exp. Brain Res.* 124:474–480, 1999.

Muscle Tone

Baldissera, F., et al. Motor neuron "bistability": a pathogenetic mechanism for cramps and myokymia. *Brain* 117:929–939, 1994.

Chleboun, G.S., et al. Relationship between muscle swelling and stiffness after eccentric exercise. *Med. Sci. Sports Exerc.* 30:529–535, 1998.

Dietz, V., Sinkjaer, T. Spastic movement disorder: impaired reflex function and altered muscle mechanics. *Lancet Neur.* 6:725–733, 2007.

Futagi, Y., et al. Primitive reflex profiles in infants: differences based on categories of neurological abnormality. *Brain Dev.* 14:294–298, 1992.

Gerrits, H.L., et al. Contractile properties of the quadriceps muscle in individuals with spinal cord injury. *Muscle Nerve* 22:1249–1256, 1999.

Horowits, R. Passive force generation and titin isoforms in mammalian skeletal muscle. *Biophys. J.* 61:392–398, 1992.

Hultborn, H. Plateau potentials and their role in regulating motoneuronal firing. *Progr. Brain Res.* 123:39–48, 1999.

Khan, S.I., Burne, J.A. Reflex inhibition of normal cramp following electrical stimulation of the muscle tendon. *J. Neurophysiol.* 98:1102–1107, 2007.

Kiehn, O., Eken, T. Functional role of plateau potentials in vertebrate motor neurons. *Curr. Opin. Neurobiol.* 8:746–752, 1998.

Löscher, W.N., et al. Excitatory drive to the α-motoneuron pool during fatiguing submaximal contraction in man. *J. Physiol. (Lond.)* 491:271–280, 1996.

Pisano, F., et al. Quantitative evaluation of normal muscle tone. *J. Neurol. Sci.* 135:168–172, 1996.

Ross, B.H., Thomas, C.K. Human motor unit activity during induced muscle cramp. *Brain* 118:983–993, 1995.

Sakai, F., et al. Pericranial muscle hardness in tension-type headache: a non-invasive measurement method and its clinical application. *Brain* 118:523–531, 1995.

Schwellnus, M.P. Cause of exercise associated muscle cramps (EAMC)—altered neuromuscular control, dehydration or electrolyte depletion? *Brit. J. Sports Med.* 43:401–408, 2009.

Simons, D., Mense, S. Understanding and measurement of muscle tone as related to clinical muscle pain. *Pain* 75:1–17, 1998.

Taylor, J. L., Gandevia, S.C. Transcranial magnetic stimulation and human muscle fatigue. *Muscle & Nerve* 24:18–29, 2001.

Van der Meché, F.G.A., Van Gijn, J. Hypotonia: an erroneous clinical concept? *Brain* 109:1169–1178, 1986.

Regeneration of Peripheral Nerves

Asensio-Pinilla, E., et al. Electrical stimulation combined with exercise increase axonal regeneration after peripheral nerve injury. *Exp. Neurol.* 219:258–265, 2009.

Brushart, T.M.E. Motor axons preferentially reinnervate motor pathways. *J. Neurosci.* 13:2730–2738, 1993.

Chen, Z.-L., et al. Peripheral regeneration. *Annu. Rev. Neurosci.* 30:209–233, 2007.

Cope, T.C., Clark, B.D. Motor-unit recruitment in self-reinnervated muscle. *J. Neurophysiol.* 70:1787–1796, 1993.

Davis, K., et al. Nerve injury triggers changes in the brain. *Neuroscientist* 17:407–422, 2011.

Hallin, R.G., et al. Spinal cord implantation of avulsed ventral roots in primates: correlation between restored motor function and morphology. *Exp. Brain Res.* 124:304–310, 1999.

Höke, A., Brushart, T. Introduction to special issue: challenges and opportunities for regeneration in the peripheral nervous system. *Exp. Neurol.* 223:1–4, 2010.

Krarup, C., et al. Factors that influence peripheral nerve regeneration: an electrophysiological study of the monkey median nerve. *Ann. Neurol.* 51:69–81, 2002.

Lang, E.M., et al. Effects of root replantation and neurotrophic factor treatment on long-term motoneuron survival and axonal regeneration after C7 spinal root avulsion. *Exp. Neurol.* 194:341–354, 2005.

Rafuse, V.F., et al. Proportional enlargement of motor units after partial denervation of cat triceps surae muscles. *J. Neurophysiol.* 68:1261–1276, 1992.

Swash, M., et al. Focal loss of anterior horn cells in the cervical cord in motor neuron disease. *Brain* 109:939–952, 1986.

Tuszynski, M.H., Steward, O. Concepts and methods for the study of axonal regeneration in the CNS. *Neuron* 74:777–791, 2012.

Chapter 22: The Motor Cortical Areas and Descending Pathways

Descending Motor Tracts

Baker, S.N. The primate reticulospinal tract, hand function and functional recovery. *J. Physiol.* 589:5603–5612, 2011.

Biber, M.P., et al. Cortical neurons projecting to the cervical and lumbar enlargements of the spinal cord in young and adult rhesus monkeys. *Exp. Neurol.* 59:492–508, 1978.

Bortoff, G.A., Strick, P.L. Corticospinal terminations in two new-world primates: further evidence that corticomotoneuronal connections provide part of the neural substrate for manual dexterity. *J. Neurosci.* 13:5105–5118, 1993.

Capaday, C., et al. Studies on the corticospinal control of human walking: I. Responses to focal transcranial magnetic stimulation of the motor cortex. *J. Neurophysiol.* 81:129–139, 1999.

Danek, A., et al. Tracing of neuronal connections in the human brain by magnetic resonance imaging *in vivo. Eur. J. Neurosci.* 2:112–115, 1990.

Dum, R.P., Strick, P.L. The origin of corticospinal projections from the premotor areas in the frontal lobe. *J. Neurosci.* 11:667–689, 1990.

Englander, R.N., et al. The location of human pyramidal tract in the internal capsule: anatomic evidence. *Neurology* 25:823–826, 1975.

Esposito, M.S., et al. Brainstem nucleus MdV mediates skilled forelimb motor tasks. *Nature* 508:351–356, 2014.

Foerster, O. Motorische Felder und Bahnen. In: *Hdb. d. Neurol,* Vol. 6. Heidelberg: Springer Verlag, 1936.

He, S.-Q., et al. Topographic organization of corticospinal projections from the frontal lobe: motor areas on the lateral surface of the hemisphere. *J. Neurosci.* 13:952–980, 1993.

Hicks, T.P., Onodera, S. The mammalian red nucleus and its role in motor systems, including the emergence of bipedalism and language. *Progr. Neurobiol.* 96:165–175, 2012.

Holstege, J.C. The ventro-medial medullary projections to spinal motoneurons: ultrastructure, transmitters and functional aspects. *Prog. Brain Res.* 107:160–181, 1996.

Jacobs, B.L., Fornal, C.A. Serotonin and motor activity. *Curr. Opin. Neurobiol.* 7:820–825, 1997.

Luppino, G., et al. Corticospinal projections from mesial frontal and cingulate areas in the monkey. *NeuroReport* 5:2545–2548, 1994.

Maier, M.A., et al. Differences in corticospinal projection from primary motor cortex and supplementary motor area to Macaque upper limb motoneurons: an anatomical and electrophysiological study. *Cereb. Cortex* 12:281–296, 2002.

Matsuyama, K., et al. Multi-segmental innervation of single pontine reticulospinal axons in the cervico-thoracic region of the cat: anterograde PHA-L tracing study. *J. Comp. Neurol.* 377:234–250, 1997.

Morecraft, R.J., et al. Terminal distribution of the corticospinal projection from the hand/arm region of the primary motor cortex to the cervical enlargement in rhesus monkey. *J. Comp. Neurol.* 521:4205–4235, 2013.

Nathan, P.W., Smith, M.C. The rubrospinal and central tegmental tracts in man. *Brain* 105:223–269, 1982.

Nathan, P.W., et al. The corticospinal tracts in man: course and location of fibres at different segmental levels. *Brain* 113:303–324, 1990.

Nathan, P.W., et al. Vestibulospinal, reticulospinal and descending propriospinal nerve fibres in man. *Brain* 119:1809–1833, 1996.

Nudo, R.J., Masterton, R.B. Descending pathways to the spinal cord: III. Sites of origin of the corticospinal tract. *J. Comp. Neurol.* 296:559–583, 1990.

Ralston, D.D., Ralston, H.J. III. The terminations of corticospinal tract axons in the macaque monkey. *J. Comp. Neurol.* 242:325–337, 1985.

Sherman, S.J., et al. Hyper-reflexia without spasticity after unilateral infarct of the medullary pyramid. *J. Neurol. Sci.* 175:145–155, 2000.

Strutton, P.H., et al. Corticospinal activation of internal oblique muscles has a strong ipsilateral component and can be lateralised in man. *Exp. Brain Res.* 158:474–479, 2004.

Turton, A., Lemon, R. The contribution of fast corticospinal input to the voluntary activation of proximal muscles in normal subjects and in stroke patients. *Exp. Brain Res.* 129:559–572, 1999.

Control of Posture and Automatic Movements

Allum, J.H.J., Honegger, F. Interactions between vestibular and proprioceptive inputs triggering and modulating human balance-correcting responses differ across muscles. *Exp. Brain Res.* 121:478–494, 1998.

Armstrong, D.M. The supraspinal control of mammalian locomotion. *J. Physiol.* 405:1–37, 1988.

Berger, W. Characteristics of locomotor control in children with cerebral palsy. *Neurosci. Biobehav. Rev.* 22:579–582, 1998.

Bloem, B.R., et al. Is lower leg proprioception essential for triggering human automatic postural responses? *Exp. Brain Res.* 130:375–391, 2000.

Brenière, Y., Bril, B. Development of postural control of gravity forces in children during the first 5 years of walking. *Exp. Brain Res.* 121:255–262, 1998.

Buccino, G., et al. Action observation activates premotor and parietal areas in a somatotopic manner: an fMRI study. *Eur. J. Neurosci.* 13:400–404, 2001.

Calancie, B., et al. Involuntary stepping after chronic spinal cord injury: evidence for a central rhythm generator for locomotion in man. *Brain* 117:1143–1159, 1994.

Capaday, C. The special nature of human walking and its neural control. *Trends Neurosci.* 25:370–376, 2002.

Caronni, A., Cavallari, P. Anticipatory postural adjustments stabilise the whole upper-limb prior to a gentle index finger tap. *Exp. Brain Res.* 194:59–66, 2009.

Cordo, P.J., Gurfinkel, V.S. Motor coordination can be fully understood only by studying complex movements. *Prog. Brain Res.* 143:29–38, 2004.

Deliagina, T.G., et al. Spinal and supraspinal postural networks. *Brain Res. Rev.* 57:212–221, 2008.

Dietz, V. Evidence for a load receptor contribution to the control of posture and locomotion. *Neurosci. Biobehav. Rev.* 22:495–499, 1998.

Dietz, V., et al. Level of spinal cord lesion determines locomotor activity in spinal man. *Exp. Brain Res.* 128:405–409, 1999.

Drew, T., Marigold, D.S. Taking the next step: cortical contributions to the control of locomotion. *Curr. Opin. Neurobiol.* 33:25–33, 2015.

Esposito, M.S., et al. Brainstem nucleus MdV mediates skilled forelimb motor tasks. *Nature* 508:351–356, 2014.

Fitzpatrick, R.C., et al. Ankle stiffness of standing humans in response to imperceptible perturbation: reflex and task-dependent components. *J. Physiol.* 454:533–547, 1992.

Forssberg, H. Neural control of human motor development. *Curr. Opin. Neurobiol.* 9:676–682, 1999.

Frigon, A. Central pattern generators of the mammalian spinal cord. *Neuroscientist* 18:56–69, 2012.

Grasso, R., et al. Development of anticipatory orienting strategies during locomotor tasks in children. *Neurosci. Biobehav. Rev.* 22:533–539, 1998.

Grillner, S., Wallén, P. Innate versus learned movements—a false dichotomy? *Brain Res.* 143:297–309, 2004.

Grillner, S., et al. Neural basis of goal-directed locomotion in vertebrates—an overview. *Brain Res. Rev.* 57:2–12, 2008.

Ito, Y., et al. The functional effectiveness of neck muscle reflexes for head-righting in response to sudden fall. *Exp. Brain Res.* 117:266–272, 1997.

Ivanenko, Y.P., et al. Distributed neural networks for controlling human locomotion: lessons from normal and SCI subjects. *Brain Res. Bull.* 78:13–21, 2009.

Kavounoudias, A., et al. From balance regulation to body orientation: two goals for muscle proprioceptive information processing? *Exp. Brain Res.* 124:80–88, 1999.

Kuo, A.D., et al. Effect of altered sensory conditions on multivariate descriptions of human postural sway. *Exp. Brain Res.* 122:185–195, 1998.

Lackner, J.R., DiZio, P.A. Aspects of body self-calibration. *Trends Cogn. Sci.* 4:279–288, 2000.

Lacour, M., et al. Sensory strategies in human postural control before and after unilateral vestibular neurotomy. *Exp. Brain Res.* 115:300–310, 1997.

Lacquaniti, F., et al. Posture and movement: coordination and control. *Arch. Ital. Biol.* 135:353–367, 1997.

Lemon, R.N., et al. Direct and indirect pathways for corticospinal control of upper limb motoneurons in the primate. *Prog. Brain Res.* 143:263–279, 2004.

Malouin, F., et al. Brain activations during motor imagery of locomotor-related tasks: a PET study. *Hum. Brain Imag.* 19:47–62, 2003.

Massion, J., et al. Why and how are posture and movement coordinated? *Prog. Brain Res.* 143:13–27, 2004.

McCrea, D.A., Rybak, I.A. Organization of mammalian locomotor rhythm and pattern generation. *Brain Res. Rev.* 57:134–146, 2008.

McLean, D.L., Dougherty, K.J. Peeling back the layers of locomotor control in the spinal cord. *Curr. Opin. Neurobiol.* 33:63–70, 2015.

Mergner, T., Rosemeier, T. Interaction of vestibular, somatosensory and visual signals for postural control and motion perception under terrestrial and microgravity conditions: a conceptual model. *Brain Res. Rev.* 28:118–135, 1998.

Muir, G.D., Stevens J.D. Sensorimotor stimulation to improve locomotor recovery after spinal cord injury. *Trends Neurosci.* 20:72–77, 1997.

Pearson, K.G. Generating the walking gait: role of sensory feedback. *Prog. Brain Res.* 143:123–129, 2004.

Perennou, D.A., et al. The polymodal sensory cortex is crucial for controlling lateral postural stability: evidence from stroke patients. *Brain Res. Bull.* 53:359–365, 2000.

Perrier, J.-F., Cotel, F. Serotonergic modulation of spinal motor control. *Curr. Opin. Neurobiol.* 33:1–7, 2015.

Pettersen, T.H., et al. Cortical involvement in anticipatory postural reactions in man. *Exp. Brain Res.* 193:161–171, 2009.

Runge, C.F., et al. Role of vestibular information in initiation of rapid postural responses. *Exp. Brain Res.* 122:403–412, 1998.

Schiepatti, M., Nardone, A. Group II spindle afferent fibers in humans: their possible role in reflex control of stance. *Prog. Brain Res.* 123:461–472, 1999.

Schmitz, C., et al. Building of anticipatory postural adjustment during childhood: a kinematic and electromyographic analysis of unloading in children from 4 to 8 years of age. *Exp. Brain Res.* 142:354–364, 2002.

Stapley, P., et al. Investigating centre of mass stabilisation as the goal of posture and movement coordination during human whole body reaching. *Biol. Cybern.* 82:161–172, 2000.

Wu, A.M., et al. Anticipatory postural adjustments in stance and grip. *Exp. Brain Res.* 116:122–130, 1997.

Wu, G., Chiang J.-H. The significance of somatosensory stimulations to the human foot in the control of postural reflexes. *Exp. Brain Res.* 114:163–169, 1997.

Zaaimi, B., et al. Changes in descending motor pathway connectivity after corticospinal tract lesion in macaque monkey. *Brain* 135:2277–2289, 2012.

Cortical Motor Areas and Voluntary Movements

Abe, M., Hanakawa, T. Functional coupling underlying motor and cognitive functions of the dorsal premotor cortex. *Behav. Brain Res.* 198:13–23, 2009.

Afshar, A., et al. Single-trial neural correlates of arm movement preparation. *Neuron* 71:555–564, 2011.

Alstermark, B., Isa, T. Circuits for skilled reaching and grasping. *Annu. Rev. Neurosci.* 35:559–578, 2012.

Ansuini, C., et al. Breaking the flow of action. *Exp. Brain Res.* 192:287–292, 2009.

Ashe, J., et al. Cortical control of motor sequences. *Curr. Opin. Neurobiol.* 16:213–221, 2006.

Assal, F., et al. Moving with or without will: functional neural correlates of alien hand syndrome. *Ann. Neurol.* 62:301–306, 2007.

Bizzi, E., Mussa-Ivaldi, F.A. Neural basis of motor control and its cognitive implication. *Trends Cogn. Sci.* 2:97–102, 1998.

Boecker, H., et al. Role of human rostral supplementary motor area and the basal ganglia in motor sequence control: investigations with H_2 ^{15}O PET. *J. Neurophysiol.* 79:1070–1080, 1998.

Bush, G., et al. Dorsal anterior cingulate cortex: a role in reward-based decision making. *Proc. Natl. Acad. Sci. USA* 99:523–528, 2002.

Carramazza, A., et al. Embodied cognition and mirror neurons: a critical assessment. *Annu. Rev. Neurosci.* 37:1–15, 2014.

Castiello, U. The neuroscience of grasping. *Nat. Rev. Neurosci.* 6:726–736, 2005.

Chouinard, P.A., Paus, T. Ther primary motor and premotor areas of the human cerebral cortex. *Neuroscientist* 12:143–152, 2006.

Culham, J.C., Valyear, K.F. Human parietal cortex in action. *Curr. Opin. Neurobiol.* 16:205–212, 2006.

Deiber, M.-P., et al. Cerebral structures participating in motor preparation in humans: a positron emission tomography study. *J. Neurophysiol.* 75:233–247, 1996.

Della-Maggiore, V., et al. Sensorimotor adaptation: multiple forms of plasticity in motor circuits. *Neuroscientist* 21:109–125, 2015.

Dushanova, J., Donoghue, J. Neurons in primary motor cortex engaged during action observation. *Eur. J. Neurosci.* 31:386–398, 2010.

Ehrsson, H.H., et al. That's my hand! Activity in premotor cortex reflects feeling of ownership of a limb. *Science* 305:875–877, 2004.

Fadiga, L., et al. Human motor cortex excitability during the perception of other's action. *Curr. Opin. Neurobiol.* 15:213–218, 2005.

Flanders, M. Functional somatotopy in sensorimotor cortex. *NeuroReport* 16:313–316, 2005.

Fogassi, L., et al. Parietal lobe: from action organization to intention understanding *Science* 308:662–667, 2005.

Gentili, R., et al. Improvement and generalization of arm motor performance through motor imagery practice. *Neuroscience* 137:761–772, 2005.

Georgopoulos, A.P., Carpenter, A.F. Coding of movements in the motor cortex. *Curr. Opin. Neurobiol.* 33:34–39, 2015.

Grafton, S.T., et al. Functional anatomy of pointing and grasping in humans. *Cereb. Cortex* 6:226–237, 1996.

Graziano, M.S., et al. Complex movements evoked by microstimulation of precentral cortex. *Neuron* 34:841–851, 2002.

Graziano, M.S., Aflalo, T.N. Rethinking cortical organization: moving away from discrete areas arranged in hierarchies. *Neuroscientist* 13:138–2007, 2007.

Halsband, U., et al. The role of the premotor cortex and the supplementary motor area in the temporal control of movement in man. *Brain* 116:243–266, 1993.

Harrison, T.C., Murphy, T.H. Motor maps and the cortical control of movement. *Curr. Opin. Neurobiol.* 24:88–94, 2014.

Hikosaka, O., et al. Differential roles of the frontal cortex, basal ganglia, and cerebellum in visuomotor sequence learning. *Neurobiol. Learn. Mem.* 70:137–149, 1998.

Hoshi, E., Tanji, J. Distinctions between dorsal and ventral premotor areas: anatomical connectivity and functional properties. *Curr. Opin. Neurobiol.* 17:234–242, 2007.

Kawato, M. Internal models for motor control and trajectory planning. *Curr. Opin. Neurobiol.* 9:718–727, 1999.

Keller, A. Intrinsic synaptic organization of the motor cortex. *Cereb. Cortex* 3:430–441, 1993.

Lacquaniti, F., Carminiti, R. Visuo-motor transformations for arm reaching. *Eur. J. Neurosci.* 10:195–203, 1998.

Loeb, G.E. What might the brain know about muscles, limbs and spinal circuits? *Prog. Brain Res.* 123:405–409, 1999.

Luria, A.R. *Higher cortical functions in man*, 2nd ed. New York: Consultants Bureau, 1980.

Macchi, G., Jones, E.G. Toward an agreement on terminology of nuclear and subnuclear subdivisions of the motor thalamus. *J. Neurosurg.* 86:670–685, 1997.

Marsden, J.F., et al. Organization of cortical activities related to movements in humans. *J. Neurosci.* 15:2307–2314, 2000.

Morecroft, R.J., et al. Cytoarchitecture and cortical connections of the anterior cingulate and adjacent somatomotor fields in the rhesus monkey. *Brain Res. Bull.* 87:457–497, 2012.

Mountcastle, V.B., et al. Posterior parietal association cortex of the monkey: command functions for operations within extrapersonal space. *J. Neurophysiol.* 38:871–908, 1975.

Nachev, P., et al. Functional role of the supplementary motor areas. *Nat. Rev. Neurosci.* 9:856–869, 2008.

Orban de Xivry, J.J., Ethier, V. Neural correlates of internal models. *J. Neurosci.* 28:7931–7932, 2008.

Overduin, S.A., et al. Microstimulation activates a handful of muscle synergies. *Neuron* 76:1071–1077, 2012.

Paus, T., et al. Role of the human anterior cingulate cortex in the control of oculomotor, manual, and speech responses: a positron emission tomography study. *J. Neurophysiol.* 70:453–469, 1993.

Pearce, A.J., et al. Functional reorganisation of the corticomotor projection to the hand in skilled racquet players. *Exp. Brain Res.* 130:238–243, 2000.

Penfield, W., Rasmussen, T. *The cerebral cortex of man.* New York: Macmillan, 1950.

Phillips, C.G. *Movements of the hand.* Liverpool, UK: Liverpool University Press, 1986.

Phillips, C.G., Porter, R. *Corticospinal neurones: their role in movement.* New York: Academic Press, 1977.

Picard, N., Strick, P.L. Motor areas of the medial wall: a review of their location and functional activation. *Cereb. Cortex* 6:342–353, 1996.

Prochazka, A. Sensorimotor gain control: a basic strategy of motor systems? *Prog. Neurobiol.* 33:281–307, 1989.

Rademacher, J., et al. Variability and asymmetry in the human pre-central motor system: a cytoarchitectonic and myeloarchitectonic brain mapping study. *Brain* 124:2232–2258, 2001.

Rao, S.M., et al. Somatotopic mapping of the human motor cortex with functional magnetic resonance imaging. *Neurology* 45:919–924, 1995.

Rathelot, J.-A., Strick, P.L. Subdivisions of primary motor cortex based on cortico-motoneuronal cells. *Proc. Natl. Acad. Sci. USA* 106:918–923, 2009.

Rioult-Pedotti, M.-S., et al. Strengthening of horizontal cortical connections following skill learning. *Nat. Rev. Neurosci.* 1:230–234, 1998.

Rizzolatti, G., et al. Motor and cognitive functions of the ventral premotor cortex. *Curr. Opin. Neurobiol.* 12:149–154, 2002.

Rowe, J.B., Frackowiak, R.S.J. The impact of brain imaging technology on our understanding of motor function and dysfunction. *Curr. Opin. Neurobiol.* 9:728–734, 1999.

Rushworth, M.F.S., et al. Parietal cortex and movement: I. Movement selection and reaching. *Exp. Brain Res.* 117:292–310, 1997.

Sanes, J.N., Donoghue, J.P. Plasticity and primary motor cortex. *Annu. Rev. Neurosci.* 23:393–415, 2000.

Schieber, M.H. How might the motor cortex individuate movements? *Trends Neurosci.* 13:440–445, 1990.

Schluter, N.D., et al. Temporary interference in human lateral premo-tor cortex suggests dominance for the selection of movements: a study using transcranial magnetic stimulation. *Brain* 121:785–799, 1998.

Serrien, D.J., et al. The missing link between action and cognition. *Prog. Neurobiol.* 82:95–107, 2007.

Sessle, B.J., Wiesendanger, M. Structural and functional definition of the motor cortex in the monkey (*Macaca fascicularis*). *J. Physiol.* 323:245–265, 1982.

Shenoy, K.V., et al. Cortical control of arm movements: a dynamical perspective. *Annu. Rev. Neurosci.* 36:337–359, 2013.

Shima, K., Tanji, J. Both supplementary and presupplementary motor areas are crucial for the temporal organization of multiple movements. *J. Neurophysiol.* 80:3247–3260, 1998.

Shindo, K., et al. Spatial distribution of thalamic projections to the supplementary motor area and the primary motor cortex: a multiple retrograde labeling study in the macaque monkey. *J. Comp. Neurol.* 357:98–116, 1995.

Stanley, J., Krakauer, J.W. Motor skill depends on knowledge of facts. *Front.Hum.Neurosci.* 7:503. doi:10.3389/fnhum.2013.00503, 2013.

Stephan, K.M., et al. The role of ventral medial wall motor areas in bimanual co-ordination: a combined lesion and activation study. *Brain* 122:351–368, 1999.

Sumner, P., Husain, M. At the edge of consciousness: automatic motor activation and voluntary control. *Neuroscientist* 14:474–486, 2008.

Tanji, J., Hoshi, E. Premotor areas: medial. In: Squire, L. (Ed.), *Encyclopedia of neuroscience* (pp. 925–933). Philadelphia: Elsevier, 2009.

Todorov, E. Direct cortical control of muscle activation in voluntary arm movements: a model. *Nat. Rev. Neurosci.* 3:391–398, 2000.

Tokuno, H., et al. Reevaluation of ipsilateral corticocortical inputs to the orofacial region of the primary motor cortex in the macaque monkey. *J. Comp. Neurol.* 389:34–48, 1997.

Tsakiris, M., et al. Having a body versus moving your body: neural signatures of agency and body-ownership. *Neuropsychol.* 48:2740–2749, 2010.

Wilson, S.A., et al. Transcranial magnetic stimulation mapping of the motor cortex in normal subjects: the representation of two intrinsic hand muscles. *J. Neurol. Sci.* 118:134–144, 1993.

Woolsey, C.N. Organization of somatic sensory and motor areas of the cerebral cortex. In: Harlow, H.F., Woolsey, C.N. (Eds.), *Biological and biochemical bases of behavior* (pp. 63–81). Madison: University of Wisconsin Press, 1958.

Xiao, J. Premotor neuronal plasticity in monkeys adapting to a new dynamic environment. *Eur. J. Neurosci.* 22:3266–3280, 2005.

Yue, G.H., et al. Brain activation during finger extension and flexion movements. *Brain Res.* 856:291–300, 2000.

Motor Learning, Imagery, and Mirror Neurons

Berger, S.E., Adolph, K.E. Learning and development in infant locomotion. *Prog. Brain Res.* 164:237–255, 2007.

Carramazza, A., et al. Embodied cognition and mirror neurons: a critical assessment. *Annu. Rev. Neurosci.* 37:1–15, 2014.

Catmur, C., et al. Through the looking glass: countermirror activation following incomparable sensorimotor learning. *Eur. J. Neurosci.* 28:1208–1215, 2008.

Decety, J., Grezes J. The power of simulation: imaging one's own and other's behavior. *Brain Res.* 1079:4–14, 2006.

Gazzola, V., et al. The anthropomorphic brain: the mirror neuron system responds to human and robotic actions. *NeuroImage* 25:1674–1684, 2007.

Gentili, R., et al. Improvement and generalization of arm motor performance through motor imagery practice. *Neuroscience* 137:761–772, 2005.

Huber, D., et al. Multiple dynamic representations in the motor cortex during sensorimotor learning. *Nature* 484:473–478, 2012.

Jacob, P., Jeannerod, M. The motor theory of social cognition. *Trends Cogn. Sci.* 9:21–25, 2005.

Jeannerod, M., Frak, V. Mental imaging of motor activity in humans. *Curr. Opin. Neurobiol.* 9:735–739, 1999.

Krakauer, J.W., Mazzoni, P. Human sensorimotor learning: adaptation, skill and beyond. *Curr. Opin. Neurobiol.* 21:636–644, 2011.

Laforce, R., Doyon, J. Distinct contribution of the striatum and cerebellum in motor learning. *Brain Cogn.* 45:189–211, 2001.

Lalazar, H., Vaadia, E. Neural basis of sensorimotor learning: modifying internal models. *Curr. Opin. Neurobiol.* 18:573–581, 2008.

Li, S., et al. The effect of motor imagery on spinal segmental excitability. *J. Neurosci.* 24:9624–9680, 2004.

Münzert, J., Zentgraf, K. Motor imagery and its implications for understanding the motor system. *Progr. Brain Res.* 174:219–229, 2009.

Naito, E., et al. Internally simulated sensations during motor imagery activate cortical motor areas and the cerebellum. *J. Neurosci.* 22:3683–3691, 2002.

Oztop, E., et al. Mirror neurons and imitation: a computationally guided review. *Neural Netw.* 19:254–271, 2006.

Pascual-Leone, A., et al. Modulation of muscle responses evoked by transcranial magnetic stimulation during the acquisition of new fine motor skills. *J. Neurophysiol.* 74:1037–1045, 1995.

Pearce, A.J., et al. Functional reorganisation of the corticomotor projection to the hand in skilled racquet players. *Exp. Brain Res.* 130:238–243, 2000.

Rioult-Pedotti, M.-S., et al. Strengthening of horizontal cortical connections following skill learning. *Nature Neurosci.* 1:230–234, 1998.

Rizzolatti, G., Fabbri-Destro, M. Mirror neurons: from discovery to autism. *Exp. Brain Res.* 200:223–237, 2010.

Sanes, J.N., Donoghue, J.P. Plasticity and primary motor cortex. *Annu. Rev. Neurosci.* 23:393–415, 2000.

Shmuelof, L., Zohary, E. Mirror-image representation of action in the anterior parietal cortex. *Nat. Rev. Neurosci.* 11:1267–1269, 2008.

Solodkin, A., et al. Fine modulation in network activation during motor execution and motor imagery. *Cereb. Cortex* 14:146–1255, 2004.

Stoeckel, M.C., et al. Congenitally altered motor experience alters somatotopic organization of human primary motor cortex. *Proc. Natl. Acad. Sci. USA* 106:2395–2400, 2009.

Taylor, J.A., Ivry, R.B. The role of strategies in motor learning. *Ann. NY Acad. Sci.* 1251:1–12, 2012.

Wang, Y., et al. Motor learning changes GABAegic terminals on spinal motoneurons. *Eur. J. Neurosci.* 23:141–150, 2006.

Wilson, M., Knoblich, G. The case for motor involvement in perceiving conspecifics. *Psychol. Bull.* 131:460–473, 2005.

Winkler, T., et al. Spinal and cortical activity-dependent plasticity following learing of complex arm movements in humans. *Exp. Brain Res.* 219:267–274, 2012.

Wolpert, D.M., et al. Perspectives and problems in motor learning. *Trends Cogn. Sci.* 5:487–494, 2001.

Injury of Central Motor Pathways (Upper Motor Neurons)

Adams, M.M., Hicks, A.L. Spasticity after spinal cord injury. *Spinal Cord* 43:577–586, 2005.

Beer, R., et al. Disturbances of voluntary movement coordination in stroke: problems of planning or execution? *Prog. Brain Res.* 123:455–460, 1999.

Bennett, D.J., et al. Evidence for plateau potentials in tail motoneurons of awake chronic spinal rats with spasticity. *J. Neurophysiol.* 86:1972–1982, 2002.

Burke, D., et al. Pathophysiology of spasticity in stroke. *Neurology* 80:S20–S26, 2013.

Burne, J.A., et al. The spasticity paradox: movement disorder or disorder of resting limbs? *J. Neurol. Neurosurg. Psychiatry* 76:47–54, 2005.

Classen, J., et al. The motor syndrome associated with exaggerated inhibition within the primary motor cortex of patients with hemi-paretic stroke. *Brain* 120:605–619, 1997.

Cleland, C.L., et al. Neural mechanisms underlying the clasp-knife reflex in the cat: stretch-sensitive muscular-free nerve endings. *J. Neurophysiol.* 64:1319–1330, 1990.

Dietz, V., Sinkjaer, T. Spastic movement disorder: impaired reflex function and altered muscle mechanics. *Lancet Neurol.* 6:725–733, 2007.

Eyre, J.A. Corticospinal tract development and its plasticity after perinatal injury. *Neurosci. Biobehav. Rev.* 31:1136–1149, 2007.

Faist, M., et al. Impaired modulation of quadriceps tendon jerk reflex during spastic gait: differences between spinal and cerebral lesions. *Brain* 117:1449–1455, 1994.

Freund, H.-J., Hummelsheim, H. Lesions of premotor cortex in man. *Brain* 108:697–733, 1985.

Grey, M., et al. Post-activation depression of soleus stretch reflexes in healthy and spastic humans. *Exp. Brain Res.* 185:189–197, 2008.

Lance, J.W. The Babinski sign. *J. Neurol. Neurosurg. Psychiatry* 73:360–362, 2202.

Landau, W.M. Muscle tone: hypertonus, spasticity, rigidity. In: Adelman, G. (Ed.), *Encyclopedia of neuroscience* (pp. 721–723). Boston: Birkhauser, 1987.

Latash, M.L., Anson, J.G. What are "normal movements" in atypical populations? *Behav. Brain Sci.* 19:55–106, 1996.

Leon, F.E., Dimitrijyevic, M.R. Recent concepts in the pathophysiology and evaluation of spasticity. *Invest. Clin.* 38:155–162, 1997.

Levin, M.F. Interjoint coordination during pointing movements is disrupted in spastic hemiparesis. *Brain* 119:281–293, 1996.

Lorentzen, J., et al. Distinguishing active from passive components of ankle plantar flexor stiffness in stroke, spinal cord injury and multiple sclerosis. *Clin. Neurophsyiol.* 121:1939–1951, 2010.

Mayer, N.H. Clinicophysiologic concepts of spasticity and motor dysfunction in adults with an upper motoneuron lesion. *Muscle Nerve* 20(Suppl. 6):S1–S13, 1997.

Malhotra, S. et al. Spasticity, an impairment that is poorly defined and poorly measured. *Clin. Rehab.* 23:651–658, 2009.

Monrad-Krohn, G.H. *The clinical examination of the nervous system*, 10th. ed. London: H.K. Lewis, 1954.

Mottram, C.J., et al. Origins of abnormal excitability in biceps brachii motoneurons of spastic-paretic stroke victims. *J. Neurophysiol.* 102:2026–3038, 2009.

Murray, K.C., et al. Motoneuron excitability and muscle spasms are regulated by 5-HT$_{2B}$ and 5-HT$_{2C}$ receptor activity. *J. Neurophysiol.* 105:731–748, 2011.

Nathan, P.W. Effects on movement of surgical incisions into the human spinal cord. *Brain* 117:337–346, 1994.

Nielsen, J.B., et al. The spinal pathophysiology of spasticity—from a basic science point of view. *Acta Physiol.* 189:171–180, 2007.

Nudo, R.J. Recovery after damage to motor cortical areas. *Curr. Opin. Neurobiol.* 9:740–747, 1999.

Ropper, A.H., et al. Pyramidal infarction in the medulla: a cause of pure motor hemiplegia sparing the face. *Neurology* 29:91–95, 1979.

Sharma, N., et al. Motor imagery: a backdoor to the motor system after stroke? *Stroke* 37:1941–1952, 2006.

Sherman, S.J., et al. Hyper-reflexia without spasticity after unilateral infarct of the medullary pyramid. *J. Neurol. Sci.* 175:145–155, 2000.

Sinkjær, T., et al. Non-reflex and reflex mediated ankle joint stiffness in multiple sclerosis patients with spasticity. *Muscle Nerve* 16:69–76, 1993.

Turton, A., Lemon R.N. The contribution of fast corticospinal input to the voluntary activation of proximal muscles in normal subjects and in stroke patients. *Exp. Brain Res.* 129:559–572, 1999.

Wilson, L.R., et al. Muscle spindle activity in the affected upper limb after a unilateral stroke. *Brain* 122:2079–2088, 1999.

Wirth, B., et al. Ankle dexterity remains intact in patients with incomplete spinal cord injury in contrast to stroke patients. *Exp. Brain Res.* 191:353–361, 2008.

Woallacott, A., Burne, J. The tonic stretch reflex and spastic hypertonia after spinal cord injury. *Exp. Brain Res.* 174:386–396, 2006.

Zadikoff, C., Lang, A.E. Apraxia in movement disorders. *Brain* 128:1480–1497, 2005.

Chapter 23: The Basal Ganglia

Structure, Connections, and Physiology

Adler, A., et al. Neurons in both pallidal segments change their firing properties similarly prior to closure of the eyes. *J. Neurophysiol.* 103:346–359, 2010.

Alexander, G.E., et al. Parallel organization of functionally segregated circuits linking basal ganglia and cortex. *Annu. Rev. Neurosci.* 9:357–381, 1986.

Averbeck, B.B., et al. Estimates of projection overlap and zones of convergence within frontal-striatal circuits. *J. Neurosci.* 34:9497–9505, 2014.

Bradfield, L.A., et al. The thalamostriatal pathway and cholinergic control of goal-directed action: interlacing new with existing learning in the striatum. *Neuron* 79:153–156, 2013.

Brittain, J.-S., Brown, P. Oscillations and the basal ganglia: motor control and beyond. *NeuroImage* 85:637–647, 2014.

Bromberg-Martin, E.S., et al. A pallidus-habenula-dopamine pathway signals inferred stimulus values. *J. Neurophysiol.* 104:1068–1076, 2010.

Chevalier, G., Deniau, J.M. Disinhibition as a basic process in the expression of striatal functions. *Trends Neurosci.* 13:277–280, 1990.

Crittenden, J.R., Graybiel, A.M. Basal ganglia disorders associated with imbalances in the striatal striosome and matrix compartments. *Front. Neuroanat.* 5:59. doi:10.3389/fnana.2011.00059, 2011.

Draganski, B., et al. Evidence of segregated and integrative connectivity patterns in the human basal ganglia. *J. Neurosci.* 28:7143–7152, 2008.

Flaherty, A.W., Graybiel, A.M. Input–output organization of the sensorimotor striatum in the squirrel monkey. *J. Neurosci.* 14:599–610, 1994.

Gerfen, C.R. The neostriatal mosaic: multiple levels of compartmental organization. *Trends Neurosci.* 15:133–138, 1992.

Gerfen, C.R. Basal ganglia. In: Paxinos, G. (Ed.), *The rat nervous system*, 3rd ed. (pp. 455–508). Philadelphia: Elsevier Academic Press, 2004.

Goldberg, J.A., Wilson, C.J. The cholinergic interneurons of the striatum: intrinsic properties underlie multiple discharge patterns. In: Steiner,H., Tseng, K. (Eds.), *Handbook of Basal Ganglia Structure and Function* (pp. 133–149). London: Academic Press, 2010.

Gonzales, K.K., et al. GABAergic inputs from direct and indirect striatal projection neurons onto cholinergic interneurons in the primate putamen. *J. Comp. Neurol.* 521:2502–2522, 2013.

Graveland, G.A., Difiglia, M. The frequency and distribution of medium-sized neurons with indented nuclei in the primate and rodent neostriatum. *Brain Res.* 327:307–311, 1985.

Graveland, G.A., et al. A Golgi study of the human neostriatum: neurons and afferent fibers. *J. Comp. Neurol.* 234:317–333, 1985.

Groenewegen, H.J., et al. Organization of the output of the ventral striatopallidal system in the rat: ventral pallidal afferents. *Neuroscience* 57:113–142, 1993.

Haber, S., Calzavara, R. The cortico-basal ganglia integrative network: the role of the thalamus. *Brain Res. Bull.* 78:69–74, 2009.

Haber, S.N., et al. The basal ganglia. In: Mai, J.K., Paxinos, G. (Eds.), *The human nervous system*, 3rd. ed. (pp. 678–738). San Diego: Elsevier Academic Press, 2012.

Kimura, M., et al. What does the habenula tell dopamine neurons? *Nat. Neurosci.* 10:677–678, 2007.

Lavoie, B., Parent, A. Pedunculopontine nucleus in the squirrel monkey: projections to the basal ganglia as revealed by anterograde tract-tracing methods. *J. Comp. Neurol.* 344:210–231, 1994.

Levesque, M., Parent, A. The striatofugal fiber system in primates: a reevaluation of its organization based on single-axon tracing studies. *Proc. Nat. Acad. Sci. USA* 102:11888–11893, 2005.

McFarland, N.R., Haber, S.N. Convergent inputs from thalamic motor nuclei and frontal cortical areas to the dorsal striatum in the primate. *J. Neurosci.* 20:3798–3813, 2000.

Meck, W.H., et al. Cortico-striatal representation of time in animals and humans. *Curr. Opin. Neurobiol.* 18:145–152, 2008.

Mena-Segovia, J., et al. Pedunculopontine nucleus and basal ganglia: distant relatives or part of the same family? *Trends Neurosci.* 27:585 589, 2004.

Middleton, F.A., Strick, P.L. Basal ganglia and cerebellar loops: motor and cognitive circuits. *Brain Res. Rev.* 31:236–250, 2000.

Munro-Davies, L.E., et al. The role of the pedunculopontine region in basal-ganglia mechanisms of akinesia. *Exp. Brain Res.* 129:511–517, 1999.

Obeso, J. A., et al. Functional organization of the basal ganglia: therapeutic implications for Parkinson's disease. *Mov. Disord.* 23(Suppl. 3):S548–S549, 2008.

Postuma, R.B., Dagher, A. Basal ganglia functional connectivity based on a meta-analysis of 126 positron emission tomography and functional magnetic resonance imaging publications. *Cereb. Cortex* 16:1508–1521, 2006.

Roberts, R.C., et al. Synaptic organization of the human striatum: a postmortem ultrastructural study. *J. Comp. Neurol.* 374:523–534, 1996.

Romanelli, P., et al. Somatotopy in the basal ganglia: experimental and clinical evidence for segregated sensorimotor channels. *Brain Res. Rev.* 48:112–128, 2005.

Sadikot, A.F., Rymar, V.V. The primate centromedian-parafascicular complex: anatomical organization with a note on neuromodulation. *Brain Res. Bull.* 78:122–130, 2009.

Selemon, L.D., et al. Islands and striosomes in the neostriatum of the rhesus monkey: non-equivalent compartments. *Neuroscience* 58:183–192, 1994.

Shimamoto, S.A., et al. Physiological identification of the human pedunculopontine nucleus. *J. Neurol. Neurosurg. Psychiatry* 81:80–86. 2010.

Shink, E., et al. Efferent connections of the internal globus pallidus in the squirrel monkey: II. Topography and synaptic organization of pallidal efferents to the pedunculopontine nucleus. *J. Comp. Neurol.* 382:348–363, 1997.

Sidibé, M., et al. Efferent connections of the internal globus pallidus in the squirrel monkey: I. Topographic and synaptic organization of the pallidothalamic projection. *J. Comp. Neurol.* 382:323–347, 1997.

Smith, Y., et al. The thalamostriatal systems: anatomical and functional organization in normal and parkinsonian states. *Brain Res. Bull.* 78:60–68, 2009.

Tepper, J.M., et al. Feedforward and feedback inhibition in neostriatal GABAergic spiny neurons. *Brain Res. Rev.* 58:272–281, 2008.

Thevathasan, W., et al. Alpha oscillations in the pedunculopontine nucleus correlates with gait performance in Parkinsonism. *Brain* 135:148–160, 2012.

Voorn, P., et al. Putting a spin on the dorsal-ventral divide of the striatum. *Trends Neurosci.* 27:468–474, 2005.

Watabe-Uchida, M., et al. Whole-brain mapping of direct inputs to midbrain dopamine neurons. *Neuron* 74:858–873, 2012.

Wichmann, T., et al. The primate subthalamic nucleus: I. Functional properties in intact animals. *J. Neurophysiol.* 72:494–506, 1994.

Wilson, C.J. Striatum: internal physiology. In: Squire, L. (Ed.), *Encyclopedia of neuroscience* (pp. 563–572). Philadelphia: Elsevier, 2009.

Wiswanath, H., et al. The medial habenula: still neglected. *Front. Hum. Neurosci.* 7:931. doi:10.3389/fnhum. 2013.00931, 2014.

Neurotransmitters and Receptors

Aizman, O., et al. Anatomical and physiological evidence for D1 and D2 dopamine receptor colocalization in neostriatal neurons. *Nat. Rev. Neurosci.* 3:226–230, 2000.

Alcaro, A., et al. Behavioral functions of the mesolimbic dopaminergic system: an affective neuroethological perspective. *Brain Res. Rev.* 56:283–321, 2007.

Aosika, T., et al. Acetylcholine-dopamine balance hypothesis in the striatum: an update. *Geriatr. Gerontol. Int.* 10(Suppl. 1):S148–157, 2010.

Aubert, I., et al. Phenotypical characterization of the neurons expressing the D1 and D2 dopamine receptors in the monkey striatum. *J. Comp. Neurol.* 418:22–32, 2000.

Calabresi, P., et al. Acetylcholine-mediated modulation of striatal function. *Trends Neurosci.* 23:120–126, 2000.

Georges, F., Aston-Jones, G. Activation of ventral tegmental area cells by the bed nucleus of the stria terminalis: a novel excitatory amino acid input to midbrain dopaminergic neurons. *J. Neurosci.* 22:5173–5187, 2002.

Hong, S. Dopamine system: manager of neural pathways. *Front. Hum. Neurosci.* 7:854. doi:10.3389/fnhum.2013.00854, 2013.

Horvitz, J.C. Mesolimbocortical and nigrostriatal dopamine response to salient non-reward events. *Neuroscience* 96:651–656, 2000.

Joel, D., Weiner I. The connections of the dopaminergic system with the striatum in rats and primates: an analysis with respect to the functional and compartmental organization of the striatum. *Neuroscience* 96:451–474, 2000.

Kitai, S.T., et al. Afferent modulation of dopamine neuron firing patterns. *Curr. Opin. Neurobiol.* 9:690–697, 1999.

Kranz, G.S., et al. Reward and the serotonergic system. *Neuroscience* 166:1023–1035, 2010.

Matsumoto, M., Takada, M. Distinct representations of cognitive and motivational signals in midbrain dopamine neurons. *Neuron* 79:1011–1034, 2013.

McNab, F., et al. Changes in cortical dopamine D1 receptor binding associated with cognitive training. *Science* 323:800–802, 2009.

Nicola, S.M., et al. Dopaminergic modulation of neuronal excitability in the striatum and nucleus accumbens. *Annu. Rev. Neurosci.* 23:185–215, 2000.

Pakhotin, P., Bracci, E. Cholinergic interneurons control the excitatory input to the striatum. *J. Neurosci.* 27:391–400, 2007.

Pisani, A., et al. Re-emergence of striatal cholinergic interneurons in movement disorders. *Trends Neurosci.* 30:545–553, 2007.

Redgrave, P., et al. What is reinforced by phasic dopamine signals? *Brain Res. Rev.* 58:322–339, 2008.

Rice, M.E., et al. Dopamine release in the basal ganglia. *Neuroscience* 198:112–137, 2011.

Schultz, W. Behavioral dopamine signals. *Trends Neurosci.* 30:203–210, 2007.

Soiza-Reilly, M., et al. Different D_1 and D_2 receptors expression after motor activity in the striatal critical period. *Brain Res.* 1004:217–221, 2004.

Surmeier, D.J., et al. Are neostriatal dopamine receptors co-localized? *Trends Neurosci.* 16:299–305, 1993.

Tepper, J.M., et al. GABAergic microcircuits in the neostriatum. *Trends Neurosci.* 27:662–669, 2004.

Threlfell, S., et al. Striatal muscarinic receptors promote activity dependence of dopamine transmission via distinct receptor subtypes on cholinergic interneurons in ventral versus dorsal striatum. *J. Neurosci.* 30:3398–3408, 2010.

Wise, R.A. Dopamine, learning and motivation. *Nat. Rev. Neurosci.* 5:483–494, 2004.

Functions

Allman, M.J., Meck, W.H. Pathophysiological distortions in time perception and timed performance. *Brain* 135:656–677, 2012.

Bhatia, K.P., Marsden, C.D. The behavioral and motor consequences of focal lesions of the basal ganglia in man. *Brain* 117:859–876, 1994.

Calebresi, P., et al. The neostriatum beyond the motor function: experimental and clinical evidence. *Neuroscience* 78:39–60, 2002.

Desmurget, M., Turner, R.S. Testing basal ganglia motor functions through reversible inactivations in the posterior internal globus pallidus. *J. Neurophysiol.* 99:1057–1076, 2007.

Doya, K. Complementary roles of basal ganglia and cerebellum in learning and motor control. *Curr. Opin. Neurobiol.* 10:732–739, 2000.

Grahn, J.A., et al. The role of the basal ganglia in learning and memory: neuropsychological studies. *Behav. Brain Res.* 199:53–60, 2009.

Graybiel, A.M. The basal ganglia: learning new tricks and loving it. *Curr. Opin. Neurobio.* 15:638–644, 2005.

Grillner, S., et al. Mechanisms for selection of basic motor programs—roles for the striatum and pallidum. *Trends Neurosci.* 28:364–370, 2005.

Hikosaka, O., Isoda, M. Switching from automatic to controlled behavior: cortico-basal ganglia mechanisms. *Trends Cogn. Sci.* 14:154–161, 2010.

Jin, X., Costa, R.M. Start/stop signals emerge in nigrostriatal circuits during sequence learning. *Nature* 466:457–462, 2010.

Jog, M.S., et al. Building neural representations of habits. *Science* 286:1745–1748, 1999.

Marsden, C.D., Obeso, J.A. The functions of the basal ganglia and the paradox of stereotaxic surgery in Parkinson's disease. *Brain* 117:877–897, 1994.

Meck, W.H., et al. Cortico-striatal representation of time in animals and humans. *Curr. Opin. Neurobiol.* 18:145–152, 2008.

Nambu, A. Seven problems on the basal ganglia. *Curr. Opin. Neurobiol.* 18:595–604, 2008.

Nelson, A.B., Kreitzer, A.C. Reassessing models of basal ganglia function and dysfunction. *Annu. Rev. Neurosci.* 37:117–135, 2014.

Packard, M.G., Knowlton, B.J. Learning and memory functions of the basal ganglia. *Annu. Rev. Neurosci.* 25:563–593, 2002.

Redgrave, P., et al. The basal ganglia: a vertebrate solution to the selection problem? *Neuroscience* 89:1009–1023, 1999.

Stevens, M.C., et al. Functional neural circuits for timekeeping. *Hum. Brain Mapp.* 28:394–408, 2007.

Takakusaki, K., et al. Role of basal ganglia-brainstem systems in the control of postural muscle tone and locomotion. *Prog. Brain Res.* 143:231–237, 2004.

Temel, Y., et al. The functional role of the subthalamic nucleus in cognitive and limbic circuits. *Prog. Neurobiol.* 76:393–413, 2005.

Zweifel, L.S., et al. Disruption of NMDAR-dependent burst firing by dopamine neurons provides selective assessment of phasic dopamine-dependent behavior. *Proc. Natl. Acad. Sci. USA* 106:7281–7288, 2009.

Ventral Striatopallidum

Breiter, H.C., Rosen, B.R. Functional magnetic resonance imaging of brain reward circuitry in the human. *Ann. NY Acad. Sci.* 877:523–547, 1999.

Cannon, C.M., Palmiter, R.D. Reward without dopamine. *J. Neurosci.* 23:10827–10831, 2003.

Day, J.J., et al. Nucleus accumbens neurons encode predicted and ongoing reward costs in rats. *Eur. J. Neurosci.* 33:308–321, 2011.

de Olmos, J.S., Heimer, L. The concepts of the ventral striatopallidal system and extended amygdala. *Ann. NY Acad. Sci.* 877:1–32, 1999.

Der-Aviakan, A., Markou, A. The neurobiology of anhedonia and other reward-related deficits. *Trends Neurosci.* 35:68–77, 2012.

Ellison, G. Stimulant-induced psychosis, the dopamine theory of schizophrenia, and the habenula. *Brain Res. Rev.* 19:223–239, 1994.

Ersche, K.D., et al. Abnormal brain structure implicated in stimulant drug addiction. *Science* 335:601–604, 2012.

Floresco, S.B., et al. Dissociable roles for the nucleus accumbens core and shell in regulating set shift. *J. Neurosci.* 26:2449–2457, 2006.

Geisler, S. The lateral habenula: no longer neglected. *CNS Spectr.* 13:484–489, 2008.

Goto, Y., Grace, A.A. Limbic and cortical information processing in the nucleus accumbens. *Trends Neurosci.* 31:552–558, 2008.

Groenewegen, H.J., et al. Convergence and segregation of ventral striatal inputs and outputs. *Ann. NY Acad. Sci.* 877:49–63, 1999.

Hikosaka, O. New insights on the subcortical representation of reward. *Curr. Opin. Neurobiol.* 18:203–208, 2008.

Kelley, A.E. Nicotinic receptors: addiction's smoking gun? *Nat. Med.* 8:447–449, 2002.

Koob, G.F. The neurocircuitry of addiction: implications for treatment. *Clin. Neurosci. Res.* 5:89–101, 2005.

Koob, G.F., et al. Neuroscience of addiction. *Neuron* 21:467–476, 1998.

McCann, U.D., et al. Long-lasting effects of recreational drugs of abuse on the central nervous system. *Neuroscientist* 3:399–411, 1997.

Nestler, E.J., et al. Drug addiction: a model for the molecular basis of neural plasticity. *Neuron* 11:995–1006, 1993.

Nutt, D.J., et al. The dopamine theory of addiction: 40 years of high and lows. *Nature Rev. Neurosci.* 16:305–3012, 2015.

O'Doherty, J., et al. Dissociable roles of ventral and dorsal striatum in instrumental conditioning. *Science* 304:452–454, 2004.

Okun, M.S., et al. Deep brain stimulation in the internal capsule and nucleus accumbens region: responses observed during active and sham programming. *J. Neurol. Neurosurg. Psychiatry* 78:310–314, 2007.

Parkinson, J.A., et al. Dissociation in effects of lesions of the nucleus accumbens core and shell on appetitive pavlovian approach behavior and the potentiation of conditioned reinforcement and locomotor behavior by D-amphetamine. *J. Neurosci.* 19:2401–2411, 1999.

Pennartz, C.M.A., et al. The hippocampal-striatal axis in learning, prediction and goal-directed behavior. *Trends Neurosci.* 34:548–559, 2011.

Root, D.H., et al. The ventral pallidum: subregion-specific functional anatomy and roles in motivated behaviors. *Progr. Neurobiol.* 130:29–70, 2015.

Ruff, C.C., Fehr, E. The neurobiology of rewards and values in social decision making. *Nature Rev. Neurosci.* 15:549–562, 2014.

Sartorius, A., Henn, F.A. Deep brain stimulation of the lateral habenula in treatment resistant major depression. *Med. Hypotheses* 69:1305–1308, 2007.

Spanagel, R., Weiss F. The dopamine hypothesis of reward: past and current status. *Trends Neurosci.* 22:521–527, 1999.

Volkov, N., Li, T.K. The neuroscience of addiction. *Nat. Neurosci.* 8:1429–1430, 2005.

Weiss, F., Porrino, L.J. Behavioral neurobiology of alcohol addiction: recent advances and challenges. *J. Neurosci.* 22:3332–3337, 2002.

Diseases of the Basal Ganglia

Ackermans, L., et al. Deep brain stimulation in Tourette's syndrome. *Neurotherapeutics* 5:339–344, 2008.

Albin, R.L., Mink, J.W. Recent advances in Tourette syndrome research. *Trends Neurosci.* 29:175–182, 2006.

Ali, F., et al. Stem cells and the treatment of Parkinson's disease. *Exp. Neurol.* 260:3–11, 2014

Antonini, A., et al. The metabolic anatomy of tremor in Parkinson's disease. *Neurology* 51:803–810, 1998.

Barker, R.A., Dunnett, S.B. Functional integration of neural grafts in Parkinson's disease. *Nat. Rev. Neurosci.* 2:1047–1048, 1999.

Baron, M.S., et al. Effects of transient focal inactivation of the basal ganglia in parkinsonian primates. *J. Neurosci.* 22:592–599, 2002.

Belujon, P., Grace, A.A. Reorganization of striatal inhibitory microcircuits leads to pathological synchrony in the basal ganglia. *Neuron* 71:766–768, 2011.

Bezard, E., Gross, C.E. Compensatory mechanisms in experimental and human parkinsonism: towards a dynamic approach. *Prog. Neurobiol.* 55:1–24, 1998.

Björklund, A., Lindvall, G. Cell replacement therapies for central nervous system disorders. *Nat. Rev. Neurosci.* 3:537–544, 2000.

Brandt, J., Butters, N. The neuropsychology of Huntington's disease. *Trends Neurosci.* 9:118–120, 1986.

Breakfield, X.O., et al. The pathophysiological basis of dystonias. *Nat. Rev. Neurosci.* 9:222–234, 2208.

Brown, P. Abnormal oscillatory synchronization in the motor system leads to impaired movement. *Curr. Opin. Neurobiol.* 17:656–664, 2007.

Brown, R.G., Marsden, C.D. Cognitive function in Parkinson's disease: from description to theory. *Trends Neurosci.* 13:21–29, 1990.

Buttery, P.C., Barker, R.A. Treating Parkinson's disease in the 21st century: can stem cell transplantation compete? *J. Comp. Neurol.* 522:2802–2826, 2014.

Cattaneo, E., et al. Normal huntingtin function: an alternative approach to Huntington's disease. *Nat. Rev. Neurosci.* 6:919–930, 2005.

Centonze, D., et al. Subthalamic nucleus lesion reverses motor abnormalities and striatal glutamatergic overactivity in experimental parkinsonism. *Neuroscience* 133:831–840, 2005.

Chiken, S., Nambu, A. Disrupting neuronal transmission: mechanism of DBS? *Front. Syst. Neurosci.* 8:33. doi:10.3389/fnsys.2014.00033, 2014.

Cody, F.W.J. Observations on the genesis of the stretch reflex in Parkinson's disease. *Brain* 109:229–249, 1986.

Collier, T.J. Rebuilding the nigrostriatal dopamine pathway: 30 years and counting. *Exp. Neurol.* 256:21–24, 2014.

Edwards, R.H. Molecular analysis of Parkinson's disease. In: Martin, J.B. (Ed.), *Molecular neurology* (pp. 155–174). New York: Scientific American, 1998.

Gil, J.A., Rego, A.C. Mechanisms of neurodegeneration in Huntington's disease. *Eur. J. Neurosci.* 27:2803–2820, 2008.

Gorman, D.A., Abi-Jaoude, E. Uncovering the complexity of Tourette syndrome, little by little. *Brit. J. Psychiat.* 204:6–8, 2014.

Gray, J.M., et al. Impaired recognition of disgust in Huntington's disease gene carriers. *Brain* 120:2029–2038, 1997.

Hagar, L., et al. High and low frequency stimulation of the subthalamic nucleus induce prolonged changes in subthalamic and globus pallidus neurons. *Front. Syst. Neurosci.* 7:73. doi:10.3389/fnsys.2013.00073, 2013.

Hilker, R., et al. Disease progression continues in patients with advanced Parkinson's disease and effective subthalamic nucleus stimulation. *J. Neurol. Neurosurg. Psychiatry* 76:1217–1221, 2005.

Hutchison, W.D., et al. Neuronal oscillations in the basal ganglia and movement disorders: evidence from whole animal and human recordings. *J. Neurosci.* 24:9240–9243, 2004.

Jankovic, J. Parkinson's disease: clinical features and diagnosis. *J. Neurol. Neurosurg. Psychiatry* 79:368–376, 2008.

Jellinger, K.A. Pathology of Parkinson's disease: changes other than the nigrostriatal pathway. *Mol. Chem. Neuropathol.* 14:153–197, 1991.

Levy, R., et al. Re-evaluation of the functional anatomy of the basal ganglia in normal and parkinsonian states. *Neuroscience* 76:335–343, 1997.

Levy, R., et al. Dependence of subthalamic nucleus oscillations on movement and dopamine in Parkinson's disease. *Brain* 125:1196–1209, 2002.

Lindvall, O., et al. Stem cell therapy for human neurodegenerative disorders—how to make it work. *Nat. Med.* 10:S42–S50, 2004.

Lozano, A.M., Kalia, S.K. New movements in Parkinsons's. *Sci. Am.* 293:68–75, 2005.

Magnin, M., et al. Single-unit analysis of the pallidum, thalamus and subthalamic nucleus in parkinsonian patients. *Neuroscience* 96:549–564, 2000.

Moore, D.J., et al. Molecular pathophysiology of Parkinson's disease. *Annu. Rev. Neurosci.* 28:57–87, 2005.

Obeso, J.A., et al. Basal ganglia pathophysiology: a critical review. In: Obesa, J.A., et al. (Eds.), *The basal ganglia and new surgical approaches for Parkinson's disease* (pp. 3–18). Advances in Neurology 74. New York: Lippincott-Raven, 1997.

Obeso, J.A., et al. The globus pallidus pars externa and Parkinson's disease: ready for prime time? *Exp. Neurol.* 202:1–7, 2006.

Pahapill, P.A., Lozano, A.M. The pedunculopontine nucleus and Parkinson's disease. *Brain* 123:1767–1783, 2000.

Pfann, K.D., et al. Pallidotomy and bradykinesia: implications for basal ganglia function. *Neurology* 51:796–803, 1998.

Raoul, S., et al. Subthalamic nucleus stimulation reverses spinal motoneuron activity in parkinsonian patients. *Brain* 135:139–147, 2012.

Reddy, P.H., et al. Recent advances in understanding the pathogenesis of Huntington's disease. *Trends Neurosci.* 22:248–255, 1999.

Riaz, S.S., Bradford, H.F. Factors involved in the determination of the neurotransmitter phenotype of developing neurons of the CNS: applications in cell replacement treatment for Parkinson's disease. *Prog. Neurobiol.* 76:257–278, 2005.

Robertson, M.M. Tourette syndrome, associated conditions and the complexity of treatment. *Brain* 123:425–462, 2000.

Rodriguez-Oroz, M.C., et al. The subthalamic nucleus in Parkinson's disease: somatotopic organization and physiological characteristics. *Brain* 124:1777–1790, 2001.

Rodriguez-Oroz, M.C., et al. Bilateral deep brain stimulation in Parkinson's disease: a multicentre study with 4 years follow-up. *Brain* 128:2240–2249, 2005.

Ross, C.A., Tabrizi, S.J. Huntington's disease: from molecular pathogenesis to clinical treatment. *Lancet Neurol.* 10:83–98, 2011.

Sacks, O. *The man who mistook his wife for a hat.* New York: Picador, 1986.

Schrock, L.E., et al. Tourette syndrome deep brain stimulation: a review and updated recommendations. *Mov. Disord.* 30:448–471, 2015.

Sheppard, D.M., et al. Tourette's and comorbid syndromes: obsessive compulsive and attention deficit hyperactivity disorder. A common etiology? *Clin. Psychol. Rev.* 19:531–532, 1999.

Singer, H.S. Tourette's syndrome: from behaviour to biology. *Lancet Neurol.* 4:149–159, 2005.

Stefanova, N., et al. Multiple system atrophy: an update. *Lancet Neurol.* 8:1172–1178, 2009.

Stephens, B. Evidence of a breakdown of corticostriatal connections in Parkinson's disease. *Neuroscience* 132:741–754, 2005.

Timmermann, L., Fink, G.R. Pathological network activity in Parkinson's disease: from neural activity and connectivity to causality? *Brain* 134:332–334, 2011.

Weiss, D., et al. Subthalamic nucleus stimulation restores the efferent cortical drive to muscle in parallel to functional motor improvement. *Eur. J. Neurosci.* 35:896–908, 2012.

Weiss, D., et al. Subthalamic stimulation modulates cortical motor network activity and synchronization in Parkinson's disease. *Brain* 138:679–693, 2015.

Wittfoth, M., et al. Lateral frontal cortex volume reduction in Tourette syndrome revealed by VBM. *BMC Neurosci.* 13:17, 2012.

York, M.K. Cognitive declines following bilateral subthalamic nucleus deep brain stimulation for the treatment of Parkinson's disease. *J. Neurol. Neurosurg. Psychiatry* 79:789–795, 2008.

Young, A.B. Huntington's disease and other trinucleotide repeat disorders. In: Martin, J.B. (Ed.), *Molecular neurology* (pp. 35–54). New York: Scientific American, 1998.

Chapter 24: The Cerebellum

Structure, Connections, and Physiology

Alstermark, B., Ekerot, C.-F. The lateral reticular nucleus: a precerebellar centre providing the cerebellum with overview and integration of motor functions at systems level. A new hypothesis. *J. Physiol.* 591:5453–5458, 2013.

Andersen, B.B., et al. A quantitative study of the human cerebellum with unbiased stereological techniques. *J. Comp. Neurol.* 326:549–560, 1992.

Apps, R. Movement-related gating of climbing fibre input to cerebellar cortical zones. *Prog. Neurobiol.* 57:537–562, 1999.

Apps, R., Garwicz, M. Anatomical and physiological foundations of cerebellar information processing. *Nat. Rev. Neurosci.* 6:297–311, 2005.

Azim, E., Alstermark, B. Skilled forelimb movements and internal copy motor circuits. *Curr. Opin. Neurobiol.* 33:16–24, 2015.

Baizer, J.S. Unique features of the human brainstem and cerebellum. *Front. Hum. Neurosci.* 8:202. doi:10.3389/fnhum.2014.00202, 2014.

Bengtsson, F., Hesslow, G. Cerebellar control of the inferior olive. *Cerebellum* 5:7–14, 2006.

Bloedel, J.R., Bracha, V. Current concepts of climbing fiber function. *Anat. Rec. (New Anat.)* 253:118–126, 1998.

Bosco, G., Poppele, R.E. Representation of multiple kinematic parameters of the cat hindlimb in spinocerebellar activity. *J. Neurophysiol.* 78:1421–1432, 1997.

Brodal, P., Bjaalie, J.G. Salient anatomic features of the cortico-ponto-cerebellar pathway. *Prog. Brain Res.* 114:227–249, 1997.

Cerminara, N.I., et al. An internal model of a moving target in the lateral cerebellum. *J. Physiol.* 587:429–442, 2009.

Dow, R.S., Moruzzi, G. *The physiology and pathology of the cerebellum.* Minneapolis: University of Minnesota Press, 1958.

Eccles, J.C., et al. *The cerebellum as a neuronal machine.* New York: Springer-Verlag, 1967.

Garwicz, M., et al. Organizational principles of cerebellar neuronal circuitry. *News Physiol. Sci.* 13:26–32, 1998.

Gauck, V., Jaeger, D. The control of rate and timing of spikes in the deep cerebellar nuclei by inhibition. *J. Neurosci.* 20:3006–3016, 2000.

Glickstein, M., et al. Functional localization in the cerebellum. *Cortex* 47:59–80, 2011.

Grodd, W., et al. Sensorimotor mapping of the human cerebellum: fMRI evidence of somatotopic organization. *Hum. Brain Mapp.* 13:55–73, 2001.

Hawkes, R., Mascher, C. The development of molecular compartmentation in the cerebellar cortex. *Acta Anat.* 151:139–149, 1994.

Hoshi, E., et al. The cerebellum communicates with the basal ganglia. *Nat. Rev. Neurosci.* 8:1491–1493, 2005.

Huang, C.C., et al. Convergence of pontine and proprioceptive streams onto multimodal cerebellar granule cells. *Elife.* 2:e00400, 2013.

Ito, M. *The cerebellum and neural control.* New York: Raven Press, 1984.

Jacobsen, G.A., et al. A model of the of olivo-cerebellar system as a temporal pattern generator. *Trends Neurosci.* 31:617–625, 2008.

Jahnsen, H. Electrophysiological characteristics of neurones in the guinea-pig deep cerebellar nuclei *in vitro. J. Physiol.* 372:129–147, 1986.

Jankowska, E., Puczynska, A. Interneuron activity in reflex pathways from group II muscle afferents is monitored by dorsal spinocere-bellar tract neurons in the cat. *J. Neurosci.* 28:3615–3622, 2008.

Jörntell, H., et al. Cerebellar molecular layer interneurons—computational properties and roles in learning. *Trends Neurosci.* 33:524–532, 2010.

King, J.S. *New concepts in cerebellar neurobiology.* New York: Alan R. Liss, 1987.

Lang, E.J., et al. Patterns of spontaneous Purkinje cell complex spike activity in the awake rat. *J. Neurosci.* 19:2728–2739, 1999.

Larouche, M., Hawkes, R. From clusters to stripes: the developmental origins of adult cerebellar compartmentation. *Cerebellum* 5:77–88, 2006.

Llinás, R., Sugimori, M. The electrophysiology of the cerebellar Purkinje cell revisited. In: Llinás, R., Sotelo, C. (Eds.), *The cerebellum revisited* (pp. 167–181). New York: Springer-Verlag, 1992.

Lu, X., et al. Topographic distribution of output neurons in cerebellar nuclei and cortex to somatotopic map of primary motor cortex. *Eur. J. Neurosci.* 25:2374–2382, 2007.

Macchi, G., Jones, E.G. Toward an agreement on terminology of nuclear and subnuclear divisions of the motor thalamus. *J. Neurosurg.* 86:670–685, 1997.

Manni, E., Petrosini, L. A century of cerebellar somatotopy: a debated representation. *Nat. Rev. Neurosci.* 5:241–249, 2004.

Middleton, F.A., Strick, P.L. Cerebellar projections to the prefrontal cortex of the primate. *J. Neurosci.* 21:700–712, 2001.

Nietschke, M.F., et al. The cerebellum in the cerebro-cerebellar network for the control of eye and hand movements—an fMRI study. *Progr. Brain Res.* 148:151–164, 2005.

Odeh, F., et al. Pontine maps linking somatosensory and cerebellar cortices are in register with climbing fiber somatotopy. *J. Neurosci.* 15:5680–5690, 2005.

Person, A.L., Raman, I.M. Synchrony and neural coding in cerebellar circuits. *Front. Neural Circuits* 6:97. doi:10.3389/fncir.2012.00097, 2012.

Ramnani, N. The primate cortico-cerebellar system: anatomy and function. *Nat. Rev. Neurosci.* 7:511–522, 2006.

Sakai, K., et al. Separate cerebellar areas for motor control. *NeuroReport* 9:2359–2363, 1998.

Sakai, S.T., et al. Comparison of cerebellothalamic and pallidothalamic projections in the monkey (*Macaca fuscata*): a double anterograde labeling study. *J. Comp. Neurol.* 368:215–228, 1996.

Sultan, F., et al. The human dentate nucleus: a complex shape untangled. *Neuroscience* 167:965–968, 2010.

Thach, W.T., et al. Cerebellar output: multiple maps and modes of control in movement coordination. In: Llinas, R., Sotelo, C. (Eds.), *The cerebellum revisited* (pp. 283–300). New York: Springer-Verlag, 1992.

Their, P., Möck, M. The oculomotor role of the pontine nuclei and the nucleus reticularis tegmenti pontis. *Prog. Brain Res.* 151:293–2320, 2006.

Valle, M., et al. Cerebellar cortical activity in the cat anterior lobe during hindlimb stepping. *Exp. Brain Res.* 187:359–372, 2008.

Voogd, J. What we do not know about cerebellar systems neuroscience. *Front. Syst. Neurosci.* 8:227. doi:10.3389/fnsys.2014.00227, 2014.

Voogd, J., Ruigrok, T.J.H. Transverse and longitudinal pattern in the mammalian cerebellum. *Prog. Brain Res.* 114:21–37, 1997.

Welker, W. Spatial organization of somatosensory projections to granule cell cerebellar cortex: functional and connectional implications of fractured somatotopy. In: King, J.S. (Ed.), *New concepts in cerebellar neurobiology* (pp. 239–280). New York: Alan R. Liss, 1987.

Wiesendanger, R., Wiesendanger, M. Cerebello-cortical linkage in the monkey as revealed by transcellular labeling with the lectin wheat germ agglutinin conjugated to the marker horseradish peroxidase. *Exp. Brain Res.* 59:105–117, 1985.

Cerebellum and Learning

Anderson, B.J., et al. Motor-skill learning: changes in synaptic organization of the rat cerebellar cortex. *Neurobiol. Learn. Mem.* 66:221–229, 1996.

Asanuma, H., Pavlides, C. Neurobiological basis of motor learning in mammals. *NeuroReport* 8:i–vi, 1997.

Bracha, V., et al. The human cerebellum and associative learning: dissociation between the acquisition, retention and extinction of conditioned eyeblinks. *Brain Res.* 860:87–94, 2000.

Catz, N., et al. Cerebellar-dependent motor learning is based on pruning of a Purkinje cell population response. *Proc. Natl. Acad. Sci. USA* 105:7309–7314, 2008.

D'Angelo, E., De Zeeuw, C.I. Timing and plasticity in the cerebellum: focus on the granular layer. *Trends Neurosci.* 32:30–40, 2008.

De Zeeuw, C.I., et al. Causes and consequences of oscillations in the cerebellar cortex. *Neuron* 58:655–658, 2008.

Hesslow, G., et al. Learned movements elicited by direct stimulation of cerebellar mossy fiber afferents. *Neuron* 24:179–185, 1999.

Ilg, W., et al. The influence of focal cerebellar lesions on the control and adaptation of gait. *Brain* 131:2913–2927, 2008.

Ioffe, M.E., et al. Role of cerebellum in learning postural tasks. *Cerebellum* 6:87–94, 2007.

Ito, M. Bases and implications of learning in the cerebellum—adaptive control and internal model mechanisms. *Prog. Brain Res.* 148:95–107, 2005.

Jirenhed, D.-A., et al. Acquisition, extinction and reacquisition of a cerebellar cortical memory trace. *J. Neurosci.* 27:2493–2502, 2007.

Kassardjian, C.D., et al. The site of a motor memory shifts with consolidation. *J. Neurosci.* 25:7979–7985, 2005.

Ke, M.C., et al. Elimination of climbing fiber instructive signals during motor learning. *Nature Neurosci.* 12:1171–1180, 2009.

Kleim, J.A., et al. Structural stability within the lateral cerebellar nucleus of the rat following complex motor learning. *Neurobiol. Learn. Mem.* 69:290–306, 1998.

Krakauer, J.W., Mazzoni, P. Human sensorimotor learning: adaptation, skill, and beyond. *Curr. Opin. Neurobiol.* 21:636–644, 2011.

Lisberger, S.G. Cerebellar LTD: a molecular mechanism of behavioral learning? *Cell* 92:701–704, 1998.

Llinás, R., Welsh, J.P. On the cerebellum and motor learning. *Curr. Opin. Neurobiol.* 3:958–965, 1993.

Medina, J.F., Lisberger, S.G. Links from complex spikes to local plasticity and motor learning in the cerebellum of awake-behaving monkeys. *Nat. Rev. Neurosci.* 11:1185–1192, 2008.

Molinari, M., et al. Cerebellum and procedural learning: evidence from focal cerebellar lesions. *Brain* 120:1753–1762, 1997.

Nixon, P.D., Passingham, R.E. Predicting sensory events: the role of the cerebellum in motor learning. *Exp. Brain Res.* 138:251–257, 2001.

Optican, L.M., Robinson, D.A. Cerebellar-dependent adaptive control of primate saccadic system. *J. Neurophysiol.* 44:1058–1076, 1978.

Pascual-Leone, A., et al. Procedural learning in Parkinson's disease and cerebellar degeneration. *Ann. Neurol.* 34:594–602, 1993.

Pritchett, D., Carey, M. A matter of trial and error for motor learning. *Trends Neurosci.* 37:465–466, 2014.

Raymond, J.L., et al. The cerebellum: a neuronal learning machine? *Science* 272:1126–1131, 1996.

Sacchetti, B., et al. Cerebellar role in fear-conditioning consolidation. *Proc. Natl. Acad. Sci. USA* 99:8406–8411, 2002.

Thach, W.T. On the specific role of the cerebellum in motor learning and cognition: clues from PET activation and lesion studies in man. *Behav. Brain Sci.* 19:411–431, 1996.

Thompson, R.F., et al. The nature of reinforcement in cerebellar learning. *Neurobiol. Learn. Mem.* 70:150–176, 1998.

Welsh, J.P., Harvey J.A. Acute inactivation of the inferior olive blocks associative learning. *Eur. J. Neurosci.* 10:3321–3332, 1998.

Werner, S., et al. The effect of cerebellar cortical degeneration on adaptive plasticity and movement control. *Exp. Brain Res.* 193:189–196, 2009.

Yang, Y., Lisberger, S.G. Role of plasticity at different sites across the time course of cerebellar motor learning. *J. Neurosci.* 34:7077–7090, 2014.

Cerebellum and Cognitive Functions

Ackermann, H., et al. Does the cerebellum contribute to cognitive aspects of speech production? A functional magnetic resonance imaging (fMRI) study in humans. *Neurosci. Lett.* 247:187–190, 1998.

Andreasen, N.C., et al. "Cognitive dysmetria" as an integrative theory of schizophrenia: a dysfunction in cortical-subcortical-cerebellar circuitry? *Schizophr. Bull.* 24:203–218, 1998.

Copeland, D.R., et al. Neurocognitive development of children after a cerebellar tumor in infancy: a longitudinal study. *J. Clin. Oncol.* 17:3476–3486, 1999.

Frank, B., et al. Aphasia, neglect and extinction are no prominent clinical signs in children and adolescents with acute surgical cerebellar lesions. *Exp. Brain Res.* 184:511–519, 2008.

Gottwald, B., et al. Evidence for distinct cognitive deficits after focal cerebellar lesions. *J. Neurol. Neursosurg. Psychiatry* 75:1524–1531, 2004.

Hoppenbrouwers, S.S., et al. The role of the cerebellum in the pathophysiology and treatment of neuropsychiatric disorders. *Brain Res. Rev.* 59:185–200, 2008.

Ioannides, A.A., Fenwick, P.B.C. Imaging cerebellum activity in real time with magnetoencephalographic data. *Prog. Brain Res.* 148:139–150, 2005.

Ito, M. Control of mental activities by internal models in the cerebellum. *Nat. Rev. Neurosci.* 9:304–313, 2008.

Ivry, R.B., Schlerf, J.E. Dedicated and intrinsic models of time perception. *Trends Cogn. Sci.* 12:273–280, 2008.

Kim, S.-G., et al. Activation of a cerebellar output nucleus during cognitive processing. *Science* 265:949–951, 1994.

Le, T.H., et al. 4T-fMRI study of nonspatial shifting of selective attention: cerebellar and parietal contributions. *J. Neurophysiol.* 79:1535–1548, 1998.

Mangels, J.A., et al. Dissociable contributions of the prefrontal and neocerebellar cortex to time perception. *Cogn. Brain Res.* 7:15–39, 1998.

Mukhopadhyay, P., et al. Identification of neuroanatomical substrates of set-shifting ability: evidence from patients with focal brain lesions. *Prog. Brain Res.* 168:95–104, 2008.

Nixon, P.D., Passingham, R.E. The cerebellum and cognition: cerebellar lesions do not impair spatial working memory or visual associative learning in the monkey. *Eur. J. Neurosci.* 11:4070–4080, 1999.

O'Reilly, J.X., et al. The cerebellum predicts the timing of perceptual events. *J. Neurosci.* 28:2252–2260, 2008.

Ravizza, S.M., et al. Cerebellar damage produces selective deficits in verbal working memory. *Brain* 129:306–320, 2006.

Schmahmann, J.D., Sherman, J.C. The cerebellar cognitive affective syndrome. *Brain* 121:561–579, 1998.

Stodley, C.J. The cerebellum and cognition: evidence from functional imaging studies. *Cerebellum* 11:352–365, 2012.

Strick, P.L., et al. Cerebellum and nonmotor function. *Annu. Rev. Neurosci.* 32:413–434, 2009.

Tedesco, A.M., et al. The cerebellar cognitive profile. *Brain* 134:3672–3686, 2011.

Timmann, D., et al. The human cerebellum contributes to motor, emotional and cognitive associative learning: a review. *Cortex* 46:845–857, 2007.

Townsend, J., et al. Spatial attention deficits in patients with acquired or developmental cerebellar abnormality. *J. Neurosci.* 19:5632–5643, 1999.

Cerebellar Function and Symptoms in Disease

Alexander, M.P., et al. Cognitive impairments due to focal cerebellar injuries in adults. *Cortex* 48:980–990, 2012.

Balsters, J., et al. Bridging the gap between functional and anatomical features of cortico-cerebellar circuits using meta-analytic connectivity modeling. *Hum. Brain Mapp.* 35:3152–3169, 2014.

Bastian, A.J. Learning to predict the future: the cerebellum adapts feedforward movement control. *Curr. Opin. Neurobiol.* 16:645–649, 2006.

Blakemore, S.J., et al. The cerebellum is involved in predicting the sensory consequences of action. *NeuroReport* 12:1879–1885, 2001.

Bower, J.M. Is the cerebellum sensory for motor's sake, or motor for sensory's sake: the view from the whiskers of a rat? *Prog. Brain Res.* 114:463–497, 1997.

Braitenberg, V., et al. The detection and generation of sequences as a key to cerebellar function. *Behav. Brain Sci.* 20:229–277, 1997.

Cerri, G., et al. Coupling hand and foot voluntary oscillations in patients suffering cerebellar ataxia: different effect of lateral and medial lesions on coordination. *Prog. Brain Res.* 148:227–241, 2005.

Ghelarducci, B., Sebastiani, L. Contributions of the cerebellar vermis to cardiovascular control. *J. Auton. Nerv. Syst.* 56:149–156, 1996.

Glickstein, M., et al. Cerebellum and finger use. *Cerebellum* 4:189–197, 2005.

Gorassani, M., et al. Cerebellar ataxia and muscle spindle sensitivity. *J. Neurophysiol.* 70:1853–1862, 1993.

Grimaldi, G., Manto, M. Topography of cerebellar deficits in humans. *Cerebellum* 11:336–351, 2012.

Habas, C., et al. In Vivo structural and functional imaging of the human rubral and inferior olivary nuclei: a mini-review. *Cerebellum* 9:167–173, 2010.

Holmes, G. The cerebellum. In: Phillips, C.G. (Ed.), *Selected papers of Gordon Holmes* (pp. 186–247). Oxford: Oxford University Press, 1979.

Imamizu, H., et al. Human cerebellar activity reflecting an acquired internal model of a new tool. *Nature* 403:192–195, 2000.

Kawato, M. Internal models for motor control and trajectory planning. *Curr. Opin. Neurobiol.* 9:718–727, 1999.

Keele, S.W., Ivry, R. Does the cerebellum provide a common computation for diverse tasks? *Ann. NY Acad. Sci.* 608:179–207, 1990.

Liu, Y., et al. The human red nucleus and lateral cerebellum in supporting roles for sensory information processing. *Hum. Brain Mapp.* 10:147–159, 2000.

Luft, A.R., et al. Comparing motion- and imagery-related activation in the human cerebellum: a functional MRI study. *Hum. Brain Mapp.* 6:105–113, 1998.

Marti, S., et al. A model-based theory on the origin of downbeat nystagmus. *Exp. Brain Res.* 188:613–631, 2008.

Merchant, H., et al. Neural basis of the perception and estimation of time. *Annu. Rev. Neurosci.* 36:313–336, 2013.

Morton, S.M., Bastian, A.J. Cerebellar control of balance and locomotion. *Neuroscientist* 10:247–259, 2004.

Müller, F., Dichgans, J. Dyscoordination of pinch and lift forces during grasp in patients with cerebellar lesions. *Exp. Brain Res.* 101:485–492, 1994.

Ohyama, T., et al. What the cerebellum computes. *Trends Neurosci.* 26:222–227, 2003.

Palliyath, S., et al. Gait in patients with cerebellar ataxia. *Mov. Disord.* 13:958–964, 1998.

Paulin, M.G. The role of the cerebellum in motor control and perception. *Brain Behav. Evol.* 41:39–50, 1993.

Pekhletski, R., et al. Impaired cerebellar synaptic plasticity and motor performance in mice lacking the mGluR4 subtype of metabotropic glutamate receptor. *J. Neurosci.* 16:6364–6373, 1996.

Robinson, F.R., Fuchs, A.F. The role of the cerebellum in voluntary eye movements. *Annu. Rev. Neurosci.* 24:981–1004, 2001.

Richter, S., et al. Patients with chronic focal cerebellar lesions show no cognitive abnormalities in a bedside test. *Neurocase* 13:25–36, 2007.

Straube, A., et al. Unilateral cerebellar lesions affect initiation of ipsilateral smooth pursuit eye movements in humans. *Ann. Neurol.* 42:891–898, 1997.

Takagi, M., et al. Effects of lesions of the oculomotor cerebellar vermis on eye movements in primate: smooth pursuit. *J. Neurophysiol.* 83:2047–2062, 2000.

Timmann, D., et al. Classically conditioned withdrawal reflex in cerebellar patients: 1. Impaired conditioned responses. *Exp. Brain Res.* 130:453–470, 2000.

Walker, M.F., Zee, D.S. Directional abnormalities of vestibular and optokinetic responses in cerebellar disease. *Ann. NY Acad. Sci.* 871:205–220, 1999.

Welsh, J.P., Harvey, J.A. The role of the cerebellum in voluntary and reflexive movements: history and current status. In: Llinás, R., Sotelo, C. (Eds.), *The cerebellum revisited* (pp. 301–334). New York: Springer-Verlag, 1992.

Werner, S., et al. The effect of cerebellar cortical degeneration on adaptive plasticity and movement control. *Exp. Brain Res.* 193:189–196, 2009.

Wolpert, D.M., et al. Internal models in the cerebellum. *Trends Cogn. Sci.* 2:338–347, 1998.

Chapter 25: Control of Eye Movements

Eye Muscles and Eye Movements

Bui Quoc, E., Milleret, C. Origins of strabismus and loss of binocular vision. *Front. Integr. Neurosci.* 8:71. doi:10.3389/fnint.2014.00071, 2014.

Büttner-Ennever, J.A., et al. Sensory control of extraocular muscles. *Prog. Brain Res.* 151:81–93, 2006.

Coubard, O.A. Saccade and vergence eye movements: a review of motor and premotor commands. *Eur. J. Neurosci.* 38:3348–3397, 2013.

Donaldson, I.M. The functions of proprioceptors of the eye muscles. *Philos. Trans. R. Soc. Lond. B Biol. Sci.* 355:1685–1754, 2000.

Erichsen, J.T., et al. Morphology and ultrastructure of medial rectus subgroup motoneurons in the macaque monkey. *J. Comp. Neurol.* 522:626–641, 2014.

Gilchrist, I.D. Saccades without eye movements. *Nature* 390:130–131, 1997.

Goldberg, S.J., Shall, M.S. Motor units of extraocular muscles: recent findings. *Prog. Brain Res.* 123:221–232, 1999.

Hayhoe, M., Ballard, D. Eye movements in natural behavior. *Trends Cogn. Sci.* 9:188–194, 2005.

Jampel, R.S. The function of the extraocular muscles, the theory of the coplanarity of fixation planes. *J. Neurol. Sci.* 280:1–9, 2009.

Lewis, R.F., et al. Oculomotor function in the rhesus monkey after deafferentation of the extraocular muscles. *J. Exp. Brain Res.* 141:349–358, 2001.

Ruff, R.L. More than meets the eye: extraocular muscle is very distinct from extremity skeletal muscles. *Muscle Nerve* 25:311–313, 2002.

Spencer, R.F., Porter, J.D. Biological organization of the extraocular muscles. *Prog. Brain Res.* 151:43–80, 2006.

Tang, X., et al. Internal organization of medial rectus and inferior rectus muscle neurons in the C-group of the oculomotor nucleus in monkey. *J. Comp. Neurol.* 523:1809–1823, 2015.

Brain Stem and Cerebellum

Büttner-Ennever, J.A. Mapping the oculomotor system. *Prog. Brain Res.* 171:3–11, 2008.

Büttner, U., Büttner-Ennever, J.A. Present concepts of oculomotor organization. *Prog. Brain Res.* 151:1–42, 2006.

Curthoys, I.S. Generation of the quick phase of horizontal vestibular nystagmus. *Exp. Brain Res.* 143:397–405, 2002.

Dean, P., et al. Event or emergency? Two systems in the mammalian superior colliculus. *Trends Neurosci.* 12:137–147, 1989.

duLac, S., et al. Learning and memory in the vestibulo-ocular reflex. *Annu. Rev. Neurosci.* 18:409–441, 1995.

Filippopulos, F., et al. Deficits of cortical oculomotor mechanisms in cerebellar atrophy patients. *Exp. Brain Res.* 224:541–550, 2013.

Gaymard, B., et al. Smooth pursuit eye movement deficits after pontine nuclei lesions in humans. *J. Neurol. Neurosurg. Psychiatry* 56:799–807, 1993.

Grosbras, M.H., et al. Human cortical networks for new and familiar sequences of saccades. *Cereb. Cortex* 11:936–945, 2001.

Grüsser, O.-J., et al. Vestibular neurones in the parieto-insular cortex of monkeys (*Macaca fascicularis*): visual and neck receptor responses. *J. Physiol.* 430:559–583, 1990.

Grüsser, O.-J., et al. Cortical representation of head-in-space movement and some psychophysical experiments on head movement. In: Berthoz, A., et al. (Eds.), *The head-neck sensory motor system* (pp. 497–509). Oxford: Oxford University Press, 1992.

Horn, A.K.E., Adamczyk, C. Reticular formation: eye movements, gaze and blinks. In: Mai, J., Paxinos, G. (Eds.), *The human nervous system,* 3rd ed. (pp. 328–366). San Diego: Elsevier Academic Press, 2012.

Ilg, U.J. Slow eye movements. *Prog. Neurobiol.* 53:293–329, 1997.

Ito, M. *The cerebellum and neural control.* New York: Raven Press, 1984.

Kawano, K. Ocular tracking: behavior and neurophysiology. *Curr. Opin. Neurobiol.* 9:467–473, 1999.

Kennard, C., Clifford Rose, F. *Physiological aspects of clinical neuro-ophthalmology.* New York: Chapman & Hall, 1988.

Kowler, E. Eye movements: The past 25 years. *Vision Res.* 51:1457–1483, 2011.

Lempert, T., et al. Effect of otolith dysfunction: impairment of visual acuity during linear head motion in labyrinthine defective subjects. *Brain* 120:1005–1013, 1997.

Lisberger, S.G., et al. Visual motion processing and sensory-motor integration of smooth pursuit eye movements. *Annu. Rev. Neurosci.* 10:97–129, 1987.

Martinez-Conde, S., et al. The role of fixational eye movements in visual perception. *Nat. Rev. Neurosci.* 5:229–240, 2004.

Müri, R.M. MRI and fMRI analysis of oculomotor function. *Prog. Brain Res.* 151:503–526, 2006.

Panouillères, M.T.N., et al. The role of the posterior cerebellum in saccadic adaptation: a transcranial direct current stimulation study. *J. Neurosci.* 35:5471–5479, 2015.

Pritchett, D., Carey, M. A matter of trial and error for motor learning. *Trends Neurosci.* 37:465–466, 2014.

Prsa, M., Thier, P. The role of the cerebellum in saccadic adaptation as a window into neural mechanisms of motor learning. *Eur. J. Neurosci.* 33:2114–2128, 2011.

Quaia, C., et al. Model for the control of saccades by superior colliculus and cerebellum. *J. Neurophysiol.* 82:999–1018, 1999.

Raphan, T., Cohen, B. The vestibulo-ocular reflex in three dimensions. *Exp. Brain Res.* 145:1–27, 2002.

Robinson, F.R. The role of the cerebellum in voluntary eye movements. *Annu. Rev. Neurosci.* 24:981–1004, 2001.

Rüb, U., et al. Functional neuroanatomy of human premotor oculo-motor brainstem nuclei: insights from postmortem and advanced in vivo imaging studies. *Exp. Brain Res.* 187:167–180, 2008.

Scudder, C.A., et al. The brainstem burst generator for saccadic eye movements: a modern synthesis. *Exp. Brain Res.* 142:439–462, 2002.

Shinoda, Y., et al. Neural circuits for triggering saccades in the brain-stem. *Prog. Brain Res.* 171:79–85, 2008.

Sparks, D.L. Conceptual issues related to the role of the superior colliculus in the control of gaze. *Curr. Opin. Neurobiol.* 9:698–707, 1999.

Suzuki, D.A., et al. Smooth-pursuit eye movement deficits with chemical lesions in macaque nucleus reticularis tegmenti pontis. *J. Neurophysiol.* 82:1178–1186, 1999.

Thier, P., Ilg, U.J. The neural basis of smooth-pursuit eye movements. *Curr. Opin. Neurobiol.* 15:645–652, 2005.

Thier, P., Möck, M. The oculomotor role of the pontine nuclei and the nucleus reticularis tegmenti pontis. *Prog. Brain Res.* 151:293–2320, 2006.

Waterston, J.A., et al. A quantitative study of eye and head movements during smooth pursuit in patients with cerebellar disease. *Brain* 115:1343–1358, 1992.

Yang, Y., Lisberger, S.G. Role of plasticity at different sites across the time course of cerebellar motor learning. *J. Neurosci.* 34:7077–7090, 2014.

Cortical Level

Amiez, C., Petrides, M. Anatomical organization of the eye fields in the human and non-human primate frontal cortex. *Progr. Neurobiol.* 89:220–230, 2009.

Andersen, R.A., et al. Evidence for the lateral intraparietal area as the parietal eye field. *Curr. Opin. Neurobiol.* 2:840–846, 1992.

Anderson, T.J., et al. Cortical control of saccades and fixation in man: a PET study. *Brain* 117:1073–1084, 1994.

Corbetta, M., et al. A common network of functional areas for attention and eye movements. *Neuron* 71:761–773, 1998.

Cullen, K.E., Van Horn, M.R. The neural control of fast vs. slow vergence eye movements. *Eur. J. Neurosci.* 33:2147–2154, 2011.

Heide, W., et al. Deficits of smooth pursuit eye movements after frontal and parietal lesions. *Brain* 119:1951–1969, 1996.

Hikosaka, O., Isoda, M. Brain mechanisms for switching from automatic to controlled eye movements. *Prog. Brain Res.* 171:375–382, 2008.

Krauzlis, R.J., Stone, L.S. Tracking with the mind's eye. *Trends Neurosci.* 22:544–550, 1999.

Latto, R. The role of the inferior parietal cortex and the frontal eye-fields in visuospatial discriminations in the macaque monkey. *Behav. Brain Res.* 22:41–52, 1986.

Leff, A.P., et al. The planning and guiding of reading saccades: a repetitive transcranial magnetic stimulation study. *Cereb. Cortex* 11:918–923, 2001.

Lisberger, S.G. Visual guidance of smooth-pursuit eye movements: sensation, action, and what happens in between. *Neuron* 66:477–491, 2010.

Liversedge, S.P., Findlay, J.M. Saccadic eye movements and cognition. *Trends Cogn. Sci.* 4:6–14, 1999.

Martinez-Conde, S., et al. The impact of microsaccades on vision: towards a unified theory of saccadic function. *Nature Rev. Neurosci.* 14:83–96, 2013.

Medendorp, W.P., et al. Parietofrontal circuits in goal-oriented behaviour. *Eur. J. Neurosci.* 33:2017–2027, 2011.

Rosenthal, C.R., et al. Supplementary eye field contributions to the execution of saccades to remembered target locations. *Prog. Brain Res.* 171:419–423, 2008.

Sweeney, J.A., et al. Positron emission tomography study of voluntary saccadic eye movements and spatial working memory. *J. Neurophysiol.* 75:454–468, 1996.

Yang, S., et al. Supplementary eye field activity reflects a decision rule governing smooth pursuit but not the decision. *J. Neurophysiol.* 103:2458–2469, 2010.

Zhang, M., et al. Monkey primary somatosensory cortex has a proprioceptive representation of eye position. *Prog. Brain Res.* 171:37–45, 2008.

Chapter 26: The Reticular Formation: Premotor Networks, Consciousness, and Sleep

Structure and Physiology

Argyropoulos, S.V., et al. Inhalation of 35% CO_2 results in activation of the HPA axis in healthy volunteers. *Psychoneuroendocrinology* 27:715–729, 2002.

Azmitia, E.C. Serotonin neurons, neuroplasticity, and homeostasis of neural tissue. *Neuropsychopharmacology* 21(Suppl.):33S–45S, 1999.

Baker, S.N. The primate reticulospinal tract, hand function and functional recovery. *J. Physiol.* 598:5603–5612, 2011.

Barlow, J.S. *The electroencephalogram: its patterns and origins.* Cambridge, MA: MIT Press, 1993.

Blessing, W.W., Benarroch, E.E. Lower brainstem regulation of visceral, cardiovascular, and respiratory function. In: Mai, J., Paxinos, G. (Eds.), *The human nervous system*, 3rd ed. (pp. 1058–1073). San Diego: Elsevier Academic Press, 2012.

Brodal, A. *The reticular formation of the brain stem: anatomical aspects and functional correlations.* Edinburgh, UK: Oliver & Boyd, 1957.

Bruinstroop, E., et al. Spinal projections of the A5, A6 (Locus coeruleus) and A7 noradrenergic cell groups in rats. *J. Comp. Neurol.* 520:1985–2001, 2012.

Dobbins, E.G., Feldman J.L. Brainstem network controlling descending drive to phrenic motoneurons in rat. *J. Comp. Neurol.* 347:64–86, 1994.

Feldman, J.L., Del Negro, C.A. Looking for inspiration: new perspectives on respiratory rhythm. *Nat. Rev. Neurosci.* 7:232–242, 2006.

Foote, S.L., Morrison, J.H. Extrathalamic modulation of cortical function. *Annu. Rev. Neurosci.* 10:67–95, 1987.

Garzia, A.J. III, et al. Networks within networks: the neuronal control of breathing. *Progr. Brain Res.* 188:31–50, 2011.

Grantyn, A., et al. Tracing premotor brain stem networks of orienting movements. *Curr. Opin. Neurobiol.* 3:973–981, 1993.

Jordan, L.M., et al. Control of functional systems in the brainstem and spinal cord. *Curr. Opin. Neurobiol.* 2:794–801, 1992.

Kerman, I. Organization of brain somatomotor-sympathetic circuits. *Exp. Brain Res.* 187:1–16, 2008.

Korn, H., Faber, D.S. Escape behavior: brainstem and spinal cord circuitry and function. *Curr. Opin. Neurobiol.* 6:826–832, 1996.

Lagercrantz, H. Neuromodulators and respiratory control during development. *Trends Neurosci.* 10:368–372, 1987.

Lund, J.P., et al. Brainstem mechanisms underlying feeding behaviors. *Curr. Opin. Neurobiol.* 8:718–724, 1998.

Miller, K.W. Are lipids or proteins the target of general anaesthetic action? *Trends Neurosci.* 9:49–51, 1986.

Mironov, S. Respiratory circuits: function, mechanisms, topology, and pathology. *Neuroscientist* 15:194–208, 2009.

Moruzzi, G., Magoun, H.W. Brain stem reticular formation and activation of the EEG. *Electroencephalogr. Clin. Neurophysiol.* 1:455–473, 1949.

Müller, C.M., et al. Structures mediating cholinergic reticular facilitation of cortical structures in the cat: effects of lesions in immunocytochemically characterized projections. *Exp. Brain Res.* 96:8–18, 1993.

Paxinos, G., et al. Organization of brainstem nuclei. In: Mai, J., Paxinos, G. (Eds.), *The human nervous system*, 3rd ed. (pp. 260–327). San Diego: Elsevier Academic Press, 2012.

Ramirez, J.-M., Richter, D.W. The neuronal mechanisms of respiratory rhythm generation. *Curr. Opin. Neurobiol.* 6:817–825, 1996.

Rho, M.-J., et al. Organization of the projection from the pericruciate cortex to the pontomedullary reticular formation of the cat: a quantitative retrograde tracing study. *J. Comp. Neurol.* 388:228–249, 1997.

Richter, D.W., Spyer, K.M. Studying rhythmogenesis of breathing: comparison of *in vivo* and *in vitro* models. *Trends Neurosci.* 24:464–472, 2002.

Scheibel, M.E., Scheibel, A.B. Structural substrates for integrative patterns in the brain stem reticular core. In: Jasper, H.H., et al. (Eds.), *Reticular formation of the brain* (pp. 31–55). Boston: Little, Brown, 1958.

Schwarzacher, S.W., et al. Neuroanatomical characteristics of the human pre-Bötzinger complex and its involvement in neurodegenerative brainstem diseases. *Brain* 134:24–35, 2011.

Sergeyev, V., et al. Serotonin and substance P co-exist in dorsal raphe neurons of the human brain. *NeuroReport* 10:3967–3970, 1999.

Simpson, K.L., et al. Projection patterns from the raphe nuclear complex to the ependymal wall of the ventricular system in the rat. *J. Comp. Neurol.* 399:61–72, 1998.

Steriade, M. Impact of network activities on neuronal properties in corticothalamic systems. *J. Neurophysiol.* 86:1–39, 2001.

Tononi, G., et al. Complexity and coherence: integrating information in the brain. *Trends Cogn. Sci.* 2:474–484, 1998.

Locus Coeruleus and Raphe Nuclei

Amat, J., et al. Medial frontal cortex determines how stressor controllability affects behavior and dorsal raphe nucleus. *Nat. Rev. Neurosci.* 8:365–371, 2005.

Aston-Jones, G., Cohen, J.D. An integrative theory of locus coeruleus-norepinephrine function: adaptive gain and optimal performance. *Annu. Rev. Neurosci.* 28:403–450, 2005.

Berridge, C.W., Foote, S.L. Effects of locus coeruleus activation on electroencephalographic activity in neocortex and hippocampus. *J. Neurosci.* 11:3135–3145, 1991.

Bouret, S., Sara, S.J. Network reset: a simplified overarching theory of locus coeruleus noradrenaline function. *Trends Cogn. Sci.* 28:574–582, 2005.

Cirelli, C., Tononi, G. Locus coeruleus control of state-dependent gene expression. *J. Neurosci.* 24:5410–5419, 2004.

Commons, K.G. Two major network domains in the dorsal raphe nucleus. *J. Comp. Neurol.* 523:1488–1504, 2015.

Counts, S.E., Mufson, E.J. Locus coeruleus. In: Mai, J., Paxinos, G. (Eds.), *The human nervous system*, 3rd ed. (pp. 425–438). San Diego: Elsevier Academic Press, 2012.

Fost, J.W. Neural rhythmicity, feature binding, and serotonin: A hypothesis. *Neuroscientist* 5:79–85, 1999.

Hamel, E. Serotonin and migraine: biology and clinical implications. *Cephalalgia*, 27:1295–1300, 2007.

Hornung, J.-P. Raphe nuclei. In: Mai, J., Paxinos, G. (Eds.), *The human nervous system*, 3rd ed. (pp. 401–424). San Diego: Elsevier Academic Press, 2012.

Jacobs, B.L., Fornal, C.A. Serotonin and motor activity. *Curr. Opin. Neurobiol.* 7:820–825, 1997.

Kobayashi, K., et al. Modest neuropsychological deficits caused by reduced noradrenaline metabolism in mice heterozygous for a mutated tyrosine hydroxylase gene. *J. Neurosci.* 20:2418–2426, 2000.

Levy, L. Migraine pain and nociceptor activation—where do we stand? *Headache* 50:909–916, 2010.

Lovick, T.A. The medullary raphe nuclei: a system for integration and gain control in autonomic and somatomotor responsiveness? *Exp. Physiol.* 82:31–41, 1997.

Richerson, G.B. Serotonergic neurons as carbon dioxide sensors that maintain pH homeostasis. *Nat. Rev. Neurosci.* 5:449–461, 2004.

Saper, C.B. Function of the locus coeruleus. *Trends Neurosci.* 10:343–344, 1987.

Sara, S.J. The locus coeruleus and noradrenergic modulation of cognition. *Nat. Rev. Neurosci.* 10:211–223, 2009.

Sergeyev, V., et al. Serotonin and substance P co-exist in dorsal raphe neurons of the human brain. *NeuroReport* 10:3967–3970, 1999.

Somogyi, J., Llewellyn-Smith, J. Patterns of colocalization of GABA, glutamate and glycine immunoreactivities in terminals that synapse on dendrites of noradrenergic neurons in rat locus coeruleus. *Eur. J. Neurosci.* 14:219–228, 2001.

Tully, K., Bolshakov, V. Emotional enhancement of memory: how norepinephrine enables synaptic plasticity. *Mol. Brain* 3:15, 2010.

Van Dongen, P.A.M. The human locus coeruleus in neurology and psychiatry. *Prog. Neurobiol.* 17:97–139, 1981.

Vecchia, D., Pietrobon, D. Migraine: a disorder of brain excitatory–inhibitory balance? *Trends Neurosci.* 35:507–520, 2012.

Consciousness and Attention

Baars, B.J., et al. Brain, conscious experience and the observing self. *Trends Neurosci.* 26:671–675, 2003.

Bargh, J.A., Morzella, E. The unconscious mind. *Perspect. Psychol. Sci.* 3:73–79, 2008.

Bauer, G., et al. Varieties of the locked-in syndrome. *J. Neurol.* 221:77–91, 1979.

Bennett, M.R., Hacker, P.M.S. *The philosophical foundations of neuroscience.* Oxford: Blackwell, 2003.

Brown, E.N., et al. General anesthesia, sleep, and coma. *N. Engl. J. Med.* 363:2638–2650, 2010.

Berlucchi, G. One or many arousal systems? Reflections on some of Guiseppe Moruzzi's foresights and insights about the intrinsic regulation of brain activity. *Arch. Ital. Biol.* 135:5–14, 1997.

Cannon, J., et al. Neurosystems: brain rhythms and cognitive processing. *Eur. J. Neurosci.* 39:705–719, 2014.

Cattaneo, L., et al. Pathological yawning as a presenting symptom of brain stem ischaemia in two patients. *J. Neurol. Neurosurg. Psychiatry* 77:98–100, 2006.

Crick, F.C., Koch, C. Consciousness and neuroscience. *Cereb. Cortex* 8:97–107, 1998.

Cruse, D., et al. Bedside detection of awareness in the vegetative state: a cohort study. *Lancet* 378:2088–2094, 2011.

Daquin, G., et al. Yawning. *Sleep Med. Rev.* 5:299–312, 2001.

Dehaene, S., et al. Conscious, preconscious, and subliminal processing: a testable taxonomy. *Trends Cogn. Sci.* 10:204–211, 2006.

Dijksterhuis, A., Aarts, H. Goals, attention, and (un)conscioiusness. *Annu. Rev. Psychol.* 61:467–490, 2010.

Franks, N.P. General anaesthesia: from molecular targets to neuronal pathways of sleep and arousal. *Nat. Rev. Neurosci.* 9:370–386, 2008.

Gazzaniga, M.S. Brain mechanisms and conscious experience. *Ciba Found. Symp.* 174:247–262, 1993.

Guldenmund, P., et al. Thalamus, brainstem and salience network connectivity changes during propofol-induced sedation and unconsciousness. *Brain Connect.* 3:273–285, 2013.

Hesslow, G. Conscious thought as simulation of behaviour and perception. *Trends Cogn. Sci.* 6:242–247, 2002.

Jennett, B. The vegetative state. *J. Neurol. Neurosurg. Psychiatry* 73:355–357, 2002.

Kaada, B. Site of action of myanesin (mephenesin, tolserol) in the central nervous system. *J. Neurophysiol.* 13:89–104, 1950.

Kinomura, S., et al. Activation by attention of the human reticular formation and thalamic intralaminar nuclei. *Science* 271:512–515, 1996.

Knudsen, E.I. Fundamental components of attention. *Annu. Rev. Neurosci.* 30:57–78, 2007.

Koch, C., Tsuchiya, N. Attention and consciousness: two distinct brain processes. *Trends Cogn. Sci.* 11:16–22, 2006.

Kurthen, M., et al. Will there be a neuroscientific theory of consciousness? *Trends Cogn. Sci.* 2:229–234, 1998.

Laureys, S. The neural correlate of (un)awareness: lessons from the vegetative state. *Trends Cogn. Sci.* 9:556–559, 2005.

Llinas, R., Ribary, U. Consciousness and the brain: the thalamocortical dialogue in health and disease. *Ann. NY Acad. Sci.* 929:166–175, 2001.

Lopez da Silva, F. EEG and MEG: relevance to neuroscience. *Neuron* 80:1112–1128, 2013.

MacDonald, A.A. Anesthesia and neuroimaging: investigating the neural correlates of unconsciousness. *Trends Cogn. Sci.* 19:100–107, 2015.

Malmivuo, J. Comparison of the properties of EEG and MEG in detecting the electric activity of the brain. *Brain Topogr.* 25:1–19, 2013.

Naccache, L. Is she conscious? *Science* 313:1395–1396, 2006.

Nelson, L.E., et al. The sedative component of anesthesia is mediated by GABA$_A$ receptors in an endogenous sleep pathway. *Nat. Neurosci.* 5:979–984, 2002.

Nosek, B.A., et al. Implicit social cognition: from measures to mechanisms. *Trends Cogn. Sci.* 15:151–159, 2011.

Overgaard, M. How can we know if patients in coma, vegetative state or minimally conscious state are conscious? *Progr. Brain Res.* 177:11–19, 2009.

Owen, A.M., Coleman, M.R. Functional neuroimaging of the vegetative state. *Nat. Rev. Neurosci.* 9:235–243, 2008.

Peltier, S.J., et al. Functional connectivity changes with concentration of sevoflurane anesthesia. *NeuroReport* 16:285–288, 2005.

Perry, E., et al. Acetylcholine in mind: neurotransmitter correlate of consciousness? *Trends Neurosci.* 22:273–280, 1999.

Petrenko, A.B., et al. Defining the role of NMDA receptors in anesthesia: are we there yet? *Eur. J. Pharmacol.* 723:29–37, 2014.

Pfaff, D.W., et al. Origins of arousal: roles for medullary reticular neurons. *Trends Neurosci.* 35:468–476, 2012.

Platek, S.M., et al. Contagious yawning and the brain. *Cogn. Brain Res.* 23:448–452, 2005.

Raz, A., Buhle, J. Typologies of attentional networks. *Nat. Rev. Neurosci.* 7:367–379, 2006.

Rodriguez, E., et al. Perception's shadow: long-distance synchronization of human brain activity. *Nature* 397:430–433, 1999.

Rudolph, U., Antkowiak, B. Molecular and neuronal substrates for general anaesthetics. *Nat. Rev. Neurosci.* 5:709–720, 2004.

Sarter, M., Bruno, J.P. Cortical cholinergic inputs mediating arousal, attentional processing and dreaming: differential afferent regulation of the basal forebrain by telencephalic and brainstem afferents. *Neuroscience* 95:933–952, 2000.

Searle, J.R. Consciousness. *Annu. Rev. Neurosci.* 23:557–578, 2000.

Shipp, S. The brain circuitry of attention. *Trends Cogn. Sci.* 8:223–230, 2004.

Singer, W. Consciousness and the binding problem. *Ann. NY Acad. Sci.* 929:123–146, 2001.

Smith, E., Delargy, M. Locked-in syndrome. *BMJ* 330:406–409, 2005.

Steriade, M. Thalamocortical oscillations in the sleeping and aroused brain. *Science* 262:679–685, 1993.

Sumner, P., Husain, M. At the age of consciousness: automatic motor activation and voluntary control. *Neuroscientist* 14:474–486, 2008.

Uhrig, L., et al. Cerebral mechanisms of general anesthesia. *Ann. Franc. d'Anest. Réanim.* 33:72–82, 2014.

van Boxtel, J.J.A., et al. Consciousness and attention: on sufficiency and necessity. *Front. Psychol.* 1:217, 2010.

Velman, M. How to separate conceptual issues from empirical ones in the study of consciousness. *Prog. Brain Res.* 168:1–9, 2008.

Weiskrantz, L. *Consciousness lost and found: a neuropsychological exploration.* New York: Oxford University Press, 1997.

Wilkes, K.V. Is consciousness important? *Brit. J. Phil. Sci.* 35:223–243, 1984.

Womelsdorf, T., Fries, P. The role of neuronal synchronization in selective attention. *Curr. Opin. Neurobiol.* 17:154–160, 2007.

Zeki, S. The disunity of consciousness. *Prog. Brain Res.* 168:11–18, 2008.

Sleep and Dreaming

Aldrich, M.S. Narcolepsy. *Neurology* 42(Suppl. 6):34–43, 1992.

Alexandre, C., et al. Control of arousal by the orexin neurons. *Curr. Opin. Neurobiol.* 23:752–759, 2014.

Antonenko, D., et al. Napping to renew learning capacity: enhanced encoding after stimulation of sleep slow oscillations. *Eur. J. Neurosci.* 37:1142–1151, 2013.

Brown, R.E., et al. Control of sleep and wakefulness. *Physiol. Rev.* 92:1087–1187, 2012.

Dickelman, S., Born, J. The memory function of sleep. *Nat. Rev. Neurosci.* 11:114–126, 2010.

Domhoff, G.W. Dreaming and the default network: a review, synthesis, and counterintuitive research proposal. *Conscious. Cogn.* 33:342–353, 2015.

Fort, P., et al. Alternative vigilance states: new insights regarding neuronal networks and mechanisms. *Eur. J. Neurosci.* 29:1741–1753, 2009.

Geraschenko, D., et al. Identification of a population of sleep-active cerebral cortex neurons. *Proc. Natl. Acad. Sci. USA* 105:10227–10232, 2008.

Gottesmann, C. Noradrenaline involvement in basic and higher integrated REM sleep processes. *Prog. Neurobiol.* 85:237–272, 2008.

Hobson, J.A. The neuropsychology of REM sleep dreaming. *NeuroReport* 9:R1–R14, 1998.

Huber, R., et al. Local sleep and learning. *Nature* 430:78–81, 2004.

Jha, S.K., et al. Sleep-dependent plasticity requires cortical activity. *J. Neurosci.* 25:9266–9274, 2005.

Joly-Mascheroni, R., et al. Dogs catch human yawns. *Biol. Lett.* 4:446–448, 2008.

Jouvet, M. Sleep and serotonin: an unfinished story. *Neuropsychopharmacology* 21(Suppl.):24S–27S, 1999.

Kavanau, J.L. Dream contents and failing memories. *Arch. Ital. Biol.* 140:109–127, 2002.

Krueger, J.M., et al. Sleep as a fundamental property of neuronal assemblies. *Nat. Rev. Neurosci.* 9:910–919, 2008.

Massimini, M., et al. Breakdown of cortical effective connectivity during sleep. *Science* 309:2228–2232, 2005.

Massimini, M., et al. Slow waves, synaptic plasticity and information processing: insights from transcranial magnetic stimulation and high-density EEG experiments. *Eur. J. Neurosci.* 29:1761–1770, 2009.

Mednick, S.C. The restorative effects of naps on perceptual deterioration. *Nat. Neurosci.* 5:677–681, 2002.

Mölle, M., Born, J. Hippocampus whispering in deep sleep to pre-frontal cortex—for good memories? *Neuron* 61:496–498, 2009.

Nishino, S., Mignot, E. Neurobiology of narcolepsy. *Neuroscientist* 4:133–143, 1998.

Oishi, Y., et al. Adenosine in the tuberomammillary nucleus inhibits the histaminergic system via A1 receptors and promotes non-rapid eye movement sleep. *Proc. Natl. Acad. Sci. USA* 105:19992–19997, 2008.

Platek, S.M., et al. Contagious yawning and the brain. *Cogn. Brain Res.* 23:448–452, 2005.

Pose, I., et al. Cuneiform neurons activated during cholinergically induced active sleep in the cat. *J. Neurosci.* 20:3319–3327, 2000.

Porkka-Heiskanen, T. Sleep homeostasis. *Curr. Opin. Neurobiol.* 23:799–805, 2013.

Rasch, B., et al. Odor cues during slow-wave sleep prompt declarative memory consolidation. *Science* 315:1426–1429, 2007.

Sakai, K., et al. Pontine structures and mechanisms involved in the generation of paradoxical (REM) sleep. *Arch. Ital. Biol.* 139:93–107, 2001.

Sakurai, T. Orexin deficiency and narcolepsy. *Curr. Opin. Neurobiol.* 23:760–766, 2013.

Sándor, P., et al. Ontogeny of dreaming a review of empirical studies. *Sleep Med. Rev.* 18:435–449, 2014.

Sarter, M., Bruno, J.P. Cortical cholinergic inputs mediating arousal, attentional processing and dreaming: differential afferent regulation of the basal forebrain by telencephalic and brainstem afferents. *Neuroscience* 95:933–952, 2000.

Scharf, M.T., et al. The energy hypothesis of sleep revisited. *Prog. Neurobiol.* 86:264–280, 2008.

Schenk, C.H., Mahowald, M.W. REM sleep behavior disorder: clinical, developmental, and neuroscience perspectives 16 years after its formal identification in SLEEP. *Sleep* 25:120–138, 2002.

Siegel, J.M. The stuff dreams are made of: anatomical substrates of REM-sleep. *Nat. Rev. Neurosci.* 9:721–722, 2006.

Siegel, J.M. Do all animals sleep? *Trends Neurosci.* 31:208–213, 2008.

Singer, O.C., et al. Yawning in acute anterior circulation stroke. *J. Neurol. Neurosurg. Psychiatry* 78:1253–1254, 2007.

Steriade, M. Sleep, epilepsy and thalamic reticular neurons. *Trends Neurosci.* 28:317–324, 2005.

Stickgold, R., Walker, M.P. Memory consolidation and reconsolidation: what is the role of sleep?. *Trends Neurosci.* 28:408–415, 2005.

Taheri, S., et al. The role of the hypocretins (orexins) in sleep regulation and narcolepsy. *Annu. Rev. Neurosci.* 25:283–313, 2002.

Tononi, G., Cirelli, C. Sleep and the price of plasticity: from synaptic and cellular homeostasis to memory consolidation and integration. *Neuron* 81:12–34, 2014.

Vassalli, A., Dijk, D.-J. Sleep function: current questions and new approaches. *Eur. J. Neurosci.* 29:1830–1841, 2009.

van den Pol, A.N. Narcolepsy: a neurodegenerative disease of the hypocretin system? *Neuron* 27:415–418, 2000.

Winson, J. The meaning of dreams. *Sci. Am.* 263:42–48, 1990.

Yoon, J.M.D., Tennie, C. Contagious yawning: a reflection of empathy, mimicry, or contagion? *Animal Behav.* 79:e1–e3, 2010.

Xie, L., et al. Sleep drives metabolic clearance from the adult brain. *Science* 342:373–377, 2013.

Chapter 27: The Cranial Nerves

Craig, A.D. How do you feel? Interoception: the sense of the physiological condition of the body. *Nat. Rev. Neurosci.* 3:655–666, 2002.

Farkas, E., et al. Periaqueductal gray matter projection to vagal preganglionic neurons and the nucleus tractus solitarius. *Brain Res.* 764:257–261, 1997.

Fay, R.A., Norgren, R. Identification of rat brainstem multisynaptic connections to the oral motor nuclei using pseudorabies virus: II. Facial muscle motor system. *Brain Res. Rev.* 25:276–290, 1997.

Goadsby, P.J., et al. Stimulation of the greater occipital nerve increases metabolic activity in the trigeminal nucleus caudalis and cervical drosal horn of the cat. *Pain* 73:23–28, 1997.

Haxhiu, M.A., Loewy, A.D. Central connections of the motor and sensory vagal systems innervating the trachea. *J. Auton. Nerv. Syst.* 57:49–56, 1996.

Knox, A.P., et al. The central connections of the vagus nerve in the ferret. *Brain Res. Bull.* 33:49–63, 1994.

Kozicz, T., et al. The Edinger-Westphal nucleus: a historical, structural, and functional perspective on a dichotomous terminology. *J. Comp. Neurol.* 519:1413–1434, 2011.

Kubota, K., et al. Central projection of proprioceptive afferents arising from maxillo-facial regions in some animals studied by HRP-labeling technique. *Anat. Anz.* 165:229–251, 1988.

Lawrence, A.J., Jarrott, B. Neurochemical modulation of cardiovascular control in the nucleus tractus solitarius. *Prog. Neurobiol.* 48:21–53, 1996.

Lazarov, N.E. Neurobiology of orofacial proprioception. *Brain Res. Rev.* 56:362–383, 2007.

Lee, B.H., et al. Calcitonin gene-related peptide in nucleus ambiguus motoneurons in rat: viscerotopic organization. *J. Comp. Neurol.* 320:531–543, 1992.

Love, S., Coakham, H.B. Trigeminal neuralgia: pathology and pathogenesis. *Brain* 124:2347–2360, 2001.

Morecraft, R.J., et al. Cortical innervation of the hypoglossal nucleus in the non-human primate (Macaca mulatta). *J. Comp. Neurol.* 522:3456–3484, 2014.

Réthelyi, M., et al. Distribution of neurons expressing calcitonin gene-related peptide mRNAs in the brain stem, spinal cord and dorsal root ganglia of rat and guinea-pig. *Neuroscience* 29:225–239, 1989.

Reynolds, S.M., et al. The pharmacology of couch. *Trends Pharmacol. Sci.* 25:569–576, 2004.

Strominger, N.L., et al. The connectivity of the area postrema in the ferret. *Brain Res. Bull.* 33:33–47, 1994.

Terao, S., et al. Course and distribution of facial corticobulbar tract fibres in the lower brain stem. *J. Neurol. Neurosurg. Psychiatry* 69:262–265, 2000.

Urban, P.P., et al. The course of corticofacial projections in the human brainstem. *Brain* 124:1866–1876, 2001.

Vilensky, J.A., et al. *The clinical anatomy of the cranial nerves: the nerves of "On old Olympus towering top."* Oxford: Wiley-Blackwell, 2015.

Zhuo, H., et al. Neurochemistry of the nodose ganglion. *Prog. Neurobiol.* 52:79–107, 1997.

Clinical

Amarenco, P., Hauw, J.-J. Cerebellar infarction in the territory of the anterior and inferior cerebellar artery. *Brain* 113:139–155, 1990.

Brazis, P.W. Isolated palsies of cranial Nerves III, IV, and VI. *Semin. Neurol.* 29:14–28, 2009.

Combarros, O., et al. Isolated unilateral hypoglossal nerve palsy: nine cases. *J. Neurol.* 245:98–100, 1998.

Deluca,C., et al. Ataxia in posterior circulation stroke: clinical-MRI correlations. *J. Neurol. Sci.* 300:39–46, 2011.

Eviston, T.J., et al. Bell's palsy: aetiology, clinical features and multidisciplinary care. *J. Neurol. Neurosurg. Psychiatry*. doi:10.1136/jnnp-2014-309563, 2015.

Kumral, E., et al. Clinical spectrum of pontine infarction: clinical-MRI correlations. *J. Neurol.* 249:1659–1670, 2003.

Malandraki, G., Robbins, J. Dysphagia. In: Barnes, M.P., Good, D.C. (Eds.), *Handbook of clinical neurology*, Vol. 110 (pp. 255–271). New York: Elsevier, 2013.

Mumenthaler, M. *Neurologie*, 6th ed. Stuttgart: Thieme Verlag, 1979.

Monrad-Krohn, G.H. *The clinical examination of the nervous system*, 10th ed. London: H. K. Lewis, 1954.

Oliveri, R.L., et al. Pontine lesion of the abducens fasciculus producing so-called posterior internuclear ophthalmoplegia. *Eur. J. Neurol.* 37:67–69, 1997.

Pearce, J.M.S. Wallenberg's syndrome. *J. Neurol. Neurosurg. Psychiatry* 68:570–571, 2000.

Samii, M., Janetta, P.J. *The cranial nerves: anatomy, pathology, pathophysiology, diagnosis, treatment.* New York: Springer-Verlag, 1981.

Silverman, I.E., et al. The crossed paralyses: the original brainstem syndromes of Millard-Gubler, Foville, Weber, and Raymond-Cestan. *Arch. Neurol.* 52:635–638, 1995.

Uzawa, A., et al. Laryngeal abductor paralysis can be a solitary manifestation of multiple system atrophy. *J. Neurol. Neurosurg. Psychiatry* 76:1739–1741, 2005.

Chapter 28: Visceral Efferent Neurons: The Sympathetic and Parasympathetic Divisions

Sympathetic and Parasympathetic Systems

Andrew, J., Nathan, P.W. Lesions of the anterior frontal lobes and disturbances of micturition and defaecation. *Brain* 87:233–262, 1964.

Appel, N.M., Elde, R.P. The intermediolateral cell column of the thoracic spinal cord is comprised of target-specific subnuclei: evidence from retrograde transport studies and immunohistochemistry. *J. Neurosci.* 8:1767–1775, 1988.

Appenzeller, O. *The autonomic nervous system: an introduction to basic and clinical concepts.* Philadelphia: Elsevier, 1990.

Appenzeller, O., et al. *The autonomic nervous system.* Part II: *Dysfunctions.* Philadelphia: Elsevier, 2001.

Berntson, G.G., et al. Autonomic space and psychophysical response. *Psychophysiology* 31:44–61, 1994.

Blessing, W.W. Inadequate frameworks for understanding bodily homeostasis. *Trends Neurosci.* 20:235–239, 1997.

Burnstock, G. The changing face of autonomic neurotransmission. *Acta Physiol. Scand.* 126:67–91, 1986.

Cheng, Z., Powley, T.L. Nucleus ambiguus projections to cardiac ganglia of rat atria: an anterograde tracing study. *J. Comp. Neurol.* 424:588–606, 2000.

Critchley, H.D., Harrison, N.A. Visceral influences on brain and behavior. *Neuron* 77:624–638, 2013.

Elfvin, L.-G., et al. The chemical neuroanatomy of sympathetic ganglia. *Annu. Rev. Neurosci.* 16:471–504, 1993.

Farkas, E., et al. Periaqueductal gray matter input to cardiac-related sympathetic premotor neurons. *Brain Res.* 792:179–192, 1998.

Fowler, C.J. Neurological disorders of micturition and their treatment. *Brain* 122:1213–1231, 1999.

Gabella, G. *Structure of the autonomic nervous system.* New York: Chapman & Hall, 1976.

Gibbins, I. Peripheral autonomic pathways. In: Mai, J.K., Paxinos, G. (Eds.), *The human nervous system*, 3rd. ed. (pp. 141–181). San Diego: Elsevier Academic Press, 2012.

Giuliano, F., Rampin, O. Central regulation of penile erection. *Neurosci. Biobehav. Rev.* 24:517–533, 2000.

Goldstein, D.S. *The autonomic nervous system in health and disease.* New York: Marcel Dekker, 2001.

Gourine, A.V., et al. Purinergic signalling in autonomic control. *Trends Neurosci.* 32:241–248, 2009.

Guyenet, P.G. The sympathetic control of blood pressure. *Nat. Rev. Neurosci.* 7:335–346, 2006.

Hakusui, S., et al. Postprandial hypotension: microneurographic analysis and treatment with vasopressin. *Neurology* 41:712–715, 1991.

Haymaker, W., Woodhall, B. *Peripheral nerve injuries: principles of diagnosis.* Philadelphia: W.B. Saunders, 1945.

Hirst, G.D.S., Edwards, F.R. Sympathetic neuroeffector transmission in arteries and arterioles. *Physiol. Rev.* 69:546–604, 1989.

Jänig, W. *The integrative action of the autonomic nervous system: neurobiology of homeostasis.* Cambridge, UK: Cambridge University Press, 2006.

Jänig, W., McLachlan, E.M. Characteristics of function-specific pathways in the sympathetic nervous system. *Trends Neurosci.* 15:475–481, 1992.

Kaufmann, H., et al. Vestibular control of sympathetic activity: an otolith-sympathetic reflex in humans. *Exp. Brain Res.* 143:463–469, 2002.

Kellogg, D.L. Jr. In vivo mechanisms of cutaneous vasodilation and vasoconstriction in humans during thermoregulatory challenges. *J. Appl. Physiol.* 100:1709–1718, 2006.

Kerman, I. Organization of brain somatomotor-sympathetic circuits. *Exp. Brain Res.* 187:1–16, 2008.

Laskey, W., Polosa, C. Characteristics of the sympathetic preganglionic neuron and its synaptic input. *Prog. Neurobiol.* 31:47–84, 1988.

Miolan, J.P., Niel, J.P. The mammalian sympathetic prevertebral ganglia: integrative properties and role in the nervous control of digestive tract motility. *J. Auton. Nerv. Syst.* 58:125–138, 1996.

Nour, S., et al. Cerebral activation during micturition in normal men. *Brain* 123:781–789, 2000.

Paton, J.F.R., et al. The yin and yang of cardiac autonomic control: vago-sympathetic interactions revisited. *Brain Res. Rev.* 49:555–565, 2005.

Pick, J. *The autonomic nervous system: morphological, comparative, clinical and surgical aspects.* Philadelphia: Lippincott, 1970.

Pyner, S., Coote, J.H. Evidence that sympathetic preganglionic neurones are arranged in target-specific columns in the thoracic spinal cord of the rat. *J. Comp. Neurol.* 342:15–22, 1994.

Rossi, P., et al. Stomach distension increases efferent muscle sympathetic nerve activity and blood pressure in healthy humans. *J. Neurol. Sci.* 161:148–155, 1998.

Sartor, D.M., Verberne, A.J.M. Abdominal vagal signalling: a novel role for cholecystokinin in circulatory control? *Brain Res. Rev.* 59:140–154, 2008.

Seifert, T., Secher, N.H. Sympathetic influence on cerebral blood flow and metabolism during exercise in humans. *Prog. Neurobiol.* 95:406–426, 2011.

Simmons, M.A. The complexity and diversity of synaptic transmission in the prevertebral sympathetic ganglia. *Prog. Neurobiol.* 24:43–93, 1985.

Spalteholz, W. *Handatlas der Anatomie des Menschen: III.* Stuttgart: Hirzel Verlag, 1933.

Standish, A., et al. Central neuronal circuit innervating the rat heart defined by transneuronal transport of pseudorabies virus. *J. Neurosci.* 15:1998–2012, 1995.

Sugiyama,Y., et al. Role of the rostral ventrolateral medulla (RVLM) in the patterning of vestibular system influences on sympathetic nervous system outflow to the upper and lower body. *Exp. Brain Res.* 210:515–527, 2011.

Travagli, R.A., et al. Brainstem circuits regulating gastric function. *Annu. Rev. Physiol.* 68:279–305, 2006.

Wallin, B.G., Fagius, J. The sympathetic nervous system in man: aspects derived from microelectrode recordings. *Trends Neurosci.* 9:63–67, 1986.

Wallin, B.G., et al. Coherence between the sympathetic drives to relaxed and contracting muscles of different limbs of human subjects. *J. Physiol.* 455:219–233, 1992.

Westerhaus, M.J., Loewy, A.D. Central representation of the sympathetic nervous system in the cerebral cortex. *Brain Res.* 903:117–127, 2001.

Zhuo, H., et al. Neurochemistry of the nodose ganglion. *Prog. Neurobiol.* 52:79–107, 1997.

The Enteric Nervous System

Furness, J.B. The enteric nervous system and neurogastroenterology. *Nat. Rev. Gastroenterol. Hepatol.* 9:282–294, 2012.

Furness, J.B., et al. Roles of peptides in transmission in the enteric nervous system. *Trends Neurosci.* 15:66–71, 1992.

Goyal, R.K., Hirano, I. The enteric nervous system. *N. Engl. J. Med.* 334:1106–1115, 1996.

Grundy, D., Schemann, M. Enteric nervous system. *Curr. Opin. Gastroenterol.* 23:121–126, 2007.

Holst, M.C., et al. Vagal preganglionic projections to the enteric nervous system characterized with *Phaseolus vulgaris* leucoagglutinin. *J. Comp. Neurol.* 381:81–100, 1997.

Kunze, W.A.A., Furness, J.B. The enteric nervous system and regulation of intestinal motility. *Annu. Rev. Physiol.* 61:117–142, 1999.

McLean, P.G., et al. 5–HT in the enteric nervous system: gut function and neuropharmacology. *Trends Neurosci.* 30:9–13, 2007.

Wood, J.D. Application of classification schemes to the enteric nervous system. *J. Auton. Nerv. Syst.* 48:17–19, 1994.

Chapter 29: Sensory Visceral Neurons and Visceral Reflexes

Andersson, K. Alpha 1-adrenoceptors and bladder function. *Eur. Urol.* 36(Suppl. 1):96–102, 1999.

Arendt-Nielsen, L., et al. Referred pain as an indicator for neural plasticity. *Prog. Brain Res.* 129:343–356, 2000.

Argiolas, A., Melis, M.R. Central control of penile erection: role of the paraventricular nucleus of the hypothalamus. *Prog. Neurobiol.* 76:1–21, 2005.

Bajaj, P., et al. Osteoarthritis and its association with muscle hyperal-gesia: an experimental controlled study. *Pain* 93:107–114, 2001.

Bernard, J.F., et al. The parabrachial area: electrophysiological evidence for an involvement in visceral nociceptive processes. *J. Neurophysiol.* 71:1646–1660, 1994.

Blackshaw, L.A., et al. Sensory transmission in the gastrointestinal tract. *Neurogastroenterol. Motil.* 19(Suppl. 1):1–19, 2007.

Blok, B.F., et al. Brain activation during micturition in women. *Brain* 121:2033–2042, 1998.

Bogduk, N. On the definitions and physiology of back pain, referred pain, and radicular pain. *Pain* 147:17–19, 2009.

Carro-Juárez, M., Rodriguez-Manzo, G. The spinal pattern generator for ejaculation. *Brain Res. Rev.* 58:106–120, 2008.

Cervero, F. Visceral pain: mechanisms of peripheral and central sensitization. *Ann. Med.* 27:235–239, 1995.

Charles, A. Migraine is not primarily a vascular disorder. *Cephalalgia* 32:431–432, 2012.

Cope, Z. *The early diagnosis of the acute abdomen.* New York: Oxford University Press, 1968.

Critchley, H.D., Harrison, N.A. Visceral influences on brain and behavior. *Neuron* 77:624–638, 2013.

Davis, K.D., et al. Visceral pain evoked by thalamic microstimulation in humans. *NeuroReport* 6:369–374, 1995.

DeGroat, W.C., et al. Neural control of the urethra. *Scand. J. Urol. Nephrol.* (Suppl.):35–43, 2001.

Drake, M.J., et al. Neural control of the lower urinary and gastrointestinal tracts: supraspinal CNS mechanisms. *Neurourol. Urodynam.* 29:119–127, 2010.

Dunckley, P., et al. A comparison of visceral and somatic pain processing in the human brainstem using functional magnetic resonance imaging. *J. Neurosci.* 25:7333–741, 2005.

Elsenbruch, S. Abdominal pain in irritable bowel syndrome: a review of putative psychological, neural and neuro-immune mechanisms. *Brain, Behav. Immun.* 25:386–394, 2011.

Fowler, C.J., et al. The neural control of micturition. *Nat. Rev. Neurosci.* 9:453–466, 2008.

Fugère, F., Lewis, G. Coeliac plexus block for chronic pain syndromes. *Can. J. Anaesth.* 40:954–963, 1993.

Giamberardino, M.A., et al. Viscero-visceral hyperalgesia: characterization in different clinical models. *Pain* 151:307–322, 2010.

Gybels, J.M., Sweet, W.H. *Neurosurgical treatment of persistent pain: physiological and pathological mechanisms of human pain.* Basel: Karger, 1989.

Hubscher, C.H. Ascending spinal pathways from sexual organs: effects of chronic spinal lesions. *Prog. Brain Res.* 152:401–420, 2006.

Jänig, W. Neurobiology of visceral afferent neurons: neuroanatomy, functions, organ regulations and sensations. *Biol. Psychol.* 42:29–51, 1996.

Jänig, W. Autonomic nervous system and pain. In: Basbaum, A.I. (Ed.), *The senses: a comprehensive reference*, Vol. 5 (pp. 193–225). Amsterdam: Elsevier, 2008.

Jänig, W. Visceral pain—still an enigma? *Pain* 151:239–240, 2010.

Karlsson, A.-K. Autonomic dysfunction in spinal cord injury: clinical presentation of symptoms. *Prog. Brain Res.* 152:1–8, 2006.

Kemp, W.J. III. The innervation of the cranial dura mater: neurosurgical case correlates and a review of the literature. *World Neurosurg.* 78:505–510, 2012.

Knowles, C.H., Aziz, Q. Basic and clinical aspects of gastrointestinal pain. *Pain* 141:191–209, 2009.

Kuhtz-Buschbeck, J.P., et al. Cortical representation of the urge to void: a functional magnetic resonance imaging study. *J. Urol.* 174:1477–1481, 2005.

Lee, L.-Y., Pisarri, T.E. Afferent properties and reflex functions of bronchopulmonary C-fibers. *Respir. Physiol.* 125:47–65, 2001.

Mayer, E.A., et al. Differences in brain responses to visceral pain between patients with irritable bowel syndrome and ulcerative colitis. *Pain* 115:398–409, 2005.

McMahon, S.B. Are there fundamental differences in the peripheral mechanisms of visceral and somatic pain? *Behav. Brain Sci.* 20:381–391, 1997.

Meller, S.T., Gebhart, G.F. A critical review of afferent pathways and the potential chemical mediators involved in cardiac pain. *Neuroscience* 48:501–524, 1992.

Napadow, V., et al. The brain circuitry underlying the temporal evolution of nausea in humans. *Cereb. Cortex* 23:806–813, 2013.

Paintal, A.S. Sensations from J receptors. *News Physiol. Sci.* 10:238–243, 1995.

Palaček, J. The role of the dorsal column pathway in visceral pain. *Physiol. Res.* 53(Suppl. 1):S125–S130, 2004.

Raj, H., et al. How does lobeline injected intravenously produce a couch? *Respir. Physiol. Neurobiol.* 145:79–90, 2005.

Rosen, S.D. From heart to brain: the genesis and processing of cardiac pain. *Can. J. Cardiol.* 28:S7–S19, 2012.

Russo, A., Conte, B. Afferent and efferent branching axons from the rat lumbo-sacral spinal cord project both to the urinary bladder and the urethra as demonstrated by double retrograde neuronal labeling. *Neurosci. Lett.* 219:155–158, 1996.

Saper, C.B. The central autonomic nervous system: conscious visceral perception and autonomic pattern generation. *Annu. Rev. Neurosci.* 25:433–469, 2002.

Sartor, D.M., Verberne, A.J.M. Abdominal vagal signalling: a novel role for cholecystokinin in circulatory control? *Brain Res. Rev.* 59:140–154, 2008.

Sullivan, M.D., Leach, A. Looking beyond myocardial ischemia in chest pain treatment. *Pain* 152:707–708, 2011.

Treede, R.-D., et al. The plasticity of cutaneous hyperalgesia during sympathetic ganglion blockade in patients with neuropathic pain. *Brain* 115:607–621, 1992.

Willis, W.D., et al. A visceral pain pathway in the dorsal column of the spinal cord. *Proc. Nat. Acad. Sci. USA* 96:7675–7679, 1999.

Chapter 30: The Central Autonomic System: Hypothalamus

Structure, Connections, General Organization

Bandler, R., et al. Central circuits mediating patterned autonomic activity during active vs. passive emotional coping. *Brain Res. Bull.* 53:95–104, 2000.

Blessing, W.W., Benarroch, E.E. Lower brainstem regulation of visceral, cardiovascular, and respiratory function. In: Mai, J., Paxinos, G. (Eds.), *The human nervous system*, 3rd ed. (pp. 1058–1073). San Diego: Elsevier Academic Press, 2012.

Cameron, A.A., et al. The efferent projections of the periaqueductal gray in the rat: a *Phaseolus vulgaris*–leucoagglutinin study: II. Descending projections. *J. Comp. Neurol.* 351:585–601, 1995.

Clark, Le Gros W.E., et al. *The hypothalamus: morphological, functional, clinical, and surgical aspects.* London: Oliver & Boyd, 1936.

Giesler, G.J., et al. Direct spinal pathways to the limbic system for nociceptive information. *Trends Neurosci.* 17:244–250, 1994.

Kostarczyk, E., et al. Spinohypothalamic tract neurons in the cervical enlargement of rats: locations of antidromically identified ascending axons and their collateral branches in the contralateral brain. *J. Neurophysiol.* 77:435–451, 1997.

Mtui, E.P., et al. Medullary visceral reflex circuits: local afferents to nucleus tractus solitarii synthesize catecholamines and project to thoracic spinal cord. *J. Comp. Neurol.* 351:5–26, 1995.

Risold, P.Y., et al. The structural organization of connections between hypothalamus and cerebral cortex. *Brain Res. Rev.* 24:197–254, 1997.

Saper, C.B. The central autonomic nervous system: conscious visceral perception and autonomic pattern generation. *Annu. Rev. Neurosci.* 25:433–469, 2002.

Saper, C.B. The hypothalamus. In: Mai, J.K., Paxinos, G. (Eds.), *The human nervous system*, 3rd ed. (pp. 1058–1073). San Diego: Elsevier Academic Press, 2012.

Smith, O., DeVito, J.L. Central neural integration for the control of autonomic responses associated with emotion. *Annu. Rev. Neurosci.* 7:43–65, 1984,

Swanson, L.W. The neural basis of motivated behavior. *Acta Morphol. Neerl. Scand.* 26:165–176. 1989.

Vann, S.D., Aggleton, J.P. The mammillary bodies: two memory systems in one? *Nat. Rev. Neurosci.* 5:35–44, 2004.

Westerhaus, M.J., Loewy, A.D. Central representation of the sympathetic nervous system in the cerebral cortex. *Brain Res.* 903:117–127, 2001.

Hypothalamus and the Endocrine System

Bethlehem, R.A.I., et al. The oxytocin paradox. *Front. Behav. Neurosci.* 8:48. doi:10.3389/fnbeh. 2014.00048, 2014.

Brunton, P.J., Russel, J.A. The expectant brain: adapting for motherhood. *Nat. Rev. Neurosci.* 9:11–25, 2008.

Cclcc, P., et al. On the effects of testosterone on brain behavioral functions. *Front. Neurosci.* 9:12. doi:10.3389/fnins.2015.00012, 2015.

De Kloet, E.R., et al. Stress and cognition: are corticosteroids good or bad guys? *Trends Neurosci.* 22:422–426, 1999.

De Voogd, T.J. Androgens can affect the morphology of mammalian CNS neurons in adulthood. *Trends Neurosci.* 10:341–342, 1987.

Donaldson, Z.R., Young, L.J. Oxytocin, vasopressin, and the neuro-genetic of sociality. *Science* 322:900–904, 2008.

Ericsson, A., et al. A functional anatomical analysis of central pathways subserving effects of interleukin-1 on stress-related neuroendocrine neurons. *J. Neurosci.* 14:897–913, 1994.

Herman, J.P., Cullinan, W.E. Neurocircuitry of stress: central control of the hypothalamo-pituitary-adrenocortical axis. *Trends Neurosci.* 20:78–84, 1997.

Landgraf, R., Neumann, I.D. Vasopressin and oxytocin release within the brain: a dynamic concept of multiple and variable modes of neuropeptide communication. *Front. Neuroendocrinol.* 25:150–176, 2004.

Lee, H.-J., et al. Oxytocin: the great facilitator of life. *Prog. Neurobiol.* 88:127–151, 2009.

Ludwig, M., Leng G. Dendritic peptide release and peptide-dependent behaviors. *Nat. Rev. Neurosci.* 7:127–136, 2006.

Meyer-Lindenberg, A., et al. Oxytocin and vasopressin in the human brain: social neuropeptides for translational medicine. *Nature Rev. Neurosci.* 12:524–538, 2011.

Park, C.R. Cognitive effects of insulin in the central nervous system. *Neurosci. Biobehav. Rev.* 25:311–323, 2001.

Ulrich-Lai, Y.M., Herman, J.P. Neural regulation of endocrine and autonomic stress responses. *Nat. Rev. Neurosci.* 10:397–409, 2009.

Yoshimura, F., Gorbman, A. *Pars distalis of the pituitary gland: structure, function and regulation.* Philadelphia: Elsevier, 1986.

Thermoregulation, Sleep, and Circadian Rhythms

Alexandre, C., et al. Control of arousal by the orexin neurons. *Curr. Opin. Neurobiol.* 23:752–759, 2013.

Aston-Jones, G., et al. A neural circuit for circadian regulation of arousal. *Nat. Neurosci.* 4:732–738, 2001.

Buijs, R.M., et al. Organization of circadian functions: interaction with the body. *Prog. Brain Res.* 153:341–350, 2006.

Falcon, J. Cellular circadian clocks in the pineal. *Prog. Neurobiol.* 58:121–162, 1999.

Foster, R.G. Shedding light on the biological clock. *Neuron* 20:829–832, 1998.

Gao, X.-B., Horvath, T. Function and dysfunction of hypocretin/orexin: an energetics point of view. *Annu. Rev. Neurosci.* 37:101–116, 2014.

Haas, H., Panula P. The role of histamine and the tuberomammillary nucleus in the nervous system. *Nat. Rev. Neurosci.* 4:121–130, 2003.

Harrison, N.A. Neural origins of human sickness in interoceptive responses to inflammation. *Biol. Psychiat.* 66:415–422, 2009.

Ibata, Y., et al. The suprachiasmatic nucleus: a circadian oscillator. *Neuroscientist* 3:215–225, 1997.

Kondratova, A.A., Kondratov, R.V. The circadian clock and pathology of the ageing brain. *Nature Rev. Neurosci.* 13:325–335, 2012.

Maywood, E.S. Circadian timing in health and disease. *Prog. Brain Res.* 253–265, 2006.

Mohawk, J.A., et al. Central and peripheral circadian clocks in mammals. *Annu. Rev. Neurosci.* 35:445–462, 2012.

Moore, R.Y., et al. The retinohypothalamic tract originates from a distinct subset of retinal ganglion cells. *J. Comp. Neurol.* 352:351–366, 1995.

Morin, L.P. The circadian visual system. *Brain Res. Rev.* 67:102–127, 1994.

Nagashima, K., et al. Neuronal circuitries involved in thermoregulation. *Auton. Neurosci.* 85:18–25, 2000.

Nakamura, K., Morrison, S.F. A thermosensory pathway that controls body temperature. *Nat. Rev. Neurosci.* 11:62–71, 2008.

O'Neill, J.S., et al. Cellular mechanisms of the circadian pacemaking: beyond transcriptional loops. In: Kramer, A, Merrow, M. (Eds.), *Circadian clocks* (pp. 67–103). Heidelberg: Springer, 2013.

Pandi-Perumal, S.R., et al. Physiological effects of melatonin: role of melatonin receptors and signal transduction pathways. *Prog. Neurobiol.* 85:335–353, 2008.

Romanovsky, A.A. Thermoregulation: some concepts have changed. Functional architecture of the thermoregulatory system. *Am. J. Physiol. Regul. Integr. Comp. Physiol.* 292:R37–R46, 2007.

Sakurai, T. The neural circuit of orexin (hypocretin): maintaining sleep and wakefulness. *Nat. Rev. Neurosci.* 8:171–181, 2007.

Sakurai, T. Orexin deficiency and narcolepsy. *Curr. Opin. Neurobiol.* 23:760–766, 2013.

Saper, C.B., et al. The sleep switch: hypothalamic control of sleep and wakefulness. *Trends Neurosci.* 24:726–731, 2002.

Saper, C.B. The central circadian timing system. *Curr. Opin. Neurobiol.* 23:747–751, 2013.

Thannickal, T.C., et al. Reduced number of hypocretin neurons in human narcolepsy. *Neuron* 27:469–474, 2000.

Vanecek, J. Cellular mechanisms of melatonin action. *Physiol. Rev.* 78:687–721, 1998.

Osmoregulation, Feeding, and Energy Balance

Beaver, J.D., et al. Individual differences in reward drive predict neural responses to images of food. *J. Neurosci.* 26:5160–5166, 2006.

Bergh, C., Söderström, P. Anorexia nervosa, self-starvation and the reward of stress. *Nat. Med.* 2:21–22, 1996.

Berthoud, H.-R. Metabolic and hedonic drives in the neural control of appetite: who is the boss? *Curr. Opin. Neurobiol.* 21:888–896, 2011.

Bourque, C.W. Central mechanisms of osmosensation and systemic osmoregulation. *Nat. Rev. Neurosci.* 9:519–531, 2008.

Cone, R., Simerly R. Leptin grows up and gets a neural network. *Neuron* 71:4–6, 2011.

Diano, S., et al. Ghrelin controls hippocampal spine synapse density and memory performance. *Nature Neurosci.* 9:381–388. 2006.

Elmquist, J.K., et al. From lesions to leptin: hypothalamic control of food intake and body weight. *Neuron* 22:221–232, 1999.

Inui, A. Feeding and body-weight regulation by hypothalamic neuro-peptides: mediation of the actions of leptin. *Trends Neurosci.* 22:62–67, 1999.

Jauch-Chara, K., Oltmanns, K.M. Obesity—a neuropsychological disease? Systematic review and neuropsychological model. *Progr. Neurobiol.* 114:84–101, 2014.

Jobst, E.E., et al. The electrophysiology of feeding circuits. *Trends Endocrinol. Metab.* 15:497–499, 2004.

Knecht, S., et al. Obesity in neurobiology. *Prog. Neurobiol.* 84:85–103, 2008.

Lawrence, C.B. Hypothalamic control of feeding. *Curr. Opin. Neurobiol.* 9:778–783, 1999.

Saper, C.B., et al. The need to feed: homeostatic and hedonic control of eating. *Neuron* 36:199–211, 2002.

Seeley, R.J., Woods, S.C. Monitoring of stored and available fuel by the CNS: implications for obesity. *Nat. Rev. Neurosci.* 4:901–909, 2003.

Uher, R., Treasure, J. Brain lesions and eating disorders. *J. Neurol. Neurosurg. Psychiatry* 76:852–857, 2005.

van den Top, M., Spanswick, D. Integration of metabolic stimuli in the hypothalamic arcuate nucleus. *Prog. Brain Res.* 153:141–152, 2006.

van Praag, H., et al. Exercise, energy intake, glucose homeostasis, and the brain. *J. Neurosci.* 34:15139–15149, 2014.

Willie, J.T. To eat or sleep? Orexin in the regulation of feeding and wakefulness. *Annu. Rev. Neurosci.* 24:429–458, 2001.

Sexual Behavior and Sex Differences

Angiolas, A., Melis, M.R. Neuropeptides and central control of sexual behaviour from the past to the present: a review. *Progr. Neurobiol.* 108:80–107, 2013.

Arnold, A.P., Gorski, R.A. Gonadal steroid induction of structural sex differences in the central nervous system. *Annu. Rev. Neurosci.* 7:413–442, 1984.

Celec, P., et al. On the effects of testosterone on brain behavioral functions. *Front. Neurosci.* 9:12. doi:10.3389/fnins.2015.00012, 2015.

Cooke, B.M., et al. A brain sexual dimorphism controlled by adult circulating androgens. *Proc. Natl. Acad. Sci. USA* 96:7538–7540, 1999.

De Voogd, T.J. Androgens can affect the morphology of mammalian CNS neurons in adulthood. *Trends Neurosci.* 10:341–342, 1987.

De Vries, G.J. Sex differences in vasopressin and oxytocin innervation of the brain. *Prog. Brain Res.* 170:17–27, 2008.

Federman, D.D. The biology of human sex differences. *N. Engl. J. Med.* 354:1507–1514, 2006.

Lasco, M.S., et al. A lack of dimorphism of sex or sexual orientation in the human anterior commissure. *Brain Res.* 936:95–98, 2002.

McEwen, B.S. Permanence of brain sex differences and structural plasticity of the adult brain. *Proc. Natl. Acad. Sci. USA* 96:7128–7130, 1999.

Morgan, M.A., et al. Estrogens and non-reproductive behaviors related to activity and fear. *Neurosci. Biobehav. Rev.* 28:55–63, 2004.

Morris, J.A., et al. Sexual differences of the vertebrate nervous system. *Nat. Neurosci.* 7:1034–1039, 2004.

Pfaus, J.G. Neurobiology of sexual behavior. *Curr. Opin. Neurobiol.* 9:751–758, 1999.

Schwaab, D.F., et al. Structural and functional sex differences in the human hypothalamus. *Horm. Behav.* 40:93–98, 2001.

Semaan, S.J., Kauffman, A.S. Sexual differentiation and development of forebrain reproductive circuits. *Curr. Opin. Neurobiol.* 20:424–431, 2010.

Simerly, R.B. Wired for reproduction: organization and development of sexually dimorphic circuits in the mammalian forebrain. *Annu. Rev. Neurosci.* 25:507–536, 2002.

Sisk, C.L., Foster D.L. The neural basis of puberty and adolescence. *Nat. Rev. Neurosci.* 7:1040–1047, 2004.

Van Furth, W.R., et al. Regulation of masculine sexual behavior: involvement of brain opioids and dopamine. *Brain Res. Rev.* 21:162–184, 1995.

Hypothalamus and the Immune System

Banks, W.A., et al. Passage of cytokines across the blood–brain barrier. *Neuroimmunomodulation* 2:241–248, 1995.

Borsody, M.K., Weiss, J.M. The subdiaphragmatic vagus nerves mediate activation of locus coeruleus neurons by peripherally administered microbial substances. *Neuroscience* 131:235–245, 2005.

Cohen, N. The uses and abuses of psychoneuroimmunology: a global overview. *Brain Behav. Immunol.* 20:99–112, 2006.

Cohen, S., Herbert, T.B. Health psychology: psychological factors and physical disease from the perspective of human psychoneuroimmunology. *Annu. Rev. Psychol.* 47:113–142, 1996.

Dantzer, R., Kelley, K.W. Twenty years of research on cytokine-induced sickness behavior. *Brain Behav. Immun.* 21:153–160, 2007.

Dantzer, R., et al. From inflammation to sickness and depression: when the immune system subjugates the brain. *Nat. Rev. Neurosci.* 9:46–57, 2008.

Dowlati, Y., et al. A meta-analysis of cytokines in major depression. *Biol. Psychiat.* 67:446–457, 2010.

Fagundes, C.P., et al. Stressful early life experiences and immune dysregulation across the lifespan. *Brain Behav. Immun.* 27:8–12, 2013.

Felten, D.L. Direct innervation of lymphoid organs: substrate for neurotransmitter signaling of cells of the immune system. *Neuropsychobiology* 28:110–112, 1993.

Goehler, L.E., et al. Interleukin-1b in immune cells of the abdominal vagus nerve: a link between the immune and nervous system? *J. Neurosci.* 19:2799–2806, 1999.

Harrison, N.A., et al. Central autonomic network mediates cardiovascular response to acute inflammation: relevance to increased cardiovascular risk in depression? *Brain Behav. Immun.* 31:189–196, 2013.

Hori, T., et al. The autonomic nervous system as a communication channel between the brain and the immune system. *Neuroimmunomodulation* 2:203–215, 1995.

Kavelaars, A., Heijnen, C.B. Stress, genetics and immunity. *Brain Behav. Immun.* 20:313–316, 2006.

Kemeny, M.E. Psychobiological responses to social threat: evolution of a psychological model in psychoneuroimmunology. *Brain Behav. Immun.* 23:1–9, 2009.

Koh, K.B., et al. Counter-stress effects of relaxation on pro-inflammatory and anti-inflammatory cytokines. *Brain Behav. Immun.* 22:1130–1137, 2008.

Konsman, J.P., et al. Cytokine-induced sickness behaviour: mechanisms and implications. *Trends Neurosci.* 25:117–127, 2001.

LaCroix, S., Rivest, S. Functional circuitry in the brain of immune-challenged rats: partial involvement of prostaglandins. *J. Comp. Neurol.* 387:307–324, 1997.

Lagercrantz, H. Neuromodulators and respiratory control during development. *Trends Neurosci.* 10:368–372, 1987.

Madden, K.S., et al. Sympathetic nervous system modulation of the immune system. *J. Neuroimmunol.* 49:77–87, 1994.

Marazziti, D., et al. Immune cell imbalance in major depressive and panic disorders. *Neuropsychobiology* 26:23–26, 1992.

Pariante, C.M. Chronic fatigue syndrome and the immune system: "findings in search of meanings." *Brain Behav. Immun.* 23:325–326, 2009.

Pavlov, V.A., Tracey, K.J. The cholinergic anti-inflammatory pathway. *Brain Behav. Immun.* 19:493–499, 2005.

Piriano, B., et al. Genetic associations of fatigue and other symptom domains of the acute sickness response to infection. *Brain Behav. Immun.* 26:552–558, 2012.

Rinner, I., Schauenstein, K. The parasympathetic nervous system takes part in the immuno-neuroendocrine dialogue. *J. Neuroimmunol.* 34:165–172, 1991.

Salzet, M., et al. Crosstalk between nervous and immune systems through the animal kingdom: focus on opioids. *Trends Neurosci.* 23:550–555, 2000.

Sanders, V.M. Interdisciplinary research: noradrenergic regulation of adaptive immunity. *Brain Behav. Immun.* 20:1–8, 2006.

Schedlowski, M., et al. Endotoxin-induced experimental systemic inflammation in humans: a model to disentangle immune-to-brain communication. *Brain Behav. Immun.* 35:1–8, 2014.

Sloan, E.K., et al. Social stress enhances sympathetic innervation of primate lymph nodes: mechanisms for viral pathogenesis. *J. Neurosci.* 27:8857–8865, 2007.

Steptoe, A., et al. Positive affect and health-related neuroendocrine, cardiovascular and inflammatory processes. *Proc. Natl. Acad. Sci. USA* 102:6508–6512, 2005.

Sundgren-Andersson, A.K., et al. Neurobiological mechanisms of fever. *Neuroscientist* 4:113–121, 1998.

Watkins, L., Maier, S.F. Implications of immune-to-brain communication for sickness and pain. *Proc. Natl. Acad. Sci. USA* 96:7710–7713, 1999.

Stress and Psychosomatic Relations

Aggarwal, V.R., et al. The epidemiology of chronic syndromes that are frequently unexplained: do they have common associated factors? *Int. J. Epidem.* 35:468–476, 2006.

Amat, J., et al. Medial prefrontal cortex determines how stressor controllability affects behavior and dorsal raphe nucleus. *Nat. Neurosci.* 8:365–371, 2005.

Arnsten, A.F.T. Stress signalling pathways that impair prefrontal cortex structure and function. *Nat. Rev. Neurosci.* 10:410–422, 2009.

Borsook, D., et al. Understanding migraine through the lens of maladaptive stress responses: a model disease of allostatic load. *Neuron* 73:219–234, 2012.

Crombez, G., et al. The unbearable lightness of somatization: a systematic review of the concept of somatization in empirical studies of pain. *Pain* 145:31–35, 2009.

Dantzer, R. Somatization: a psychoneuroimmune perspective. *Psychoneuroendocrinology* 30:947–952, 2005.

de Kloet, E.R., et al. Stress and the brain: from adaptation to disease. *Nat. Rev. Neurosci.* 6:463–475, 2005.

De Waal, F.B.M. What is an animal emotion? *Ann. NY Acad. Sci.* 1224:191–206, 2011.

Feder, A., et al. Psychobiology and molecular genetics of resilience. *Nat. Rev. Neurosci.* 10:446–457, 2009.

Friedman, H.S., Kern, M.L. Personality, well-being, and health. *Annu. Rev. Psychol.* 65:719–742, 2014.

Gunnar, M., Quevedo, K. The neurobiology of stress and development. *Annu. Rev. Psychol.* 58:145–173, 2007.

Hines, L.A., et al. Posttraumatic stress disorder post Iraq and Afghanistan: prevalence among military subgroups. *Can. J. Psychiat.* 59:468–479, 2014.

Joëls, M., Baram, T.Z. The neuro-symphony of stress. *Nat. Rev. Neurosci.* 10:459–466, 2009.

Joëls, M., et al. Learning under stress: how does it work? *Trends Cogn. Sci.* 10:152–158, 2006.

Karatsoreos, I.N., McEwen, B.S. Annual research review: the neurobiology and physiology of resilience and adaptation across the life course. *J. Child Psychol. Psychiat.* 54:337–347, 2013.

Kellner, R. Psychosomatic syndromes, somatization and somatoform disorders. *Psychother. Psychosom.* 61:4–24, 1994.

Krishnan, V. Defeating the fear: new insights into the neurobiology of stress susceptibility. *Exp. Neurol.* 261:412–416, 2014.

Liston, C., et al. Stress-induced alterations in prefrontal cortical dendritic morphology predict selective impairments in attentional set-shifting. *J. Neurosci.* 26:7870–7874, 2006.

Liston, C., et al. Psychosocial stress reversibly disrupts prefrontal processing and attentional control. *Proc. Natl. Acad. Sci. USA* 106:912–917, 2009.

McEwen, B., Wingfield, J.C. What is in a name? Integrating homeostasis, allostasis and stress. *Hormon. Behav.* 57:105–111, 2010.

Miller, G., et al. Health psychology: developing biologically plausible models linking the social world and physical health. *Annu. Rev. Psychol.* 60:501–524, 2009.

Rief, W., Barsky, A.J. Psychobiological perspectives on somatoform disorders. *Psychoneuroendocrinology* 30:996–1002, 2005.

Segerstrom, S.Z. Optimism and immunity: do positive thoughts always lead to positive effects? *Brain Behav. Immun.* 19:195–200, 2005.

Shariff, A.F., Tracy, J.L. What are emotion expressions for? *Curr. Dir. Psychol. Sci.* 20:395–399, 2011.

Sousa, N., Almeida, O.F.X. Disconnection and reconnection: the morphological basis of (mal)adaptation to stress. *Trends Neurosci.* 35:742–751, 2012.

Steptoe, A., et al. Positive affect and health-related neuroendocrine, cardiovascular, and inflammatory processes. *Proc. Natl. Acad. Sci. USA* 102:6508–6512, 2005.

Thayer, J.F., Brosschat, J.F. Psychosomatics and psychopathology: looking up and down from the brain. *Psychoneuroendocrinology* 30:1050–1058, 2005.

Ursin, H., Eriksen, H.R. The cognitive activation theory of stress. *Psychoneuroendocrinology* 29:567–592, 2004.

Wu, G. Understanding resilience. *Front. Behav. Neurosci.* 7:10. doi:10.3389/fnbeh.2013.00010, 2013.

Zhou, Q., et al. Central and peripheral hypersensitivity in the irritable bowel syndrome. *Pain* 148:454–461, 2010.

Chapter 31: The Amygdala and Other Neuronal Groups With Relation to Emotion

Barrett, L.F., Satpute, A.B. Large-scale brain networks in affective and social neuroscience: towards an integrative functional architecture of the brain. *Curr. Opin. Neurobiol.* 23:361–372, 2013.

Dalgleish, T., et al. Affective neuroscience: past, present, and future. *Emotion Rev.* 1:355–368, 2009.

Damasio, A. Toward a neurobiology of emotion and feeling: operational concepts and hypotheses. *Neuroscientist* 1:19–25, 1995.

Davidson, R.J., Irwin, W. The functional neuroanatomy of emotion and affective style. *Trends Cogn. Sci.* 3:11–21, 1999.

Davidson, R.J., Sutton, S.K. Affective neuroscience: the emergence of a discipline. *Curr. Opin. Neurobiol.* 5:217–224, 1995.

Dijksterhuis, A. Think different: the merits of unconscious thought in preference development and decision making. *J. Person. Social Psychol.* 87:586–598, 2004.

Ekman, P. Expression and the nature of emotion. In: Scherer, K.R., Ekman, P. (Eds.), *Approaches to emotion* (pp. 319–343). Mahwah, NJ: Lawrence Erlbaum, 1984.

Ekman, P. Facial expression and emotion. *Am. Psychologist* 48:376–379, 1993.

Grossman, S.P. Behavioral functions of the septum: a reanalysis. In: DeFrance, J.F. (Ed.), *The septal nuclei* (pp. 361–422). New York: Plenum Press, 1976.

Hamman, S. Mapping discrete and dimensional emotions onto the brain: controversies and consensus. *Trends Cogn. Sci.* 458–466, 2012.

LaBar, K.S., Cabeza R. Cognitive neuroscience of emotional memory. *Nat. Rev. Neurosci.* 7:54–64, 2006.

LeDoux, J.E. Emotion circuits in the brain. *Annu. Rev. Neurosci.* 23:155–184, 2000.

LeDoux, J.E. Rethinking the emotional brain. *Neuron* 73:653–676, 2012.

Papez, J.W. A proposed mechanism for emotion. *Arch. Neurol.* 38:725–743, 1937.

Pessoa, L. On the relationship between emotion and cognition. *Nat. Rev. Neurosci.* 9:148–158, 2008.

Phan, K.L., et al. Functional neuroanatomy of emotion: a meta-analysis of emotion activation studies in PET and fMRI. *NeuroImage* 16:331–348, 2002.

Price, J.L., Drevets, W.C. Neural circuits underlying the pathophysiology of mood disorders. *Trends Cogn. Sci.* 16:61–71, 2012.

Rolls, E.T. *The brain and emotion.* Oxford: Oxford University Press, 1999.

Amygdala

Adolphs, R. Fear, faces, and the human amygdala. *Curr. Opin. Neurobiol.* 18:166–172, 2008.

Adolphs, R., et al. A mechanism for impaired fear recognition after amygdala damage. *Nature* 433:68–72, 2005.

Alvarez, R.P., et al. Contextual fear conditioning in humans: cortical-hippocampal and amygdala contributions. *J. Neurosci.* 28:6211–6219, 2008.

Anderson, A.K., Phelps, E.A. Is the human amygdala critical for the subjective experience of emotion? Evidence of intact dispositional affect in patients with amygdala lesions. *J. Cogn. Neurosci.* 14:709–720, 2002.

Bancaud, J., et al. Anatomical origin of *déjà vu* and vivid "memories" in human temporal lobe epilepsy. *Brain* 117:71–90, 1994.

Barrett, L.F., et al. The experience of emotion. *Annu. Rev. Psychol.* 58:373–403, 2007.

Bauman, M.D., et al. The development of mother–infant interactions after neonatal amygdala lesions in rhesus monkeys. *J. Neurosci.* 21:711–721, 2004.

Bechara, A., et al. Different contributions of the human amygdala and ventromedial prefrontal cortex to decision-making. *J. Neurosci.* 19:5473–5481, 1999.

Bergado, J.A., et al. Emotional tagging—a simple hypothesis in a complex reality. *Progr. Neurobiol.* 94:64–76, 2011.

Bernard, J.F., et al. Nucleus centralis of the amygdala and the globus pallidus ventralis: electrophysiological evidence for an involvement in pain processes. *J. Neurophysiol.* 68:551–569, 1992.

Berton, O., Nestler, E.J. New approaches to antidepressant drug discovery: beyond monoamines. *Nat. Rev. Neurosci.* 7:137–151, 2006.

Buchanan, T.W., et al. Emotional autobiographical memories in amnesic patients with temporal lobe damage. *J. Neurosci.* 25:3151–3160, 2005.

Callagher, M., Schoenbaum, G. Functions of the amygdala and related forebrain areas in attention and cognition. *Ann. NY Acad. Sci.* 877:397–411, 1999.

Costafreda, S.G., et al. Predictors of amygdala activation during the processing of emotional stimuli: a meta-analysis of 385 PET and fMRI studies. *Brain Res. Rev.* 58:57–70, 2008.

Dapretto, M., et al. Understanding emotions in others: mirror neuron dysfunction in children with autism spectrum disorders. *Nat. Neurosci.* 9:28–30, 2006.

Heilig, M., et al. Corticotropin-releasing factor and neuropeptide Y: role in emotional integration. *Trends Neurosci.* 17:80–85, 1994.

Heimburger, R.F., et al. Stereotactic amygdalotomy for convulsive and behavioral disorders. *Appl. Neurophysiol.* 41:43–51, 1978.

Herry, C., et al. Switching on and off fear by distinct neuronal circuits. *Nature* 454:600–608, 2008.

Holland, P.C., Callagher, M. Amygdala circuitry in attentional and representational processes. *Trends Cogn. Sci.* 3:65–73, 1999.

Hooker, C.I., et al. Amygdala response to facial expressions reflects emotional learning. *J. Neurosci.* 26:8915–8922, 2006.

Jacobson, R. Disorders of facial recognition, social behaviour and affect after combined bilateral amygdalotomy and subcaudate tractotomy: a clinical and experimental study. *Psychol. Med.* 16:439–450, 1986.

Kalin, N.H., et al. The role of the central nucleus of the amygdala in mediating fear and anxiety in the primate. *J. Neurosci.* 24:5506–5515, 2004.

Klavir, O., et al. Functional connectivity between amygdala and cingulate cortex for adaptive aversive learning. *Neuron* 80:1290–1300, 2013.

Korpelainen, J.T., et al. Asymmetrical skin temperature in ischemic stroke. *Stroke* 26:1543–1547, 1995.

LaLumiere, R.T. Optogenic dissection of amygdala functioning. *Front. Behav.Neurosci.* 8:107. doi:10.3389/fnbeh.2014.00107, 2014.

LeDoux, J.E. Emotion: clues from the brain. *Annu. Rev. Psychol.* 46:209–235, 1995.

Machado, C.J., et al. Bilateral neurotoxic amygdala lesions in rhesus monkeys (*Macaca mulatta*): consistent pattern of behavior across different social contexts. *Behav. Neurosci.* 122:251–266, 2008.

McDonald, A.J. Cortical pathways to the mammalian amygdala. *Prog. Neurobiol.* 55:257–332, 1998.

Morrison, S.E., Salzman, C.D. Re-valuing the amygdala. *Curr. Opin. Neurobiol.* 20:221–230, 2010.

Murray, E.A. The amygdala, reward, and emotion. *Trends Cogn. Sci.* 11:490–497, 2007.

Narabayashi, H., et al. Stereotactic amygdalectomy for behavior disorders. *Arch. Neurol.* 9:11–26, 1963.

Ono, T., et al. Amygdala role in associative learning. *Prog. Neurobiol.* 46:401–422, 1995.

Ousdal, O.A., et al. The human amygdala is involved in general behavioral relevance detection: evidence from an event-related functional magnetic resonance imaging go-nogo task. *Neuroscience* 156:450–455, 2008.

Paton, J.J., et al. The primate amygdala represents the positive and negative value of visual stimuli during learning. *Nature* 439:865–870, 2006.

Phelps, E.A. Human emotion and memory: interactions of the amygdala and hippocampal complex. *Curr. Opin. Neurobiol.* 14:198–202, 2004.

Pitkänen, A., et al. Intrinsic connections of the rat amygdaloid complex: projections originating in the lateral nucleus. *J. Comp. Neurol.* 356:288–310, 1995.

Rich, E.L., Wallis, J.D. Prefrontal-amygdala interactions underlying value coding. *Neuron* 80:1344–1346, 2013.

Roozendaal, B., et al. Stress, memory, and the amygdala. *Nat. Rev. Neurosci.* 10:423–433, 2009.

Schafe, G.E., et al. Tracking the fear engram: the lateral amygdala is an essential locus of fear memory. *J. Neurosci.* 25:10010–10015, 2005.

Schiller, D., Johansen, J. Prelimbic prefrontal neurons drive fear expression: a clue for extinction–reconsolidation interactions. *J. Neurosci.* 29:13432–13434, 2009.

Seymour, B., Dolan, R. Emotion, decision making, and the amygdala. *Neuron* 58:662–671, 2008.

Shaikh, M.B., et al. Basal amygdaloid facilitation of midbrain periaq-ueductal gray elicited defensive rage behavior in the cat mediated trough NMDA receptors. *Brain Res.* 635:187–195, 1994.

Shaw, P., et al. The impact of early and late damage to the human amygdala on "theory of mind" reasoning. *Brain* 127:1535–1548, 2004.

Swanson, L.W., Petrovich, G.D. What is the amygdala? *Trends Neurosci.* 21:323–331, 1998.

Vuilleumier, P. How brains beware: neural mechanisms of emotional attention. *Trends Cogn. Sci.* 9:585–594, 2005.

Young, A.W., et al. Facial expression processing after amygdalotomy. *Neuropsychologia* 34:31–39, 1996.

Cortical Areas Related to Autonomic Functions and Emotions

Adolphs, R. Neural systems for recognition of emotion. *Curr. Opin. Neurobiol.* 12:169–177, 2002.

Allman, J.M., et al. The anterior cingulate cortex: the evolution of an interface between emotion and cognition. *Ann. NY Acad. Sci.* 935:107–117, 2001.

Boksem, M.A.S., Tops, M. Mental fatigue: costs and benefits. *Brain Res. Rev.* 59:125–139, 2008.

Botvinik, M.M., et al. Conflict monitoring and anterior cingulate cortex: an update. *Trends Cogn. Sci.* 8:539–546, 2004.

Bush, G., et al. Dorsal anterior cingulate cortex: a role in reward-based decision making. *Proc. Natl. Acad. Sci. USA* 99:523–528, 2002.

Calder, A.J., et al. Neurospychology of fear and loathing. *Nat. Rev. Neurosci.* 2:352–363, 2001.

Carmichael, S.T., Price, J.L. Limbic connections of the orbital and medial prefrontal cortex in macaque monkeys. *J. Comp. Neurol.* 363:615–641, 1995.

Chu, C.-C., et al. The autonomic-related cortex: pathology in Alzheimer's disease. *Cereb. Cortex* 7:86–95, 1997.

Cohen, R.A., et al. Impairments of attention after cingulotomy. *Neurology* 53:819–824, 1999.

Damasio, A., et al. Persistence of feelings and sentience after bilateral damage of the insula. *Cereb. Cortex* 23:833–846, 2013.

Davis, K.D., et al. Human anterior cingulate cortex neurons encode cognitive and emotional demands. *J. Neurosci.* 25:8402–8406, 2005.

Devinsky, O., et al. Contributions of the anterior cingulate cortex to behavior. *Brain* 118:279–306, 1995.

Engen, H.G., Singer, T. Empathy circuits. *Curr. Opin. Neurobiol.* 23:275–282, 2013.

Gu, X., et al. Anterior insular cortex and emotional awareness. *J. Comp. Neurol.* 521:3371–3388, 2013.

Immordino-Yang, M.H., et al. Neural correlates of admiration and compassion. *Proc. Natl. Acad. Sci. USA* 106:8021–8026, 2009.

Izquierdo, A., et al. Comparison of the effects of bilateral orbital prefrontal cortex lesions and amygdala lesions on emotional responses in rhesus monkeys. *J. Neurosci.* 25:8534–8542, 2005.

Kensinger, E.A. Remembering the details: effects of emotion. *Emotion Rev.* 1:99–113, 2009.

Lamm, C., Singer, T. The role of the anterior insular cortex in social emotions. *Brain Struct. Funct.* 214:579–591, 2010.

Likhtik, E., et al. Prefrontal control of the amygdala. *J. Neurosci.* 25:7429–7437, 2005.

Oppenheimer, S.M., et al. Cardiovascular effects of human insular cortex stimulation. *Neurology* 42:1727–1732, 1992.

Phan, K.L., et al. Functional neuroanatomy of emotion: a meta-analysis of emotion activation studies in PET and fMRI. *NeuroImage* 16:331–348, 2002.

Price, J.L. Prefrontal cortical networks related to visceral function and mood. *Ann. NY Acad. Sci.* 877:383–396, 1999.

Reekie, Y.L., et al. Uncoupling of behavioral and autonomic responses after lesions of the primate orbitofrontal cortex. *Proc. Natl. Acad. Sci. USA* 105:9787–9792, 2008.

Richter, E.O., et al. Cingulotomy for psychiatric disease: microelec-trode guidance, a callosal reference system for documenting lesion location, and clinical results. *Neurosurgery* 54:622–630, 2004.

Roy, M., et al. Ventromedial prefrontal-subcortical systems and the generation of affective meaning. *Trends Cogn. Sci.* 16:147–156, 2012.

Salzman, C.D., Fusi, S. Emotion, cognition, and mental state representation in amygdala and prefrontal cortex. *Annu. Rev. Neurosci.* 33:173–202, 2010.

Vogt, B.A. Pain and emotion interactions in subregions of the cingulate gyrus. *Nat. Rev. Neurosci.* 6:533–544, 2005.

Wager, T.D., et al. Prefrontal-subcortical pathways mediating successful emotion regulation. *Neuron* 59:1037–1050, 2008.

The Basal Forebrain

Adhikari, A. Distributed circuits underlying anxiety. *Front. Behav. Neurosci.* 8:112. doi:10.3389/fnbeh.2014.00112, 2014.

Alheid, G.F., Heimer, L. New perspectives in basal forebrain organization of special relevance for neuropsychiatric disorders: the striatopallidal, amygdaloid, and corticopetal components of substantia innominata. *Neuroscience* 27:1–39, 1988.

Baxter, M.G., Chiba, A.A. Cognitive functions of the basal forebrain. *Curr. Opin. Neurobiol.* 9:178–183, 1999.

de Olmos, J.S., Heimer, L. The concepts of the ventral striatopallidal system and extended amygdala. *Ann. NY Acad. Sci.* 877:1–32, 1999.

Fudge, J.L., Haber, S.N. Bed nucleus of the stria terminalis and the extended amygdala inputs to dopamine subpopulations in primates. *Neuroscience* 104:807–827, 2001.

Ghashghaei, H.T., Barbas, H. Neural interaction between the basal forebrain and functionally distinct prefrontal cortices in the rhesus monkey. *Neuroscience* 103:593–614, 2001.

Gray, T.S. Functional and anatomical relationships among the amygdala, basal forebrain, ventral striatum, and cortex: an integrative discussion. *Ann. NY Acad. Sci.* 877:439–444, 1999.

Hohmann, C.F., Berger-Sweeney, J. Cholinergic regulation of cortical development and plasticity: new twists to an old story. *Perspect. Dev. Neurobiol.* 5:401–425, 1998.

Holland, P.C., Gallagher, M. Differential roles for amygdala central nucleus and substantia innominata in the surprise-induce enhancement of learning. *J. Neurosci.* 26:3791–3797, 2006.

Koob, G.F. The neurocircuitry of addiction: implications for treatment. *Clin. Neurosci. Res.* 5:89–101, 2005.

McLin, D.E. III, et al. Induction of behavioral associative memory by stimulation of the nucleus basalis. *Proc. Natl. Acad. Sci. USA* 99:4002–4007, 2002.

Mesulam, M.M. The cholinergic innervation of the human cerebral cortex. *Progr. Brain Res.* 145:67–78, 2004.

Mesulam, M.M. Cholinergic circuitry of the human nucleus basalis and its fate in Alzheimer's disease. *J. Comp. Neurol.* 521:4124–4144, 2013.

Morris, M.K., et al. Amnesia following a discrete basal forebrain lesion. *Brain* 115:1827–1847, 1992.

Reynolds, S.M., Zahm, D.S. Specificity in the projections of the prefrontal and insular cortex to ventral striatopallidum and the extended amygdala. *J. Neurosci.* 25:11757–11767, 2005.

Selden, N.R., et al. Trajectories of cholinergic pathways within the cerebral hemispheres of the human brain. *Brain* 121:2249–2257, 1998.

Wright, C.I., et al. Basal amygdaloid complex afferents to the rat nucleus accumbens are compartmentally organized. *J. Neurosci.* 16:1877–1893, 1996.

Zaborsky, L., et al. The basal forebrain corticopetal system revisited. *Ann. NY Acad. Sci.* 877:339–367, 1999.

Chapter 32: The Hippocampal Formation: Learning and Memory

Hippocampal Formation

Alvarez, P., et al. Damage limited to the hippocampal region produces long-lasting memory impairment in monkeys. *J. Neurosci.* 15:3796–3807, 1995.

Amaral, D.G. Emerging principles of intrinsic hippocampal organization. *Curr. Opin. Neurobiol.* 3:225–229, 1993.

Andersen, P., et al. Lamellar organization of excitatory hippocampal pathways. *Exp. Brain Res.* 13:222–238, 1971.

Andersen, P., et al. (Eds.) *The hippocampus book.* New York: Oxford University Press, 2006.

Battaglia, F.P., et al. The hippocampus: hub of brain network communication for memory. *Trends Cogn. Sci.* 15:310–318, 2011.

Bear, M.F., Abraham, W.C. Long-term depression in hippocampus. *Annu. Rev. Neurosci.* 19:437–462, 1996.

Bird, C.M., Burgess, N. The hippocampus and memory: insights from spatial processing. *Nat. Rev. Neurosci.* 9:182–194, 2008.

Blatt, G., Rosene, D.L. Organization of direct hippocampal efferent projections to the cerebral cortex of the rhesus monkey. *J. Comp. Neurol.* 392:92–114, 1998.

Buzsáki, G. The hippocampo-neocortical dialogue. *Cereb. Cortex.* 6:81–92, 1996.

Colgin, L.L. Mechanisms and functions of the theta rhythms. *Annu. Rev. Neurosci.* 36:295–312, 2013.

Hafting, T., et al. Microstructure of a spatial map in the entorhinal cortex. *Nature* 436:801–806, 2005.

Holland, P.C., Bouton, M.E. Hippocampus and context in classical conditioning. *Curr. Opin. Neurobiol.* 9:195–202, 1999.

Insausti, R., Amaral, D.G. Hippocampal formation. In: Mai, J.K., Paxinos, G. (Eds.), *The human nervous system*, 3rd ed. (pp. 896–942). San Diego: Elsevier Academic Press, 2012.

Insausti, R., Muños, M. Cortical projections of the non-entorhinal hippocampal formation in the cynomolgus monkey (*Macaca fascicularis*). *Eur. J. Neurosci.* 14:435–451, 2001.

Jacobs, J., et al. Direct recordings of grid-like neuronal activity in human spatial navigation. *Nature Neurosci.* 16:1188–1190, 2013.

Ji, D.M., Wilson, A. Coordinated memory replay in the visual cortex and the hippocampus during sleep. *Nat. Neurosci.* 10:100–107, 2007.

Kentros, C. Hippocampal place cells: the "where" of episodic memory? *Hippocampus* 16:743–754, 2006.

Klintsova, A.Y., Greenough, W.T. Synaptic plasticity in cortical systems. *Curr. Opin. Neurobiol.* 9:203–208, 1999.

Colgin, L.L. Mechanisms and functions of theta rhythms. *Annu. Rev. Neurosci.* 36:295–312, 2013.

Lim, C., et al. Connections of the hippocampal formation in humans: I. The mossy fiber pathway. *J. Comp. Neurol.* 385:325–351, 1997.

Maguire, E.A., et al. Human spatial navigation: cognitive maps, sexual dimorphism, and neuronal substrates. *Curr. Opin. Neurobiol.* 9:171–177, 1999.

Martin, S.J., Clark, R.E. The rodent hippocampus and spatial memory: from synapses to systems. *Cell. Mol. Life Sci.* 64:401–431, 2007.

McNaughton, B.L., et al. Path integration and the neural basis of the "cognitive map." *Nature Rev. Neurosci.* 7:663–678, 2006.

Meunier, M., et al. Effects of rhinal cortex lesions combined with hippocampectomy on visual recognition memory in rhesus monkeys. *J. Neurophysiol.* 75:1190–1205, 1996.

Monteggia, L.M., et al. Essential role of brain-derived neurotrophic factor in adult hippocampal function. *Proc. Natl. Acad. Sci. USA* 101:10827–10832, 2004.

Morris, R.G.M. Elements of a neurobiological theory of hippocampal function: the role of synaptic plasticity, synaptic tagging and schemas. *Eur. J. Neurosci.* 23:2829–2846, 2006.

Moser, E. I., Moser, M.-B. Grid cells and neural coding in high end cortices. *Neuron* 80:765–774, 2013.

Muños, M., Insausti, R. Cortical projections of the entorhinal cortex and the adjacent parahippocampal region in the monkey (*Macaca fascicularis*). *Eur. J. Neurosci.* 14:435–451, 2001.

O'Keefe, J., Nadel, L. *The hippocampus as a cognitive map.* Oxford: Clarendon Press, 1978.

Roman, F.S., et al. Correlations between electrophysiological observations of synaptic plasticity modifications and behavioral performance in mammals. *Prog. Neurobiol.* 58:61–87, 1999.

Saunders, R.C., Aggleton, J.P. Origin and topography of fibers contributing to the fornix in macaque monkeys. *Hippocampus* 17:396–411, 2007.

Shastri, L. Episodic memory and cortico-hippocampal interactions. *Trends Cogn. Sci.*; 6:162–168, 2002.

Suzuki, W.A., Amaral, D.G. Perirhinal and parahippocampal cortices of the macaque monkey: cortical afferents. *J. Comp. Neurol.* 350:497–533, 1994.

Suzuki, W.A., Naya, Y. The perirhinal cortex. *Annu. Rev. Neurosci.* 37:39–53, 2014.

Van Strien, N.M., et al. The anatomy of memory: an interactive overview of the parahippocampal-hippocampal network. *Nat. Rev. Neurosci.* 10:272–282, 2009.

Vinogradova, O.S. Expression, control, and probable functional significance of the neuronal theta-rhythm. *Prog. Neurobiol.* 45:523–583, 1995.

Learning and Memory

Alain, C., et al. A distributed network for auditory sensory memory in humans. *Brain Res.* 812:23–37, 1998.

Alberini, C.M. Mechanisms of memory stabilization: are consolidation and reconsolidation similar processes? *Trends Neurosci.* 28:51–56, 2005.

Baddeley, A. Working memory: theories, models, and controversies. *Annu. Rev. Psychol.* 63:1–29, 2012.

Battaglia, F.P., et al. The hippocampus: hub of brain network communication for memory. *Trends Cogn. Sci.* 15:310–318, 2011.

Baxter, M.G. Involvement of medial temporal lobe structures in memory and perception. *Neuron* 12:667–677, 2009.

Bennett, M.R., Hacker, P.M.S. *Philosophical foundations of neuroscience.* Oxford: Blackwell, 2003.

Binder, J.R., Desai, R.H. The neurobiology of semantic memory. *Trends Cogn. Sci.* 15:527–536, 2011.

Blakemore, S.-J., Frith, U. *The learning brain: lessons for education.* Oxford: Blackwell, 2005.

Buckner, R.L., et al. Frontal cortex contributes to human memory formation. *Nat. Neurosci.* 2:311–314, 1999.

Cabeza, R., et al. Brain regions differentially involved in remembering what and when: a PET study. *Neuron* 19:863–870, 1997.

Cabeza, R., St. Jacques, P. Functional neuroimaging of autobiographical memory. *Trends Cogn. Sci.* 11:219–227, 2007.

Costa-Mattioli, M., et al. Translational control of long-lasting synaptic plasticity and memory. *Neuron* 15:10–26, 2009.

Cowan, N. What are the differences between long-term, short-term and working memory? *Progr. Brain Res.* 169:323-338, 2007.

Damasio, A.R., Tranel, D. Knowledge systems. *Curr. Opin. Neurobiol.* 2:186–190, 1992.

De Haan, M., et al. Human memory development and its dysfunction after early hippocampal injury. *Trends Neurosci.* 29:374–381, 2006.

Düzel, E., et al. Brain oscillations and memory. *Curr. Opin. Neurobiol.* 20:143–149, 2010.

Elgersma, Y., Silva, A.J. Molecular mechanisms of synaptic plasticity and memory. *Curr. Opin. Neurobiol.* 9:209–213, 1999.

Epstein, R.A. Parahippocampal and retrosplenial contributions to human spatial navigation. *Trends Cogn. Sci.* 12:388–396, 2008.

Frackowiak, R.S.J. Functional mapping of verbal memory and language. *Trends Neurosci.* 17:109–114, 1994.

Gaffan, D. Widespread cortical networks underlie memory and attention. *Science* 309:2172–2173, 2005.

Gaffan, D., Parker, A. Mediodorsal thalamic function in scene memory in rhesus monkeys. *Brain* 123:816–827, 2000.

Gilboa, A., et al. Remembering our past: functional neuroanatomy of recollection of recent and very remote personal events. *Cereb. Cortex* 14:1214–1225, 2004.

Hasselmo, M.E., McClelland, J.L. Neural models of memory. *Curr. Opin. Neurobiol.* 9:184–188, 1999.

Howe, M.L. Memory development: implications for adults recalling childhood experiences in the courtroom. *Nature Rev. Neurosci.* 14:869–876, 2013.

Kim, J.J., Baxter, M.G. Multiple memory systems: the whole does not equal the sum of its parts. *Trends Neurosci.* 24:324–330, 2001.

Leutgeb, S., et al. Independent codes for spatial and episodic memory in hippocampal neuronal ensembles. *Science* 309:619–623, 2005.

Lisman, J.E. Relating hippocampal circuitry to function: recall of memory sequences by reciprocal dentate–CA3 interactions. *Neuron* 22:233–242, 1999.

Martin, S.J., et al. Synaptic plasticity and memory: an evaluation of the hypothesis. *Annu. Rev. Neurosci.* 23:649–711, 2000.

Maguire, E.A., et al. London taxi drivers and bus drivers: a structural MRI and neuropsychological analysis. *Hippocampus* 16:1091–1101, 2006.

Mottaghy, F.M., et al. Neuronal correlates of encoding and retrieval in episodic memory during a pair-word association learning task: a functional magnetic resonance imaging study. *Exp. Brain Res.* 128:332–342, 1999.

Nadel, L., Moskowitch, M. The hippocampal complex and long-term memory revisited. *Trends Cogn. Sci.* 5:228–230, 2002.

Nader, K., Hardt, O. A single standard for memory: the case for reconsolidation. *Nat. Rev. Neurosci.* 10:224–234, 2009.

Nee, D.E., et al. Neuroscientific evidence about the distinction between short- and long-term memory. *Curr. Dir. Psychol. Sci.* 17:102–106, 2008.

Neves, G., et al. Synaptic plasticity, memory, and the hippocampus: a neural network approach to causality. *Nat. Rev. Neurosci.* 9:65–75, 2008.

Polyn, S.M., Kahana, M.J. Memory search and the neural representation of context. *Trends Cogn. Sci.* 12:24–30, 2007.

Raymond, C.R. LTP forms 1, 2 and 3: different mechanisms for the "long" in long-term potentiation. *Trends Neurosci.* 30:167–174, 2007.

Schnider, A., Ptak, R. Spontaneous confabulators fail to suppress currently irrelevant memory traces. *Nat. Neurosci.* 2:677–680, 1999.

Shastri, L. Episodic memory and cortico-hippocampal interactions. *Trends Cogn. Sci.* 6:162–168, 2002.

Shrager, Y., et al. Neural basis of the cognitive map: path integration does not require hippocampus or entorhinal cortex. *Proc. Natl. Acad. Sci. USA* 105:12034–12038, 2008.

Stanley, J., Krakauer, J.W. Motor skills depends on knowledge of facts. *Front. Hum.Neurosci.* 7:503. doi:10.3389/fnhum.2013.00503, 2013.

Svoboda, E., et al. The functional neuroanatomy of autobiographical memory: a meta-analysis. *Neuropsychologia* 44:2189–2208, 2006.

Tronson, N.C., Taylor, J.R. Molecular mechanisms of memory consolidation. *Nat. Rev. Neurosci.* 8:262–275, 2007.

Tsivilis, D., et al. A disproportionate role for the fornix and mammillary bodies in recall versus recognition memory. *Nat. Neurosci.* 11:834–842, 2008.

Tulving, E., Markowitsch, H.J. Memory beyond the hippocampus. *Curr. Opin. Neurobiol.* 7:209–216, 1997.

Vann, S.D. Re-evaluating the role of the mammillary bodies in memory. *Neuropsychol.* 48:2316–2327, 2010.

Vargha-Khadem, F., et al. Differential effects of early hippocampal pathology on episodic and semantic memory. *Science* 277:376–380, 1997.

Woolf, N.J. A structural basis for memory storage in mammals. *Prog. Neurobiol.* 55:59–77, 1998.

Amnesia

Aggleton, J.P., et al. Differential cognitive effects of colloid cysts in the third ventricle that spare or compromise the fornix. *Brain* 123:800–815, 2000.

Alvarez, P., et al. Damage limited to the hippocampal region produces long-lasting memory impairment in monkeys. *J. Neurosci.* 15:3796–3807, 1995.

Bayley, P.J., et al. The fate of old memories after medial temporal lobe damage. *J. Neurosci.* 26:13311–13317, 2006.

Cipolotti, L., et al. Long-term retrograde amnesia: the crucial role of the hippocampus. *Neurospsychology* 39:151–172, 2001.

Corkin, S., et al. H.M.'s medial temporal lobe lesion: findings from magnetic resonance imaging. *J. Neurosci.* 17:3964–3979, 1997.

Dusoir, H., et al. The role of diencephalic pathology in human memory disorder: evidence from a penetrating paranasal brain injury. *Brain* 113:1695–1706, 1990.

Eichenbaum, H. What H.M. taught us. *J. Cogn. Neurosci.* 25:14–21, 2012.

Gaffan, D., Gaffan, E.A. Amnesia in man following transection of the fornix. *Brain* 114:2611–2618, 1991.

Gilboa, A., et al. Mechanisms of spontaneous confabulations: a strategic retrieval account. *Brain* 129:1399–1414, 2006.

Harding, A., et al. Degeneration of anterior thalamic nuclei differentiates alcoholics with amnesia. *Brain* 123:141–154, 2000.

Kopelman, M.D. The Korsakoff syndrome. *Br. J. Psychiatry* 166:154–173, 1995.

Mishkin, M., et al. Amnesia and the organization of the hippocampal system. *Hippocampus* 8:212–216, 1998.

Morris, M.K., et al. Amnesia following a discrete basal forebrain lesion. *Brain* 115:1827–1847, 1992.

Schnider, A., Ptak, R. Spontaneous confabulators fail to suppress currently irrelevant memory traces. *Nat. Rev. Neurosci.* 2:677–680, 1999.

Scoville, W.B., Milner, B. Loss of recent memory after bilateral hippocampal lesions. *J. Neurol. Neurosurg. Psychiatry* 20:11–21, 1957.

Stuss, D.T., et al. An extraordinary form of confabulation. *Neurology* 28:1166–1172, 1978.

Zola-Morgan, S., et al. Human amnesia and the medial temporal region: enduring memory impairment following a bilateral lesion limited to field CA1 of the hippocampus. *J. Neurosci.* 6:2950–2967, 1986.

Chapter 33: The Cerebral Cortex: Intrinsic Organization and Connections

Creutzfeldt, O., Creutzfeldt, M. *Cortex cerebri: performance, structural and functional organisation of the cortex.* Oxford: Oxford University Press, 1995.

Rakic, P., Singer, W. *Neurobiology of neocortex.* New York: John Wiley & Sons, 1988.

Zilles, K., Amunts, K. Architecture of the cerebral cortex. In: Mai, J.K., Paxinos, G. (Eds.), *The human nervous system*, 3rd ed. (pp. 836–895). San Diego: Elsevier Academic Press, 2012.

Intrinsic Structure and Physiology

Ainsworth, M., et al. Rates and rhythms: a synergistic view of frequency and temporal coding in neuronal networks. *Neuron* 75:572–583, 2012.

Bear, M.F., Kirkwood, A. Neocortical long-term potentiation. *Curr. Opin. Neurobiol.* 3:197–202, 1993.

Brodmann, K. *Vergleichende lokalisationslehre der Grosshirnrinde.* Leipzig: J.A. Barth, 1909.

Bullmore, E., Sporns, O. The economy of brain network organization. *Nature Rev. Neurosci.* 13:336–349, 2012.

Egger, V., et al. Coincidence detection and changes of synaptic efficacy in spiny stellate neurons in rat barrel cortex. *Nat. Neurosci.* 2:1098–1103, 1999.

Fjell, A.M., et al. Multimodal imaging of the self-regulating developing brain. *Proc. Natl. Acad. Sci. USA* 109:19620–19625, 2012.

Foote, S.L., Morrison, J.H. Extrathalamic modulation of cortical function. *Annu. Rev. Neurosci.* 10:67–95, 1987.

Gilbert, C.D. Horizontal integration and cortical dynamics. *Neuron* 9:1–13, 1992.

Hendry, S.F.C., Jones, E.G. The organization of pyramidal and non-pyramidal cell dendrites in relation to thalamic afferent terminations in the monkey somatic sensory cortex. *J. Neurocytol.* 12:277–298, 1983.

Herculana-Houzel, S., et al. The basic nonuniformity of the cerebral cortex. *Proc. Natl. Acad. Sci. USA* 105:12593–12598, 2008.

Hornung, J.-P., De Tribolet, N. Distribution of GABA-containing neurons in human frontal cortex: a quantitative immunocytochemical study. *Anat. Embryol. (Berl.)* 189:139–145, 1994.

Hutsler, J.J., et al. Individual variation of cortical surface area asymmetries. *Cereb. Cortex* 8:11–17, 1998.

Isaacson, J.S., Scanziani, M. How inhibition shapes cortical activity. *Neuron* 72:231–243, 2011.

Jones, E.G. Anatomy of cerebral cortex: columnar input–output relations. In: Schmidt, F.O., et al. (Eds.), *The cerebral cortex* (pp. 199–235). Cambridge, MA: MIT Press, 1981.

Kanai, R., Rees, G. The structural basis of inter-individual differences in human behaviour and cognition. *Nature Rev. Neurosci.* 12:231–242, 2011.

Klntsova, A.Y., Greeough, W.T. Synaptic plasticity in cortical systems. *Curr. Opin. Neurobiol.* 9:203–208, 1999.

Krnjević, K. Synaptic mechanisms modulated by acetylcholine in cerebral cortex. *Prog. Brain Res.* 145:81–93, 2004.

Kubota, Y. Untangling GABAergic wiring in the cortical microcircuit. *Curr. Opin. Neurobiol.* 26:7–14, 2014.

Larkum, M. A cellular mechanism for cortical associations: an organizing principle for the cerebral cortex. *Trends Neurosci.* 36:141–151, 2013.

Majewska, A.K., Sur, M. Plasticity and specificity of cortical processing networks. *Trends Neurosci.* 29:323–328, 2006.

Markram, H., et al. Interneurons of the neocortical inhibitory system. *Nat. Rev. Neurosci.* 5:793–807, 2004.

McCormick, D.A., et al. Neurotransmitter control of neocortical neuronal activity and excitability. *Cereb. Cortex* 3:387–398, 1993.

Mesulam, M.-M. The cholinergic innervation of the cerebral cortex. *Prog. Brain Res.* 145:67–78, 2004.

Mountcastle, V.B. The columnar organization of the neocortex. *Brain* 120:701–722, 1997.

Parnavelas, J.G., Papadopolous, G.C. The monoaminergic innervation of the cerebral cortex is not diffuse and nonspecific. *Trends Neurosci.* 12:315–319, 1989.

Passingham, R.E., et al. The anatomical basis of functional localization in the cortex. *Nat. Rev. Neurosci.* 3:606–616, 2002.

Penfield, W., Rasmussen, T. *The cerebral cortex of man.* New York: Macmillan, 1950.

Peters, A., Jones, E.G. (Eds.) *Cerebral cortex:* Vol. 1. *Cellular components of the cerebral cortex.* New York: Plenum Press, 1984.

Peters, A., Jones, E.G. (Eds.) *Cerebral cortex:* Vol. 7. *Development and maturation of the cerebral cortex.* New York: Plenum Press, 1988.

Pucak, M.L., et al. Patterns of intrinsic and associational circuitry in monkey prefrontal cortex. *J. Comp. Neurol.* 376:614–630, 1996.

Rakic, P., et al. Decision by division: making cortical maps. *Trends Neurosci.* 32:291–301, 2009.

Ranganath, C., Rainer, G. Neural mechanisms for detecting and remembering novel events. *Nat. Rev. Neurosci.* 4:193–202, 2003.

Rockel, A.J., et al. The basic uniformity in structure of the neocortex. *Brain* 103:221–244, 1980.

Rowland, D.C., Moser, M. B. From cortical modules to memories. *Curr. Opin. Neurobiol.* 24:22–27, 2014.

Šimić, G., Hof, P.R. In search of the definitive Brodmann's map of cortical areas in human. *J. Comp. Neurol.* 523:5–14, 2015.

Uylings, H.B.M. Consequences of large interindividual variability for human brain atlases: converging macroscopical imaging and microscopical neuroanatomy. *Anat. Embryol.* 210:423–431, 2005.

Verhoog, M.B., et al. Mechanisms underlying the rules for associative plasticity at adult human neocortical synapses. *J. Neurosci.* 33:17197–17208, 2013.

Wall, J.T. Variable organization in cortical maps of the skin as an indication of the lifelong adaptive capacities of the circuits in the mammalian brain. *Trends Neurosci.* 11:549–558, 1988.

West, M. Stereological methods for estimating the total number of neurons and synapses: issues of precision and bias. *Trends Neurosci.* 22:51–61, 1999.

Zador, A., Dobrunz, M. Dynamic synapses in the cortex. *Neuron* 19:1–4, 1997.

Zilles, K., Amunts, K. Centenary of Brodmann's map—conception and fate. *Nature Rev. Neurosci.* 11:139–145, 2010.

Thalamus

Benarroch, E.E. Pulvinar: associative role in cortical function and clinical correlations. *Neurology* 84:738–747, 2015.

Briggs, F., Usrey, W.M. Emerging views of corticothalamic function. *Curr. Opin. Neurosci.* 18:403–407, 2008.

Crick, F. Function of the thalamic reticular complex: the searchlight hypothesis. *Proc. Natl. Acad. Sci. USA.* 81:4586–4590, 1984.

Ergenzinger, E.R., et al. Cortically induced thalamic plasticity in the primate somatosensory system. *Nat. Neurosci.* 1:226–229, 1998.

Grieve, K.L., et al. The primate pulvinar nuclei: vision and action. *Trends Neurosci.* 23:35–39, 2000.

Jones, E.G. *The thalamus*, 2nd ed. Cambridge, UK: Cambridge University Press 2007.

Lee Robinson, D., Petersen, S.E. The pulvinar and visual salience. *Trends Neurosci.* 15:127–132, 1992.

Llinás, R.R., et al. Temporal binding via cortical coincidence detection of specific and nonspecific thalamocortical inputs: a voltage dependent dye-imaging study in mouse brain slices. *Proc. Natl. Acad Sci. USA* 99:449–454, 2002.

Macchi, G., Bentivoglio, M. Is the "nonspecific" thalamus still "nonspecific"? *Arch. Ital. Biol.* 137:201–226, 1999.

McAlonan, K., et al. Attentional modulation of thalamic reticular neurons. *J. Neurosci.* 26:4444–4450, 2006.

Miniamimoto, T., et al. Complementary process to response bias in the centromedian nucleus of the thalamus. *Science* 308:1798–1801, 2005.

Mitchell, A.S., et al. Advances in understanding mechanisms of thalamic relays in cognition and behavior. *J. Neurosci.* 34:15340–15346, 2014.

Percheron, G. Thalamus. In: Paxinos, G., Mai, J.K. (Eds.), *The human nervous system*, 2nd ed. (pp. 592–675). Philadelphia: Elsevier Academic Press, 2004.

Pinault, D. The thalamic reticular nucleus: structure, function and concept. *Brain Res. Rev.* 46:1–31, 2004.

Schmid, M.C., et al. Thalamic coordination of cortical communication. *Neuron* 75:551–552, 2012.

Sherman, S.M. Thalamic relays and cortical functioning. *Prog. Brain Res.* 149:107–126, 2005.

Sherman, S.M. The thalamus is more than just a relay. *Curr. Opin. Neurosci.* 17:417–422, 2007.

Sherman, S.M., Guilllery, R.W. *Exploring the thalamus and its role in cortical function.* Cambridge, MA: MIT Press, 2005.

Shipp, S. Pulvinar structure and circuitry in primates. In: Squire, L. (Ed.), *Encyclopedia of neuroscience* (pp. 1233–1244). Philadelphia: Elsevier, 2009.

Trageser, J.C., Keller, A. Reducing the uncertainty: gating of peripheral inputs by the Zona incerta. *J. Neurosci.* 24:8911–8915, 2004.

Wilke, M., et al. Pulvinar inactivation disrupts selection of movement plans. *J. Neurosci.* 30:8650–8659, 2010.

Corticocortical Connections

Chavis, D.A., Pandya, D.N. Further observations on corticofrontal connections in the rhesus monkey. *Brain Res.* 117:369–386, 1976.

Cippoloni, P.B., Pandya, D.N. Cortical connections of the frontoparietal opercular areas in the rhesus monkey. *J. Comp. Neur.* 403:431–458, 1999.

Croxson, P.L., et al. Quantitative investigation of connections of the prefrontal cortex in the human and macaque using probabilistic diffusion tractography. *J. Neurosci.* 28:8854–8866, 2005.

Di Virgilio, G., et al. Cortical regions contributing to the anterior commissure in man. *Exp. Brain Res.* 124:1–7, 1999.

Gong, G., et al. Mapping anatomical connectivity patterns of human cerebral cortex using in vivo diffusion tensor imaging tractography. *Cereb. Cortex.* 19:524–536, 2009.

Jones, E.G., Powell, T.P.S. An anatomical study of converging sensory pathways within the cerebral cortex of the monkey. *Brain* 93:793–820, 1970.

Man, K., et al. Neural convergence and divergence in the mammalian cerebral cortex: from experimental neuroanatomy to functional neuroimaging. *J. Comp. Neurol.* 521:4097–4111, 2013.

Markov, N.T., et al. Anatomy of hierarchy: feedforward and feedback pathways in macaque visual cortex. *J. Comp. Neurol.* 522:225–259, 2014.

Matelli, M., et al. Superior area 6 afferents from the superior parietal lobule in the macaque monkey. *J. Comp. Neurol.* 402:327–352, 1998.

Pandya, D.N., Kuypers, H.G. Cortico-cortical connections in the rhesus monkey. *Brain Res.* 13:13–36, 1969.

Pandya, D.N., Yeterian, E.H. Comparison of prefrontal architecture and connections. *Philos. Trans. R. Soc. Lond. B. Biol. Sci.* 351:1423–1432, 1996.

Petrides, M., Pandya, D.N. The frontal cortex. In: Mai, J., Paxinos, G. (Eds.), *The human nervous system*, 3rd ed. (pp. 988–1011). San Diego: Elsevier Academic Press, 2012.

Pucak, M.L., et al. Patterns of intrinsic and associational circuitry in monkey prefrontal cortex. *J. Comp. Neurol.* 376:614–630, 1996.

Rockland, K.S. Collateral branching of long-distance cortical projections in the monkey. *J. Comp. Neurol.* 521:4112–4123, 2013.

Seltzer, B., Pandya, D.N. Parietal, temporal, and occipital projections to cortex of the superior temporal sulcus in the rhesus monkey: a retrograde tracer study. *J. Comp. Neur.* 343:445–463, 1994.

Van Hoesen, G. The modern concept of association cortex. *Curr. Opin. Neurobiol.* 3:150–154, 1993.

Wang, Z., et al. Understanding structural-functional relationships in the human brain: a large-scale network perspective. *Neuroscientist* 21:290–305, 2015.

Chapter 34: Functions of the Neocortex

Association Areas and Networks

Adolphs, R. Neural systems for recognition of emotion. *Curr. Opin. Neurol.* 12:169–177, 2002.

Berlucchi, G., Aglioti, S. The body in the brain: neural bases of corporeal awareness. *Trends Neurosci.* 20:560–564, 1997.

Blood, A.J., et al. Emotional responses to pleasant and unpleasant music correlate with activity in paralimbic brain regions. *Nat. Neurosci.* 2:382–387, 1998.

Bolz, J., et al. Pharmacological analysis of cortical circuitry. *Trends Neurosci.* 12:292–296, 1989.

Christoff, K., et al. Experience sampling during fMRI reveals default network and executive system contributions to mind wandering. *Proc. Nat. Acad. Sci. USA* 106:8719–8724, 2009.

Cocchi, L., et al. Dynamic cooperation and competition between brain systems during cognitive control. *Trends Cogn. Sci.* 17:493–501, 2013.

Colby, C.L. Action-oriented spatial reference frames in cortex. *Neuron* 20:15–24, 1998.

Deary, I.J. Human intelligence differences: a recent history. *Trends Cogn. Sci.* 5:127–130, 2001.

Diamond, A. Executive functions. *Annu. Rev. Neurosci.* 64:135–168, 2013.

Fair, D.A., et al. The maturing architecture of the brain's default network. *Proc. Natl. Acad. Sci. USA* 105:4028–4032, 2008.

Flint, J. The genetic basis of cognition. *Brain* 122:2015–2031, 1999.

Fox, M.D., et al. The human brain is intrinsically organized into dynamic, anticorrelated functional networks. *Proc. Natl. Acad. Sci. USA* 102:9673–9678, 2005.

Friston, K. Beyond phrenology: what can neuroimaging tell us about distributed circuitry? *Annu. Rev. Neurosci.* 25:221–250, 2002.

Gaffan, D. Widespread cortical networks underlie memory and attention. *Science* 309:2172–2173, 2005.

Gauthier, I., et al. Expertise for cars and birds recruits brain areas involved in face recognition. *Nat. Neurosci.* 3:191–197, 2000.

Gisiger, T., et al. Computational models of association cortex. *Curr. Opin. Neurobiol.* 10:250–259, 2000.

Goldman-Rakic, P.S. Topography of cognition: parallel and distributed networks in primate association cortex. *Annu. Rev. Neurosci.* 11:137–156, 1988.

Gross, C.G., Graziano, M.S.A. Multiple representations of space in the brain. *Neuroscientist* 1:43–50, 1995.

Halder, B., McCormick, D.A. Rapid neocortical dynamics: cellular and network mechanisms. *Neuron* 62:171–189, 2009.

Harrison, B.J., et al. Consistency and functional specialization in the default mode brain network. *Proc. Natl. Acad. Sci. USA* 105:9781–9786, 2008.

Haynes, J.-D., Rees, G. Decoding mental states from brain activity in humans. *Nat. Rev. Neurosci.* 7:523–534, 2006.

Heeger, D.J., Ress, D. What does fMRI tell us about neuronal activity? *Nat. Rev. Neurosci.* 3:142–151, 2002.

Menon, V. Large-scale brain networks and psychopathology: a unifying triple network model. *Trends Cogn. Sci.* 15:483–506, 2011.

Hofmann, W., et al. Executive functions and self-regulation. *Trends Cogn. Sci.* 16:174–180, 2012.

Horwitz, B., et al. Neural modeling, functional brain imaging, and cognition. *Trends Cogn. Sci.* 3:91–98, 1999.

Hummel, F., Gerloff, C. Larger interregional synchrony is associated with greater behavioral success in a complex sensory integration task in humans. *Cereb. Cortex* 15:670–678, 2005.

Libet, B., et al. Control of the transition from sensory detection to sensory awareness in man by the duration of a thalamic stimulus: the cerebral "time-on" factor. *Brain* 114:1731–1757, 1991.

Marois, R., Ivanoff, J. Capacity limits of information processing in the brain. *Trends Cogn. Sci.* 9:296–305, 2005.

Mesulam, M.-M. From sensation to cognition. *Brain* 121:1013–1052, 1998.

Norman, K.A., et al. Beyond mind-reading: multi-voxel pattern analysis of fMRI data. *Trends Cogn. Sci.* 10:424–430, 2006.

Ojeman, G.A., et al. Lessons from the human brain: neuronal activity related to cognition. *Neuroscientist* 4:285–300, 1998.

Owen, A.M. Cognitive planning in humans: neuropsychological, neuroanatomical and neuropharmacological perspectives. *Prog. Neurobiol.* 53:431–450, 1997.

Peron, S., et al. Comprehensive imaging of cortical networks. *Curr. Opin. Neurobiol.* 32:115–123, 2015.

Poldrack, R.A. Can cognitive processes be inferred from neuroimaging data? *Trends Cogn. Sci.* 10:59–63, 2006.

Posner, M.I., Dehaene, S. Attentional networks. *Trends Neurosci.* 17:75–79, 1994.

Rauschecker, J.P., Korte, M. Auditory compensation for early blindness in cat cerebral cortex. *J. Neurosci.* 13:4538–4548, 1993.

Sacks, O. To see and not see. In: Sacks, O., *An anthropologist on Mars* (pp. 102–144). New York: Picador, 1995.

Schindler, I., et al. Neck muscle vibration induces lasting recovery in spatial neglect. *J. Neurol. Neurosurg. Psychiatry* 73:412–419, 2002.

Scharpf, K.R., et al. The brain's relevance detection network operates independently of stimulus modality. *Behav. Brain Res.* 210:16–23, 2010.

Shafi, M.M., et al. Exploration and modulation of brain network interactions with noninvasive brain stimulation in combination with neuroimaging. *Eur. J. Neurosci.* 35:805–825, 2012.

Shammi, P., Stuss, D.T. Humor appreciation: a role of the right frontal lobe. *Brain* 122:657–666, 1999.

Shaw, P., et al. Intellectual ability and cortical development in children and adolescents. *Nature* 440:676–679, 2006.

Singer, W. Neuronal synchrony: a versatile code for the definition of relations? *Neuron* 24:111–125, 1999

Singer, W. Cortical dynamics revisited. *Trends Cogn. Sci.* 17:616–629, 2013.

Smith, S.M., et al. Temporally independent functional modes of spontaneous brain activity. *Proc. Natl. Acad. Sci. USA* 109:3131–3136, 2012.

Sridharan, D., et al. A critical role for the right fronto-insular cortex in switching between central-executive and default-mode networks. *Proc. Nat. Acad. Sci. USA* 105:12569–12574, 2008.

Tovée, M.J. Is face processing special? *Neuron* 21:1239–1242, 1998.

Varela, F., et al. The brainweb: phase synchronization and large scale integration. *Nat. Rev. Neurosci.* 2:251–262, 2001.

Zanto, T.P., Gazzaley, A. Fronto-parietal network: flexible hub of cognitive control. *Trends Cogn. Sci.* 17:602–603, 2013.

Symptoms after Damage to Association Areas

Andersen, R.A., et al. Optic ataxia: from Balint's syndrome to the parietal reach region. *Neuron* 81:967–983, 2014.

Buxbaum, L.J., et al. Critical brain regions for tool-related and imitative actions: a componential analysis. *Brain* 137:1971–1985, 2014.

Committeri, G., et al. Neural bases of personal and extrapersonal neglect in humans. *Brain* 130:431–441, 2007.

Corbetta, M., Shulman, G.L. Spatial neglect and attention networks. *Annu. Rev. Neurosci.* 34:569–599, 2011.

Coslett, H.B. Neglect in vision and visual imagery: a double dissociation. *Brain* 120:1163–1171, 1997.

Farah, M.J. Agnosia. *Curr. Opin. Neurobiol.* 2:162–164, 1992.

Greene, J.D.W. Apraxia, agnosias, and higher visual function abnormalities. *J. Neurol. Neurosurg. Psychiatry* 76(Suppl V):v25–v34, 2005.

Halligan, P.W., et al. Spatial cognition: evidence from visual neglect. *Trends Cogn. Sci.* 7:125–133, 2003.

Konen, C.S., et al. The functional neuroanatomy of object agnosia: a case study. *Neuron* 71:49–60, 2011.

Orfei, M.D., et al. Unawareness of illness in neuropsychiatric disorders: phenomenological certainty versus etiopathogenic vagueness. *Neuroscientist* 14:203–222, 2008.

Petreska, B., et al. Apraxia: a review. *Prog. Brain Res.* 164:61–83, 2007.

Pouget, A., Driver, J. Relating unilateral neglect to the neural coding of space. *Curr. Opin. Neurobiol.* 10:242–249, 2000.

Rafal, R.D. Neglect. *Curr. Opin. Neurobiol.* 4:231–236, 1994.

Ramachandran, V.S. What neurological syndromes can tell us about human nature: some lessons from phantom limbs, Capgras syndrome, and anosognosia. The Dorcas Cummings Lecture. *Cold Spring Harbor Symposia* 61:115–134, 1996.

Roiser, J. What has neuroscience ever done for us? *Psychologist* 28:284–287, 2015.

Rusconi, E., Kleinschmidt, A. Gerstmann's syndrome: where does it come from and what does it tell us? *Fut. Neurol.* 6:23–32, 2010.

Schindler, I., et al. Neck muscle vibration induces lasting recovery in spatial neglect. *J. Neurol. Neurosurg. Psychiatry* 73:412–419, 2002.

Zadikoff, C., Lang, A.E. Apraxia in movement disorders. *Brain* 128:1489–1497, 2005.

Networks and Mental Illness

Abi-Dargam, A., et al. Prefrontal dopamine D1 receptors and working memory in schizophrenia. *J. Neurosci.* 22:3708–3719, 2002.

Altar, C.A. Neurotrophins and depression. *Trends Pharmacol. Sci.* 20:59–62, 1999.

Anderson, S.W., et al. Impairment of social and moral behavior related to early damage in human prefrontal cortex. *Nature Neurosci.* 2:1032–1037, 1999.

Andreasen, N.C. Pieces of the schizophrenia puzzle fall into pieces. *Neuron* 16:697–700, 1996.

Beauregard, M. Mind does really matter: evidence from neuroimaging studies of emotional self-regulation, psychotherapy, and placebo effect. *Prog. Neurobiol.* 81:218–236, 2007.

Belzung, C., et al. Neuropeptides in psychiatric diseases: an overview with particular focus on depression and anxiety disorders. *CNS Neurol. Disord. Drug Targets* 5:135–145, 2006.

Castrén, E. Is mood chemistry? *Nat. Rev. Newurosci.* 6:251–246, 2005.

Cotter, D., et al. Reduced neuronal size and glial cell density in area 9 of the dorsolateral prefrontal cortex in subjects with major depressive disorder. *Cereb. Cortex* 12:386–394, 2002.

Drzyzga, L., et al. Cytokines in schizophrenia and the effects of antipsychotic drugs. *Brain Behav. Immun.* 20:532–545, 2006.

Egan, M.F., Weinberger, D. Neurobiology of schizophrenia. *Curr. Opin. Neurobiol.* 7:701–707, 1997.

Fallon, J.H., et al. The neuroanatomy of schizophrenia: circuitry and neurotransmitter systems. *Clin. Neurosci. Res.* 3:77–107, 2003.

Flint, J., Kendler, K.S. The genetics of major depression. *Neuron* 81:484–503, 2014.

Gogtay, N., et al. Three-dimensional brain growth abnormalities in childhood-onset schizophrenia visualized by using tensor-based morphometry. *Proc. Natl. Acad. Sci. USA* 105:15979–15984, 2008.

Goodwin, F.K. Neurobiology of manic-depressive illness. *Clin. Neurosci.* 1:157–162, 1993.

Hahn, C.-G., et al. Altered neuregulin 1–erbB4 signaling contributes to NMDA receptor hypofunction in schizophrenia. *Nat. Med.* 12:824–828, 2006.

Hariri, A.R., Holmes, A. Genetics of emotional regulation: the role of the serotonin transporter in neural function. *Trends Cogn. Neurosci.* 10:182–191, 2006.

Harrison, P.J. The neuropathology of schizophrenia: a critical review of the data and their interpretation. *Brain* 122:593–624, 1999.

Henn, F.A. Animal models of depression. *Clin. Neurosci.* 1:152–156, 1993.

Kristiansen, L.V., et al. Changes in NMDA receptor subunits and interacting PSD proteins in dorsolateral prefrontal and anterior cingulated cortex indicate abnormal regional expression in schizophrenia. *Mol. Psychiatry* 11:737–747, 2006.

Kuperberg, G., Heckers, S. Schizophrenia and cognitive function. *Curr. Opin. Neurobiol.* 10:205–210, 2000.

Kupfer, D.J., et al. Major depressive disorder: new clinical, neurobiological, and treatment perspectives. *Lancet* 379:1054–1055, 2012.

Lewis, D.A., et al. Cortical inhibitory neurons and schizophrenia. *Nat. Rev. Neurosci.* 6:312–324, 2005.

Linden, D.E.J. The challenges and promise of neuroimaging in psychiatry. *Neuron* 73:8–22, 2012.

Marx, C.E., et al. Neuroactive steroids are altered in schizophrenia and bipolar disorder: relevance to pathophysiology and therapeutics. *Neuropsychopharmacology* 31:1249–1263, 2006.

Narr, K.L., et al. Mapping cortical thickness and gray matter concentrations in first episode of schizophrenia. *Cereb. Cortex* 15:708–719, 2005.

Need, A., Goldstein, D.B. Schizophrenia genetics comes of age. *Neuron* 83:760–763, 2014.

Palaniyappan, L., et al. Neural primacy of the salience processing system in schizophrenia. *Neuron* 79:814–828, 2013.

Rolls, E.T., et al. Computational models of schizophrenia and dopamine modulation in the prefrontal cortex. *Nat. Rev. Neurosci.* 9:696–709, 2008.

Scarr, E., et al. Cortical glutamatergic markers in schizophrenia. *Neuropsychopharmacology* 30:1521–1531, 2005.

Sharp, F.R. Psychosis: pathological activation of limbic thalamocortical circuits by psychomimetics and schizophrenia? *Trends Neurosci.* 24:330–334, 2001.

Sheline, Y.I. Neuroanatomical changes with unipolar major depression. *Neuroscientist* 4:331–334, 1998.

Styner, M., et al. Morphometric analysis of lateral ventricles in schizophrenia and healthy controls regarding genetic and disease-specific factors. *Proc. Natl. Acad. Sci. USA* 102:4872–4877, 2005.

Tost, H., Meyer-Lindenberg, A. Schizophrenia, social environment and the brain. *Nature Med.* 18:211–213, 2012.

Uhlhaas, P.J., Singer, W. Neuronal dynamics and neuropsychiatric disorders: toward a translational paradigm for dysfunctional large-scale networks. *Neuron* 75:963–980, 2012.

Vaidya, V.A., Duman, R.S. Depression: emerging insights from neurobiology. *Br. Med. Bull.* 57:61–79, 2001.

Weinberger, D., et al. Evidence for dysfunction of the prefrontal-limbic network in schizophrenia: a magnetic resonance imaging and regional blood flow study of discordant monozygotic twins. *Am. J. Psychiatry* 149:890–897, 1992.

Parietal Cortex

Andersen, R.A., Bueno, C.A. Intentional maps in posterior parietal cortex. *Annu. Rev. Neurosci.* 25:189–220, 2002.

Beachamp, M.S. See me, hear me, touch me: multisensory integration in lateral occipital-temporal cortex. *Curr. Opin. Neurobiol.* 15:145–153, 2005.

Brannon, E.M. The representation of numerical magnitude. *Curr. Opin. Neurobiol.* 16:222–229, 2006.

Caspers, S., et al. Posterior parietal cortex: mulitmodal association cortex. In: Mai, J., Paxinos, G. (Eds.), *The human nervous system*, 3rd ed. (pp. 1036–1055). San Diego: Elsevier Academic Press, 2012.

Critchley, M. *The parietal lobes.* London: Edward Arnold, 1953.

Desmurget, M., et al. Movement intention after parietal cortex stimulation in humans. *Science* 324:811–813, 2009.

Fogassi, L., et al. Parietal lobe: from action organization to intention understanding. *Science* 308:662–666, 2005.

Gottlieb, J. From thought to action: the parietal cortex as a bridge between perception, action, and cognition. *Neuron* 53:9–16, 2007.

Husain, M., Nachev, P. Space and the parietal cortex. *Trends Cogn. Sci.* 11:30–36, 2006.

Hyvärinen, J. *The parietal cortex of monkey and man.* New York: Springer-Verlag, 1982.

Iriki, A. The neural origins and implications of imitation, mirror neurons ans tool use. *Curr. Opin. Neurobiol.* 16:660–667, 2006.

Luria, A.R. *The man with a shattered world.* Cambridge, MA: Harvard University Press, 1987.

Matshashi, M., Hallett, M. The timing of the conscious intention to move. *Eur. J. Neurosci.* 28:2344–2351, 2008.

Medendorp, W.P., et al. Parietofrontal circuits in goal-directed behavior. *Eur. J. Neurosci.* 33:2017–2027, 2011.

Mountcastle, V.B., et al. Posterior parietal association cortex of the monkey: command functions for operations within extrapersonal space. *J. Neurophysiol.* 38:871–908, 1975.

Rizzolatti, G., Fabbri-Destro, M. The mirror system and its role in social cognition. *Curr. Opin. Neurobiol.* 18:179–184, 2008.

Romo, R., de Lafuente, V. Conversion of sensory signals into perceptual decisions. *Progr. Neurobiol.* 103:41–75, 2013.

Sack, A.T. Parietal cortex and spatial cognition. *Behav. Brain Res.* 202:153–161, 2009.

Sereno, M.I., Huang, R.-S. Multisensory maps in the parietal cortex. *Curr. Opin. Neurobiol.* 24:39–46, 2014.

Shadlen, M.N., Newsome, W.T. Neural basis of a perceptual decision in the parietal cortex (area LIP) of the rhesus monkey. *J. Neurophysiol.* 86:1916–1936, 2001.

Texeira, S., et al. Integrative parietal cortex processes: neurological and psychiatric aspects. *J. Neurol. Sci.* 338:12–22, 2014.

Vandeberghe, R., Gillebert, C.R. Parcellation of parietal cortex: convergence between lesion-symptom mapping and mapping of the intact functioning brain. *Behav. Brain Res.* 199:171–182, 2009.

Wheaton, L., et al. Synchronization of parietal and premotor areas during preparation and execution of praxis hand movements. *Clin. Neurophysiol.* 116:1382–1390, 2005.

Wilke, M., et al. Functional imaging reveals rapid reorganization of cortical activity after parietal inactivation in monkeys. *Proc. Nat. Acad. Sci. USA* 109:8274–8279, 2012.

Prefrontal Cortex

Amodio, D.M., Frith, C.D. Meeting of minds: the medial frontal cortex and social cognition. *Nat. Rev. Neurosci.* 7:268–277, 2006.

Anderson, S.W., et al. Impairment of social and moral behavior related to early damage in human prefrontal cortex. *Nat. Neurosci.* 2:1032–1037, 1999.

Badre, D. Cognitive control, hierarchy, and the rostro-caudal organization of the frontal lobes. *Trends Cogn. Sci.* 12:193–200, 2008.

Brass, M., Haggard, P. The what, when, whether model of intentional action. *Neuroscientist* 14:319–325, 2008.

Engen, H.G., Singer, T. Empathy circuits. *Curr. Opin. Neurobiol.* 23:275–282, 2013.

Fletcher, P.C., Henson, R.N.A. Frontal lobes and human memory: insights from functional neuroimaging. *Brain* 124:849–881, 2001.

Frith, C.D., Frith, U. Mechanisms of social cognition. *Annu. Rev. Psychol.* 63:287–313, 2011.

Gehring, W.J., Fencsik, D.E. Functions of the medial frontal cortex in the processing of conflict and errors. *J. Neurosci.* 21:9430–9437, 2001.

Genovesio, A., et al. Prefrontal-parietal function: from foraging to foresight. *Trends Cogn. Sci.* 18:72–81, 2014.

Gray, J.R., Thompson, P.M. Neurobiology of intelligence: science and ethics. *Nat. Rev. Neurosci.* 5:471–482, 2004.

Haggard, P. Decision time for free will. *Neuron* 69:404–406, 2011.

Hauser, M.D. Perseveration, inhibition and the prefrontal cortex: a new look. *Curr. Opin. Neurobiol.* 9:214–222, 1999.

Hein, G., Singer, T. I feel how you feel but not always: the emphatic brain and its modulation. *Curr. Opin. Neurobiol.* 18:153–158, 2008.

Jeon, H.-A., Friederici, D.A. Degree of automaticity and the prefrontal cortex. *Trends Cogn. Sci.* 19:244–250, 2015.

Koster-Hale, J., Saxe, R. Theory of mind: a neural prediction problem. *Neuron* 79:836–848, 2013.

Mansouri, F.A., et al. Conflict-induced behavioural adjustment: a clue to the executive functions of the prefrontal cortex. *Nat. Rev. Neurosci.* 10:141–152, 2009.

Miller, E.K. The prefrontal cortex: complex neural properties for complex behavior. *Neuron* 22:15–17, 1999.

Munakata, Y., et al. A unified framework for inhibitory control. *Trend Cogn. Sci.* 15:453–459, 2011.

Price, J.L. Prefrontal cortical networks related to visceral function and mood. *Ann. NY Acad. Sci.* 877:383–396, 1999.

Procyk, E., Goldman-Rakic, P.M. Modulation of dorsolateral prefrontal delay activity during self-organized behavior. *J. Neurosci.* 26:11313–1323, 2006.

Ramnani, N., Owen, A.M. Anterior prefrontal cortex: insights into function from anatomy and neuroimaging, *Nat. Rev. Neurosci.* 5:184–194, 2004.

Roberts, A.C. Primate orbitofrontal cortex and adaptive behaviour. *Trends Cogn. Sci.* 10:83–90, 2006.

Rolls, E.T., Grabenhorst, F. The orbitofrontal cortex: from affect to decision-making. *Prog. Neurobiol.* 86:216–244, 2008.

Rossi, A.F., et al. The prefrontal cortex and the executive control of attention. *Exp. Brain Res.* 192:489–497, 2009.

Roy, M., et al. Ventromedial prefrontal-subcortical systems and the generation of affective meaning. *Trends Cogn. Sci.* 16:147–156, 2012.

Sakagami, M., Pan, X. Functional role of the ventrolateral prefrontal cortex in decision making. *Curr. Opin. Neurobiol.* 17:228–233, 2007.

Seitz, R.J., et al. Value judgment and self-control of action: the role of the medial frontal action. *Brain Res. Rev.* 60:368–378, 2009.

Shammi, P., Stuss, D.T. Humor appreciation: a role of the right frontal lobe. *Brain* 122:657–666, 1999.

Stoet, G., Snyder, L.H. Neural correlates of executive control functions in the monkey. *Trends Cogn. Sci.* 13:228–234, 2009.

Teffer, K., Semendeferi, K. Human prefrontal cortex: evolution, development, and pathology. *Progr. Brain Res.* 195:191–218, 2012.

Thompson-Schill, S.L., et al. The frontal lobes and the regulation of mental activity. *Curr. Opin. Neurobiol.* 15:219–224, 2005.

Tsujimoto, S., et al. Frontal pole cortex: encoding ends at the end of the endbrain. *Trends Cogn. Sci.* 15:169–176, 2011.

Vendetti, M.S., Bunge, S.A. Evolutionary and developmental changes in the lateral frontoparietal network: a little goes a long way for higher-level cognition. *Neuron* 84:906–917, 2014.

Wallis, J.D., et al. Single neurons in prefrontal cortex encode abstract rules. *Nature* 411:953–956, 2001.

White, I.M., Wise, S.P. Rule-dependent neuronal activity in the prefrontal cortex. *Exp. Brain Res.* 126:315–335, 1999.

Wilson, C.R.E., et al. Functional localization within the prefrontal cortex: missing the forest for the trees? *Trends Neurosci.* 33:533–540, 2010.

Temporal Cortex

Barnes, C.L., Pandya, D.N. Efferent cortical connections of multi-modal cortex of the superior temporal sulcus in the rhesus monkey. *J. Comp. Neur.* 318:222–244, 1992.

Beachamp, M.S. See me, hear me, touch me: multisensory integration in lateral occipital-temporal cortex. *Curr. Opin. Neurobiol.* 15:145–153, 2005.

Binder, J.B., et al. Where is the semantic system? A critical review and meta-analysis of 120 functional neuroimaging studies. *Cereb. Cortex* 19:2767–2796, 2009.

Carr, L., et al. Neural mechanisms for empathy in humans: a relay from neural systems for imitation to limbic areas. *Proc. Natl. Acad. Sci. USA* 100:5497–5501, 2003.

Farrer, C., et al. Modulating the experience of agency: a positron emission tomographic study. *NeuroImage* 18:324–333, 2003.

Gauthier, I., et al. Expertise for cars and birds recruits brain areas involved in face recognition. *Nat. Neurosci.* 3:191–197, 2000.

Grill-Spector, K., Weiner, K.S. The functional architecture of the ventral temporal cortex and its role in categorization. *Nature Rev. Neurosci.* 15:536–548, 2014.

Haxby, J.V., et al. Distributed and overlapping representations of faces and objects in ventral temporal cortex. *Science* 293:2425–2430, 2001.

Insausti, R. Comparative neuroanatomical parcellation of the human and the non-human temporal pole. *J. Comp. Neurol.* 521:4163–4176, 2013.

Klüver, H., Bucy, P.C. Psychic blindness and other symptoms following bilateral temporal lobectomy in rhesus monkeys. *Am. J. Physiol.* 119:352–353, 1937.

Levy, D.A., et al. The anatomy of semantic knowledge: medial vs. lateral temporal lobe. *Proc. Natl. Acad. Sci. USA* 101:6710–6715, 2004.

Messinger, A., et al. Neuronal representations of stimulus associations develop in the temporal lobe during learning. *Proc. Natl. Acad. Sci. USA* 98:12239–12244, 2001.

Olson, I.R., et al. The enigmatic temporal pole: a review of findings on social and emotional processing. *Brain* 130:1718–1731, 2007.

Schwarzlose, R.F., et al. Separate face and body selectivity on the fusiform gyrus. *J. Neurosci.* 23:11055–11059, 2005.

Tovée, M.J. Is face processing special? *Neuron* 21:1239–1242, 1998.

Insula

Afif, A., et al. Anatomofunctional organization of the insular cortex: a study using intracerebral electrical stimulation in epileptic patients. *Epilepsia* 51:2305–2315, 2010.

Augustine, J.R. Circuitry and functional aspects of the insular lobe in primates including humans. *Brain Res. Rev.* 22:229–244, 1996.

Baumgärtner, U., et al., Laser-evoked potentials are graded and somatotopically organized anteroposteriorly in the operculoinsular cortex of anesthetized monkeys. *J. Neurophysiol.* 96:2802–2808, 2006.

Craig, A.D. How do you feel now? The anterior insula and human awareness. *Nat. Rev. Neurosci.* 10:59–70, 2009.

Critchley, H.D., et al. Neural systems supporting interoceptive awareness. *Nat. Rev. Neurosci.* 7:189–195, 2004.

Damasio, A., et al. Persistence of feelings and sentience after bilateral damage of the insula. *Cereb. Cortex* 23:833–846, 2013.

Gallay, D.S., et al. The insula of Reil revisited: multiarchitectonic organization in macaque monkeys. *Cereb. Cortex.* 22:175–190, 2012.

Gu, X., et al. Anterior insular cortex and emotional awareness. *J. Comp. Neurol.* 521:3371–3388, 2013.

Harrison, N.A., et al. Neural origins of human sickness in interoceptive responses to inflammation. *Biol. Psychiat.* 66:415–422, 2009.

Jones, C.L., et al. The neuropsychological impact of insular cortex lesions. *J. Neurol. Neurosurg. Psychiatry* 81:611–618, 2010.

Karnath, H.O., et al. Awareness of the functioning of one's own limbs mediated by the insular cortex? *J. Neurosci.* 25:7134–7138, 2005.

Lovero, K.L., et al. Anterior insular cortex anticipates impending stimulus significance. *NeuroImage* 45:976–983, 2009.

Naqvi, N.H., et al. Damage to the insula disrupts addiction to cigarette smoking. *Science* 315:531–534, 2007.

Nieuwenhuys, R. The insular cortex: a review. *Progr. Brain Res.* 195:123–163, 2012.

Ostrowsky, K., et al. Representation of pain and somatic sensation in the human insula: a study of responses to direct electrical cortical stimulation, *Cereb. Cortex* 12:376–385, 2002.

Language and Music

Bavelier, D., et al. Brain and language: a perspective from sign language. *Neuron* 21:275–278, 1998.

Belin, P., et al. Recovery from nonfluent aphasia after melodic intonation therapy: a PET study. *Neurology* 47:1504–1511, 1996.

Bookheimer, S. Functional MRI of language: new approaches to understanding the cortical organization of semantic processing. *Annu. Rev. Neurosci.* 25:151–188, 2002.

Brust, J.C.M. Music and language: musical alexia and agraphia. *Brain* 103:367–392, 1980.

Crinion, J., et al. Language control in the bilingual brain. *Science* 312:1537–1540, 2006.

Dehaene-Lambertz, G., et al. Nature and nurture in language acquisition: anatomical and functional brain-imaging studies in infants. *Trends Neurosci.* 29:367–373, 2006.

Evers, S., et al. The cerebral haemodynamics of music perception: a transcranial Doppler sonography study. *Brain* 122:75–85, 1999.

Feredoes, E., et al. The neural bases of the short-term storage of verbal information are anatomically variable across individuals. *J. Neurosci.* 27:11003–11008, 2007.

Fiez, J.A. Sound and meaning: how native language affects reading strategies. *Nat. Rev. Neurosci.* 3:3–5, 2000.

Friederici, A.D. The brain basis of language processing: from structure to function. *Physiol. Rev.* 91:1357–1392, 2011.

Friederici, A.D., Gierhan, S.M.E. The language network. *Curr Opin. Neurobiol.* 23:250–254, 2013.

Geranmayeh, F., et al. Overlapping networks engaged during spoken language production and its cognitive control. *J. Neurosci.* 34:8728–8740, 2014.

Geva, S., et al. The neural correlates of inner speech defined by voxel-based lesion-symptom mapping. *Brain* 134: 3071–3082, 2011.

Greenfield, P.M. Language, tools and brain: the ontogeny and phylogeny of hierarchially organized sequential behavior. *Behav. Brain Sci.* 14:531–595, 1991.

Hagoort, P. On Broca, brain, and binding: a new framework. *Trends Cogn. Sci.* 9:416–423, 2005.

Halpern, A.R., Zatorre, R.J. When that tune runs through your head: a PET investigation of auditory imagery for familiar melodies. *Cereb. Cortex* 9:697–704, 1999.

Hannon, E.E., Trainor, L.J. Music acquisition: effects of enculturation and formal training on development. *Trends Cogn. Sci.* 11:466–472, 2007.

Hickok, G., Poeppel, D. The cortical organization of speech processing. *Nat. Rev. Neurosci.* 8:393–402, 2007.

Hinke, R.M., et al. Functional magnetic resonance imaging of Broca's area during internal speech. *NeuroReport* 4:675–678, 1993.

Howard, D., et al. The cortical localization of the lexicons: positron emission tomography evidence. *Brain* 115:1769–1782, 1992.

Koelsch, S. Brain correlates of music-evoked emotions. *Nature Rev. Neurosci.* 15:170–180, 2014.

Koelsch, S., Siebel, W.A. Towards a neural basis of music perception. *Trends Cogn. Sci.* 9:578–584, 2005.

Kuhl, P.K. Early language acquisition: cracking the speech code. *Nat. Rev. Neurosci.* 5:831–843, 2004.

Lecours, A.R., et al. *Aphasiology*. London: Bailliere Tindall, 1983.

Leitman, D.L. "It's not what you say, but how you say it": a reciprocal temporo-frontal network for affective prosody. *Front. Hum. Neurosci.* 4:19. doi:10.3389/fnhum.2010.00019, 2010.

Levithin, D.L. What does it mean to be musical? *Neuron* 73:633–637, 2012.

Lotto, A.J., et al. Reflections on mirror neurons and speech perception. *Trends Cogn. Sci.* 13:110–114, 2008.

Nobre, A.C., Plunkett, K. The neural system of language: structure and development. *Curr. Opin. Neurobiol.* 7:262–268, 1997.

Onishi, T., et al. Functional anatomy of musical perception in musicians. *Cereb. Cortex* 11:754–760, 2001.

Patterson, K., Ralph, M.A.L. Selective disorders of reading? *Curr. Opin. Neurobiol.* 9:235–239, 1999.

Pell, M.D. Judging emotion and attitudes from prosody following brain damage. *Prog. Brain Res.* 156:303–315, 2006.

Penfield, W., Roberts, L. *Speech and brain mechanisms*. Princeton, NJ: Princeton University Press, 1959.

Price, C.J. The functional anatomy of word comprehension and production. *Trends Cogn. Sci.* 2:281–288, 1998.

Pulvermüller, F. Brain mechanisms linking language and action. *Nat. Rev. Neurosci.* 6:576–582, 2005.

Sammler, D., et al. Prosody meets syntax: the role of the corpus callosum. *Brain* 133:2643–2655, 2010.

Schirmer, A., Kotz, S.A. Beyond the right hemisphere: brain mechanisms mediating vocal emotional processing. *Trends Cogn. Sci.* 10:24–30, 2006.

Schuppert, M., et al. Receptive amusia: evidence for cross-hemispheric networks underlying music processing strategies. *Brain* 123:546–559, 2000.

Sergent, J. Music, the brain and Ravel. *Trends Neurosci.* 16:168–172, 1993.

Shalom, D.B., Poeppel, D. Functional anatomic models of language: assembling the pieces. *Neuroscientist* 14:119–127, 2008.

Springer, J.A., et al. Language dominance in neurologically normal and epilepsy subjects: a functional MRI study. *Brain* 122:2033–2045, 1999.

Stewart, L., et al. Music and the brain: disorder of musical listening. *Brain* 129:2533–2553, 2006.

Trost, W., et al. Mapping aesthetic musical emotions in the brain. *Cereb. Cortex* 22:2769–2783, 2012.

Weiskrantz, L. *Thought without language*. Oxford: Oxford University Press, 1988.

Willems, R.M., Hagoort, P. Neural evidence for the interplay between language, gesture, and action: a review. *Brain. Lang.* 101:278–289, 2007.

Willmes, K., Poeck, K. To what extent can aphasic syndromes be localized? *Brain* 116:1527–1540, 1993.

Woods, B.T. Is the left hemisphere specialized for language at birth? *Trends Neurosci.* 6:115–117, 1983.

Zatorre, R.J., Salimpoor, V.N. From perception to pleasure: music and its neural substrates. *Proc. Nat. Acad. Sci. USA* 110:10430–10437, 2013.

Corpus Callosum and Lateralization

Annett, M. Cerebral asymmetry in twins: predictions of the right shift theory. *Neuropsychology* 41:469–479, 2003.

Bryden, M.P., et al. Handedness is not related to self-reported disease incidence. *Cortex* 27:605–611, 1991.

Canli, T. Hemispheric asymmetry in the experience of emotion: a perspective from functional imaging. *Neuroscientist* 5:201–207, 1999.

Catani, M., ffytche, D.H. The rises and falls of disconnection syndromes. *Brain* 128:2224–2239, 2005.

Corballis, M.C. Lateralization of the human brain. *Progr. Brain Res.* 195:103–121, 2012.

Davidson, R.J. Hemispheric asymmetry and emotion. In: Scherer, K.R., Ekman, P. (Eds.), *Approaches to emotion* (pp. 39–57). Mahwah, NJ: Lawrence Erlbaum, 1984.

Frost, J.A., et al. Language processing is strongly left lateralized in both sexes. *Brain* 122:199–208, 1999.

Gazzaniga, M.S. Principles of human brain organization derived from split-brain studies. *Neuron* 14:217–228, 1995.

Glass, A. *Individual differences in hemispheric specialization.* New York: Plenum Press, 1987.

Hervé, P.-Y., et al. Revisiting human hemispheric specialization with neuroimaging. *Trends Cogn. Sci.* 17:69–80, 2013.

Jäncke, L., et al. The relationship between corpus callosum size and forebrain volume. *Cereb. Cortex* 7:48–56, 1997.

Kim, S.-G., et al. Functional magnetic resonance imaging of motor cortex: hemispheric asymmetry and handedness. *Science* 261:615–617, 1993.

Knecht, S. et al. Language lateralization in healthy right-handers. *Brain* 123:74–81, 2000.

Kotz, S.A., et al. Lateralization of emotional prosody in the brain: an overview and synopsis on the impact of study design. *Prog. Brain Res.* 156:285–294, 2006.

Lent, R., Schmidt, S.L. The ontogenesis of the forebrain commissures and the determination of brain asymmetries. *Prog. Neurobiol.* 40:249–276, 1993.

Moffat, S.D., et al. Morphology of the planum temporale and corpus callosum in left handers with evidence of left and right hemisphere speech representation. *Brain* 121:2369–2379, 1998.

Mohr, C., et al. Brain state-dependent functional hemispheric specialization in men but not in women. *Cereb. Cortex.* 15:1451–1458, 2005.

Myers, R.E. Phylogenetic studies of commissural connexions. In: Ettinger, E.G., et al. (Eds.), *Functions of the corpus callosum* (pp. 138–142). New York: Churchill Livingstone, 1965.

Paul, L.K., et al. Agenesis of the corpus callosum: genetic, developmental and functional aspects of connectivity. *Nat. Rev. Neurosci.* 8:287–299, 2007.

Pujol, J., et al. Cerebral lateralization of language in normal left-handed people studied by functional MRI. *Neurology* 52:1038–1043, 1999.

Sammler, D., et al. Prosody meets syntax: the role of the corpus callosum. *Brain* 133:2643–2655, 2010.

Sperry, R.W. Lateral specialization in the surgically separated hemispheres. In: Schmidt, F.O., Worden, F.G. (Eds.), *The neurosciences: third study program* (pp. 5–19). Cambridge, MA: MIT Press, 1974.

Springer, S.P., Deutsch, G. *Left brain, right brain: perspectives from cognitive neuroscience*, 5th. ed. New York: W.H. Freeman, 1997.

Stone, V.E., et al. Left hemisphere representations of emotional facial expressions. *Neuropsychologia* 34:23–29, 1996.

Sun, T., Walsh, C.A. Molecular approaches to brain asymmetry and handedness. *Nat. Rev. Neurosci.* 7:655–662, 2006.

Toga, A.W., Thompson, P.M. Mapping brain asymmetry. *Nat. Rev. Neurosci.* 4:37–48, 2003.

Cognitive Gender Differences

Aboitiz, F., et al. Morphometry of the sylvian fissure and the corpus callosum, with emphasis on sex differences. *Brain* 115:1521–1541, 1992.

Allen, J.S., et al. Sexual dimorphism and asymmetries in the gray-white composition of the human cerebrum. *NeuroImage* 18:880–894, 2003.

Baron-Cohen, S., et al. Sex differences in the brain: implications for explaining autism. *Science* 310:819–823, 2005.

Benbow, C.P. Sex differences in mathematical reasoning ability in intellectually talented preadolescents: their nature, effects, and possible causes. *Behav. Brain Sci.* 11:169–232, 1988.

Bleier, R., et al. Can the corpus callosum predict gender, handedness, or cognitive differences? *Trends Neurosci.* 9:391–394, 1986.

Celec, P., et al. On the effects of testosterone on brain behavioral functions. *Front. Neurosci.* 9:12. doi:10.3389/fnins.2015.00012, 2015.

Cooke, B.M., Woolley, C.S. Sexually dimorphic synaptic organization of the medial amygdala. *J. Neurosci.* 16:10759–10767, 2005.

de Courten-Myers, G.M. The human cerebral cortex: gender differences in structure and function. *J. Neuropathol. Exp. Neurol.* 58:217–226, 1999.

Eliot, L. *Pink brain, blue brain: how small differences grow into troublesome gaps—and what we can do about it.* Boston: Houghton Mifflin Harcourt, 2009.

Eliot, L. The trouble with sex differences. *Neuron* 72:895–898, 2011.

Federman, D.D. The biology of human sex differences. *N. Engl. J. Med.* 354:1507–1514, 2006.

Grön, G., et al. Brain activation during human navigation: gender different neural networks as substrate of performance. *Nat. Neurosci.* 3:404–408, 2000.

Holden, C. Parsing the genetics of behavior. *Science* 322:892–895, 2008.

Hyde, J.S. Gender similarities and differences. *Annu. Rev. Psychol.* 65:373–398, 2014.

Janowsky, J.S. Thinking with your gonads: testosterone and cognition. *Trends Cogn. Sci.* 10:77–82, 2006.

Kimura, D. Sex, sexual orientation and sex hormones influence human cognitive function. *Curr. Opin. Neurobiol.* 6:259–263, 1996.

Landis, S., Insel, T.R. The "neuro" in neurogenetics. *Science* 322:821, 2008.

Leonard, C.M., et al. Size matters: cerebral volume influences sex differences in neuroanatomy. *Cereb. Cortex.* 18:2920–2931, 2008.

Luders, E., Toga, A.W. Sex differences in brain anatomy. *Progr. Brain Res.* 186:2–12, 2010.

McCarthy, M.M., Konkle, A.T.M. When is a sex difference not a sex difference? *Front. Neuroendocrinol.* 26:85–102, 2005.

Miller, D.I., Halpern, D.F. The new science of cognitive sex differences. *Trends Cogn. Sci.* 18:37–45, 2014.

Moffat, S.D., et al. Navigation in a "virtual" maze: sex differences and correlation with psychometric measures of spatial abilities. *Evol. Hum. Behav.* 9:73–87, 1999.

Mohr, C., et al. Brain state-dependent functional hemispheric specialization in men but not in women. *Cereb. Cortex* 15:1451–1458, 2005.

Shors, T.J. Stress and sex effects on associative learning: for better or for worse. *Neuroscientist* 4:353–364, 1998.

Sowell, E., et al. Sex differences in cortical thickness mapped in 176 healthy individuals between 7 and 87 years of age. *Cereb. Cortex* 17:1550–1560, 2007.

Sullivan, E.V., et al. Sex differences in corpus callosum size: relationship to age and intracranial size. *Neurobiol. Aging* 22:603–611, 2001.

Watson, N.V. Sex differences in throwing: monkeys having a fling. *Trends Cogn. Sci.* 5:98–99, 2001.

Index

Note: Page numbers followed by italicized letters indicate *figures* or *tables*.